NUTRITION HANDBOOK

For Nursing Practice

Second Edition

NUTRITION HANDBOOK

For Nursing Practice

Second Edition

Susan G. Dudek, R.D., B.S.

Consultant Dietitian
Bertrand Chaffee Hospital
Jennie B. Richmond Nursing Home
Springville, New York

Formerly Nutrition and Diet Therapy Instructor
Sisters of Charity Hospital of Buffalo
School of Nursing
Buffalo, New York

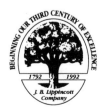

J. B. Lippincott Company
Philadelphia

Sponsoring Editor: Donna L. Hilton, R.N., B.S.N.
Coordinating Editorial Assistant: Susan Perry
Project Editor: Barbara Ryalls
Indexer: Victoria Boyle
Design Coordinator: Kathy Kelley-Luedtke
Interior Designer: Susan Hess Blaker
Cover Art: Jerry Cable
Production Manager: Helen Ewan
Production Coordinator: Nannette Winski
Compositor: Circle Graphics
Printer/Binder: R. R. Donnelley & Sons
Cover Printer: John Pow

2nd Edition

6 5 4 3 2

Library of Congress Cataloging-in-Publication Data

Dudek, Susan G.
    Nutrition handbook for nursing practice / Susan G. Dudek :
reviewers, Margaret A. Borquist, Colleen Gullickson, Irene Anne
Taylor, Jeanne C. Scherer. — 2nd ed.
        p.   cm.
    Includes bibliographical references and index.
    ISBN 0-397-54928-8
    1. Diet therapy. 2. Nutrition. 3. Nursing. I. Title.
    [DNLM: 1. Diet Therapy—handbooks. 2. Diet Therapy—nurses'
instruction. 3. Health Promotion—handbooks. 4. Health Promotion—
nurses' instruction. 5. Nutrition—handbooks. 6. Nutrition—
nurses' instruction. WB 39 D845n]
    RM216.863 1993
    615.8'54—dc20
    DNLM/DLC
    for Library of Congress   92-49654
                                                                                    CIP

Any procedure or practice described in this book should be applied by the healthcare practitioner under appropriate supervision in accordance with professional standards of care used with regard to the unique circumstances that apply in each practice situation. Care has been taken to confirm the accuracy of information presented and to describe generally accepted practices. However, the authors, editors, and publisher cannot accept any responsibility for errors or omissions or for any consequences from application of the information in this book and make no warranty express or implied, with respect to the contents of the book.

Every effort has been made to ensure drug selections and dosages are in accordance with current recommendations and practice. Because of ongoing research, changes in government regulations and the constant flow of information on drug therapy, reactions and interactions, the reader is cautioned to check the package insert for each drug for indications, dosages, warnings and precautions, particularly if the drug is new or infrequently used.

For my parents, Charles and Annie Maedl, who have given
me a lifetime of support and love

and

Joseph—without him none of my dreams would ever
come true.

Reviewers

Margaret A. Borquist, RN, BSN
Nursing Instructor
Olympic College
Bremerton, Washington

Colleen Gullickson, RN, PhD
Assistant Professor
School of Nursing
University of Wisconsin—Madison
Madison, Wisconsin

Jeanne C. Scherer
Instructor
Former Assistant Director and Medical-Surgical Coordinator
Sisters of Charity Hospital
School of Nursing
Buffalo, New York

Irene Anne Taylor, RN, BSN
Practical Nursing Instructor
Bellingham Technical College
Bellingham, Washington

Preface

Because nutrition is a basic human need, ever-changing throughout the life cycle and along the wellness–illness continuum, it is a vital and integral component of nursing care. Knowledge of nutrition principles and the ability to apply that knowledge are required of nurses, whether they are involved in some or all of the stages of nutritional care (assessment, planning, implementation, and evaluation).

NUTRITION HANDBOOK FOR NURSING PRACTICE, 2nd edition, is a comprehensive handbook that may be used as a core or supplemental text by students from a variety of educational backgrounds, or as a reference manual by practicing nurses. Using the nursing process format, it provides easily accessible, practical information to facilitate the integration of nutrition into nursing care plans. Tables are used extensively throughout the book for concise presentation of material. Current nutrition topics, including some that are controversial, are featured under the heading *Food for Thought*. Where applicable, *Drug Alert*s have been included, which highlight possible adverse nutritional side effects of commonly used medications and specify appropriate actions to alleviate those effects. Special displays of *sample menus* and *specific modified diets* allow the reader to see, at a glance, how nutritional needs are met in specific situations. Besides providing the most recent current nutrition information and most recent revision of the RDA tables, the new Food Pyramid, and up-to-date diet recommendations from leading health organizations, this edition also features other significant changes such as a stronger nursing process format that includes nursing diagnoses, and the addition of "newer" health concerns such as AIDS and Alzheimer's disease.

Section One: Principles of Nutrition presents the fundamentals of nutrition. Topics covered include carbohydrates, protein, lipids, energy balance and weight control, vitamins, minerals, and fluid and electrolytes. Background data on nutrient functions, sources, and requirements are augmented by brief overviews of nutrient or body metabolism. Potential adverse side effects of deficient and excessive intakes, and current intake recommendations are discussed. Consumption trends and future areas of research are presented where applicable.

Section Two: Nutrition in Health Promotion focuses on optimal nutrition for the "well" population at various stages of the life cycle and is presented in the nursing process format. Where appropriate, alterations in health that commonly occur only at certain stages of the life cycle (*i.e.*, during pregnancy, infancy, and childhood) are discussed, along with recommended dietary interventions.

Building on the foundation laid in Sections One and Two, **Section Three: Nutrition in Clinical Practice** combines the knowledge and application for nutrition in clinical practice. Alterations in health are presented, which range from stress and surgery to oncology. For each particular disorder, background information regarding etiology, complications, treatment, and diet therapy objectives is reviewed. Assessment data follows: Please note that the focus of this information is on the nutritional and dietary implications of each specific disorder and, therefore, should not be viewed as a complete nursing assessment guide. A sample, or generic, nursing diagnosis is given for each clinical disorder to illustrate how nutrition can be incorporated into nursing care plans. It should be noted that in *practice*, actual nursing diagnoses are formulated only after all pertinent assessment data is gathered and analyzed. For any given individual, the sample diagnoses may be incomplete or inappropriate. Although, in practice, Planning and Implementation are two distinct steps, they are grouped together for the sake of written presentation. As with the assessment data, client goals and nursing interventions, including Diet Management, Client Teaching, and Monitoring, focus only on nutrition. Evaluation projects optimal client outcomes.

Throughout Section Three, specific modified diets are presented in tabular form and emphasize potential problems, the rationale, nursing interventions, and client teaching.

Finally, Appendices provide a wealth of useful reference material such as food composition tables, the American Diabetes Association/American Dietetic Association Exchanges Lists, generalizations about diet and drugs, and a composite of selected enteral formulas.

Susan G. Dudek, R.D., B.S.

Acknowledgments

I am grateful for the support and help of all the people whose efforts contributed to the development and production of this book. Because of the dedication and professionalism of the people at J. B. Lippincott, the challenge of writing has been a satisfying and pleasurable experience.

I especially thank:

Donna L. Hilton, Nursing Editor, who directed and nurtured this project with her innovative insights and ideas and seemingly ceaseless energy.

Susan Perry, Editorial Assistant, for always having an answer or finding one. I appreciate all her efforts in coordinating and guiding the production of this book.

Barbara Ryalls, Project Editor, for her outstanding competence in editing and meticulous attention to detail.

Mark Jacobson, for his patience, perseverance, and computer expertise.

All the behind-the-scenes design and production people at JBL whose combined efforts transformed an ugly duckling into a beautiful swan.

The readers of the first edition and the reviewers of the second edition, whose thoughtful comments and suggestions broadened my perspective and helped shape, in my opinion, a new and improved edition.

Jeanne Scherer, author and editor of nursing textbooks, who has been my mentor and inspiration. I am forever indebted to her for her guidance, confidence, and unselfish support.

My family, Joseph, Christopher, Kaitlyn, and Kara, for the joy and meaning they bring to my life, and the sacrifices they made for this book.

Contents

Contents

NUTRITION
HANDBOOK
For Nursing Practice

Second Edition

I
Principles of Nutrition

1 *The Study of Energy*

1 Carbohydrates

Carbohydrates, commonly known as sugars and starches, provide the major source of energy in almost all human diets. Americans consume 40% to 45% of their calories in the form of carbohydrates (CHO). People in developing countries may obtain as much as 80% to 90% of total calories from CHO.

Carbohydrates are found mainly in plants. Compared to raising animals for food, plants are easy to grow, have a high energy yield per unit of land, are easy to store after harvesting, and are therefore relatively inexpensive. As such, CHO intake and income have an inverse relationship—as income goes up, CHO intake decreases, and the intake of protein and fat (more expensive forms of energy) increases.

SYNTHESIS

Through the process of photosynthesis, all green plants trap energy from the sun, water from the soil, and carbon dioxide from the air to make CHO. Plants store CHO as either sugar (*i.e.*, fruit and sugar beets) or starch (*i.e.*, root and tuber vegetables, dried peas and beans, and cereal grains). As some plants ripen and mature, they become less sweet as

5

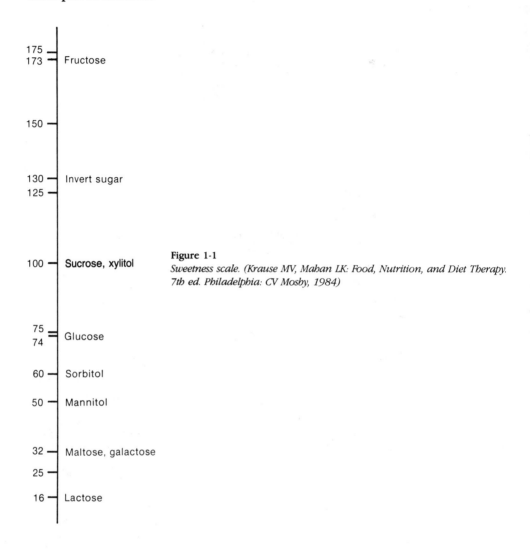

Figure 1-1
Sweetness scale. (Krause MV, Mahan LK: Food, Nutrition, and Diet Therapy. 7th ed. Philadelphia: CV Mosby, 1984)

sugar is converted to starch (*i.e.*, peas, corn, and carrots). Conversely, fruit becomes more sweet as it ripens because starch is converted to sugar.

Chemically, all CHO are composed of the elements carbon (C), hydrogen (H), and oxygen (O). Like water (H_2O), CHO have twice as many hydrogen atoms as oxygen atoms. Because each particular CHO has a distinct chemical arrangement, sweetness (Fig. 1-1) and other physical properties vary.

CLASSIFICATIONS

The two major classifications of carbohydrates are simple carbohydrates (sugars) and complex carbohydrates (starches and fiber). *Simple carbohydrates* are composed of one or two sugar, or saccharide, molecules; they are known as monosaccharides and disaccharides, respectively. This group includes naturally occurring sugars that do not taste sweet (*i.e.*, lactose, maltose), as well as sugar sweeteners, like sucrose and fructose, which are known as *nutritive* sweeteners because they provide calories. (*Non-nutritive* sweeteners, like aspartame and saccharin, are considered noncaloric, high-intensity, or alternative sweeteners;[1] they are not true carbohydrates.)

Complex carbohydrates, or polysaccharides, are made of long chains of many (poly) sugar (saccharide) molecules. Because of the way their sugar molecules are arranged, polysaccharides do not taste sweet. Starch, dextrins, glycogen, and fiber belong to this category.

Monosaccharides: Simple Sugars

Monosaccharides are the simplest type of CHO because they cannot be hydrolyzed (broken down) into smaller molecules, instead, they are absorbed directly into the bloodstream without undergoing digestion. Depending on the number of carbon atoms contained in each sugar molecule, monosaccharides may be classified as trioses, tetroses, pentoses, or hexoses (three, four, five, and six carbon atoms, respectively). The hexoses, specifically glucose, fructose, and galactose, are the only monosaccharides abundant in food and nutritionally significant (Table 1-1). Mannose is a hexose of limited nutritional importance.

Glucose: D-glucose, Dextrose, Grape Sugar, Blood Sugar

Glucose is the major fuel of the body and the form of CHO to which all other CHO are converted in order to be transported through the blood or utilized for energy. Because of this, glucose is the only sugar found in the body in significant amounts. Normal blood glucose levels range from 70 mg/dl to 100 mg/dl and are regulated by hormones (Table 1-2).

Fructose: Fruit Sugar, Levulose

Fructose is the sweetest simple sugar and is particularly effective at sweetening high-acid and cold foods. When used in other foods, it may not produce a sweeter taste. Pure

Table 1-1
The Common Hexoses and Their Sources

Hexose	Sources
Glucose	Fruits, vegetables, honey, and corn syrup; made commercially from the hydrolysis of starch or corn through the action of heat, acid, or enzymes
Fructose	Fruits, vegetables, corn syrup, and honey; commercially available from the hydrolysis of sucrose or natural extraction from fruit
Galactose	Not found freely in food, but is combined with glucose to form the disaccharide lactose
Mannose	Found in small amounts in peaches, apples, and oranges

Table 1-2
The Effect of Hormones on Blood Glucose Levels

Hormone	Effect on Blood Glucose Level	Mechanism
Insulin: produced by the β cells of the islets of Langerhans in the pancreas	Decrease	Enhances the uptake of glucose by muscle and adipose cells
		Promotes the conversion of glucose to glycogen in the liver and muscle cells (glycogenesis)
		Enhances the conversion of glucose to fat in the liver and adipose cells (lipogenesis)
Glucagon: produced by the α cells of the islets of Langerhans in the pancreas	Increase	Stimulates the synthesis of glucose from non-CHO sources (gluconeogenesis)
		Promotes the breakdown of glycogen to release glucose (glycogenolysis)
Epinephrine: produced by the adrenal medulla	Increase	Stimulates glycogenolysis
		Decreases the release of insulin
Glucocorticoids: produced by the adrenal medulla	Increase	Stimulate gluconeogenesis
		Cause the tissue to be insensitive to the action of insulin
Thyroxine: produced by the thyroid gland	Increase	Stimulates glycogenolysis in the liver
		Stimulates gluconeogenesis
		Increases the rate of intestinal absorption of the hexoses

crystalline fructose produces a flatter insulin response and smaller increase in blood glucose levels than sucrose. As such, small amounts of fructose can be used by diabetics, but calories and CHO must be considered. Like other sugars, fructose is converted to glucose in the liver. Fructose is widely used both in the pharmaceutical industry and in food processing.

Galactose

Galactose is not found freely in food but is combined with glucose in the disaccharide lactose. It is also converted to glucose in the liver.

Monosaccharide Derivatives: Sugar Alcohols

Sugar alcohols, of which sorbitol, mannitol, and xylitol are the most common, are produced when an aldehyde group is changed to an alcohol. Although sugar alcohols provide the same amount of calories per unit of measure as other sugars, they are not completely absorbed, and therefore their calorie content may be slightly less. They are used most commonly as sugar substitutes in dietetic products because they are slowly absorbed and produce less of an effect on blood glucose levels and insulin secretion than sucrose. However, when consumed in significant amounts, sugar alcohols can produce osmotic diarrhea and other side effects. Sources of sugar alcohols appear in Table 1-3.

Table 1-3
Sugar Alcohols and Their Sources

Sugar Alcohol	Sources
Sorbitol	Apples, cherries, pears, and plums
	Hard candy, sugarless gum, jams, jellies
	Made commercially from glucose and used as a sweetener in many dietetic products
Mannitol	Pineapples, olives, asparagus, carrots, and sweet potatoes
	Used as a drying agent in some foods
Xylitol	Raspberries, strawberries, spinach, cauliflower, cereals, and seaweed
	Made commercially from birch tree chips and used in dietetic chewing gum and other dietetic products

Disaccharides

Disaccharides are double sugars made from the chemical union of one molecule of glucose and one other monosaccharide (Table 1-4).

Sucrose: Sugar, Table Sugar

Sucrose is the least expensive and most common sugar in the diet, accounting for 52% of all sugars used.[1] Daily sucrose consumption in the United States ranges from 14 g to 60 g, with an average of 41 g/day (¼ cup).[1] Sucrose provides, on average, approximately 7% to 11% of total calorie intake. As sucrose intake has declined over the last decade, the intake of corn-derived sweeteners and non-nutritive sweeteners has increased. It is estimated that the amount of per capita carbohydrate sweeteners available for consumption in the United States is 127 pounds/year.[2] Unfortunately, there is no difference in caloric or nutritional value between sucrose and all other nutritive sweeteners (see box, The Many Tastes of "Sugar"), so that no particular one is any healthier.

Table 1-4
Disaccharides: Their Composition and Common Food Sources

Disaccharide	Composition	Sources
Sucrose	Glucose + fructose	Sugar cane, sugar beets, molasses, maple syrup, bananas, dates, ripe pineapple, peas, and sweet potatoes
Lactose	Glucose + galactose	Milk and milk products
Maltose	Glucose + glucose	Produced in the malting and fermentation of grains (*i.e.,* present in malted food products and beer)
		Insignificant as a dietary source of CHO

The Many Tastes of "Sugar"

Blackstrap molasses: the syrup remaining after the third and final extraction of sugar from the boiled juice of sugar cane or beets. It is very dark and bitter and is barely sweet.

Brown sugar ("sugar with a suntan"): partly purified white sugar (sucrose) that contains molasses. The lighter the color, the more purified the sugar.

Cane sugar: a concentrated syrup of mixed sugars made by boiling cane sap.

Corn syrup: a syrup produced by hydrolyzing cornstarch with acids. Glucose is the major sugar.

Date sugar: ground dates, which are high in natural sugars and very sweet.

High-fructose corn syrup (HFCS): a commercially made sweetener made by treating regular corn syrup with enzymes to break down the glucose to fructose, which is much sweeter; HFCS is used extensively in soft drinks, canned foods, and other processed foods because it is cheaper than sucrose. It is estimated that the average American consumes about 39 lb of HFCS yearly.

Honey: the nectar of flowers that is collected, modified, and concentrated by bees. Contains mostly glucose and fructose, and small amounts of sucrose. Honey containing more than 8% sucrose is considered adulterated.

Invert sugar: a mixture of equal amounts of glucose and fructose that forms when sucrose is hydrolyzed by enzymes or by being heated in water. It is sweeter than white sugar.

Lump sugar: sucrose pressed into a cube or tablet form.

Maple syrup: made from the concentrated sap of maple trees. May be boiled down into maple sugar.

Molasses: the residue that remains after sucrose crystals have been removed from the juices of the sugar cane or beet. Contains mostly sucrose, with smaller amounts of glucose and fructose.

Powdered sugar: made from white granulated sugar that has been machine-ground. Powdered sugar ranges in texture from coarse to extrafine: Generally the more ×s on the label, the finer the powder (i.e., 10× is finer than 6×). Cornstarch is usually added to prevent caking.

Raw sugar: coarse granulated sugar made by the evaporation of sugar cane juice. By law, impurities must be removed before raw sugar can be sold in the United States.

Sorghum: a syrup made from sorghum cane that looks like molasses. Sorghum has about the same sugar content as cane syrup.

Turbinado sugar: produced by separating raw sugar crystals and washing them with steam to remove impurities and most of the molasses contained in raw sugar. It has a slight molasses flavor and is coarser than white sugar.

Unsulfured molasses: made directly from sugar cane juice before any sugar crystals have been extracted. It is the sweetest type of molasses and is free of sulfur dioxide.

Lactose: "Milk Sugar"

Lactose is insoluble in water, is not very sweet, and is more slowly digested than sucrose. Lactose promotes the growth of friendly intestinal bacteria that produce vitamin K and enhances the absorption of calcium. It is added to infant formulas and is used by food processing and pharmaceutical industries.

Maltose: "Malt Sugar"

Maltose is not found free in food but is produced as an intermediate in starch digestion and also through the processes of malting (malted milk drinks) and brewing (beer). It is used in some infant formulas, instant foods, and bakery products in the form of maltodextrin.

Complex Carbohydrates: Polysaccharides

Polysaccharides are complex compounds composed of 10 or more glucose units. Polysaccharides are not sweet and are usually insoluble (Table 1-5).

Starch

Starch is the storage form of glucose for plants; it is composed of hundreds to thousands of glucose molecules, which may be arranged in one long chain (amylose) or in a branched chain (amylopectin). Different sources of starch (potatoes, rice, corn, and wheat) have different physical properties (solubility, thickening power, and flavor) based on the ratio of

Table 1-5
Polysaccharides: Their Composition and Sources

Polysaccharide	Composition	Sources
Starch	Hundreds to thousands of glucose molecules	Grains and grain products, legumes, potatoes and other root vegetables, and unripe fruit
Dextrin	Fragments of starch	Leaves of starch-forming plants Also formed as an intermediate in the breakdown of starch by the action of heat (*i.e.*, cooking and toasting) or enzymes
Glycogen	30 to 60 thousand glucose molecules	Not considered a significant form of CHO in the diet. After animals are slaughtered, the glycogen in their muscles quickly breaks down and virtually disappears. Oysters, scallops, and lobsters do contain some glycogen, but they are not eaten in large enough quantities to be considered significant.
Cellulose	Many glucose molecules arranged in a way that they cannot be digested by the enzymes present in the human GI tract	Skins of fruit, shells of corn kernels, the fibers of plants, the coverings of seeds, and the structural part of plants

amylose to amylopectin. Other good sources of starch include barley, dried peas and beans, and lentils.

Plants store starch in microscopic granules that swell and rupture when moist heat is applied. Cooking makes starch more digestible and slightly sweeter.

Modified food starches are natural starches that are commercially treated to improve their viscosity, stability, clarity, or solubility. They are used extensively in commercially prepared sauces, frozen fruit pies, infant foods, canned and instant puddings, and gum drops.

Dextrins

Dextrins are polysaccharide fragments, or intermediates, that form when starch is subjected to enzymes (digestion) or heat (cooking or toasting). They are more soluble and slightly sweeter than starch but do not have the thickening power of starch.

Glycogen: Animal Starch

Glycogen, the only form of CHO that animals and humans can store, is found in the liver and muscles. It is not considered a significant form of carbohydrate in the diet because only small amounts are contained in meat, and most of that is converted to lactic acid at the time of slaughter. However, it has great physiologic importance.

A typical adult can store up to three-quarters of a pound of glycogen (the primary and most readily available source of glucose and energy) or about 1400 calories—enough calories for half a day of moderate activity. Glycogen that is stored in the liver can be broken down quickly into glucose to maintain normal blood glucose levels between meals and to provide fuel for tissues. Glycogen that is stored in the muscle is used primarily as a source of energy. Athletes can almost double their storage of glycogen to increase their energy reserve for long-distance events by practicing "glycogen loading" (see Chap. 11).

Cellulose and Other Fibers

The precise definition of fiber has yet to be universally agreed on. Most commonly, fiber is defined as the portion of plant cells that cannot be digested by human enzymes and therefore cannot be absorbed from the small bowel.[14] Although only cellulose is truly fibrous, dietary fiber is the accepted group name for roughage or residue that includes cellulose, hemicellulose, pectins, lignin, gums, mucilages, and polysaccharides from algae and seaweed. Methylcellulose is a cellulose derivative that absorbs large amounts of water. It is used in low-calorie foods such as imitation syrups and salad dressings and in bulk-forming laxatives.

Because fiber is defined physiologically, it is difficult to measure accurately. In the past, *crude* fiber was used to describe what is left after a plant was treated with dilute acids and dilute alkalis, but this method greatly underestimated dietary fiber content and is not really relevant to human nutrition. *Dietary* fiber, which is what remains after a food is digested, is difficult to measure, but is estimated to be two to three times greater than the crude fiber content of foods. Unfortunately, data on fiber content are not available for all sources.

Fiber is commonly classified according to its solubility in water because insoluble and soluble fibers have different physiologic effects (Table 1-6). The most consistent benefit from fiber is the relief of constipation; however, only insoluble fibers, like hemicellulose in

Table 1-6
Major Types of Fiber: Their Sources and Physiologic Effects

Water-Soluble Fibers	*Sources*
PHYSIOLOGIC EFFECTS	
Slow gastric emptying and intestinal transit time	
Lower serum cholesterol levels	
Delay glucose absorption, which helps improve glucose tolerance in diabetics	
Gums	Oat bran and oatmeal
	Dried peas and beans
Pectin	Apples, citrus fruit, strawberries
	Dried peas
	Squash, cauliflower, cabbage, carrots, potatoes

Water-Insoluble Fibers	*Sources*
PHYSIOLOGIC EFFECTS	
Absorbs water to increase fecal bulk	
Reduces pressure within the colon	
Decreases intestinal transit time	
Little effect on serum cholesterol or glucose	
Hemicellulose	Wheat bran and whole grains and cereals
Cellulose	Whole-wheat flour and wheat bran
	Vegetables: cabbage, peas, green beans, wax beans, broccoli, brussel sprouts, root vegetables
	Apples
Lignin	Cereals and wheat bran
	Mature vegetables
	Pears, strawberries
	Eggplant, green beans

wheat bran, actually increase stool weight and promote regularity. Soluble fibers, like gums found in oatmeal, have little effect on elimination but have been shown to lower serum cholesterol and stabilize or reduce blood glucose levels in diabetics.

Because of the different effects of fiber, it is difficult to define precise need. The National Cancer Institute recommends that Americans consume 20 to 30 g of fiber daily (see box, How Much Is 20 to 30 g of Fiber?); actual average intake is 10 to 20 g/day. Except for relief of constipation, fiber supplements are not recommended.

CARBOHYDRATE FUNCTIONS

Provide Energy

The primary function of carbohydrates in the diet is to provide the major source of energy for the body. Under normal conditions, the nervous system and lung tissue rely on glucose as their sole source of energy. Glucose is also the major fuel used by muscles. Unlike

How Much Is 20 to 30 g of Fiber?

To consume an average of 20 to 30 g of fiber daily, you need to eat:

6–10 servings of whole-grain bread and cereals. One serving equals 1 slice of bread, ½ bagel, ½ cup rice or pasta

plus

3 servings of vegetables. One serving equals ½ to ⅔ cup

plus

2–3 servings of fruit. One serving equals 1 medium piece of fruit.

protein and fat, glucose is burned efficiently and completely and does not leave a toxic end product that the kidneys must eliminate.

Regardless of the source, all carbohydrates supply 4 cal/g, with the exception of undigestible fibers, which are essentially calorie-free because they cannot be broken down and absorbed. Since the amount of stored glycogen and circulating glucose is limited, carbohydrates should be eaten at frequent and regular intervals to meet the body's energy needs.

Spare Protein

For protein to be used most efficiently (*i.e.*, to carry on its specific functions such as repairing and replacing tissue), the diet must contain enough CHO calories to meet the body's energy requirements. An adequate CHO intake is particularly important any time protein requirements increase, such as after surgery or trauma, and during periods of rapid growth like infancy, pregnancy, and lactation.

If CHO intake is inadequate, the body will convert dietary protein—or break down and convert its own protein tissue—into glucose to be used for energy (gluconeogenesis). If protein is used for energy, it cannot be used to repair and replace tissue. In addition, the kidneys are taxed with excreting the nitrogenous wastes that remain after protein is degraded.

Prevent Ketosis

Some carbohydrates are needed to oxidize fat completely. When CHO intake is inadequate to meet energy needs, fat is inefficiently and incompletely broken down into ketones. The accumulation of ketones in the bloodstream leads to nausea, fatigue, loss of appetite, and ketoacidosis. Dehydration and sodium depletion may follow as the body tries to rid itself of ketones through the kidneys (ketonuria). The rapid weight loss characteristic of low-CHO fad diets is related to loss of body fluids resulting from the use of protein and fat for energy.

Combine With Other Compounds to Form Important Body Constituents

One example of such a combination is mucopolysaccharides, a group of complex compounds present in various body secretions and structures, which are composed of polysaccharides combined with protein and amino sugars. The following are common mucopolysaccharides:

- Hyaluronic acid, found in the fluid that lubricates the joints and the vitreous humor of the eyeball
- Chondroitin sulfate, found in cartilage, skin, and bone
- Heparin, the naturally occurring anticoagulant in blood
- Keratan sulfate, present in hard structures like fingernails
- Dermatan sulfate, present in the skin

HOW THE BODY HANDLES CARBOHYDRATES

Digestion

Carbohydrates are digested more quickly and completely than protein and fat (Fig. 1-2). In most diets, more than 90% of the CHO is digested; the remainder is excreted in the feces. Diets high in cellulose and other fibers are less well digested.

Cooked starch begins to undergo digestion in the slightly alkaline medium of the mouth by the action of salivary amylase, or ptyalin. Virtually no chemical digestion of starch occurs in the stomach. Some sucrose may be hydrolyzed to fructose and glucose in the presence of hydrochloric acid (HCl).

The principal site of CHO digestion is the slightly alkaline medium of the small intestine. In the duodenum, pancreatic amylase hydrolyzes complex CHO into maltose. The intestinal disaccharidases, located within the brush border of the intestine, break down the disaccharides into monosaccharides, the end products of CHO digestion.

Absorption

The monosaccharides (glucose, fructose, and galactose) are absorbed through the intestinal mucosa and transported to the liver through the portal blood circulation.

Metabolism

In the liver, fructose and galactose are converted readily to glucose.

Normally, blood glucose levels are held fairly constant by the action of hormones (see Table 1-2). As blood glucose levels rise after eating, insulin is secreted to move glucose out of the bloodstream and into the cells. Muscle cells may convert glucose to glycogen to maintain their stores. Through a complex series of metabolic reactions, cells oxidize

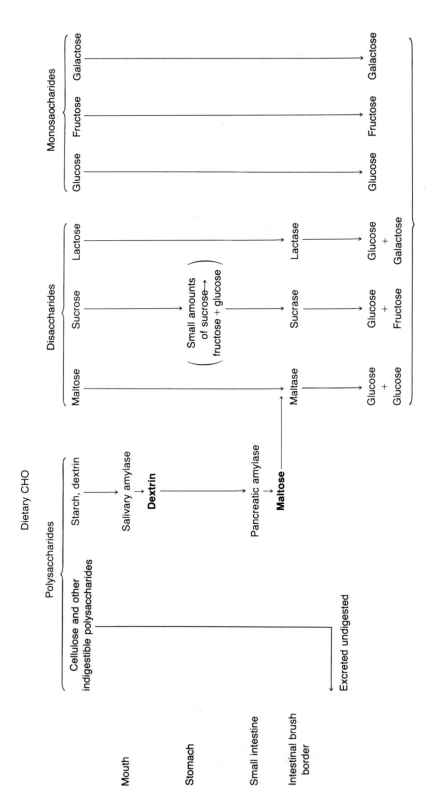

Figure 1-2
CHO digestion.

16

(burn) glucose to produce energy, carbon dioxide, and water. Depending on calorie intake and energy requirements, the time period between CHO consumption and the release of energy may vary from minutes to hours to months.

As cells take glucose out of the serum and use it for energy or storage, liver glycogen is broken down continually to maintain serum glucose levels (glycogenolysis). Even a slight drop in serum glucose triggers hunger, a signal for the body to replenish its supply of glucose. If eating is not resumed and fasting is prolonged, the body will synthesize glucose from amino acids and a component of fat (gluconeogenesis). Table 1-7 lists the signs and symptoms and possible etiology of altered blood glucose levels.

Glucose that is not needed as an immediate source of energy or to replace glycogen (glycogenesis) may be converted in the liver to other essential carbohydrates like ribose, a component of ribonucleic acid (RNA) and deoxyribonucleic acid (DNA). The liver may also break down glucose to provide a carbon stem that the body uses to make nonessential amino acids (if nitrogen and other necessary components are available).

Finally, any glucose that remains can be converted by liver and adipose cells to fatty

Table 1-7
Altered Blood Glucose Levels: Signs, Symptoms, and Possible Etiology*

	Hyperglycemia	*Hypoglycemia*
BLOOD GLUCOSE LEVEL	>140 mg/dl	<70 mg/dl
SIGNS AND SYMPTOMS	Polyphagia, polyuria, polydipsia, dehydration, glucosuria, ketonuria, blurred vision, changes in vision, weight loss, recurrent or persistent infections, weakness, fatigue, muscle wasting, and cramps	Fatigue, weakness, confusion, headache, psychosis, irritability, anxiety, rapid, shallow breathing, hunger, nausea, tingling, pallor, slurred speech, ataxia, marked personality changes, diaphoresis, dizziness, convulsions, coma, and death if untreated
POSSIBLE ETIOLOGY	Diabetes mellitus related to a relative or absolute deficiency of insulin (see Chap. 17) Excessive CHO intake, such as concentrated TPN solutions Hormone imbalances Stress Liver disease Head injuries Anesthesia Toxemia of pregnancy	Excessive insulin secretion, such as hypoglycemia secondary to postgastrectomy Excessive exogenous insulin or oral antidiabetic agents Deficient glucose production related to certain drugs Deficiency of hormones that increase blood glucose levels (*i.e.,* glucagon, epinephrine) Increased glucose utilization related to exercise, fever, renal glycosuria, and pregnancy Decreased glucose production related to diffuse liver disease

* Alterations in blood glucose levels are symptoms of underlying problems, not diseases themselves. Numerous claims that allergies, depression, hyperactivity in children, substance abuse, and criminal behavior are caused by hypoglycemia are unproven, as is the assumption that hypoglycemia is a common malady caused by eating a high-CHO diet.

acids and stored as triglycerides (fat). Calories eaten in excess of need, regardless of the source, are converted to fat, and unfortunately the body has an unlimited capacity to store fat. The body cannot rid itself of an excess carbohydrate intake through excretion.

The many reactions involved in the metabolism of CHO require adequate amounts of B vitamins, particularly thiamine, riboflavin, and niacin, which act as coenzymes.

SOURCES OF CARBOHYDRATES

Carbohydrates are found almost exclusively in plants. Complex CHO are found in grains and vegetables, including dried peas and beans. Fruits and sugar (by all its names) are sources of simple CHO. The only significant source of animal CHO is lactose, which is found in milk and dairy products.

The exchange system, developed by the American Diabetic Association and the American Dietetic Association, is a fairly simple and accurate method of estimating CHO intake, as well as the amount of protein, fat, and calories consumed. Six lists contain foods with similar CHO, protein, and fat content (see Appendix 11). Each serving of any item within a list is approximately equivalent in amounts of CHO, protein, and fat, to any other. The four groups containing CHO are listed in Table 1-8.

Sugars and *sweets* are not included in the exchange system because they are not considered appropriate for calorie- or CHO-controlled diets. They are, however, widely used and provide a significant amount of calories in the average American diet. One

Table 1-8
Sources of Carbohydrate Based on the American Diabetic Association / American Dietetic Association Exchange Lists

Group	Serving Size	CHO (g)	Protein (g)	Fat (g)
EXCHANGE LISTS CONTAINING CHO				
Starch/Bread				
Bread	1 slice	15	3	trace
Cereal, cooked	½ cup	15	3	trace
Most ready-to-eat, unsweetened cereal, dry	¾ cup	15	3	trace
Starchy vegetable, pasta	½ cup	15	3	trace
Rice	⅓ cup	0	0	0
Vegetable	½ cup cooked or 1 cup raw	5	2	0
Fruit	Varies	15	0	0
Milk				
Skim	1 cup	12	8	trace
Low-fat	1 cup	12	8	5
Whole	1 cup	12	8	8
EXCHANGE LISTS CONTAINING NO CHO				
Meat				
Lean	1 oz	0	7	3
Medium-fat	1 oz	0	7	5
High-fat	1 oz	0	7	8
Fat	Varies	0	0	5

teaspoon of sugar, eaten alone or as an ingredient in other foods, provides 4 g of CHO and 16 calories. However, with the exception of packaged cereals, which have the sugar content listed on the label (Table 1-9), the exact amount of sugar in processed foods cannot be determined. Generally, if sugar is one of the first ingredients listed on the label, it is likely that the item is a high-sugar food, unless of course there are only a few ingredients in the product. On the other hand, a product may be a high-sugar food even if sugar is listed as the last ingredient, if other sweeteners appear high on the ingredient list.

Table 1-9
The Percentage of Calories From Sucrose and Other Sugars in Ready-to-eat Cereals

	Serving Size	Calories	Sucrose and Other Sugars (g)	Calories from Sugar (%)
GENERAL MILLS				
Kix	1½ c	110	3	11
Lucky Charms	1 c	110	11	40
Total	1 c	100	3	12
Cinnamon Toast Crunch	¾ c	120	9	30
Triples	¾ c	110	3	11
Cocoa Puffs	1 c	110	13	47
Trix	1 c	110	12	44
Cheerios	1¼ c	110	1	3
Honey Nut Cheerios	¾ c	110	10	36
KELLOGGS				
Nut & Honey Crunch	⅔ c	110	9	33
Corn Pops	1 c	110	12	44
Apple Jacks	1 c	110	14	51
Frosted Flakes	¾ c	110	11	40
All Bran	⅓ c	70	5	29
Just Right	⅔ c	100	5	20
Big Mix	½ c	110	8	29
Rice Krispies	1 c	110	3	11
Crispix	1 c	110	3	11
RALSTON				
Cookie Crisp	1 c	110	13	47
Corn Chex	1 c	110	3	11
POST				
Fruity Pebbles	⅞ c	110	12	44
Cocoa Pebbles	⅞ c	110	13	47
Super Golden Crisp	⅞ c	100	15	60
Alpha-Bits	1 c	110	11	40
QUAKER OATS				
Honey Graham Oh's	1 c	120	11	37
Life	⅔ c	100	6	24
Cap'n Crunch	¾ c	120	12	40
Oat Squares	½ c	100	6	24
NABISCO				
Team Flakes	1 c	110	5	20
Spoon-size Shredded Wheat	⅔ c	90	0	0
Spoon-size Shredded Wheat N' Bran	⅔ c	90	0	0

CARBOHYDRATE REQUIREMENTS AND AVERAGE INTAKES

A recommended dietary allowance (RDA) for CHO has not been established because the body can synthesize glucose from amino acids and the glycerol component of fat. However, carbohydrate is an essential component of the diet. According to the 10th edition of *Recommended Dietary Allowances*, adults need 50 g to 100 g of CHO per day to prevent the effects of a low-CHO diet: ketoacidosis, muscle protein breakdown, sodium depletion, and dehydration.[9] However, 100 g of CHO supplies only 400 calories or about 20% of the total calories needed by most adults. Most experts agree that more than half of total calories consumed should be supplied by CHO and most of those in the form of complex CHO.

In 1985, the percentage of calories obtained from CHO in the diet of adult American men was 45.3% and 46.4% for adult women.[9] Grain products contribute the largest amount of carbohydrate calories, followed by fruits and vegetables (Fig. 1-3). Compared to the typical American CHO intake during the years 1909 to 1913 (Table 1-10), Americans are now eating fewer total calories from carbohydrates and fewer complex CHO, mostly because of a decreased intake of grains and potatoes. One reason for the decline is the widespread belief that CHO are "fattening," even though ounce-for-ounce they have the same number of calories as protein and less than half the calories of fat. And, as stated previously, excess calories from any source—CHO, protein, or fat—are converted to fat and stored in the body, so CHO do not have a greater tendency to "turn to fat" than other sources of calories.

Although Americans are eating more simple CHO in the form of sucrose and other sweeteners, the major source of our sugar intake has shifted from the sugar bowl to soft drinks and sweetened processed foods. However, with the increased popularity of sugar substitutes (see "Food for Thought") and low-sugar foods, sugar intake is beginning to decline.

RECOMMENDATIONS

The third edition of *Dietary Guidelines for Americans*, issued by the United States Department of Agriculture (USDA) and the United States Department of Health and Human Services (USDHHS), makes two recommendations concerning carbohydrate intake.[13] First, it recommends Americans choose a diet with plenty of vegetables, fruits, and grain products because of their complex carbohydrate and dietary fiber content. Second, it urges Americans to use sugars only in moderation.

Why Eat More Complex Carbohydrates?

Diets high in complex CHO are proportionately low in fat, and studies suggest that high-fat diets increase the risk of certain chronic disorders that are common in the United States. Because fats are a concentrated source of energy (9 cal/g compared to 4 cal/g for CHO), a high-fat diet increases the risk of obesity and its complications, such as type II diabetes, hypertension, and increased surgical complications. A high-fat diet is also implicated in the development of coronary heart disease and certain types of cancer, especially of the breast

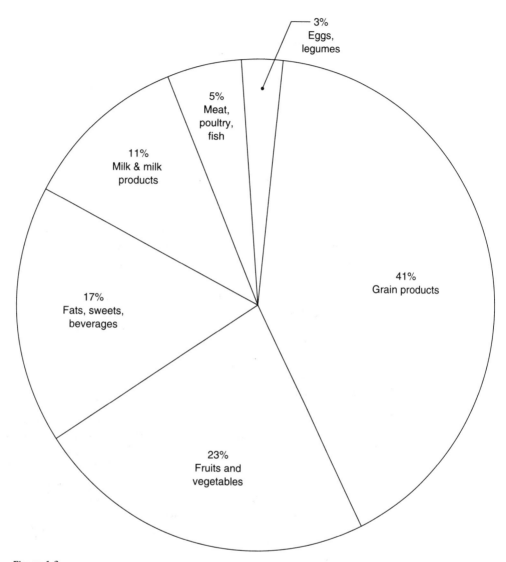

Figure 1-3
Percent of total carbohydrate calories contributed by various sources. (USDA Nationwide Food Consumption Survey 1977–78, 48 Coterminous States)

and colon. Conversely, diets high in complex CHO are not associated with any adverse health effects. In his 1988 *Report on Nutrition and Health*, the Surgeon General recommends increasing complex carbohydrate intake as the best alternative to eating fats and cholesterol.[14]

Another benefit of complex carbohydrates, especially whole grains and cereals, is that they are often a rich source of vitamins, minerals, and fiber. With the exception of vitamin B_{12}, which is found only in animal products, *whole grains* provide significant amounts of the B vitamins, several minerals, protein, and fiber. *Refined grains* are whole grains with

Table 1-10
Trends in CHO Intake

	Total Calories from CHO (%)	From Complex CHO (%)	From Simple CHO (%)
1909–1913	56	68	32
1947–1949	49	52	48
1980	46	47	53

(Welsh SO, Marston RM: Review of trends in food use in the United States, 1909 to 1980. J Am Diet Assoc 81:120, 1982)

most of the germ and bran removed; consequently, they are still high in complex carbohydrates, but many nutrients and fiber are lost (see box, High Fiber, Low Fiber). Although the Food and Drug Administration (FDA) has set minimum levels to which refined products should be enriched with iron, thiamine, riboflavin, and niacin, the other vitamins, minerals, and fiber that are removed during refining are not replaced. Although enrichment is credited with virtually eliminating once-common thiamine-, riboflavin-, and niacin-deficiency diseases, enriched products are not nutritionally equivalent to their whole grain counterparts (Table 1-11).

Why Eat More Fiber?

Many leading health organizations urge Americans to increase their intake of fiber by eating whole grain breads and cereals, and more fruits and vegetables. Potential benefits include the following:

The prevention or relief of constipation. Insoluble fibers draw water into the gut, which increases fecal bulk, stimulates peristalsis, and reduces transit time (see Chap. 15). The related decrease in pressure within the intestinal lumen also helps prevent or alleviate diverticular disease, and hemorrhoids.

A decrease in serum cholesterol levels. By one or more poorly understood mechanisms, soluble fiber lowers serum cholesterol levels, which corresponds to a lower risk of coronary heart disease.

A reduction in fasting blood glucose levels and insulin requirements in diabetics.

A decreased risk of colon cancer. However, both animal and epidemiologic studies have yielded inconsistent results.[6] Further research is needed to determine the relationship between fiber and cancer.

An aid to weight reduction. Fiber delays gastric emptying time and provides a feeling of fullness, or satiety. Studies have shown that eating a high-fiber breakfast causes people to eat fewer calories for lunch. Fiber can also help control weight by displacing calorie-dense foods. For instance, when a high-fiber cereal is chosen over bacon and eggs, fiber intake increases at the expense of fat and cholesterol intake.

A reduced incidence of dental caries when fiber replaces sugars in the diet. Fiber may also help clean the teeth.

Artificial Sweeteners: Tasty or Toxic?

Artificial, non-nutritive, or high-intensity sweeteners are man-made products intended to provide the sweet taste of sugar without the calories—a popular idea with diet-conscious Americans. Despite numerous health concerns, artificially sweetened products are in demand. Per capita consumption of sugar substitutes has tripled since 1975, and diet food and beverage sales have grown to 8 billion dollars annually.[3] In fact, more than 78 million people use low-calorie foods and beverages. However, artificial sweeteners have failed to become the panacea for weight control: The percentage of obese Americans has remained fairly constant since 1975. Although saccharin and aspartame are the prevalant artificial sweeteners used today, consumer demand and emerging technology ensure a growing market.

Saccharin

An estimated 50 to 70 million Americans are regular users of sodium saccharin, a petroleum product that is 300 to 500 times sweeter than sugar. It is most often found in low-calorie carbonated soft drinks.

In 1977, saccharin was banned because of numerous reports that it may contribute to bladder cancer and other forms of cancer. At that time, Congress enacted the Saccharin Study and Labeling Act, which requires that foods containing saccharin have warning labels and that establishments selling saccharin-containing products display warning signs. However, because safety issues remain unresolved, consumer demand is widespread, and a safe, inexpensive all-purpose replacement is not available, Congress has imposed numerous extensions to prevent the withdrawal of saccharin from the market. The current moratorium extension will expire May 1, 1997. However, recent studies indicate saccharin is probably not a human carcinogen. Some industry experts believe that the ban on saccharin will eventually be repealed.

Aspartame (NutraSweet)

More than 100 products are currently made with aspartame, a "natural" synthetic sweetener made by combining the two amino acids aspartic acid and phenylalanine. Aspartame has the same number of calories as sugar (4 cal/g), but because it is 180 to 200 times sweeter than sugar, its few calories are insignificant. Unlike saccharin, aspartame does not leave an aftertaste, and thus appeals to dieters and nondieters alike.

Unfortunately, aspartame loses its sweetening power when heated (making it unsuitable for baking), and is unstable in liquid form. Aspartame in soft drinks may decompose to methanol and formaldehyde when exposed to heat

(continued)

Artificial Sweeteners: Tasty or Toxic?

or stored for long periods of time. In addition, the American Academy of Pediatrics questions whether or not aspartame is safe for pregnant women and infants because of the possibility that toxic levels of phenylalanine may accumulate in the bloodstream. Certainly phenylketonurics, who cannot metabolize phenylalanine normally, are alerted to aspartame-containing products by warning labels. Although the American Diabetes Association has endorsed the use of aspartame for diabetics and the FDA stands by its position on the safety of aspartame, numerous consumer groups have petitioned for more hearings on its safety.

Acesulfame-K (Sunette)

Acesulfame-K is a derivative of actoacetic acid that is 200 times sweeter than sucrose. In 1988, the FDA granted approval for its use as a sugar substitute in powder and tablet form, and also for use in chewing gum, dry beverages, instant coffee and tea; dry bases of gelatine, puddings, and pudding desserts; and dry bases for dairy product analogs. Acesulfame-K retains its sweetness in liquids and soft drinks and, unlike aspartame, is suitable for baking. It requires no health warning label, does not contribute to tooth decay, can be safely used by diabetics, and is sodium- and calorie-free. Twenty-five countries have approved acesulfame-K for a variety of uses.

Future Possibilities

Two more sweeteners are expected to be approved for use by the FDA in the near future. *Alitame*, which is 2000 times sweeter than sucrose, provides no calories because only small amounts are needed to sweeten foods. Its potential uses include beverages, baked goods, toiletries, and pharmaceuticals. *Chlorosucrose (sucralose)* is a noncaloric sweetener that is 600 times sweeter than sucrose. In the future, it may be approved for use in beverages, baked goods, milk products, fruit spreads, syrups, toppings, frozen desserts, and as a table-top sweetener.

Why Eat Less Sugar?

• High-sugar foods may displace the intake of other nutrient-dense foods.

Sugars are called *empty calories* because they provide few or no nutrients other than calories. The more empty calories in the diet, the harder it is to eat a nutritionally adequate diet without exceeding calorie requirements. For instance, a child who eats half of his or her daily calorie requirement in the form of high-sugar foods (which is common) has relatively few calories remaining to meet all requirements for essential nutrients like protein, vitamins, and minerals. The child may end up not meeting his or her nutritional requirements or may have to exceed calorie requirements to consume enough nutrients.

Table 1-11
Nutritional Comparison Between Whole Wheat and Enriched Bread (per slice)

	Whole Wheat Bread	Enriched White Bread
CHO (g)	11.4	11.7
Protein (g)	2.4	2.0
Fat (g)	1.1	0.9
Fiber (g)	1.6	<1.0
NUTRIENTS ENRICHED BY LAW		
Iron (mg)	0.86	0.68
Thiamine (mg)	0.09	0.11
Riboflavin (mg)	0.05	0.07
Niacin (mg)	1.0	0.9
NUTRIENTS NOT REPLACED WITH ENRICHMENT		
Vitamin B_6 (µg)	0.05	0.01
Folacin, total (µg)	14	8
Pantothenic acid (mg)	0.18	0.10
Calcium (mg)	18	30
Magnesium (mg)	23	5
Potassium (mg)	44	27
Zinc (mg)	0.40	0.15

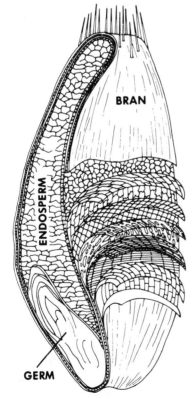

Endosperm . . . about 83% of the kernel
Source of white flour. Of the nutrients in the whole kernel the endosperm contains about

70-75% of the protein
43% of the pantothenic acid
32% of the riboflavin   B-complex
12% of the niacin   vitamins
6% of the pyridoxine
3% of the thiamine

Enriched flour products contain added quantities of riboflavin, niacin and thiamine, plus iron, in amounts equal to or exceeding whole wheat—according to a formula established on the basis of popular need of those nutrients.

Bran . . . about 14½% of the kernel
Included in whole wheat flour. Of the nutrients in whole wheat, the bran, in addition to indigestible cellulose material contains about:

86% of the niacin   42% of the riboflavin
73% of the pyridoxine   33% of the thiamine
50% of the pantothenic acid 19% of the protein

Germ . . . about 2½% of the kernel
The embryo or sprouting section of the seed, usually separated because it contains fat which limits the keeping quality of flours. Available separately as human food. Of the nutrients in whole wheat, the germ contains about:

64% of the thiamine   8% of the protein
26% of the riboflavin   7% of the pantothenic acid
21% of the pyridoxine   2% of the niacin

(Pennington JAT: Bowes and Church's Food Values of Portions Commonly Used, 15th ed. Philadelphia, JB Lippincott, 1989)

Low Fiber/High Fiber

Low Fiber "Refined"	Moderate Fiber "Whole grain"	High Fiber "Bran"
Wheat		
White flour	Whole wheat flour	Wheat bran
Pasta	Whole wheat pasta	
Cream of Wheat	Shredded Wheat cereal	
Oat		
Oat flour	Oatmeal	Oat bran
	Rolled oats	
Corn		
Cornstarch	Cornmeal	Corn bran
Cornflakes		
Rice		
White rice	Brown rice	Rice bran
Rice Krispies		

Some studies suggest that high-sugar diets, particularly diets laden with sweetened beverages, may be responsible for the beginning of thiamine deficiency.

- Fermentable carbohydrates + susceptible teeth + oral bacteria = tooth decay from an increase in acid production

Bacteria present in the mouth can ferment carbohydrates, especially sugars, which produces an acid that eats away at tooth enamel and results in dental caries. Although sticky sweets have been viewed traditionally as the major culprit, experts now believe that how often sugars are eaten and whether they are eaten alone or with meals is just as important, or perhaps more important, than their consistency (see Chap. 11 for more on diet and dental health).

- Sugar has also been blamed for causing obesity, diabetes, heart disease, and hyperactivity in children.

However, with the exception of inborn errors of carbohydrate metabolism, studies have shown that dietary sugars are not an independent risk factor for any particular disease.[1]

Obesity is caused by an excess calorie intake, not specifically by an excessive intake of sugars: People can become obese by eating too much "good" food as well as too much "junk" food. Studies also indicate that overweight people do not eat more sugar than thin people, and may even eat less, although sugar intake may decline after obesity is established.

Type II diabetes, commonly called *sugar diabetes*, also is related to an excessive calorie intake, not to an overconsumption of sweets. People who have diabetes have been treated traditionally with low-sugar diets, based on the premise that simple CHO raise blood glucose levels too rapidly and too high. Research indicates, however, that some simple sugars actually may have less of an effect on blood glucose levels than some sources of complex CHO, and that the amount of protein and fat in the meal (both of which slow the rise in blood glucose levels) may be as important as the form of CHO eaten. In the future, and as more research data become available, diabetic diets may become more flexible (see Chap. 17 for more information on diabetes).

Heart disease has been shown clearly to be related to diets high in total calories, fat, and cholesterol. No relationship between sugar intake and heart disease is apparent.

Hyperactivity in children is blamed frequently on sugar, although no scientific evidence supports this claim (see Chap. 11 for more on hyperactivity).

ALCOHOL

Ethyl alcohol (ethanol) is produced from the fermentation of CHO (glucose) by the enzymes in yeast. Other than providing 7 cal/g, or 5.6 cal/ml, alcohol has no nutritional value and therefore is not considered a nutrient.

Absorption, Metabolism, and Utilization

Alcohol is absorbed rapidly and completely from the stomach and small intestine. The presence of food in the stomach slows the rate of alcohol absorption from the stomach but does not decrease the rate of absorption from the small intestine. Because it is water-soluble, alcohol is evenly dispersed throughout the body fluids. The greater the water content of a tissue, the greater the concentration of alcohol (*i.e.*, a large amount of absorbed alcohol is found in the blood, whereas very little is present in bone and adipose tissue).

About 10% of the alcohol absorbed is excreted in the urine and expired through exhalations; the remaining 90% is oxidized by the liver at a fixed rate of about 10 ml/hour. Exercise, food, caffeine, vitamin supplements, and cold showers do not increase the rate of alcohol metabolism.

In the liver, several enzyme systems work to oxidize alcohol into acetyl-CoA, a form of energy that all tissues and muscles use. Skeletal muscles cannot initiate the metabolism of alcohol because they lack the necessary enzymes.

The liver preferentially oxidizes alcohol over glucose and fatty acids until alcohol is removed from the circulation. Because glucose and fatty acids are spared, alcohol can contribute to a positive calorie balance (see Table 1-12 for the calorie content of selected alcoholic beverages).

Alcohol abuse can lead to multiple nutritional deficiencies by several different mechanisms. Most obvious is that food intake may be inadequate—alcoholics may consume up to 50% of their calories in the form of alcohol. In addition, alcohol intake can interfere with eating by altering the senses of taste and smell, and by causing gastrointestinal upset. Nutrients that are consumed may be less well absorbed because of the toxic effect of alcohol on the intestinal mucosa. The metabolism of alcohol requires the use of nutrients, especially the B vitamins; nutrients "wasted" on the metabolism of alcohol cannot be used

Table 1-12
Alcoholic Beverages: Calorie, CHO, and Alcohol Content

Beverage	Serving Size	Calories	CHO (g)	Alcohol (g)
DISTILLED LIQUORS				
Gin, rum, vodka, whisky (rye/scotch)				
94 proof	1 ½ oz	116	0	16.7
100 proof	1 ½ oz	124	0	17.9
WINES				
Table, red	3.5 oz	72	1.4	9.6
Table, rose	3.5 oz	73	1.5	9.6
Table, white	3.5 oz	70	0.8	9.6
MALT LIQUORS (American)				
Ale	12 oz	157	11.1	15.5
Beer, light	12 oz	100	4.8	11.3
Beer	12 oz	146	13.2	12.8
COCKTAILS				
Daiquiri	1 cocktail	111	4.1	13.9
Manhattan	1 cocktail	128	1.8	17.4
Martini	1 cocktail	156	0.2	22.4
Pina colada	4.5 oz	262	39.9	14.0
Screwdriver	7 oz	174	18.4	14.1
Tequila sunrise	5.5 oz	189	14.7	18.7
Tom Collins	7.5 oz	121	3.0	16.0
Whiskey sour	3 oz	123	5.0	15.1

(Pennington JAT, Church HN: Bowes and Church's Food Values of Portions Commonly Used, 16th ed. Philadelphia, JB Lippincott, 1993)

to perform other necessary metabolic functions. Finally, alcohol can alter nutrient metabolism by decreasing storage, increasing nutrient catabolism, and increasing nutrient excretion.

Chronic alcohol abuse can affect every organ system of the body, especially the nervous system (polyneuritis, Wernicke-Korsakoff syndrome) and the liver (fatty liver → hepatitis → cirrhosis; see Chap. 15).

BIBLIOGRAPHY

1. American Dietetic Association: Position of The American Dietetic Association: Appropriate use of nutritive and non-nutritive sweeteners. J Am Diet Assoc 87:1689, 1987
2. Anderson GH: Facts and myths about sugar. Contemporary Nutrition 16(1), 1991
3. Blume E: Do artificial sweeteners help you lose weight? Nutrition Action Health Letter 14(4):1, 1987
4. Blumenthal D: A Simple Guide to Complex Carbohydrates. DHHS Publication No. (FDA) 90-2230, 1989
5. Caggiula AW: The high fiber diet: Practical advice for clients. J Am Diet Assoc 89:1737, 1989
6. Greenwald P, Lanza E, Eddy GA: Dietary fiber in the reduction of colon cancer risk. J Am Diet Assoc 87:1178, 1987

7. Hopson J: Carbohydrates: A key to health and performance. In Nutrition and Health: Hafen B, ed. New Concepts and Issues. Englewood, CO: Morton Publishing, 1985

8. Mayer J (ed): Why sugar continues to concern nutritionists. Tufts University Diet and Nutrition Letter 3:3, 1985

9. National Research Council: Recommended Dietary Allowances. 10th ed. Washington, DC: National Academy Press, 1989

10. Owen AL: The impact of future foods on nutrition and health. J Am Diet Assoc 90:1217, 1990

11. Rosauer R: Sweet and good—good and sweet. In Nutrition and Health: New Concepts and Issues. Englewood CO, Morton Publishing, 1985

12. Slavin, JL: Dietary fiber: Classification, chemical analyses, and food sources. J Am Diet Assoc 87:1164, 1987

13. United States Department of Agriculture, United States Department of Health and Human Services: Nutrition and Your Health: Dietary Guidelines for Americans. 3rd ed. Home and Garden Bulletin No. 232, 1990

14. United States Department of Health and Human Services: The Surgeon General's Report on Nutrition and Health: Summary and Recommendations. DHHS (PHS) Publication No. 88-50211, 1988

2 Protein

In Greek, *protein* means "to take first place," and indeed, life could not exist without protein. Protein is a component of every living cell: plant, animal, and even microorganism. The human body contains more than a thousand different proteins, which carry out a variety of essential functions. In the adult, protein accounts for 20% of total weight. Almost half of the body's protein is in muscles, one fifth in bone and cartilage, one tenth in skin, and the rest in other tissues and body fluids. With the exception of bile and urine, every tissue and fluid in the body contains some protein.

COMPOSITION AND STRUCTURE

Proteins are large, complex molecules composed of at least 100 individual chemical building blocks known as amino acids (Fig. 2-1). Like carbohydrates and fats, amino acids contain the elements carbon, hydrogen, and oxygen. The presence of nitrogen, which

Generic amino acid

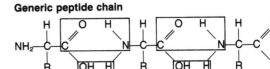

C: carbon stem
H: hydrogen
NH_2: basic amino group
COOH: acid carboxylic group
R: radical group, the chemical variable that distinguishes one amino acid from another

Figure 2-1
Amino acid and peptide structures.

Generic peptide chain

COHN: peptide bond
H_2O: water formed from the peptide bond

comprises about 16% protein, distinguishes protein from the other energy nutrients. Because amino acids contain both a basic amino group (NH_2) and an acidic carboxylic group (COOH) attached to a carbon atom, they can act as buffers to neutralize either acids or bases.

The body needs amino acids, and not protein *per se*, to build its own proteins. Of the 22 known amino acids, 9 must be supplied in the diet because they cannot be synthesized in the body. These are known as essential or indispensable amino acids. The remaining amino acids are no less important, but because they can be manufactured in the body from nitrogen and carbohydrate or fat, they are nonessential, or dispensable, in terms of dietary intake (Table 2-1).

Table 2-1
Amino Acids

Essential	Nonessential
Histidine	Alanine
Isoleucine	Arginine
Leucine	Asparagine
Lysine	Aspartic acid
Methionine	Cystine (cysteine)
Phenylalanine	Glutamic acid
Threonine	Glutamine
Tryptophan	Glycine
Valine	Hydroxyproline
	Hydroxylysine
	Proline
	Serine
	Tyrosine

Table 2-2A
Simple Proteins

Example	Occurrence
Albumin	Plasma protein
Insulin	Hormone produced by the pancreas
Histones	Cell nuclei
Globulins	Myosin, a muscle protein

Table 2-2B
Conjugated Proteins

Type	Example	Composition
Nucleoproteins	DNA (deoxyribonucleic acid) in cell nuclei	Protein + nucleic acid
Glycoproteins, mycoproteins	Mucin in mucous membrane secretions	Protein + CHO
Phosphoproteins	Casein in milk	Protein + phosphorus-containing substances other than phospholipid or nucleic acids
Chromoproteins	Hemoglobin	Protein + a nonprotein pigment
Lipoproteins	HDL (high-density lipoproteins)	Protein + a triglyceride or other lipid
Metalloproteins	Ferritin, the storage form of iron	Protein + a metal

Just as the 26 letters of the alphabet can be arranged to make an almost infinite number of words, the amino acids can be joined together by peptide bonds to form a virtually limitless variety of proteins. Based on their composition, proteins in the body may be classified as simple (proteins composed only of amino acids or their derivatives) or conjugated (simple proteins combined with a nonprotein substance) (Table 2-2). The wide variations in physical characteristics and functions among different types of protein are related to the differences in any of the following situations:

- The total number of amino acids contained in the protein
- The particular amino acids that are present in the protein molecule and how frequently they occur
- The order in which the amino acids are joined
- The actual shape of the protein molecule; that is, whether it is coiled, folded, or straight

FUNCTIONS

The major function of protein in the diet is to supply adequate amounts and proportions of amino acids for the synthesis of body proteins.

In the body, proteins are used to repair body tissues that break down from normal "wear and tear," to support growth through the synthesis of new tissues, and to provide a framework for the body. Bones, muscles, tendons, blood vessels, skin, hair, and nails are all protein-containing structures.

Protein is also used to synthesize many essential body secretions and fluids, such as hormones (*i.e.*, insulin, thyroxine, and epinephrine), plasma proteins (*i.e.*, albumin, hemoglobin), neurotransmitters (*i.e.*, serotonin, acetylcholine), all enzymes, breast milk, mucus, sperm, bile acids, and histamine. Antibodies (immunoglobins), which help the body resist infection and disease, are also made from protein.

Numerous body compounds include protein, such as opsin, the light-sensitive visual pigment in the eye, and thrombin, a protein necessary for normal blood clotting.

Specific amino acids have specific functions within the body. For instance, tryptophan is a precursor of the vitamin niacin, and tyrosine is the precursor of melanin, the pigment that colors hair and skin.

Protein has a role in regulating fluid balance by maintaining oncotic pressure. Plasma proteins, particularly albumin, help maintain proper water balance between the bloodstream and the fluid surrounding the blood vessel. A decrease in serum albumin leads to edema. Protein also helps regulate acid–base balance by buffering excess acids or bases, and works to detoxify harmful foreign substances.

Another function of protein is to transport other substances through the blood. For instance, lipoproteins transport triglycerides, cholesterol, phospholipids, and the fat-soluble vitamins; transferrin transports iron; protein-bound iodine transports iodine; and albumin transports free fatty acids, bilirubin, and many drugs.

Protein also can be oxidized to provide energy. Like CHO, protein supplies 4 cal/g. However, using protein for energy is a physiologic and economic waste, because when amino acids are used for energy, they cannot be used to synthesize protein, a function unique to amino acids. Protein oxidation is most likely to occur when protein is consumed in excess of need or when protein intake is of poor quality (*i.e.*, not all essential amino acids are present in adequate amounts), and is therefore unable to support protein synthesis. The remaining amino acids can be used only for energy. In addition, whenever protein-sparing calorie intake from carbohydrates is inadequate, protein is converted to energy to meet the body's calorie requirements.

Another disadvantage of using protein for energy is that proteins are not as efficiently and completely burned for energy as carbohydrates. The nitrogenous wastes resulting from protein metabolism burden the kidneys and require energy in order to be excreted. Protein is also more expensive to buy than CHO, and rich sources of protein are often high in fat.

Before amino acids can be used for energy, the amino group (NH_2) must be removed from the carbon stem (see Fig. 2-1). Although the amino group may be used to synthesize other compounds, most of it is converted to urea in the liver and then excreted in the urine. After the amino group is removed, the body can convert the carbon stem that remains to an intermediate to be used by the peripheral tissues for immediate energy. It can also be converted to glucose or fat and used for immediate energy or converted to fat and stored in adipose tissue.

SOURCES OF PROTEIN

According to the American Diabetic Association and American Dietetic Association exchange lists, protein is found in milk, vegetables, meat, and starches (Table 2-3). Fruits contain only trace amounts of protein, and pure fats contain none (oils, butter, shortening, and so forth).

Table 2-3
***Sources of Protein Based on the American Diabetic
Association / American Dietetic Association Exchange Lists***

Group	Serving Size	CHO (g)	Protein (g)	Fat (g)
EXCHANGE LISTS CONTAINING COMPLETE PROTEIN				
Meat				
Lean	1 oz	0	7	3
Medium-fat	1 oz	0	7	5
High-fat	1 oz	0	7	8
Milk				
Skim	1 cup	12	8	trace
Low-fat	1 cup	12	8	5
Whole	1 cup	12	8	8
EXCHANGE LISTS CONTAINING INCOMPLETE PROTEIN				
Starch/Bread				
Bread	1 slice	15	3	trace
Cereal, cooked	½ cup	15	3	trace
Most ready-to-eat unsweetened cereal, dry	¾ cup	15	3	trace
Starchy vegetable, pasta	½ cup	15	3	trace
Rice	⅓ cup			
Vegetable	½ cup cooked or 1 cup raw	5	2	
EXCHANGE LISTS CONTAINING NO PROTEIN				
Fruit	Varies	15	0	0
Fat	Varies	0	0	5

CLASSIFICATIONS OF FOOD PROTEINS

With the exception of gelatin, all dietary proteins contain some of all known amino acids. Because different proteins have different amounts, types, and ratios of amino acids, they are not all equal in terms of quality. Although most sources of protein in the diet contain all the essential amino acids, they may not all be present in adequate amounts to meet the body's needs.

Complete Proteins

Based on the relative quantities of amino acids present, dietary proteins can be classified as *complete proteins*, or high-quality proteins, if they provide all the essential amino acids in adequate amounts and proportions needed by the body for growth and tissue mainte-nance. With the exception of gelatin, all animal sources of protein (meat, fish, poultry, eggs, and dairy products) are complete proteins.

Incomplete Proteins

Dietary proteins can be classified as *incomplete proteins*, or low-quality proteins, if they are deficient in one or more essential amino acids. The essential amino acid present in the smallest amount is known as the "limiting amino acid" because it limits protein synthesis to the extent of its availability. Once it is used up, protein synthesis cannot continue, and the remaining amino acids are broken down and wasted as a source of energy.

Plant proteins (legumes, grains, nuts, and seeds) are incomplete proteins when they are eaten alone. However, because different plant proteins lack different essential amino acids, they can be combined in certain ways, or "complemented," to provide sufficient quantities and proportions of all the essential amino acids (Table 2-4). When complementary proteins are eaten in the same meal, they result in a protein of equal or higher quality

Table 2-4
Complementary Proteins

Food Group	Limiting Amino Acids	Abundant Amino Acids	Complementary Proteins

Grains	Lysine
	Isoleucine
	Threonine
		Methionine
		Tryptophan
			Grains + legumes
			  Rice + kidney beans
			  Rice + soybeans
			  Brown bread + baked beans
			  Wheat bread + peanut butter*
			  Corn tortillas + black bean soup
			  Toast + pea soup
			  Rice + lentil curry
			Grains + milk products
			  Bread pudding
			  Rice pudding
			  Cereal + milk
			  Cheese sandwich
			  Macaroni + cheese
			  Rice + cheese

Legumes	Methionine
	Tryptophan
		Lysine
		Threonine
		Isoleucine
			Legumes + grains (see above)
			Legumes + milk products
			  Lentils + cheese
			  Garbanzo beans + cheese
			  Bean soup + milk

Nuts, seeds	Lysine
	Isoleucine
		Methionine
		Tryptophan
			Nuts (seeds) + legumes
			  Sesame seeds + black-eyed peas
			  Sesame seeds + bean soups or
			    casseroles
			Nuts (seeds) + milk products
			  Sesame seeds + milk
			  Sunflower seeds + cheese

Vegetables	Methionine
	Isoleucine
		Lysine
		Tryptophan
			Vegetables + milk products
			  Broccoli + cheese
			  Cream of cauliflower soup
			  Corn pudding

Peanuts are actually legumes.

than meat. Wheat products, for example, are deficient in lysine, but have adequate amounts of methionine; legumes have adequate amounts of lysine, but are deficient in methionine. When wheat products and legumes are consumed together, the total protein intake is of higher nutritional quality than when wheat and legumes are eaten alone.

Another method of complementing proteins is to consume a small amount of a complete protein with an incomplete protein. Because complete proteins supply adequate amounts of all the essential amino acids, any complete protein (*i.e.*, milk, eggs, and meat) may be used to complement any plant protein.

EVALUATING PROTEIN QUALITY

The terms *complete* and *incomplete* are nonspecific with regard to actual protein quality. For instance, even though eggs and meat are both complete proteins, they differ in their relative amino acid composition and pattern, as well as in their digestibility. Such factors influence the extent to which proteins can be used by the body for tissue maintenance and growth. The following are more specific measurements of protein quality (Table 2-5).

Biologic Value

Biologic value refers to the percentage of absorbed nitrogen retained by the body; the higher the proportion of nitrogen supplied by the essential amino acids, the higher the biologic value (BV) of that food. Proteins with biologic values greater than 70% are considered to be high biologic value (HBV) proteins and able to support growth if calorie

Table 2-5
Measurements of Protein Quality

Protein Source	Biologic Value (BV) (%)	Net Protein Utilization (NPU) (%)	Protein Efficiency Ratio (PER)
Egg	100	94	3.92
Cow's milk	93	82	3.09
Wheat germ	75	71	2.90
Fish	75	—	3.55
Beef	75	67	2.30
Soybeans	73	61	2.32
Corn	72	36	—
Whole wheat	65	49	1.53
Oats	65	—	2.19
Peas	64	55	1.57
Polished rice	64	57	2.18
Sesame seeds	62	53	1.77
Peanuts	55	55	1.65

(Williams SR: Nutrition and Diet Therapy. 5th ed. St Louis: Times Mirror/Mosby, 1985.)

needs are met. Generally, complete proteins have a high biologic value and incomplete proteins have a low biologic value.

Net Protein Utilization (NPU)

Net protein utilization is the amount of protein that is actually available for the body to use; therefore, it is a more useful measurement than biologic value. It differs from biologic value in that the digestibility of a protein is considered. That is, the biologic value and NPU are the same for proteins that are completely digested; proteins less well digested have NPU values that are lower than the biologic value.

Protein Efficiency Ratio (PER)

Protein efficiency ratio is the gram of body weight gained by a test animal per gram of protein food eaten in an adequate diet over a specific test period.

HOW THE BODY HANDLES PROTEIN

Digestion

Chemical digestion of protein begins in the stomach, where HCl converts pepsinogen to the active enzyme pepsin (Fig. 2-2). Pepsin breaks down protein into smaller units called polypeptides.

The principal site of protein digestion is the small intestine, where protein hydrolysis

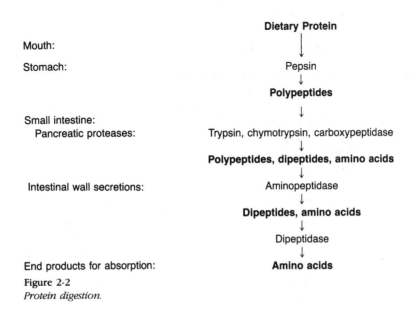

Figure 2-2
Protein digestion.

continues under the action of pancreatic proteases (a generic term for enzymes that break down protein).

Three major proteases (trypsin, chymotrypsin, carboxypeptidases) break down peptones into polypeptides, dipeptides, and free amino acids.

Two more proteases (aminopeptidase, dipeptidase) secreted by glands in the intestinal wall complete the breakdown of protein into free amino acids.

Absorption

Free amino acids are absorbed through the mucosa of the small intestine by active transport, an energy-requiring process. Amino acid absorption also requires vitamin B_6 and the mineral manganese. Once absorbed, amino acids are transported through the portal blood circulation to the liver. Some dipeptides may be absorbed and enter the portal bloodstream.

Newborns are able to absorb whole proteins, which allow breast-fed infants to absorb the protein antibodies in colostrum, thus receiving immunity from the mother.

Some amino acids remain in the intestinal mucosa, where they are used to synthesize intestinal enzymes and new intestinal cells.

Normally, only about 1% of ingested protein is excreted in the feces. Although urine contains nitrogenous wastes derived from protein metabolism, it normally is protein-free.

Metabolism

In the liver, amino acids may be used to synthesize specific proteins, that is, to make liver cells, nonessential amino acids, or specialized proteins such as plasma albumin. The liver also releases amino acids into the bloodstream for transport to tissues and cells where protein synthesis can occur.

Protein Synthesis

Like all body constituents, body proteins are in a constant state of flux. New proteins are continuously synthesized (anabolism) to replace old proteins that break down (catabolism) from normal "wear and tear." Red blood cells, for example, are broken down and replaced every 60 to 120 days and gastrointestinal cells are replaced every 2 to 3 days. Enzymes used in the digestion of food are continuously replenished. The synthesis of new proteins also occurs during periods of tissue growth and development—pregnancy and lactation, infancy, childhood, and adolescence.

The way in which amino acids are arranged in each particular type of protein is determined by the genetic code located within each cell nucleus.

The amino acids needed for protein synthesis may come from either dietary proteins (exogenous) or from the catabolism of tissue protein (endogenous). Following an "all or none" rule, protein synthesis proceeds only when all the needed amino acids are present simultaneously and in the proper ratio or pattern. When the supply of the limiting amino acid is used up, the remaining amino acids cannot be used to build proteins and are broken down for energy.

Protein Catabolism

Catabolism, the opposite reaction of anabolism, is an ongoing process of breaking down old, worn-out tissues. Normal catabolism occurs regardless of the amount of protein in the diet; however, a low-calorie or low-protein diet, as well as certain diseases, trauma, and stress, can accelerate protein catabolism.

Metabolic Pool

Amino acids, obtained from either protein digestion or tissue catabolism, are used to synthesize new proteins. Although the body cannot truly store excess amino acids for future use, a limited amount of amino acids is available in a so-called metabolic pool. These amino acids exist in a dynamic state of equilibrium because of the constant buildup and breakdown of body tissues.

Turnover refers to the cycle of anabolism and catabolism of body proteins. Although the body cannot store amino acids as protein, it can use tissue proteins to supply amino acids during a time of need. For instance, the turnover of proteins in the liver, pancreas, and small intestine is rapid, and during starvation, these tissues supply amino acids for protein synthesis or energy. The turnover of muscle proteins is slower, but because muscle mass is so large, a considerable amount of amino acids is derived from muscles during starvation. The turnover in the brain and nervous system is negligible.

NITROGEN BALANCE

$$\text{Nitrogen intake} - \text{Nitrogen excretion} = \text{State of nitrogen balance}$$

$$\frac{\text{Protein intake (g)}}{6.25} - (24 \text{ hr urine urea nitrogen (g)} + 4) = \text{State of nitrogen balance}$$

Nitrogen balance is a measure of the degree of protein anabolism and catabolism. Although protein synthesis and breakdown occur simultaneously and continuously within every cell, the net effect of these processes determines the state of nitrogen balance. Hormones that influence nitrogen balance are outlined in Table 2-6.

Table 2-6
Hormonal Influences on Protein Metabolism

ANABOLIC HORMONES (Stimulate Protein Synthesis)
Growth hormone (GH)
Insulin
Testosterone (stimulates protein synthesis during growth only)
Thyroxine (in normal amounts; excess thyroxine stimulates protein catabolism)

CATABOLIC HORMONES (Stimulate Protein Breakdown)
Glucocorticoids

Nitrogen Intake

Protein, the only energy nutrient that contains nitrogen, is approximately 16% nitrogen by weight. Therefore, 1 g of nitrogen equals 6.25 g of protein. Nitrogen intake can be determined by dividing the grams of protein consumed by 6.25.

Nitrogen Excretion

Nitrogen is lost continuously through the urine (urine–urea nitrogen), feces, hair, nails, and skin. To account for the nitrogen lost in the feces, hair, nails, and skin, a coefficient of 4 is usually added to the amount of urea collected in a 24-hour urine sample.

States of Nitrogen Balance

Nitrogen Equilibrium

Nitrogen equilibrium exists when nitrogen intake equals nitrogen excretion, indicating that protein buildup is occurring at approximately the same rate as protein breakdown (Fig. 2-3). Healthy adults who consume a diet adequate in calories and all the essential amino acids are in a state of nitrogen equilibrium.

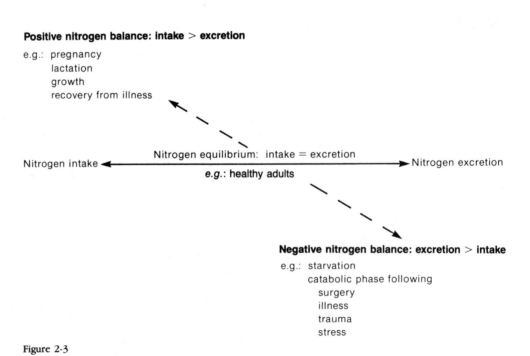

Positive nitrogen balance: intake > excretion

e.g.: pregnancy
      lactation
      growth
      recovery from illness

Nitrogen intake ←————— Nitrogen equilibrium: intake = excretion —————→ Nitrogen excretion

e.g.: healthy adults

Negative nitrogen balance: excretion > intake

e.g.: starvation
      catabolic phase following
          surgery
          illness
          trauma
          stress

Figure 2-3
States of nitrogen balance.

Positive Nitrogen Balance
(Nitrogen Intake > Nitrogen Excretion)

A positive nitrogen balance exists when the rate of tissue synthesis exceeds the rate of tissue breakdown, reflecting the growth of tissue. This occurs during periods of rapid growth, such as during infancy, childhood, adolescence, pregnancy, and lactation (if the protein content of the breast milk is considered). A positive nitrogen balance also occurs during the anabolic or recovery phase after surgery, burns, trauma, and stress, when tissue is being replaced.

Negative Nitrogen Balance
(Nitrogen Excretion > Nitrogen Intake)

A negative nitrogen balance occurs when the rate of tissue breakdown exceeds the rate of tissue synthesis, reflecting body wasting and the loss of body protein. This is an undesirable state, and is most likely to occur during any of the following:
- Periods of inadequate calorie and protein intake, resulting in the use of dietary and tissue protein for energy
- Starvation, infection, prolonged immobility, and stress
- Catabolic phase immediately after surgery and crush injuries

PROTEIN REQUIREMENTS AND RECOMMENDATIONS

Nitrogen balance studies are used to determine amino acid requirements and minimum total protein needs. The estimated minimum level of protein required to maintain nitrogen equilibrium in the healthy adult is 0.6 g/kg of ideal body weight, if calorie needs are met. However, the recommended dietary allowance (RDA) is set substantially higher, at 0.8 g/kg/day for both sexes, to account for wide variations in needs among individuals related to numerous factors (Table 2-7). Another reason why the RDA is higher is because the average American diet, which consists of both animal and plant proteins, has an protein utilization efficiency of 75%.

The RDAs for protein for various age groups and conditions are listed in Table 2-8. For any age, protein needs increase when calorie intake is inadequate or marginal, or when protein intake is of poor quality; that is, when there is a low percentage of net protein utilization, or when not all of the essential amino acids are supplied at the same time. Ideally, a high-quality protein or two complementary plant proteins should be consumed at every meal to supply the tissues adequately with all the essential amino acids needed for tissue synthesis. Table 2-9 lists conditions that may require adjustments in protein intake.

Most leading health organizations (i.e., American Heart Association, American Diabetes Association) recommend that protein contribute 10% to 20% of total calorie intake.

Recommendations regarding protein intake, per se, are not addressed in the third edition of Dietary Guidelines for Americans (see Chap. 8). However, suggestions for selecting a diet low in fat, saturated fat, and cholesterol recommend that Americans have two or three servings of meat, poultry, fish, dry beans, and eggs daily, for a total intake of

Table 2-7
Factors Influencing Individual Protein Requirements

Factor	Effect on Protein Requirements
Body size	The greater the size and weight of the body, the greater the protein requirements.
Age	Protein requirements per unit of body weight decrease from infancy through adulthood; however the elderly may require more protein than younger adults to maintain nitrogen equilibrium.
Sex	Although the RDA lists protein allowances for all adults at 0.8 g/kg of body weight, females actually need less protein than males of the same age and weight because of differences in body composition: Females have smaller muscle masses and a larger percentage of body fat.
Nutritional status	Undernutrition increases protein requirements.
Stress, infection, and heat	Emotional or physical stress, infection, and high environmental temperatures all increase nitrogen losses and therefore increase protein requirements.
Physical training	Physical training → increased muscle mass → increased protein requirements.

Table 2-8
RDA for Protein

Category	Age (years) or Condition	Weight (kg)	Recommended Dietary Allowance (g/kg)*	(g/day)
Both sexes	0–0.5	6	2.2	13
	0.5–1	9	1.6	14
	1–3	13	1.2	16
	4–6	20	1.1	24
	7–10	28	1.0	28
Males	11–14	45	1.0	45
	15–18	66	0.9	59
	19–24	72	0.8	58
	25–50	79	0.8	63
	51+	77	0.8	63
Females	11–14	46	1.0	46
	15–18	55	0.8	44
	19–24	58	0.8	46
	25–50	63	0.8	50
	51+	65	0.8	50
Pregnancy	1st trimester			+10
	2nd trimester			+10
	3rd trimester			+10
Lactation	1st 6 months			+15
	2nd 6 months			+12

*Amino acid score of typical U.S. diet is 100 for all age groups, except young infants. Digestibility is equal to reference proteins. Values have been rounded upward to 0.1 g/kg.

Table 2-9
Conditions Requiring Alterations in Protein Intake

Alteration	Indications
Increase total protein intake	Hypermetabolic conditions, such as burns, sepsis, and major trauma
	Protein-energy malnutrition
	Cancer cachexia
	Major surgery
	Peritoneal dialysis
	Multiple fractures
	Protein-losing renal diseases
	Hepatitis
	Malabsorption syndromes, including protein-losing enteropathy, short-bowel syndrome, inflammatory bowel diseases, and celiac disease
Maintain normal total protein intake but reduce or eliminate specific protein substances:	
Gluten-free diet	Celiac disease (see Chap. 15)
Low-phenylalanine diet	Phenylketonuria (see Chap. 11)
Low-purine diet	Gout (see Chap. 19)
Low-tyramine diet	People taking monoamine oxidase (MAO) inhibitors (Appendix 4)
Decrease total protein intake	Anuric phase of acute renal failure
	Chronic renal failure not treated with dialysis
	Cirrhosis of the liver with signs of impending coma

about 6 ounces. The guidelines also suggest occasional meatless meals. Two or three servings daily of skim milk or low-fat milk products is advised.

CONSUMPTION TRENDS IN THE UNITED STATES

According to the Nationwide Food Consumption Survey of 1977–78, 88% of all Americans consume more than 100% of the RDA for protein.[7] In the United States, the average adult protein intake is 90 to 110 g for men and 65 to 70 g for women. Although the percentage of calories from protein in the diet and the total amount of protein have remained fairly constant over the last 70 to 80 years, the source of protein has changed significantly (Table 2-10). Today, more than two thirds of the protein is derived from animal sources, whereas plant and animal sources contributed almost equally to the total protein intake during 1909 to 1913. This change can be attributed to the increase in meat, poultry, and fish consumption and the decline in the intake of grain products: Meat is the largest contributor of protein in the diet for all age–sex groups (Fig. 2-4).

America's love of protein, especially meat, is centered around several common myths and attitudes, such as:

- Protein builds muscle. Although muscle tissue is composed of protein, protein consumed in excess of need is not magically converted to muscle. Instead, excess protein,

Table 2-10
Protein Consumption Trends in the United States

	Total Calories from Protein (%)	Animal Protein (%)	Vegetable Protein (%)
1909–1913	12	52	48
1947–1949	12	64	36
1980	12	68	32

(Welsh SO, Marston RM: Review of trends in food use in the United States, 1909 to 1980. J Am Diet Assoc 81:120, 1982)

like excess CHO or fat, is converted to and stored as body fat. The only way to increase the size of muscles is by repeated use.

- Protein is nonfattening. At 4 cal/g, pure protein is just as fattening, or nonfattening, as pure CHO. But pure protein does not exist in the diet: Protein foods also contain CHO (grains, vegetables, and milk) or fat (meat, whole and low-fat milk and milk products). Some supposedly high-protein foods actually provide more calories from fat than from protein (Table 2-11).
- Protein aids in weight reduction. True, high-protein, low-CHO diets do promote weight loss, but the rapid weight lost is largely because of water loss, not fat loss. When CHO intake is inadequate to meet the body's energy requirements, protein is broken down and used for energy, resulting in the excretion of large amounts of water in order to rid the body of the nitrogenous wastes. The temporary drop in weight is regained when fluid balance is restored.
- Protein is a status food. Protein intake, namely the intake of meat, increases as income increases. Conversely, low meat intakes are associated with low socio-economic status.
- Meat is essential in order to get enough protein. Because the average American diet contains considerably more protein than the RDA, most Americans could completely eliminate meat, fish, and poultry from their diets and still meet their RDA for protein. In fact, studies show that even though lacto-ovo and strict vegetarians eat less protein than meat-eaters, they still eat more than the RDA. *Nutrients* are essential; *particular foods*, including meats, are not.

VEGETARIAN DIETS

According to a recent survey, as many as 7 million Americans consider themselves vegetarians, an increase of almost 300% over a generation ago. In addition to various religious, political, and economic reasons for becoming vegetarian, people are also abstaining from meat for health concerns. In fact, vegetarian diets come closer to the *Dietary Guidelines for Americans*[8] than the typical average American diet.

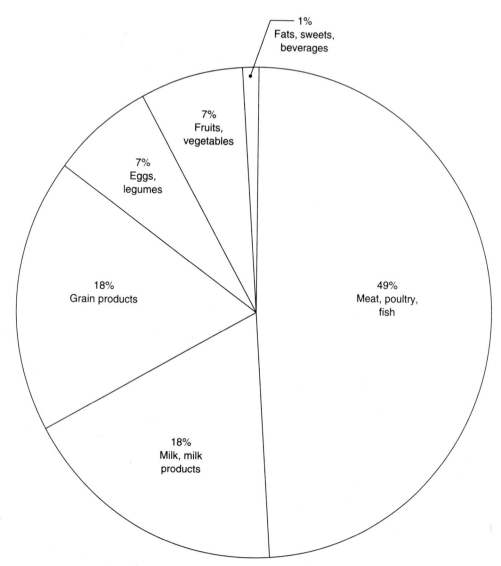

Figure 2-4
Percent contribution of various sources of protein in the average American diet. (USDA Nationwide Food Consumption Survey 1977–78, 48 Coterminous States)

Types of Vegetarian Diets

Vegetarianism is loosely defined as the abstinence from animal products. Pure vegetarians, or vegans, eat only plants; because of this, proper diet planning is essential in order to ensure adequate intakes of calories, vitamin B_{12}, vitamin D, iron, and calcium. Contrary to popular belief, protein requirements are rather easily met by vegans. As with the general population, average protein intake among vegans is well above the RDA.

Table 2-11
The Percentage of Fat Calories in Selected "Protein" Foods

	Serving Size	Calories	Calories from Fat (%)
DAIRY PRODUCTS			
Cheese			
American, pasteurized process	1 oz	105	77
Cheddar	1 oz	115	70
Cottage cheese			
Creamed	½ c	115	39
Low fat (2%)	½	100	18
Mozzarella, part skim	1 oz	80	56
Parmesan	1 T	25	72
Ricotta			
Whole milk	½ c	215	67
Low fat	½ c	170	53
Swiss	1 oz	105	68
Ice cream	1 c	270	47
Ice milk	1 c	185	29
Milk			
Whole	1 c	150	48
2%	1 c	125	36
1%	1 c	105	17
Skim	1 c	85	5
Yogurt, low fat, plain	1 c	145	25
Yogurt, low fat, fruit flavored	1 c	230	8
MEATS			
Beef			
Braised or pot roasted, chuck, lean	3 oz	230	47
Braised or pot roasted, bottom round	3 oz	190	38
Ground beef, broiled			
Lean	3 oz	230	63
Regular	3 oz	245	66
Steak, sirloin, broiled, lean only	3 oz	185	34
Lamb chops, broiled lean only	3 oz	185	39
Pork			
Bacon, fried	3 sl	110	74
Ham, roasted, lean only	3 oz	135	33
Chops, centerloin, broiled, lean only	3 oz	195	41
Veal cutlet, braised or broiled	3 oz	185	44
Sausages			
Bologna	2 oz	180	80
Frankfurters	1	145	81
Salami, cooked type	2 oz	145	68
POULTRY			
Chicken, roasted			
Dark meat without skin	3 oz	175	41
Light meat without skin	3 oz	145	25
Duck, roasted meat without skin	3 oz	170	53

(continued)

Table 2-11 (*continued*)

	Serving Size	Calories	Calories from Fat (%)
Turkey, roasted			
Dark meat without skin	3 oz	160	34
Light meat without skin	3 oz	135	20
Egg, hard cooked	1 lge	80	68
SEAFOOD			
Flounder, baked			
With butter or margarine	3 oz	120	45
Without butter or margarine	3 oz	85	11
Oyster, raw	3 oz	60	30
Shrimp, broiled or steamed	3 oz	100	9
Tuna, packed in oil, drained	3 oz	165	38
Tuna, water packed, drained	3 oz	135	7
OTHER			
Peanut butter	1 T	95	76
Peanuts, roasted, salted	½ c	420	75

(*U.S. Department of Health and Human Services, Public Health Service, National Institutes of Health: Diet, Nutrition and Cancer Prevention: A Guide to Food Choices. NIH Publication no. 87-2878. May 1987*)

Most vegetarians in the United States are classified as either lacto- or lacto-ovo vegetarians, whose diets include milk products or milk products and eggs, respectively. Their diets are not likely to be deficient in any nutrients. Many Americans consider themselves vegetarians simply because they avoid red meat.

An extreme type of vegetarian diet devised during the 1960s by the writer George Ohsawa was called the Zen-macrobiotic diet. In a series of 10 steps, the diet advances from meat-containing meals to a highly restrictive intake consisting mainly of brown rice, which supposedly is the ultimate food. The "higher" diets are dangerous and have caused severe cases of malnutrition and even death.

Nutritional Adequacy

Obviously, the more foods that are restricted, the greater the chance that the diet will be nutritionally inadequate. However, with careful planning and proper complementation of proteins (see Table 2-4), all types of vegetarian diets, including vegan diets, can be nutritionally adequate for almost all healthy adults. Table 2-12 lists good sources of minerals and vitamins that may be limited in vegan diets. A suggested meal plan appears in the box, Sample Vegetarian Meal Plan for Healthy Adults.[6] Because pregnant and lactating women, infants and children have high nutritional requirements, vegan diets may be inadequate for them. Also, special vegetarian diet planning may be needed for clients with lactose intolerance and diabetes mellitus.

Table 2-12
Good Sources of Nutrients That May Be Limited in Vegetarian Diets

Nutrient	Sources
MINERALS	
Calcium	Dark-green, leafy vegetables ("greens"), broccoli, brussels sprouts, okra, legumes, rutabaga, almonds, filberts, and calcium-fortified soybean milk
Iron	Dark-green, leafy vegetables, whole grain and enriched grains, dried fruit, winter squash, sweet peas, dried peas and beans, lentils, iron that leaches into foods cooked in uncoated cast-iron pots
Zinc	Whole grain breads and cereals, dried yeast, dry beans, and nuts
VITAMINS	
Riboflavin	Whole grains, enriched breads, fortified cereals, dark-green, leafy vegetables, broccoli, nuts, mushrooms, and avocado
Vitamin B_{12}	Fortified soybean milk, dietary supplements, yeast grown on B_{12}-enriched media, and meat analogs
Vitamin D	Sunlight, fortified soybean milk, and dietary supplements

Potential Health Benefits

A pure vegan diet is inherently low in fat, high in fiber, and cholesterol-free. The benefits of such a diet include a decreased risk of obesity, coronary heart disease, type II diabetes, constipation, and certain cancers, especially of the breast and colon. However, lacto and lacto-ovo vegetarians are not assured of either a low-fat or healthful diet, for their diets can be high in fat if whole milk, whole milk cheeses, eggs, oils and other fats, nuts, seeds, and high-fat desserts are used extensively.

Diet Recommendations for Vegetarians

While using the meal plan listed in the box as a general guide for meal planning, the following recommendations are also appropriate:

Eat a variety of foods.

Use complementary proteins whenever possible to ensure a high-quality protein intake.

Avoid "empty calorie" foods that provide few nutrients other than calories.

Eat more whole grain breads and cereals and milk products if additional calories are needed.

Include a rich source of vitamin C at every meal to maximize iron absorption.

Be aware of the potential nutrient deficiencies in a pure vegan diet. Be sure to select good sources of calcium, iron, zinc, riboflavin, vitamin B_{12}, and vitamin D (see Table 2-12). Pure vegans may need to supplement their diet with vitamin B_{12}-fortified soybean milk or take dietary supplements of vitamin B_{12} to compensate for the lack of animal products in the diet (vitamin B_{12} is found only in animal products).

Sample Vegetarian Meal Plan for Healthy Adults*

Protein Foods (2–4 servings per day)

One serving equals
    ¾ c cooked dried beans or peas
    4 oz tofu
    1 c fortified soy milk
    ¼ c almonds, cashews, walnuts, pecans
    2 tbsp peanut butter or peanuts
    1 c low-fat milk or yogurt
    1 oz cheese
    ¼ c cottage cheese
    1 egg

Whole Grains (at least 6–8 servings/day)

One serving equals
    1 slice whole wheat, rye, or whole grain bread
    1 buckwheat or whole wheat pancake or waffle
    1–2″ piece cornbread
    1 whole grain muffin or biscuit
    2 tbsp wheat germ
    1 oz wheat or oat bran
    ¼ c sunflower, sesame, or pumpkin seeds
    ¾ c wheat, bran, or corn flakes
    ½ c cooked brown rice, barley, bulghur, or corn
    ½ c whole wheat noodles, macaroni, or spaghetti

Vegetables (at least 4–6 servings/day)

Choose 2 servings/day of vitamin A-rich vegetables (1 serving equals ½ c cooked or 1 c raw)
    broccoli
    brussels sprouts
    collards
    kale
    chard
    spinach
    romaine
    cabbage
    carrots
    sweet potatoes
    winter squash
    tomatoes
Choose 2 servings/day of any other vegetable (1 serving equals ½ c cooked or 1 c raw)

Fruits (4–6 servings/day)

Choose 2 servings/day of vitamin C-rich fruits
    ¾ c berries
    ¼ cantaloupe
    1 orange
    ½ grapefruit
    1 lemon or lime
    ½ papaya
    1 slice watermelon
    ½ c orange, grapefruit, or vitamin C-enriched juice

(continued)

Sample Vegetarian Meal Plan for Healthy Adults* *(continued)*

Choose 2–4 serving/day of other fruits:
  1 small piece fresh fruit
  ¾ c grapes
  ½ c cooked fruit or canned fruit without sugar
  2 tbsp raisins, dates, or dried fruit

Fats (0–4 servings/day)

One serving equals
  1 tsp margarine, butter, or oil
  2 tsp mayonnaise or salad dressing
  1 tbsp cream cheese, gravy, or cream sauce

*This meal plan may not be adequate for pregnant or lactating women, or adults with increased nutritional requirements. Vegans need to include a vitamin B_{12} source weekly.
(Ransom R: 28 day meal plan. In Vegetarian Journal Reports. Baltimore: Vegetarian Resource Group, 1990)

PROTEIN EXCESSES

Infants have a limited capacity to tolerate protein; their immature kidneys are unable to concentrate the urine sufficiently to excrete large amounts of nitrogenous wastes that result from a high protein intake (see Chap. 11). However, protein intakes two to three times higher than the RDA appear to be harmless to healthy adults.

Diets high in protein, particularly animal protein, however, may not be optimal. If animal protein foods are consumed at the expense of adequate amounts of fruits, vegetables, and grain products, the intake of fiber and certain vitamins and minerals may be inadequate. Diets high in animal protein also tend to be high in saturated fat and cholesterol, a risk factor for atherosclerosis.

According to some studies, a high protein intake increases the excretion of calcium, which may accelerate bone loss, increase the risk of calcium renal stones, and increase the risk of osteoporosis (see Chap. 19). Chronic high protein consumption may also damage the kidneys. According to animal studies, age-related decline in kidney function can be avoided with a low-protein diet; less nitrogenous waste means less work for the kidneys.[3] Researchers believe the same may be true for people.

Lastly, diets high in animal protein generally are expensive.

PROTEIN DEFICIENCY

With the exception of the elderly, hospitalized patients, fad dieters, and people of low socioeconomic status, protein deficiency is rare in the United States and other affluent nations. However, in the developing countries, protein-energy malnutrition (PEM) is a major health concern.

Protein-energy malnutrition is estimated to cause 50% of the infant deaths in developing countries; infants and children are more susceptible to nutritional deficiencies because they have high requirements relative to their weight. Kwashiorkor and marasmus are the most severe forms of PEM. Children displaying symptoms of both diseases are said to have marasmic kwashiorkor, a less severe form of PEM.

Experts have questioned whether kwashiorkor and marasmus are actually two different problems, since the diets implicated in each are not significantly different. They hypothesize that marasmus may be a normal adaptive response to starvation, and that kwashiorkor occurs when the body cannot adapt to starvation because of a superimposed illness or infection. Such maladaptation may be responsible for the clinical and biochemical differences between kwashiorkor and marasmus.

Kwashiorkor

Kwashiorkor is a syndrome of severe protein malnutrition caused by an inadequate intake of good-quality protein; total protein intake may or may not be adequate. Starchy foods usually provide a marginal intake of calories.

In African dialect, kwashiorkor literally means "the disease of the deposed baby when the next one is born," an accurate description because it occurs most commonly after children are weaned because another child is born.

Kwashiorkor is most often seen between the ages of 1 to 4 years in areas where economic, social, and cultural factors combine to prevent an adequate protein intake, such as in 19 of the 21 countries in the Americas, India, most Middle and Far Eastern countries, and all the countries and territories of Africa south of the Sahara. In the United States, kwashiorkor most often occurs secondary to malabsorption disorders, cancer and cancer therapies, certain kidney diseases, hypermetabolic illnesses, and iatrogenic causes.

Signs and symptoms that may indicate kwashiorkor include edema and bloating related to low serum albumin; low weight, which may not be apparent because of edema; retarded growth and maturation; mental apathy; muscular wasting; depigmentation of hair and skin; and scaly, flaky skin.

Without adequate and timely nutritional intervention, protein depletion can lead to fatty infiltration of the liver and increased susceptibility to infections. Diarrhea and malabsorption develop because of the decrease in both the number of intestinal cells and the quantity of digestive enzymes secreted. Numerous nutrient deficiencies develop secondary to malabsorption, and also because the synthesis of transport proteins for the bloodstream is limited. For example, a severe vitamin A deficiency leading to permanent blindness can occur when the protein required to move vitamin A through the blood is unavailable. Other complications include growth failure severe enough to cause permanent damage to physical and mental development and a high mortality rate, usually before age 5.

Marasmus

Marasmus is a condition of chronic protein and calorie undernutrition that varies in severity. It occurs most often in 6- to 18-month-old infants whose parents are poor, uneducated, or mentally or emotionally disturbed. In addition to total food deprivation, the infant is usually lacking in emotional and physical care. Marasmus may also occur secondary to tuberculosis, malabsorption disorders, chronic infections, anorexia nervosa, and alcoholism. Isolated or hospitalized elderly patients are also at risk for PEM.

Food for Tomorrow

The Food and Agriculture Organization (FAO) of the World Health Organization (WHO) conservatively estimates that 450 million people in the world suffer from severe malnutrition. On the other end of the spectrum, Americans suffer from chronic diseases related to overnutrition: heart disease, atherosclerosis, certain types of cancer, diabetes, and cirrhosis. Affluent nations use 70% of the world's grain supply, but only 7% of this supply is actually consumed by people; the remainder is used to produce alcohol and to feed livestock.

Frances Moore Lappe, author of *Diet for a Small Planet*, maintains that eating meat for protein is as inefficient as paddling a canoe with a tennis racket.[12] According to one report, beef cattle require 10 pounds of grain in order to gain 1 pound of weight, which is a combination of both muscle (protein) and fat.[2] Pigs require 2 pounds of grain for every pound of weight gain, and chickens gain 1 pound of weight for every 1 pound of feed. It is clear that using grain to raise animals for consumption is not an efficient use of the world's food supply.

Besides more efficient use of conventional foods, new sources of food and innovative methods of food production are needed to feed the world's hungry people. Foods of tomorrow may be fortified with:

Oilseeds: Oilseed meal, residue, or cake is a by-product of cottonseed, soybean, sesame, and sunflower oils. It may be the most inexpensive source of protein and contains 40% to 50% good-quality protein. Complementing oilseeds with grains increases the overall quality by providing sufficient amounts of methionine, the limiting amino acid in oilseeds.

Soybean meal, in the form of soy flour, soy concentrate, and soy isolate, is currently used in infant formulas and foods, enteral formulas, beverages, cereals, breads, cakes, simulated milk, textured meat analogs, and meat extenders.

Fish protein concentrate (FPC): A tasteless, colorless powder that contains 80% to 90% high-quality protein. Although relatively expensive, small amounts of FPC is added to flour, infant foods, soups, livestock feed, and pet foods. Cereal with 5% to 10% FPC added has a protein composition comparable to animal protein.

Single-cell protein (SCP): A colorless, tasteless, dried powder containing 40% protein that is produced by bacteria or yeast that ferment petroleum derivatives or organic wastes. Any fermented food product, like yogurt, wine, and cheese, contains cellular organisms.

Leaf protein: Although green leaves are the largest supply of protein in the world, they are largely indigestible by humans because of their high cellulose and lignin content. However, juice extracted from the leaves contains 25% to 50% of the leaves' protein and is digestible.

Marasmus may produce the following signs and symptoms: muscle wasting and loss of subcutaneous fat, leading to an emaciated appearance; physical and mental growth impairments; apathy; and lowered body temperature. Severe growth failure and diarrhea are common complications.

Treatment and Prevention of Kwashiorkor and Marasmus

Of primary importance in the initial treatment of both kwashiorkor and marasmus is adequate fluid replacement and potassium replacement. Diuresis is expected about 7 days after the treatment of kwashiorkor begins. Clinical symptoms may disappear within 4 to 6 weeks with a diet adequate in high-quality protein, calories, and all other required nutrients; an increase of 30% above the RDA in both protein and calories is recommended. Vitamin supplements are generally indicated but not during the first 2 weeks of treatment.

Prevention of kwashiorkor and marasmus is far more effective than treatment, especially if the child is returned to the same environment and conditions after nutritional rehabilitation is completed. Prevention of both kwashiorkor and marasmus requires that broad, sweeping actions be taken:

Resolving socioeconomic and psychologic problems

Increasing education in agriculture, nutrition, and health: Breastfeeding should be encouraged for the first 6 months of life; thereafter, a nutritionally adequate diet should be initiated and continued

Implementing effective policies to improve nutrition and health care

Achieving a balance between population and food supply

Providing food aid to victims of man-made and natural disasters

Controlling infectious diseases

BIBLIOGRAPHY

1. American Dietetic Association: Position of the American Dietetic Association: Vegetarian diets. J Am Diet Assoc 88:351, 1988
2. American Dietetic Association: Vegetarian diets: Technical support paper. J Am Diet Assoc 88:352, 1988
3. Blume E: Overdosing on protein. Nutrition Action Health Letter 14(2):1, 1987
4. Chandler KB: Life without meat: The vegetarian view. In Nutrition and Health: New Concepts and Issues L, Hafen, B, ed. Englewood, CO: Morton Publishing, 1985
5. National Research Council: Recommended Dietary Allowances. 10th ed. Washington, DC: National Academy Press, 1989
6. Ransom R: 28-day meal plan. Vegetarian Journal Reports. Baltimore, MD: Vegetarian Resource Group, 1990
7. United States Department of Agriculture, Human Nutrition Information Service Consumer Nutrition Division: Nutrient Intakes: Individuals in 48 States, Year 1977–78. Nationwide Food Consumption Survey 1977–78, Report No. 1-2, 1984
8. United States Department of Agriculture, United States Department of Health and Human Services: Nutrition and Your Health: Dietary Guidelines for Americans. 3rd ed. Home and Garden Bulletin no 232, 1990

3 Lipids

Lipids, commonly referred to as *fats*, are a group of organic compounds that are insoluble in water but soluble in alcohol, ether, chloroform, and other fat solvents. Of the three major classes of lipids in the diet, triglycerides ("fats and oils") represent 95% of the total fat intake; the remaining 5% comes from phospholipids (*i.e.*, lecithin) and sterols (*i.e.*, cholesterol).

SOURCES OF FATS

In some foods (*i.e.*, butter, margarine, and oils), fat provides 100% of the total calories. In other foods, such as meat, eggs, dairy products, desserts, and sweets, the percentage of calories from fat varies.

According to the exchange lists developed by the American Diabetic Association and the American Dietetic Association, fat is found in the meat and fat groups (Table 3-1). Fats that can be easily identified, such as butter, oils, and the fat around meat, are known as *visible fats*. *Invisible fats* are hidden in foods that do not appear to be "fatty," such as the fat marbled throughout meat, and the fat in egg yolks, whole milk and whole milk products, nuts, desserts, and baked goods. As such, some items within the milk and bread groups also contain fat or "invisible" fat. Unless prepared with added fat, the fruit and vegetable groups are virtually fat-free, with the exception of avocados. The exchange lists fail to

Table 3-1
***Sources of Fat Based on the American Diabetic
Association / American Dietetic Association Exchange Lists***

Group	Serving Size	CHO (g)	Protein (g)	Fat (g)
EXCHANGE LISTS CONTAINING FAT				
Meat				
Lean	1 oz	0	7	3
Medium-fat	1 oz	0	7	5
High-fat	1 oz	0	7	8
Fat	Varies	0	0	5
EXCHANGE LISTS THAT MAY CONTAIN FAT, DEPENDING ON THE SELECTION				
Milk				
Skim	1 cup	12	8	Trace
Low-fat	1 cup	12	8	5
Whole	1 cup	12	8	8
EXCHANGE LISTS CONTAINING NO FAT (If Prepared Without Added Fat)				
Starch/Bread				
Bread	1 slice	15	3	Trace
Cereal, cooked	½ cup	15	3	Trace
Most ready-to-eat unsweetened cereal, dry	¾ cup	15	3	Trace
Starchy vegetable, pasta	½ cup	15	3	Trace
Rice	⅓ cup	15	3	Trace
Vegetable	½ cup cooked or 1 cup raw	5	2	0
Fruit	Varies	15	0	0

identify the "other" group, which commonly contains sweets, snacks, and desserts, all
traditionally high-fat items (Table 3-2).

FUNCTIONS

Supplying 9 cal/g, fats and oils are the most concentrated source of energy in the diet,
providing more than twice the fuel value of CHO and protein. With the exception of the
central nervous system and erythrocytes, which normally rely solely on glucose for energy,
all body cells can directly oxidize fatty acids to produce energy. However, because fat
metabolism is more complicated than CHO metabolism, CHO is generally the preferred
fuel.

Linoleic acid and linolenic acids are essential fatty acids (EFA) because they cannot be
synthesized by the body and must therefore be supplied in the diet. Because linoleic acid is
a precursor of arachidonic acid, arachidonic acid becomes an EFA when linoleic acid intake
is deficient. Essential fatty acids play a role in the metabolism of cholesterol, and, by some
unknown mechanism, help lower serum cholesterol levels. Essential fatty acids also help
maintain the function and integrity of capillaries and cell membranes. They are precursors
of prostaglandins, a group of hormone-like substances with various metabolic functions,

Table 3-2
Fat Content of Selected Foods From the Other Group

Item	Portion Size	Calories	Fat (g)	% Calories From Fat
CANDY				
Chocolate chips, milk chocolate	¼ c	196	8.8	40
Fudge, chocolate	1 oz	113	3.5	28
Kit Kat wafer, Hershey	1.625 oz	244	13.2	49
Peanut butter cups, Reeses	2 pieces	281	16.7	53
CHIPS AND SNACKS				
Bugles	1 oz	150	8	48
Cheese balls/curls	1 oz	160	11.0	62
Corn chips	1 oz	153	8.8	52
Popcorn, fat added	1 cup	41	2.0	44
Potato chips	1 oz	148	10.0	61
Pretzels	1 oz	111	1	8
Tortilla chips, Planters	1 oz	150	8.0	48
DESSERTS				
Brownie, fudge, from mix	2″ square	150	6	36
Cake				
Angel food, homemade	1 pc	161	0.1	1
Butter recipe, mix	¹⁄₁₂	260	12	42
Carrot, frzn, Am Hosp Co	3 oz	326	17.1	47
Cheesecake	1 pc	257	16.3	57
Coffe cake, from mix	⅙ cake	232	6.9	27
Pound, old-fashioned, homemade	1 pc	142	9	57
Yellow, homemade	1 pc	283	12.4	40
Cookies				
Animal	10 pc	112	2.4	19
Chocolate chip, homemade	1	46	2.7	53
Molasses	1	137	3.4	22
Oatmeal	1	62	2.6	38
Sugar	2	71	2.7	34
Doughnuts				
Cake	1	105	5.8	50
Chocolate coated	1	130	8.0	55
Glazed	1	230	12.0	47
Sugar	1	110	5.0	41
Pie				
Apple, homemade	⅛	282	11.9	38
Chocolate cream, homemade	⅛	301	17.3	52
Pumpkin, homemade	⅛	241	12.8	48

(Pennington JA: Bowes and Church's Food Values of Portions Commonly Used. 15th ed. Philadelphia: JB Lippincott, 1989)

and of phospholipids, the structural lipids found in cell membranes and myelin sheaths, the insulating cover around nerves that speeds the transmission of nerve impulses.

Fat improves the palatability and flavor of food and influences its texture. It delays gastric emptying time—fat may remain in the stomach for 3.5 to 4 hours after a meal, providing a feeling of fullness (satiety) and delaying the return of hunger. In addition, the presence of fat in the duodenum stimulates the release of a hormone in the stomach that

Nonfattening Fats

According to consumer polls and industry predictions, Americans are becoming increasingly concerned with nutrition and health, and clearly one area of regard is fat intake and its role in chronic diseases. Recommendations from every leading health organization stress reduced fat intake as a top priority.

In response to consumer demand for low-fat, low-calorie foods, the food industry is developing fat substitutes to replace all the fat in certain products with a virtually noncaloric substitute. The potential benefits are enormous: Millions of overweight Americans seemingly could lose weight painlessly and effortlessly, a kind of have-your-cake-and-eat-it-too scenario.

However, it is likely that once approved for use, these products will fall short of becoming a panacea for the typical American diet. As research has shown, the average American has gained weight since the advent of artificial sweeteners. So, too, may fat substitutes fail to achieve their lofty objectives if consumers overlook the obvious: Although fat calories in a food may be lessened or eliminated, there is no guarantee that total calories will follow suit.

Fat substitutes currently being developed include Olestra (Procter and Gamble), Simplesse (NutraSweet Company), and Trailblazer (Kraft).

Olestra

Olestra, chemically known as sucrose polyester, is currently being developed by the food industry to be used in margarine, butter spreads, beverages, baked goods, dressings, and frying. Composed of fatty acids and sucrose, olestra lowers serum cholesterol levels in hypercholesterolemic individuals by increasing the excretion of both exogenous (dietary) and endogenous cholesterol. It appears to have little effect on people with normal cholesterol levels, and, because it is totally nonabsorbable, it provides no calories. Although it does not alter the absorption of other fats, it may reduce the absorption of vitamins A and D.

Simplesse

Simplesse is made from milk and/or egg white protein and provides a mere 1⅓ calories/g. It was recently approved by the FDA for use in products that do not require cooking, such as dressings, mayonnaise, margarine, butter, ice cream, yogurt, sour cream dips, and cheese spreads. Products made with Simplesse contain 20% to 80% fewer calories than products made with traditional fats.

Trailblazer

Trailblazer is made from "all natural ingredients," and presumably is an egg white and skim milk derivative. Its proposed uses are frozen desserts; Trailblazer has not yet been approved for use by the FDA.

inhibits hunger contractions. The absorption of the fat-soluble vitamins A, D, and E through the intestinal mucosa depends on fat.

Like phospholipids, cholesterol is a major component of cell membranes and myelin. Cholesterol has other essential metabolic functions, including being the precursor of steroid hormones and bile (see section on Other Lipids).

Fat, in the form of triglycerides, that is not used as an immediate energy source or needed for other functions is stored in adipose tissue. White fat and brown fat are the two forms of adipose tissue. White fat, the most abundant type of fat in the body, normally accounts for 15% to 25% of total body weight. It is deposited under the skin, in the abdominal cavity, and to a lesser extent in intramuscular tissue. Its functions are to provide energy in time of need, to insulate and protect the body against cold environmental temperatures, and to support internal organs such as the kidneys and heart, protecting them against mechanical injury. Brown fat is much less abundant; the greatest amount of brown fat is present during infancy and decreases with age. Less than 1% of an adult's body weight is from brown fat. It is located only in certain areas in the body, mostly around the neck and chest. Its primary function is thermogenesis—that is, generating heat to protect against the cold. Brown fat, or the lack of it, has been theorized to play a role in the development of obesity (see Chap. 4).

COMPOSITION AND STRUCTURE

Fats are made of the elements carbon, hydrogen, and oxygen in the form of one glycerol molecule with one, two, or three fatty acids attached. Although fats contain the same elements as CHO, they have proportionately less oxygen and more hydrogen and carbon atoms, and are therefore higher in calories.

Glycerol

Glycerol is an alcohol made of a three-carbon atom stem with alcohol groups attached to each; all glycerol molecules are the same. After fat is broken down through the process of digestion into fatty acids and glycerol, the glycerol molecule is absorbed directly into the portal vein.

$$
\begin{array}{c}
H \\
| \\
H-C-OH \\
H-C-OH \\
H-C-OH \\
| \\
H
\end{array}
$$

Fatty Acids

Fatty acids are composed of a straight chain of carbon atoms with hydrogen atoms attached and an acid group at one end. Most fatty acids have an even number of carbon atoms ranging from 2 to 24 (Table 3-3). Two variables that determine the physical properties of fatty acids are the length of the carbon chain and the degree of saturation.

Table 3-3
Some Naturally Occurring Saturated and Unsaturated Fatty Acids

Fatty Acids	Number of Carbon Atoms	Food Sources
SATURATED FATTY ACIDS		
Short-chain		
Butyric acid	4	Butter
Caproic acid	6	Butter
Medium-chain		
Caprylic acid	8	Butter, coconut oil
Capric acid	10	Butter, coconut oil, and palm oil
Long-chain		
Lauric acid	12	Butter, coconut oil
Myristic acid	14	Butter, coconut oil
Palmitic acid	16	Beef, pork, lamb, and most vegetable oils
Stearic acid	18	Beef, pork, lamb, and most vegetable oils
Arachidic acid	20	Peanut oil, lard
MONOSATURATED FATTY ACIDS (1 Double Bond)		
Long-chain		
Palmitoleic acid	16	Butter, seed oils
Oleic acid	18	Meats, olive oil, and most other fats and oils
POLYUNSATURATED FATTY ACIDS		
Long-chain		
Linoleic acid	18 (2 double bonds)	Corn, cottonseed, soybean, sunflower, and safflower oils; poultry, walnuts
Linolenic acid	18 (3 double bonds)	Soybean oil, other vegetables oils, and egg yolk
Arachidonic acid	20 (4 double bonds)	Very little in foods

Carbon Chain Length

Based on the length of the carbon chain, fatty acids may be classified as *short-chain fatty acids*, which contain 6 or less carbon atoms, *medium-chain fatty acids*, which contain 8 to 10 carbon atoms, or *long-chain fatty acids*, which contain 12 or more carbon atoms. Most food fats contain predominantly long-chain fatty acids.

Degree of Saturation

The degree of saturation refers to the number of double bonds between carbon atoms. If all of the carbon atoms in a fatty acid have all four of their potential bonding sites "saturated" with bonds to either other carbon atoms or hydrogen atoms, no double bonds can exist. Such fatty acids are classified as saturated. All short- and medium-chain fatty acids are saturated; long-chain fatty acids may be either saturated or unsaturated. The major saturated fatty acids are palmitic acid and stearic acid.

Fatty acids are classified as unsaturated when one or more double bonds exist between carbon atoms; the carbon atoms are not saturated because not all four potential binding sites are used. Monounsaturated fatty acids contain only one double bond between carbon atoms.

The most prevalent monounsaturated fatty acid in the diet is oleic acid.

$$H-\underset{\underset{H}{|}}{\overset{\overset{H}{|}}{C}}-\underset{\underset{H}{|}}{\overset{\overset{H}{|}}{C}}-\underset{\underset{H}{|}}{\overset{\overset{H}{|}}{C}}-\underset{\underset{H}{|}}{\overset{\overset{H}{|}}{C}}-\underset{\underset{H}{|}}{\overset{\overset{H}{|}}{C}}-\underset{\underset{H}{|}}{\overset{\overset{H}{|}}{C}}-\underset{\underset{H}{|}}{\overset{\overset{H}{|}}{C}}-\overset{\overset{H}{|}}{C}=\overset{\overset{H}{|}}{C}-\underset{\underset{H}{|}}{\overset{\overset{H}{|}}{C}}-\underset{\underset{H}{|}}{\overset{\overset{H}{|}}{C}}-\underset{\underset{H}{|}}{\overset{\overset{H}{|}}{C}}-\underset{\underset{H}{|}}{\overset{\overset{H}{|}}{C}}-\underset{\underset{H}{|}}{\overset{\overset{H}{|}}{C}}-\underset{\underset{H}{|}}{\overset{\overset{H}{|}}{C}}-\overset{\overset{O}{\|}}{C}-O-H$$ (oleic acid)

Polyunsaturated fatty acids (PUFA) have two or more double bonds between carbon atoms. Omega-6 PUFA have their first double bond six carbon atoms from the methyl carbon. Linoleic acid, an omega-6 fatty acid, is one of the most common PUFA in plants. Omega-3 PUFA have their first double bond three carbon atoms from the methyl carbon. The most abundant omega-3 fatty acids are linolenic acid, found in plants, and the currently popular "fish oils," eicosapentaenoic acid (EPA) and docosahexaenoic acid (DHA).

$$H-C-C-C-C-C-C=C-C-C=C-C-C-C-C-C-C-C-O-H$$ (linoleic acid)

FOOD FATS: TRIGLYCERIDES

Glycerol molecules that are bound with only one fatty acid are known as monoglycerides (Fig. 3-1). When two fatty acids are attached to a glycerol molecule, they result in a diglyceride (Fig. 3-1). Both monoglycerides and diglycerides, which represent a very small percentage of the lipids in the diet, function as emulsifiers to keep fat particles dispersed and suspended in solution. For this reason, they often are used as food additives.

Triglycerides, which have three fatty acids attached to a glycerol molecule, comprise about 95% of the lipids in food. Just as amino acids can be arranged in limitless combinations to form different proteins, fatty acids can attach to glycerol molecules in various ratios and patterns to form a large variety of triglycerides within a single food fat. The types and amounts of fatty acids present determine the characteristics of triglycerides, which in turn determine the characteristics of food fats. For instance, butter tastes and acts differently than corn oil, which tastes and acts differently than lard.

Composition of Most Food Fats

Most food fats are generally made of long-chain fatty acids (*i.e.*, long-chain triglycerides); short- and medium-chain triglycerides occur less frequently. Long-chain fatty acids are more insoluble in water than shorter-chain fatty acids and also are more difficult to absorb than short- or medium-chain fatty acids.

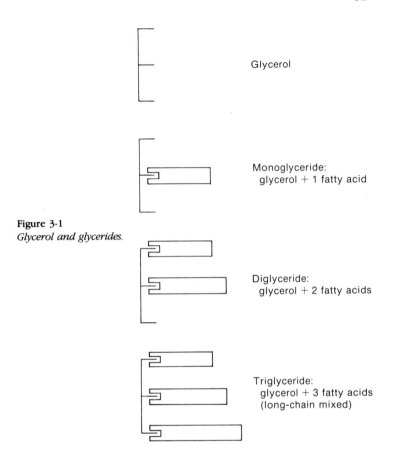

Figure 3-1
Glycerol and glycerides.

Glycerol

Monoglyceride:
glycerol + 1 fatty acid

Diglyceride:
glycerol + 2 fatty acids

Triglyceride:
glycerol + 3 fatty acids
(long-chain mixed)

Medium-chain triglycerides (MCT) containing fatty acids with 8 and 10 carbon atoms occur rarely in nature but are produced commercially from coconut oil. In powder or liquid form they are used therapeutically in the treatment of malabsorption disorders (see Chap. 15) because they are easily and quickly absorbed. Unlike long-chain triglycerides, MCT do not require emulsification with bile or digestion by pancreatic lipase because medium-chain fatty acids liberated from the glycerol molecule are absorbed directly into the portal system. Although MCT provide needed calories to patients unable to digest and absorb dietary fat, they are unpalatable, lack the essential fatty acids (EFA are long-chain, unsaturated fatty acids), and are expensive.

Most food fats also contain two or more different fatty acids, and hence are known as mixed triglycerides. The characteristics of triglycerides that contain two or more different fatty acids also are influenced by the order in which they are arranged. Simple triglycerides, which contain three molecules of the same fatty acids, are rare.

Most food fats contain both saturated and unsaturated fatty acids. When applied to individual triglycerides and sources of fat in the diet, saturated and unsaturated are not absolute terms used to describe the only type of fatty acids present; rather, they are relative descriptions of the type of fatty acids present in the largest amount (Table 3-4).

Table 3-4
The Percentage of Polyunsaturated, Monounsaturated, and Saturated Fatty Acids in Selected Fats and Oils

	% Polyunsaturated Fatty Acids	% Monounsaturated Fatty Acids	% Saturated Fatty Acids
"UNSATURATED" OILS			
Safflower	**75**	12	9
Sunflower	**66**	20	10
Corn	**59**	24	13
Soybean	**58**	23	14
Cottonseed	**52**	18	26
"MONOUNSATURATED" FATS AND OILS			
Olive oil	8	**74**	13
Stick margarine	30	**59**	19
Canola oil	33	**55**	7
Soft tub margarine	31	**47**	18
Peanut oil	32	**46**	17
"SATURATED" FATS AND OILS			
Coconut oil	2	6	**86**
Palm kernel oil	2	11	**81**
Butter	4	29	**64**
Palm oil	9	37	**49**
Beef fat	4	42	**50**

(USDHHS Public Health Service: Facts About Blood Cholesterol. National Institutes of Health Publication no. 88-2696, 1987)

Unsaturated Fats

Generally, food fats high in polyunsaturated fatty acids tend to be soft or liquid at room temperature and have low melting points—the more double bonds in a fatty acid, the lower the melting point. Poultry fat, for instance, is softer than beef fat because it has a higher percentage of unsaturated fatty acids. All vegetable oils, with the exception of coconut, palm kernel, and palm, are high in unsaturated fats (see Table 3-4). Although they are animals, chicken and freshwater fish are also high in unsaturated fat.

Polyunsaturated fats, especially the EFA, are susceptible to rancidity when exposed to light and oxygen over a prolonged period of time. The chemical change that occurs results in an offensive change in taste and smell and the loss of vitamins A and E. The two major antioxidants added to fats (*i.e.*, BHA, BHT) extend shelf life and protect vitamins A and E. Minimizing storage time and avoiding high temperatures also protects fats against rancidity.

Saturated Fats

Generally, food fats high in saturated fatty acids tend to be solid at room temperature and have high melting points. With the exception of those in poultry and freshwater fish, all animal fats are high in saturated fats (see Table 3-4). The only saturated vegetable fats are coconut, palm kernel, and palm oils.

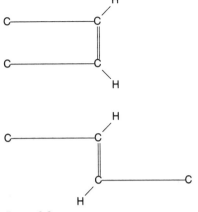

Cis-fatty acid configuration: both hydrogen atoms are on the same side of the double bond.

Trans-fatty acid: the hydrogen atoms are on opposite sides of the double bond.

Figure 3-2
Cis- *and* trans-*fatty acid configurations.*

Hydrogenated Fats

Hydrogenated fats are unsaturated vegetable oils (usually corn, soybean, cottonseed, safflower, peanut, or olive) that have hydrogen atoms added to some of the double bonds to make the fat more saturated and solid at room temperature—the more hydrogen atoms added, the more saturated and harder the resulting product. Examples of hydrogenated fats include shortening, margarine, and spreads such as cheese, butter, or cream. Although hydrogenated products are less likely to oxidize and become rancid, they bear little resemblance to the original oil.

Unfortunately, hydrogenated fats have lower unsaturated fatty acid contents than the original oil. Unsaturated fatty acids have been shown to lower serum cholesterol levels and may therefore help reduce the risk of atherosclerosis. Also, the unsaturated fatty acids that remain are structurally different from the original molecule: The double bonds in the *cis*-position, which occur naturally in nature, are converted to the *trans*-position (Fig. 3-2). Unfortunately, transpolyunsaturated fatty acids do not provide essential fatty acid function, nor are they made by the body or naturally abundant in foods. Although they are assumed to be safe, their effect on metabolism and health is unknown.

OTHER LIPIDS

The other 5% of lipids in the diet are phospholipids, of which lecithin is the most common, and sterols, including cholesterol. Lipoproteins are compound lipids that serve to transport lipids and cholesterol through the blood.

Phospholipids

Phospholipids are a group of compound lipids that are similar to triglycerides in that they contain a glycerol molecule and two fatty acids. However, in place of the third fatty acid, phospholipids have a substance containing phosphorus and nitrogen. Phospholipids are found naturally in almost all foods, and because they are soluble in both water and fat, they are used extensively by the food industry as emulsifiers.

Lecithin is the best-known phospholipid. Numerous claims that lecithin should be supplemented in the diet because it is an essential nutrient are untrue. Although lecithin does have important roles in the body, it is not required in the diet because the body synthesizes it. Also, lecithin consumed in the diet is not absorbed intact and transported throughout the body to perform super-functions. Instead, lecithin is broken down by enzymes in the intestinal tract, and its individual components are absorbed and sent to the liver to be used as necessary.

Phospholipids serve as a structural component of cell membranes and are able to transport water-soluble and fat-soluble substances across membranes. Phospholipids are precursors of prostaglandins, a group of fatty-acid derivatives with hormone-like actions that help regulate blood pressure, aid in nerve impulse transmission, regulate gastric secretions and muscular contractions of the gastrointestinal tract, stimulate uterine contractions, induce labor and abortions, and inhibit lipid catabolism.

Cholesterol

Cholesterol is a member of the sterol family, which includes bile acids, sex hormones, the adrenocortical hormones, and vitamin D. Although cholesterol performs vital functions in the body, it is not essential in the diet because it is synthesized primarily in the liver from glucose or saturated fatty acids. In fact, every day the body manufactures two to three times more cholesterol than the average diet contains.

Cholesterol is found only in animal products and is most abundant in organ meats and egg yolks (Table 3-5). Like other lipids, cholesterol is transported through the blood in lipoproteins.

Cholesterol is an essential constituent of all cell membranes and is especially abundant in brain and nerve cells. About 80% of metabolized cholesterol is used to synthesize bile acids; the cholesterol in bile acids is recycled. A high-fiber diet enhances the excretion of bile salts and, therefore, reduces cholesterol in the body. Cholesterol is a precursor of the steroid hormones and vitamin D: cholesterol in the skin + ultraviolet light = the formation of vitamin D.

The role of dietary cholesterol is widely debated in the development of atherosclerosis, a condition characterized by the formation of fatty plaques (containing mostly cholesterol) along the inside of arteries. A high serum cholesterol level is one of many risk factors associated with atherosclerosis, and diet influences serum cholesterol levels. Because most of the cholesterol circulating in the bloodstream is made by the liver from saturated fats, a high intake of saturated fat has a greater impact on serum cholesterol levels than a high intake of cholesterol. To help lower serum cholesterol levels, researchers recommend reducing total fat and saturated fat intake, replacing some saturated fat intake with PUFA and monounsaturated fats, and limiting dietary intake of cholesterol. See Chapter 16 for more on diet and heart disease.

Lipoproteins

Lipoproteins are compound lipids containing protein with various types and amounts of lipids. They are made mostly in the liver and are used to transport water-insoluble lipids

Table 3-5
Cholesterol Content of Selected Foods

	Cholesterol (mg)		Cholesterol (mg)
BEEF (3½ oz cooked)		**FISH (3½ oz cooked)**	
Kidneys	387	Haddock	74
Liver	389	Cod	55
Sirloin, lean only	76	Salmon, sockeye	87
Chuck, pot roast, lean only	101	Lobster, northern	72
Salami, cured	65	Shrimp	195
LAMB (3½ oz cooked)		**MILK (8 ounces)**	
Loin chop, lean	94	Skim	4
Arm chop, lean only	122	Buttermilk	9
PORK (3½ oz cooked)		1% Fat	10
		2% Fat	18
Liver	355	Whole	33
Kidneys	480	**CHEESE**	
Fresh ham	96	Mozzarella, 1 oz, part skim	16
Liverwurst	158	Swiss, 1 oz	26
VEAL (3½ oz cooked)		Cheddar, 1 oz	30
Rump, lean only	128	**EGGS***	
Loin chop, lean only	90	White only	0
POULTRY (3½ oz cooked)		Whole egg	213
		Yolk	213
Turkey, light meat with skin	95	**FROZEN DESSERTS (1 cup)**	
Turkey, dark meat without skin	112	Sherbet	14
Chicken, light meat without skin	75	Ice milk, hard	18
Duck, flesh only	89	Ice cream, French vanilla, soft	153
Goose, flesh only	96	Ice cream, vanilla, rich	88
Turkey bologna, 3.5 slices	99		
Chicken frankfurter, 2	101		

(USDHHS Public Health Service, National Institutes of Health: Eating to Lower Your High Blood Cholesterol. Washington DC: Government Printing Office, 1989.
* The cholesterol content of eggs was recently adjusted downward from the 274-mg figure that has been quoted since 1976. Better methods of analyzing cholesterol content are responsible, say researchers at the USDA's Nutrient Composition Laboratory)

through the blood. Elevated levels of certain kinds of lipoproteins (hyperlipoproteinemias) are risk factors for the development of atherosclerosis (see Chap. 16). The following are classifications of lipoproteins based on density:

- Chylomicrons: composed mainly of triglycerides encased in a protein and phospholipid coating, chylomicrons form to transport absorbed triglycerides from the intestines to the liver. High serum chylomicron levels do not increase the risk of atherosclerosis.
- Very-low-density lipoproteins (VLDL): contain primarily triglycerides with little protein and cholesterol. VLDL transport endogenous triglycerides from the liver to the tissues. High serum VLDL levels may increase the risk of atherosclerosis.
- Low-density lipoproteins (LDL): composed largely of cholesterol, function to transport cholesterol from the liver to the tissues. High serum LDL levels greatly increase the risk of atherosclerosis.
- High-density lipoproteins (HDL): primarily protein, with small amounts of tri-

glycerides and cholesterol, HDL transport cholesterol from the tissues to the liver to be metabolized. High serum HDL levels are protective against the development of atherosclerosis.

HOW THE BODY HANDLES FAT

Digestion

A minimal amount of chemical digestion of fat occurs in the stomach by the action of a gastric lipase on short-chain triglycerides (found in butter) into fatty acids and glycerol (Fig. 3-3).

Through a series of events, fat in the duodenum stimulates the gallbladder to contract and release bile, which is not an enzyme, but an emulsifier. Continually produced in the liver and concentrated and stored in the gallbladder, bile contains bile salts, cholesterol, phospholipids, bilirubin, and electrolytes. As an emulsifier, bile breaks down fat globules into smaller particles to increase the surface area on which pancreatic lipase can work.

Pancreatic lipase is the most important and powerful lipase, or fat-digesting enzyme. It splits off one fatty acid at a time from triglyceride molecules. Because each removal of a fatty acid becomes increasingly difficult, only one third to one half of the total fat is actually broken down completely to fatty acids and glycerol.

The end products of triglyceride digestion are fatty acids, glycerol, and mono-glycerides.

Absorption

Short- and medium-chain free fatty acids, glycerol, and medium-chain triglycerides are absorbed directly through the mucosal cells into the portal vein and are transported to the liver.

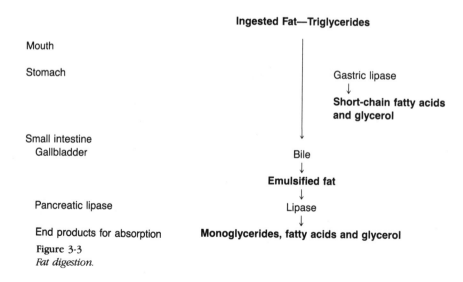

Figure 3-3
Fat digestion.

Monoglycerides and long-chain fatty acids, which are insoluble in water but dissolve in micelles, are formed from bile salts. Micelles then transport the monoglycerides and fatty acids to the mucosal cells of the villi, where they diffuse into the cells. The released bile salts return to the intestine, where most are reabsorbed in the terminal ileum, transported back to the liver, and recycled (enterohepatic circulation).

Within the mucosal cells of the small intestine, intestinal lipase breaks down monoglycerides into fatty acids and glycerol; the fatty acids and glycerol are then reformed into triglycerides. The reformed triglycerides, along with other lipids, such as cholesterol and phospholipids, become encased in protein to form chylomicrons.

Chylomicrons enter the bloodstream via the lymph system and the thoracic duct. Their destination is the liver by way of the hepatic artery.

About 95% of fat consumed is absorbed, mostly in the duodenum and jejunum. Normally, about 5 g of fat are excreted in the feces daily. Inadequate bile output, a high-fiber diet, and rapid gastrointestinal motility all decrease fat absorption and thereby increase fecal fat excretion. Steatorrhea, a condition that occurs when fecal fat excretion exceeds 6% of total fat intake, is a symptom of fat maldigestion or malabsorption disorders (see Chap. 15; see box, Conditions Requiring Alterations in Fat Intake).

Metabolism

After entering the bloodstream, lipids are transported either to the liver or adipose tissue. Fat anabolism (buildup) and catabolism (breakdown) are regulated by hormones (Table 3-6).

Fat Anabolism

The liver can synthesize lipids from an excess intake of CHO or protein through the process of lipogenesis. Through a complex series of steps, glucose is converted to glycerol and fatty acids, which may then be synthesized into triglycerides for storage in adipose tissue, or converted to lipoproteins, phospholipids, or cholesterol as needed. Ketogenic amino acids remaining after protein requirements are met can be converted to and stored as fat.

Fat Catabolism

In order for the body to use stored fat for energy, lipases within the cell first must split the triglycerides into their component parts—a glycerol molecule and fatty acids.

The glycerol molecule is converted to glucose (gluconeogenesis) and metabolized for energy, converted to glycogen, or converted to fat.

Through a complex series of reactions, fatty acids are catabolized by the liver (β oxidation) to two-carbon fragments. These fragments, known as acetyl coenzyme A (CoA), can be oxidized for energy.

During normal fat metabolism, which requires oxygen and a compound generated by glucose (CHO) metabolism, small amounts of ketone bodies are formed (ketogenesis) and used for energy. However, when fat catabolism is excessive, such as when CHO intake is inadequate or unavailable to meet the body's energy needs (as in the case of uncontrolled

Conditions Requiring Alterations in Fat Intake

LOW-FAT DIETS ARE USED FOR

Chronic pancreatitis

Cystic fibrosis

Other malabsorption syndromes

Possibly for gallbladder disease

Obesity, as part of an overall reduction in calorie intake

MODIFIED FAT DIETS (SUCH AS LOW CHOLESTEROL, LOW SATURATED FAT, INCREASED POLYUNSATURATED FAT DIETS) MAY BE USED

To treat hyperlipoproteinemias

As a preventative measure against coronary heart disease

As part of a diabetic diet as prevention against long-term complications resulting from altered fat metabolism

A HIGH-FAT DIET MAY BE USED

To induce ketosis in patients with epilepsy or other seizure disorders

diabetes), ketones accumulate in the bloodstream, leading to the condition known as *ketosis.* Normal fat catabolism cannot proceed if the supply of oxygen is inadequate, such as during strenuous exercise or respiratory disease.

FAT ALLOWANCES, RECOMMENDATIONS, AND CONSUMPTION TRENDS

Saturated fatty acids, monounsaturated fatty acids, and cholesterol can be synthesized in the body, and therefore no dietary requirement exists. Linoleic acid, which is known as "*the* EFA" because it alone can alleviate symptoms of EFA deficiency, should supply 1% to 2% of the total calorie intake in adults, or a minimum daily intake of 3 to 6 g/day. This requirement is easily met in the typical American diet; safflower, sunflower, corn, cottonseed, and soybean oils are excellent sources of EFA. It is estimated that even in a totally fat-free diet, as little as one teaspoon of corn oil would supply enough linoleic acid to meet EFA require-ments. For infants consuming 100 cal/kg of body weight/day, EFA requirement is approx-imately 0.2 g/kg.

Although only 3 to 6 g of fat/day may truly be required, additional fat may be included in the diet for energy (calorie) requirements. However, because the body can get calories

Table 3-6
Hormones Affecting Fat Metabolism

Hormone	Effect on Fat Metabolism
ACTH (adrenocorticotropic hormone)	Increases fat mobilization
Epinephrine	Increases the rate of fat mobilization
Glucagon	Increases fat mobilization; decreases fat synthesis
Glucocorticoids	Increases the rate of fat mobilization
Growth hormone	Stimulates the release of free fatty acids from adipose tissue
Insulin	Stimulates fat synthesis
Thyroxine	Increases the rate of fat mobilization

from other sources (*i.e.*, carbohydrates), a fat requirement to meet calorie needs is not necessary.

The third edition of *Dietary Guidelines for Americans* recommends that Americans choose a diet low in fat, saturated fat, and cholesterol.[7] The suggestions for implementing these recommendations appear in Chapter 8. According to *The Surgeon General's Report on Nutrition and Health*, a reduction in total fat intake, especially saturated fat, is emerging as the priority for dietary change in American diets.[6] Research indicates that diets high in fat, saturated fat, and cholesterol increase the risk of obesity, heart disease, and certain cancers (see below). Indeed, the American Cancer Society and the Food and Nutrition Board's Committee on Diet and Health recommend that all adult Americans limit fat intake to 30% of total calories or less. In addition, the American Heart Association further advises that saturated fat intake and PUFA intake each not exceed 10% of total calories. Whether or not these recommendations are appropriate for infants, children, and the elderly is debated.

Currently, the average American adult consumes 37% of total calories from fat, down from 43% in 1980. The major sources of fat in the American diet are meat, fish, poultry, milk, and dairy products (Fig. 3-4).

Although some progress is being made toward reducing and modifying fat intake, more change is needed, since average saturated fat intake is 13% of total calories and PUFA contribute 7% of total calories. To achieve the necessary changes in fat intake, Americans need to become more knowledgeable about their total fat allowance based on individual calorie requirements and must learn how to read labels to evaluate the fat content of foods eaten (see box, Figuring Fat). A general goal should be a fat intake of 30% of total calories or less; foods providing more than 30% are not necessarily contraindicated, but they should be balanced with low-fat foods so that overall intake approximates 30%.

FAT EXCESSES

An "excess of fat" is hard to define because actual fat requirement is so small. Most nutrition and health experts agree that Americans consume too much fat, which increases our risk as follows:

- Obesity. True, obesity can result from eating more calories than the body needs regardless of the source. However, because fats are a concentrated source of energy,

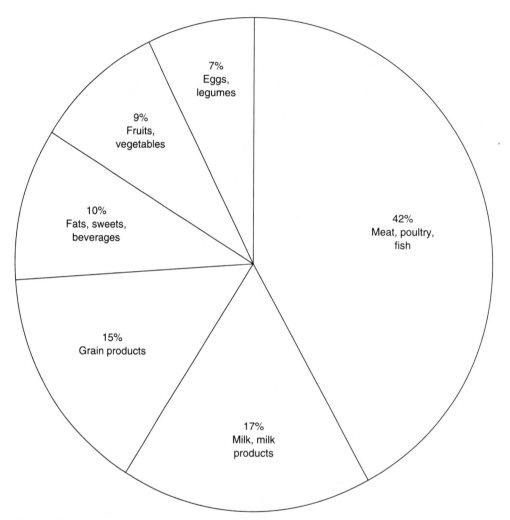

Figure 3-4
Percent contribution of various sources of fat in the average American diet. (USDA Nationwide Food Consumption Survey 1977–78, 48 Coterminous States)

eating 50 extra grams of fat (50 g × 9 cal/g = 450 calories) will cause weight gain more quickly than 50 extra grams of either CHO or protein (50 g × 4 cal/g = 200 extra calories). Whereas high-fat diets are high in calories, extremely low-fat diets tend to be unpalatable and lack satiety, that is, they leave you feeling hungry shortly after eating. An acceptable solution is a moderate fat intake (*i.e.*, 30% of calories), which eliminates excess calories but not palatability and satiety.

• Coronary heart disease. Heart disease is not a foregone conclusion for *individuals* who eat a diet rich in fat, saturated fat, and cholesterol. However, epidemiologic, animal, and clinical studies show that *population groups* who consume diets rich in fat have elevated serum cholesterol and lipoprotein levels, which are major risk factors in the development of atherosclerosis and coronary heart disease. The American Heart

Figuring Fat

To determine total daily fat allowance:
1. Multiply total number of calories in the diet by 30% (0.30) to determine the desired maximum number of calories from fat:

$$\begin{array}{r} 1800 \text{ calories} \\ \times\ 0.30 \\ \hline 540 \text{ calories from fat} \end{array}$$

2. Divide the total number of fat calories by 9 calories/g to determine the total grams of fat recommended per day:

540 fat calories divided by 9 calories/g = 60 g fat

To determine the percentage of calories provided by fat in a food item, the total number of calories/serving and the grams of fat/serving must be known (see Nutrition Information for fudge brownies below)
1. Multiply the grams of fat by 9 calories per gram to determine the number of fat calories:

7 g of fat × 9 calories/g = 63 fat calories

2. Divide the number of fat calories by the total number of calories per serving:

63 fat calories divided by 150 total calories = 0.42

3. Multiply the previous answer by 100 to determine the percent of calories provided by fat:

0.42 × 100 = 42%

Nutrition Information for fudge brownies per 2" square serving:

Calories	150
Protein (g)	1
CHO (g)	20
Fat (g)	7

Association recommends that in an effort to prevent heart and vascular diseases, adults limit their intake of total fat to 30% or less of total calories and limit saturated fat to 10% or less of total calories.

- Certain types of cancer. Although the role of diet in the development of cancer is far from clear, the American Cancer Society estimates that 30% to 35% of all cases of cancer are diet-related. Based on numerous epidemiologic and animal studies, it appears that high-fat diets increase the risk of breast and colon cancers. Although fat itself probably does not cause cancer, it seems to promote its development. In view of this, the Committee on Diet, Nutrition, and Cancer of the National Research Council/ National Academy of Sciences recommends Americans limit total fat intake to 30% of calories to reduce cancer risk. Interestingly, polyunsaturated fats seem just as likely to promote cancer as saturated fats, and cholesterol appears to have no known risk.

FAT DEFICIENCY

An EFA deficiency is rare but may develop in adults on prolonged EFA-free parenteral feedings and in infants consuming EFA-deficient formulas. Essential fatty acid-deficient infants may exhibit inadequate growth rates and decreased resistance to infection, possibly from an inadequate production of prostaglandins.

An inadequate total fat intake is not likely to occur, because the body can synthesize fats from other sources. Moreover, the average American diet contains an abundance of fat. When an inadequate intake of fat does occur, namely as an inadequate intake of calories, it is most likely related to one or more of the following problems:

- Disease or drug-induced anorexia (*i.e.*, cancer and cancer therapies)
- Anorexia nervosa, the psychological disorder of self-imposed starvation
- Altered digestion and absorption, such as pancreatic insufficiency, celiac sprue, lactose intolerance, and other malabsorption syndromes

Possible signs and symptoms of an inadequate fat intake include a thin, emaciated appearance related to the loss of subcutaneous adipose tissue; sensitivity to cold; dry, dull hair; constipation (fat in the intestine acts as a lubricant); secondary deficiencies of the fat-soluble vitamins; and secondary protein malnutrition.

BIBLIOGRAPHY

1. American Heart Association: Dietary Guidelines for Healthy American Adults: A Statement for Physicians and Health Professionals by the Nutrition Committee, American Heart Association. Dallas: American Heart Association, 1986
2. Lecos C: A compendium on fats. In Nutrition and Health: New Concepts and Issues L, Hafen, B, ed. Englewood, CO: Morton Publishing, 1985
3. Leibman B: Fish oil: Fad or find? Nutrition Action Health Letter 16:1, 1989
4. National Research Council: Recommended Dietary Allowances. 10th ed. Washington, DC: National Academy Press, 1989
5. Owens AL: The impact of future foods on nutrition and health. J Am Diet Assoc 90:1217, 1990
6. Public Health Service, United States Department of Health and Human Services: The Surgeon General's Report on Nutrition and Health: Summary and Recommendations. DHHS (PHS) Publication no. 88-50211. Washington, DC: Government Printing Office, 1988
7. United States Department of Agriculture, and United States Department of Health and Human Services: Nutrition and Your Health: Dietary Guidelines for Americans. 3rd ed. Home and Garden Bulletin no. 232, 1990

4 Energy Balance and Weight Control

ENERGY BALANCE

The body requires energy to carry on any kind of activity—whether voluntary, such as reading, eating, talking, and running, or involuntary, such as inflating the lungs, secreting enzymes, and beating the heart. The body derives energy in the form of calories from CHO, protein, fat, and also from alcohol. By comparing energy intake with output, a person's state of energy balance can be determined (Table 4-1).

Energy Intake

Units of Measure

Kilocalorie

A kilocalorie represents the amount of heat needed to raise the temperature of 1 g of water from 15°C to 16°C. It is the only unit of measure used in nutrition and is commonly abbreviated as kcal, calorie, cal, or c. In this text, kilocalories are abbreviated to "calories" and "cal." However, a kilocalorie actually is 1000 times larger than a true *calorie*, a unit of measure used only in chemistry and physics.

Kilojoule

Although calories are the unit of measure used in food composition tables and on food labels, the Committee on Nomenclature of the American Institute of Nutrition recom-

Table 4-1
State of Energy Balance

Balance	Description	Weight Status
Neutral	Calorie intake = calorie expenditure	Stable
Positive	Calorie intake > calorie expenditure	Increasing
Negative	Calorie intake < calorie expenditure	Decreasing

mended in 1970 that the unit *kilojoule* replace kilocalorie as soon as feasible. A kilojoule is a metric measurement defined as the amount of mechanical energy required when a force of 1 newton (N) moves 1 kilogram (kg) by a distance of 1 meter (m). One kilojoule equals 1000 joules and may be abbreviated as j, kJ, or KJ. Because 1 calorie equals 4.18 kilojoules, calories can be converted to kilojoules by multiplying the number of calories by 4.18.

Food Energy

To measure the calorie content of a food, a device known as a bomb calorimeter is used. In carefully controlled laboratory settings, a sample of burning food is placed in the calorimeter and its energy value is determined by measuring the rise in the temperature of the surrounding water (Fig. 4-1). Although a similar process takes place in the body when food is oxidized for energy, food actually produces less energy in the body than in the calorimeter because some food consumed is not absorbed and used for energy, but is excreted in the feces. Also, digestion, absorption, and metabolism are energy-requiring processes, and thus, some energy is used to produce energy. In addition, some absorbed nutrients may not be completely oxidized for energy.

The amount of energy available to the body from the metabolism of food has been determined to be 4 cal/g of carbohydrates, 4 cal/g of protein, 9 cal/g of fat, and 7 cal/g of alcohol. The total number of calories in a food or diet can be calculated if the total amount of CHO, protein, fat, and alcohol is known (see box, Sample Calculation). The calories and nutritional compositions of selected foods are listed in Appendix 1.

Energy Output

Total energy expenditure = resting energy expenditure (REE) + physical activity + the metabolic response to food

Resting Energy Expenditure (REE)

Resting energy expenditure is the caloric cost of staying alive, or the amount of energy required to carry on the involuntary activities of the body at rest and in the absence of fever. It is the energy required to maintain body temperature and muscle tone, produce and release secretions, propel the gastrointestinal tract, inflate the lungs, and beat the heart. Basal metabolic rate (BMR) is a more precise measurement of REE taken immediately after waking and 12 hours after the previous meal to eliminate any residual thermal effect. In practice, REE and BMR differ by less than 10%, and the terms are generally used interchangeably.

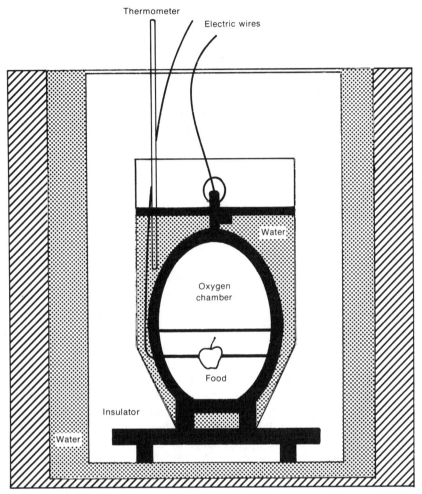

Figure 4-1
Sketch of a bomb calorimeter.

Sample Calculation of the Number of Calories in a Food Based on its CHO, Protein, and Fat Content

A piece of pumpkin pie containing 32 g CHO, 5 g protein, and 15 g fat contains

$$
\begin{aligned}
32 \text{ g CHO} \times 4 \text{ cal/g CHO} &= 128 \text{ cal of CHO} \\
5 \text{ g pro} \times 4 \text{ cal/g pro} &= 20 \text{ cal of protein} \\
15 \text{ g fat} \times 9 \text{ cal/g fat} &= \underline{135 \text{ cal of fat}} \\
&\quad\ \ 283 \text{ total calories}
\end{aligned}
$$

Unless physical activity is unusually high, REE accounts for more than half of most people's total energy requirements.[14] As physical activity decreases, the proportion of calories used for REE increases. Resting energy expenditure is generally about 1 cal/kg of body weight per hour for men and 0.9 cal/kg/hour for women. Table 4-2 gives equations for predicting REE from body weight. These values are not precise for individuals, however, and should be used only as a guide. Hyperthermia, anxiety, growth, pregnancy and lactation, and elevated levels of hormones, particularly epinephrine and thyroid hormone, increase REE. Prolonged fasting, weight loss, starvation, hypothyroidism, anesthesia, paralysis, drugs (barbiturates, narcotics, and muscle relaxants), and sleep decrease REE. Table 4-3 lists the effects of other variables on both REE and physical activity.

EXAMPLE

The number of calories spent on REE/day by a person weighing 143 lb (65 kg) is

$$\text{REE for a 65-kg man} = 65 \text{ kg} \times 1 \text{ cal/kg} \times 24 \text{ hours}$$
$$= 1560 \text{ cal/24 hours}$$
$$\text{REE for a 65-kg woman} = 65 \text{ kg} \times 0.9 \text{ cal/kg} \times 24 \text{ hours}$$
$$= 1404 \text{ cal/24 hours}$$

Physical Activity

Unfortunately, mental activity requires little energy, although it may increase REE if it increases tension—and people may be *busy* without being physically active. Since the turn of the century, work-related energy expenditure has declined for most Americans because of the increase in mechanization and proliferation of labor-saving devices.

The actual amount of energy expended on voluntary physical activity depends on the intensity and duration of the activity—the more intense and prolonged the activity, the greater the energy expended. Another factor is the weight of the person performing the activity. Heavier people, who have more weight to move, use more energy than lighter people to perform the same activity.

Table 4-2
Equations for Predicting Resting Energy Expenditure from Body Weight*

Sex and Age Range (years)	Equation to Derive REE in kcal/day	Sex and Age Range (years)	Equation to Derive REE in kcal/day
MEN		**WOMEN**	
0–3	$(60.9 \times \text{wt}\dagger) - 54$	0–3	$(61.0 \times \text{wt}) - 51$
3–10	$(22.7 \times \text{wt}) + 495$	3–10	$(22.5 \times \text{wt}) + 499$
10–18	$(17.5 \times \text{wt}) + 651$	10–18	$(12.2 \times \text{wt}) + 746$
18–30	$(15.3 \times \text{wt}) + 679$	18–30	$(14.7 \times \text{wt}) + 496$
30–60	$(11.6 \times \text{wt}) + 879$	30–60	$(8.7 \times \text{wt}) + 829$
>60	$(13.5 \times \text{wt}) + 487$	>60	$(10.5 \times \text{wt}) + 596$

(National Research Council: Recommended Dietary Allowances. 10th ed. Washington, DC: National Academy of Sciences, 1989)

*From WHO (1985). These equations were derived from BMR data.

† Weight of person in kilograms.

Table 4-3
The Impact of Variables on REE and Physical Activity

Variable	Effect on REE	Effect on Activity
Age	The amount and composition of active tissue is influenced by age. Lean body mass decreases after early adulthood by 2% to 3% per decade; REE declines proportionately.	Children are typically active. Activity generally decreases with age.
Sex	After maturity, men have a greater amount of lean body mass than women, which accounts for approximately 10% difference in REE between the sexes.	Due to an increase in women in the workplace, work-related activity requirements are now similar for men and women.
Body Size	REE is higher for people with large body size compared to smaller people of the same sex and age.	The more a person weighs, the more calories are expended per unit of time performing activities.
Climate		
Cold	Exposure to cold that induces shivering results in an increase in REE.	Calorie expenditure may increase modestly as a result of carrying extra weight of cold weather clothing and footwear.
Heat	Environmental temperatures greater than 99°F increase REE by requiring more energy be spent to regulate body temperature.	Extreme heat may result in a voluntary reduction in physical activity.

There are numerous methods available for calculating energy expenditure, based on body weight, REE, or estimations of activity level (*i.e.*, very light, light, moderate, or heavy). Table 4-4 gives calories expended per minute by the "average" man and woman for various activity levels.

Metabolic Response to Food

The metabolic response to food, sometimes referred to as "specific dynamic action" (SDA), is the amount of energy required to digest, absorb, and metabolize food. Because the metabolism of protein requires a lot of energy, high-protein meals may increase BMR by as much as 15% to 30%. However, in a normal, mixed diet, the "cost" of processing food is about 5% to 10% of the total calorie intake.[14] For instance, people consuming 1800 cal/day use about 180 calories to process their food. If actual calorie intake is unknown, SDA can be estimated by calculating 10% of the average total calories consumed.

IDEAL BODY WEIGHT

"Ideal body weight" has yet to be conclusively defined; it is an imprecise term used to describe optimal weight for optimal health. Standards for ideal body weight are often controversial: Overweight people may regard them as overly harsh, whereas people who are underweight may argue they are inflated. New evidence that heavier may be better as

| Food for Thought | **A Calorie Is a Calorie Is a Calorie . . . or Is It?** |

Compared to the turn of the century, Americans are eating fewer calories but average weight continues to climb. True, our lifestyle is generally more sedentary because an increase in mechanization has caused us to burn fewer calories at work and at play. But, we are also eating a greater percentage of our calories from fat, and research has shown that the more fat calories are consumed, the greater the tendency to gain weight, regardless of total calorie intake.

It appears that the body uses only 3% of the calories in fat to convert dietary fat into fat deposits, compared to using 23% of calories in carbohydrates to convert carbohydrate into adipose. In addition, carbohydrates appear to require more energy to be digested than previously thought, so actual available calories from carbohydrates are less. Simply stated, if two people with the same calorie requirements adhere to a 1200-calorie reduction diet, the one eating the fewest fat calories will lose weight faster. So it is not just how *much* we eat, but *what* we eat that determines body weight. And strike up another plus for complex carbohydrates.

people age, and that the distribution of weight may be just as, or more important than total weight, has prompted a change in terminology in weight recommendations as put forth in the third edition of *Dietary Guidelines for Americans*.[16] Instead of "maintain desirable weight," Americans are now urged to "maintain healthy weight," whatever that weight may be.

Table 4-4
The Amount of Calories Expended / Minute Based on Activity and Weight

Activity	Cal/Min	
	70-kg Man	*58-kg Women*
Sleeping, reclining	1.0–1.2	0.9–1.1
Very light activity: seated and standing activities, painting, auto and truck driving, laboratory work, typing, playing musical instruments, sewing, ironing, walking slowly	Up to 2.5	Up to 2.0
Light activity: level walking at 2.5 mph to 3 mph, tailoring, pressing, garage work, electrical trades, carpentry, restaurant trades, cannery workers, washing clothes, shopping with light load, golfing, sailing, table tennis, volleyball	2.5–4.9	2.0–3.9
Moderate activity: walking 3.5 mph to 4 mph, plastering, gardening, loading and stacking bales, scrubbing floors, shopping with heavy load, cycling, skiing, tennis, dancing	5.0–7.4	4.0–5.9
Heavy activity: walking with load uphill, tree felling, work with pick and shovel, basketball, swimming, climbing, football, jogging, chopping wood	7.5–12.0	6.0–10.0

(Previte JJ: Human Physiology. New York, McGraw-Hill, 1983)

Guidelines for Calculating Ideal Weight/Height

The following guidelines for determining ideal body weight are generally accepted as appropriate for populations; they may or may not be appropriate for individuals, depending on muscle mass, body frame, other physiologic factors, and age.

Infants: Based on weight/age or weight/length (see growth charts in Chap. 11)

Children: Based on weight/age (see Chap. 11)

Adults: Women

- Allow 100 lb for 5 ft of height
- Add 5 lb for each additional inch over 5 ft
- Subtract 10% for small frame; add 10% for large frame

Men

- Allow 106 lb for 5 ft of height
- Add 6 lb for each additional inch over 5 ft
- Subtract 10% for small frame; add 10% for large frame

EXAMPLE

IBW for a 5'6" adult is

	Female	Male
5' of height:	100 lb	106 lb
Per additional inch:	6" × 5 lb/" = 30 lb	6" × 6 lb/" = 36 lb
IBW equals:	130 lb ± 13 lb	142 lb ± 14 lb
	depending on frame size	depending on frame size

Metropolitan Life Insurance Tables

Initially, life insurance weight tables presented average weights of its policy holders. Periodically updated, the tables developed into "ideal" weight tables based on mortality statistics. Although the weights indicated in the most recent edition (1983) of the *Metropolitan Life Insurance Tables* are associated with the lowest mortality rate (Table 4-5), they are not labeled "ideal" and are heavier than previous tables. A guide for estimating body size has also been included (Table 4-6).

Body Mass Index (BMI)

Body mass index, defined as weight in kilograms divided by height in meters squared, is a relatively new method of evaluating body weight. Body mass index generally is interpreted as follows: normal = 20 to 25; overweight = 26 to 30; obese = 30 to 40; morbid obesity = >40.

Table 4-5
1983 Metropolitan Life Insurance Co.
Height and Weight Tables

Height	Small Frame	Medium Frame	Large Frame
	←———————————— lb ————————————→		
MEN*			
5' 2"	128–134	131–141	138–150
5' 3"	130–136	133–143	140–153
5' 4"	132–138	135–145	142–156
5' 5"	134–140	137–148	144–160
5' 6"	136–142	139–151	146–164
5' 7"	138–145	142–154	149–168
5' 8"	140–148	145–157	152–172
5' 9"	142–151	148–160	155–176
5' 10"	144–154	151–163	158–180
5' 11"	146–157	154–166	161–184
6' 0"	149–160	157–170	164–188
6' 1"	152–164	160–174	168–192
6' 2"	155–168	164–178	172–197
6' 3"	158–172	167–182	176–202
6' 4"	162–176	171–187	181–207
WOMEN†			
4' 10"	102–111	109–121	118–131
4' 11"	103–113	111–123	120–134
5' 0"	104–115	113–126	122–137
5' 1"	106–118	115–129	125–140
5' 2"	108–121	118–132	128–143
5' 3"	111–124	121–135	131–147
5' 4"	114–127	124–138	134–151
5' 5"	117–130	127–141	137–155
5' 6"	120–133	130–144	140–159
5' 7"	123–136	133–147	143–163
5' 8"	126–139	136–150	146–167
5' 9"	129–142	139–153	149–170
5' 10"	132–145	142–156	152–173
5' 11"	135–148	145–159	155–176
6' 0"	138–151	148–162	158–179

*Weights at ages 25 to 59 based on lowest mortality. Weight in pounds according to frame (in indoor clothing weighing 5 lb, shoes with 1" heels).
†Weights at ages 25 to 59 based on lowest mortality. Weight in pounds according to frame (in indoor clothing weighing 3 lb, shoes with 1" heels).
(Courtesy of Metropolitan Life Insurance Company)

Determining Body Composition

Although weight tables provide a general guideline for ideal weight for height, they do not take into consideration body composition. A football player, for instance, may greatly exceed the average ideal weight range for his height because of a large muscle mass, not because he is overfat.

Recent research indicates that the distribution of body fat may be a more important

Table 4-6
*How to Determine Your Body Frame by Elbow Breadth**

To make a simple approximation of your frame size:

Extend your arm and bend the forearm upwards at a 90° angle. Keep the fingers straight and turn the inside of your wrist toward the body. Place the thumb and index finger of your other hand on the two prominent bones on either side of your elbow. Measure the space between your fingers against a ruler or a tape measure. Compare this measurement with the measurements shown below.

These tables list the elbow measurements for men and women of medium frame at various heights. Measurements lower than those listed indicate that you have a small frame, while higher measurements indicate a larger frame.

Height (in 1" heels)	Elbow Breadth (in.)	Height (cm) (in 2.5-cm heels)	Elbow Breadth (cm)
MEN			
5'2"–5'3"	2½–2⅞	158–161	6.4–7.2
5'2"–5'7"	2⅝–2⅞	162–171	6.7–7.4
5'8"–5'11"	2¾–3	172–181	6.9–7.6
6'0"–6'3"	2¾–3⅛	182–191	7.1–7.8
6'4"	2⅞–3¼	192–193	7.4–8.1
WOMEN			
4'10"–4'11"	2¼–2½	148–151	5.6–6.4
5'0"–5'3"	2¼–2½	152–161	5.8–6.5
5'4"–5'7"	2⅜–2⅝	162–171	5.9–6.6
5'8"–5'11"	2⅜–2⅝	172–181	6.1–6.8
6'0"	2½–2¾	182–183	6.2–6.9

* *Source of basic data: Data tape, HANES I. (Courtesy of Metropolitan Life Insurance Company)*

and reliable indicator of health risk than total body fatness.[2] A high distribution of abdominal fat, as indicated by a waist : hip ratio greater than 0.95 in men, is associated with an increased risk of non-insulin-dependent diabetes mellitus and cardiovascular disease, even though no association between generalized obesity and those diseases is evident.[2] Another study indicates that women with waist : hip ratios higher than 0.8 are roughly five times more likely to have breast cancer than women whose ratios are lower.[7] Waist : hip ratio can be obtained by dividing waist measurement by the measurement of the hips taken at the widest point between the hips and buttocks.

Skinfold measurements, taken of the biceps, triceps, subscapular, or suprailiac, provide an objective measurement of subcutaneous fat stores. Unfortunately, training and skill are required to obtain reliable measurements, and equipment is needed. See Chapter 9 for the procedure and interpretation of triceps skinfold measurements.

Clinically impractical objective measurements of body fatness can be obtained through the water displacement test: The percentage of body fat can be determined by measuring the amount of water displaced when a person is weighed underwater. Radioactive potassium counting, a procedure used only for research purposes, measures lean body tissue by "counting" the radioactive potassium it emits.

Simple subjective measurements of body composition include the following:

Mirror Test: Looking in the mirror can tell a great deal about body composition, without
  taking any kind of measurements.

Pinch Test: Pinching more than 1 inch of skin between the thumb and forefinger on the back of the upper arm indicates that a person is overfat.

Ruler Test: While lying on the back, place a 12-inch ruler on the stomach with the ends pointing toward the head and toes. If both ends of the ruler do not touch the body, overfat is indicated.

Girth Test (for men): By using a belt as a measuring device, determine body size at the waist and around the chest. Overfat is indicated when the waist is larger than the chest.

ESTIMATING CALORIE REQUIREMENTS

Calorie requirements, like ideal weight, can be determined using a variety of methods. Although highly variable and individualized, average calorie requirements have been set by the National Research Council of the National Academy of Sciences (Table 4-7). Generally, calorie requirements are higher among men than among women, due to a higher proportion of body weight from muscle, which requires more energy to be

Table 4-7
Median Heights and Weights and Recommended Energy Intake

Category	Age (years) or Condition	Weight (kg)	Weight (lb)	Height (cm)	Height (in)	REE* (kcal/day)	Multiples of REE	Average Energy Allowance (kcal)† per kg	per day‡
INFANTS	0.0–0.5	6	13	60	24	320		108	650
	0.5–1.0	9	20	71	28	500		98	850
CHILDREN	1–3	13	29	90	35	740		102	1300
	4–6	20	44	112	44	950		90	1800
	7–10	28	62	132	52	1130		70	2000
MEN	11–14	45	99	157	62	1440	1.70	55	2500
	15–18	66	145	176	69	1760	1.67	45	3000
	19–24	72	160	177	70	1780	1.67	40	2900
	25–50	79	174	176	70	1800	1.60	37	2900
	51+	77	170	173	68	1530	1.50	30	2300
WOMEN	11–14	46	101	157	62	1310	1.67	47	2200
	15–18	55	120	163	64	1370	1.60	40	2200
	19–24	58	128	164	65	1350	1.60	38	2200
	25–50	63	138	163	64	1380	1.55	36	2200
	51+	65	143	160	63	1280	1.50	30	1900
PREGNANT	1st trimester								+0
	2nd trimester								+300
	3rd trimester								+300
LACTATING	1st 6 months								+500
	2nd 6 months								+500

(National Research Council: Recommended Dietary Allowances. 10th ed. Washington, DC: National Academy of Sciences, 1989)
* Calculation of REE (Resting Energy Expenditure) based on FAO equations, then rounded.
† In the range of light to moderate activity, the coefficient of variation is ±20%.
‡ Figure is rounded.

maintained than fat tissue. Calorie requirements also increase during periods of growth (infancy, childhood, adolescence, pregnancy, and lactation) and during periods of stress, illness, and recovery.

Specific calorie requirements can be calculated by measuring the total amount of calories used for REE plus physical activity plus SDA. Other ways of estimating calorie needs are as follows:

- Determining BMR based on ideal weight and adding calories for activity (Method I; see box, Three Methods of Calculating Calorie Requirements)
- Multiplying ideal body weight by a known number of calories/pound based on the degree of physical activity (Method II; see box, Three Methods of Calculating Calorie Requirements)
- Using the USDA's guidelines based on sex, activity, and ideal body weight (Method III; see box, Three Methods of Calculating Calorie Requirements)

WEIGHT CONTROL: OVERWEIGHT AND OBESITY

When energy consumption exceeds energy expenditure, a positive energy balance results, leading to a weight gain over time. This can be caused by overeating, inactivity, or, most often, a combination of both. For instance, 1 pound of body fat equals 3500 calories; therefore, eating 500 extra cal/day for 7 days will produce a 1-lb weight gain. A person will gain 2 lb/week if daily intake exceeds expenditure by 1000 cal/day. Even a seemingly insignificant 1 extra glass of soft drink that supplies 145 calories will produce a 15-lb weight gain in a year if consumed daily and if not offset with an increase in activity.

$$145 \text{ cal} \times 365 \text{ days/year} = 52,925 \text{ extra cal/year}$$

$$\frac{52,925 \text{ cal/year}}{3500 \text{ cal/lb}} = 15 \text{ lb/year}$$

Although society in general assumes obese people consume hoards of food, research has shown that many obese people actually eat less than their thin counterparts. The snowball effect of inactivity and increased weight gain perpetuates obesity—inactivity can lead to an increased weight gain, and a weight gain can lead to social isolation and further reduction in activity (Fig. 4-2). Inactivity has been identified as a major cause of obesity among Americans.[6]

Obesity is defined as excess body fat. However, because it is difficult and impractical to accurately measure body fat, weight compared to height is most often used to assess the degree of obesity.

Reportedly, 70 million Americans want to lose weight, although only 34 million are actually overweight according to the following definitions:

Desirable weight range: IBW ± 10%

Overweight: weight between 110% and 120% of desirable body weight

Mild obesity: weight 120% to 140% of desirable body weight. Of all Americans classified as obese, 90.5% are considered mildly obese.

Moderate obesity: weight 141% to 200% of desirable body weight, affecting 9% of obese Americans

Three Methods of Calculating Calorie Requirements

Method I

ADULTS

Multiply ideal body weight (IBW) (kg) × 24 hours × 1.0 cal/kg (men) or 0.9 cal/kg (women) to determine basal calorie requirements. Depending on activity level, multiply basal energy requirements by the appropriate number indicated below.

Activity	Calories
Sedentary	Basal calorie needs × 1.3
Moderate	Basal calorie needs × 1.5
Heavy	Basal calorie needs × 1.75

CHILDREN (Under 12 Years Old)

Generally allow 1000 calories plus 100 calories/year of age. For example, a 4-year-old child needs approximately 1000 + (100 calories × 4) = 1400 calories.

Method II

Depending on activity level, multiply IBW in pounds by the appropriate number of calories.

Activity	Cal/lb of IBW
Sedentary	11–12
Light	13–14
Moderate	15–16
Heavy	18–19

Method III: USDA Guidelines for Calculating Calorie Requirements

Based on activity level, multiply ideal body weight in pounds by the appropriate number of calories/pound according to sex.

Activity	Cal/lb of IBW Males	Females
Sedentary	16	14
Moderate	21	18
Heavy	26	22

Morbidly obesity: greater than 200% of desirable body weight, affecting 0.5% of the obese population

The etiology of obesity is multifactorial and differs among individuals. Numerous genetic, physiologic, environmental, and psychological causes have been proposed (see box, Genetic, Physiologic, Environmental, and Psychological Theories). It is estimated that approximately 25% of American children are obese.

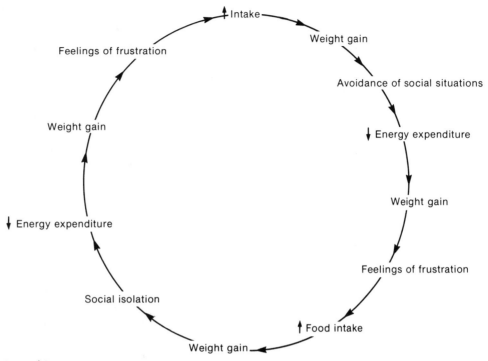

Figure 4-2
Perpetuating cycle of inactivity and weight gain.

Obesity is a serious problem because it increases the risks of hypertension, hyperlipidemia, cardiovascular diseases, non-insulin-dependent diabetes mellitus, respiratory disorders, osteoarthritis, and other chronic diseases. Obesity may increase the risk of colon and breast cancers, and increases surgical risks. Obesity also is associated with complications during pregnancy, labor, and delivery, and obese people have a higher mortality and morbidity than their thin counterparts.

Obesity also presents psychological and social disadvantages. In a society that emphasizes thinness, obesity leads to feelings of failure, desperation, frustration, and rejection. Obese people may be viewed as "bad," "dirty," and "stupid" and are often discriminated against in social, educational, and employment settings.

Unfortunately, obesity is very resistant to treatment. According to Brownell,[4] obesity is harder to "cure" than many forms of cancer, if cure is defined as attaining and maintaining ideal body weight for 5 years. Less than 20% of those who achieve desired weight loss are able to maintain their new weight. The prevention of obesity is far more effective than its treatment.

Treatment

Treatment programs vary with the degree of overweightness, although there are key components common to all successful weight control programs (Table 4-8). Conventional weight control programs stressing diet counseling, prescribed exercise, and psycho-

Genetic, Physiologic, Environmental, and Psychological Theories Related to the Etiology of Obesity

Genetic Theories

Faulty ATP production: Obese people have lower levels of ATPase, an enzyme responsible for 15% to 40% of all the energy use not associated with physical activity.[12] Because obese people have less ATPase than thin people, they use less energy performing metabolic activities.

Familial traits: The weight of natural children is highly correlated to that of their natural parents, whereas there is only a slight correlation between the weight of adopted children and their adoptive parents.

Physiologic Theories

Fat cell theory: People of normal weight have approximately 30 billion fat cells; morbidly obese people may have three to five times more. Although the biggest increase in the number of fat cells occurs from birth to age 5 and from 7 to 11, the number of fat cells can increase at any age. Once created, a fat cell exists for life. Fat cells can shrink in size when fat is broken down for energy, but the number of fat cells remains the same. Hence, obese people have extreme difficulty losing weight because of biologic pressures to keep the fat cells supplied with energy.[13]

"Set point" theory: A center in the hypothalamus determines a "set point" or ideal biologic weight for the individual. When weight falls below what the body has determined as "ideal," metabolic rate is adjusted downward to reduce energy expenditure and conserve fat stores. Weight reduction becomes increasingly difficult below an individual's set point.[6]

Brown fat: Obese people have less brown fat than people of normal weight, and therefore expend less energy producing heat through nonshivering or diet-induced thermogenesis.[10]

Insulin response: Obese people respond more readily to external cues, such as the sight, sound, or smell of food, which stimulate the release of insulin: An increase in insulin → decrease blood glucose levels → the sensation of hunger and an increase in lipogenesis (fat formation).

Hormonal imbalances: An underactive thyroid gland → inadequate secretion of thyroid hormone → low BMR → weight gain.

Environmental Theories

Food environment: An abundance of food may entice some people to overeat.

Family environment: A child with no obese parents has a 10% chance of becoming obese; with one obese parent, the chance increases to 40%; and

(continued)

Genetic, Physiologic, Environmental, and Psychological Theories Related to the Etiology of Obesity (*continued*)

if both parents are obese, children have a 80% chance of becoming obese, possibly related to familial eating patterns and attitudes regarding food and obesity.

Work environment: The mechanization of America has led to a decrease in energy expenditure. Likewise, even though work days and work weeks are generally shorter than at the turn of the century, people tend to spend their increased leisure time observing rather than participating in activities.

Psychological Theories

Obese people overeat

Because they have a compulsive behavioral disorder similar to alcoholics and drug abusers: Food controls the person's actions

As an emotional crutch

To compensate for a lack of affection, love, and companionship

To relieve boredom, tension, anxiety, and frustration

therapy, plus pleading by health professionals, have been largely ineffective, with estimates of less than 5% of the clients attaining and maintaining desired weight loss. New approaches focusing on social support, a more active lifestyle, behavior modification, and, for moderately to morbidly obese clients, rapid weight loss diets, appear to be more effective. For this population, surgery may be used as a last resort.

Table 4-8
Comparison of Treatment Components for Overweight and Obesity

	Degree of Overweightness	
Treatment Component	*Overweight →* *Mild Obesity*	*Moderate →* *Morbid Obesity*
Social support	X	X
Increase exercise	X	X
Behavior modification	X	X
Moderate calorie restricted diet	X	
Very-low-calorie diet (VLCD)		X
Surgery		+

"X" indicates appropriateness.
"+" indicates may be appropriate.

Social Support

Because social background and environment have a far greater and longer-lasting impact on an individual's food choices than a health professional, social support may be central to the success of any weight control program. Clearly, weight loss can be helped or hindered by family and friends. Areas of social support that may be developed include spousal involvement and group therapy, which is shown to be more effective than individualized therapy even though actual contact with the health professional is less. Also, there is the potential for strong social support in the work setting due to the social relationships that develop and the close, almost daily interaction among workers. For children, parental involvement and school programs may be effective.

Exercise

In response to recommendations made by leading health authorities, many Americans are adopting aerobic exercise activities for cardiovascular and weight-control benefits. Certainly, becoming more physically active may be the best way to achieve energy balance and promote well-being; dieting alone becomes less and less effective at achieving weight loss because the body lowers its metabolic rate as a compensatory mechanism when calorie intake is chronically or severely restricted. After repeated attempts at dieting, the lowered metabolic rate may not return to normal when normal calorie intake resumes. Thus dieting becomes less successful with each attempt.[2] Physical activity provides the benefit of not only burning calories during activity but also of stimulating metabolic rate.

Although some people claim that the benefits of exercise are offset by an increase in appetite, research does not support this idea. In fact, animal and human studies indicate that exercise helps suppress appetite, and that even though vigorous exercisers do increase their food intake, the increase is not enough to cause weight gain.

Exercise also changes body composition by decreasing the percentage of fat and increasing the amount of lean body mass, which requires more calories to be maintained than fat. So although initial weight loss may not be apparent because the weight of the lean body mass that develops offsets the weight of the fat lost, body dimensions improve and metabolic rate increases. Eventually the gain in lean body tissue is less than the weight of fat lost, and weight loss results.

A sustained increase in metabolic rate induced by exercise prevails even after physical activity ceases. Studies show that the body burns calories at a faster rate for 4 to 12 hours after exercising; the increase in BMR appears to be greatest among beginner exercisers. This increase in BMR can offset the natural decrease in BMR that occurs within days after calorie intake is restricted.

Lowered blood pressure and serum glucose levels, and changes in serum lipid levels are additional benefits of exercise, as is a subjective improvement in sense of well-being, reduced tension, increased agility, and improved alertness. However, exercise should be practiced with caution by people with back problems, hypertension, and insulin-dependent diabetes.

Behavior Modification

"Dieting" has negative connotations and is viewed by most people as a form of punishment or a short-term hurdle to be overcome. In order for a weight control program to be successful and long-lasting, a permanent change in eating attitudes and behaviors must occur. Unless food habits change, the perpetual cycle of weight loss followed by weight gain is inevitable.

Behavior modification, a conceptual approach to altering behavior, is widely used by many commercial programs and self-help groups such as Weight Watchers and TOPS (Take Off Pounds Sensibly). It has been shown to be more effective than any other treatment with which it has been compared, has a lower attrition rate than traditional programs, and tends to improve psychological functioning among its participants.[4] Behavior modification is an essential component of any weight loss program because it seeks to identify eating behaviors that need correcting and offer techniques on "how to" and "how not to" change eating behaviors, rather than the standard list of "do's" and "don'ts" offered to most dieters (see box, Behavior Modification Techniques). "Bad" eating behaviors are reprogrammed and "good" habits are reinforced. Positive reinforcement for achieving realistic goals is stressed.

Diet Intervention

Weight Loss Diets for the Overweight to Mildly Obese

For overweight to mildly obese clients (*i.e.*, people weighing 110% to 140% of desirable body weight), a nutritionally adequate diet mildly restricted in calories that allows for a 1- to 2-pound weight loss per week may be the safest and most effective method of achieving weight loss. Generally, calorie intake should not fall below 1000 to 1200 calories for adult women and 1200 to 1500 calories for adult men. Individually, the number of calories needed for weight loss can be calculated by determining the number of calories needed to maintain ideal body weight and subtracting 500 to 1000 cal/day for a 1- to 2-lb weight loss per week, respectively. (500 cal/day × 7 days/week = 3500 calorie deficit/ week, the equivalent of 1 lb of body weight; or 1000 cal day × 7 days/week = 7000-calorie deficit/week, the equivalent of 2 lb of body weight.)

EXAMPLE

Based on guidelines used by the USDA (see box, Three Methods of Calculating Calorie Requirements), the total calorie requirements of a sedentary woman whose IBW is 130 lb can be computed by multiplying her IBW by 14:

$$130 \text{ lb} \times 14 \text{ cal/lb} = 1820 \text{ calories}$$

To lose 1 lb/week, she must restrict her intake to 1320 cal/day:

$$1820 \text{ cal} - 500 \text{ cal/day} = 1320 \text{ cal/day}$$

To lose 2 lb/week, she would have to limit her intake to 820 cal/day, a level too restricted to be nutritionally adequate:

$$1820 \text{ cal} - 1000 \text{ cal/day} = 820 \text{ cal/day}$$

After ideal weight has been achieved, the diet can be liberalized to provide enough calories for weight maintenance. For instance, the woman in the above example should maintain her weight loss on 1820 cal/day.

There are numerous weight loss diets available, and no one approach is ideal for all people. Important criteria for evaluating any weight-reduction diet are listed in the box, Criteria for Evaluating Weight-Reduction Diets. Low-calorie diets can be achieved through the following methods.

Behavior Modification Techniques

Think Thin

- Make a list of reasons why you want to lose weight before beginning a diet.
- Set long-term goals; avoid crash dieting based on getting into a particular dress or weighing a certain weight for an upcoming event or occasion.
- Give yourself a nonfood reward like new clothes or a night of entertainment for losing weight.
- Don't talk about food.
- Enlist the support of family and friends.
- Learn to distinguish hunger from cravings.

Planning

- Keep food only in the kitchen, not scattered around the house.
- Stay out of the kitchen except when preparing meals and cleaning up.
- Avoid tasting food while cooking; don't take extra portions in order to get rid of a food.
- Place the low-calorie foods in the front of the refrigerator; keep the high-calorie foods hidden.
- Remove temptation to better resist it; "out of sight, out of mind."
- Keep forbidden foods to a minimum.
- Plan meals, snacks, and grocery shopping to help eliminate hasty decisions and impulses that may sabotage dieting.

Eating

- Wait 10 minutes before eating when you feel the urge; hunger pangs may go away if you delay eating.
- Never skip meals.
- Eat only in one designated place and devote all your attention to eating. Activities like reading and watching television can be so distracting that you may not even realize you ate.
- Serve food directly from the stove to the plate instead of family style, which can lead to large portions and second helpings.
- Eat the low-calorie foods first.
- Use a small plate to give the appearance of eating a full plate.
- Chew food thoroughly and eat slowly.
- Put utensils down between mouthfuls.
- Leave some food on your plate to help you feel in control of food, rather than having food control you.
- Eat before attending a social function that features food; while there, select low-calorie foods to nibble on.

(continued)

Behavior Modification Techniques (*continued*)

Shopping

- Never shop while hungry.
- Shop only from a list; resist impulse buying.
- Buy food only in the quantity you need.
- Don't buy foods you find tempting.
- Buy low-calorie foods for when you need a snack.

Life-Style Changes

- Keep busy with hobbies or projects that are incompatible with eating to take your mind off dieting and eating.
- Accept "diet" as it is really defined—a way of eating—not as a temporary reduction in calories that must be endured before "normal" eating habits can be resumed.
- Trim recipes of extra fat and sugar.
- Don't weigh yourself too often.
- If you eat something you shouldn't, accept it and go on with your plan. Don't let disappointment lure you into a real eating binge.
- Exercise.
- Get more sleep if fatigue triggers eating.

Counting Calories

Unfortunately, counting calories does not ensure a nutritionally adequate diet. It is possible to lose weight on a diet consisting only of soft drinks and french fries, as long as the total calorie intake is less than total calorie expenditure. In addition, counting calories does not have long-term possibilities. Who would carry around a food composition table, paper, pencil, and calculator indefinitely?

Eliminating Extras and Second Portions

This approach may produce a consistent, gradual weight loss for clients who do not have a lot of weight to lose. It may be particularly effective for children by enabling them to "outgrow" their overweightness without actually losing weight and "dieting." For some adults, this approach may rely too much on willpower and self-control to be effective.

Utilizing American Diabetic Association Exchange Lists for Meal Planning

The American Diabetic Association exchange lists and meal patterns, which are described in Chapter 17, allow flexibility. They are nutritionally adequate and they are consistent in calorie intake. A daily food allowance for a 1200-calorie and 1500-calorie diet is shown in Table 4-9. For greatest client compliance, meal patterns should correlate as closely as possible with the individual's normal pattern of eating and likes and dislikes.

Criteria for Evaluating Weight-Reduction Diets

A sound weight-reduction diet should

- Be realistic and flexible; that is, easily adaptable to your lifestyle and based on individual calorie requirements
- Suggest that a doctor be consulted
- Use food to meet nutritional requirements rather than vitamin or mineral supplements
- Encourage foods from each of the major food groups
- Meet the RDA for all nutrients
- Promote nutrition education
- Recommend exercise
- Promote a 1-lb to 2-lb weight loss/week
- Have long-term possibilities; diets recommended for only short periods of time obviously are not safe
- Be comprised of 50% to 55% CHO, approximately 15% protein, and 30% fat
- Allow nutritious, low-calorie snacks
- Emphasize portion control
- Emphasize the need for behavior modification to attain and maintain weight loss
- Offer a maintenance plan after weight loss is achieved

Self-Help Groups Such as Weight Watchers and TOPS

Group weight loss programs tend to be more successful than individual programs, even though individual time spent with a diet counselor is less. Although the cost of these programs may be a disadvantage to some, fee programs tend to have a smaller attrition rate than free programs, and deposit–refund programs are even more successful; requiring a fee or deposit tends to discourage unmotivated clients from entering and increases the motivation of those who do enroll.

Diet Programs

Diet book, magazine, and tabloid publishers have given dieters in the United States what they want—a proliferation of quick-weight-loss schemes that adds up to a $32 billion business each year.[14] Although fad diets may produce weight loss, especially diets high in protein and low in CHO, they tend to be highly restrictive, which leads invariably not only to a decrease in intake and loss of weight but also to boredom and attrition. Besides the lack of long-term staying power, many of these diets are unbalanced, providing not enough of some nutrients and excessive amounts of others. A summary of currently popular diet programs appears in Table 4-10.

Other weight loss gimmicks of questionable reliability, validity, and safety are presented in Table 4-11.

Table 4-9
Sample 1200-calorie and 1500-calorie Meal Plans*
Based on the American Diabetic Association
Exchange Lists

Food Group	Servings/Day for 1200 Calories	Servings/Day for 1500 Calories
Starch/Bread	5	7
Meat, medium fat	4 oz	5 oz
Vegetables	2	2
Fruit	3	3
2% Milk	2 cups	2 cups
Fats	2	3
Calorie-free items	as desired	as desired

*Each plan provides 50% of calories from carbohydrates, 20% from protein, 30% from fat.

Weight Loss Diets for Moderately to Morbidly Obese Clients

As indicated in Table 4-8, social support, increased exercise, and behavior modification are also appropriate approaches in the treatment of moderate to morbid obesity. However, for this population, moderate calorie-restricted diets may produce too slow a rate of weight loss, and therefore may not be the dietary treatment of choice. Very-low-calorie diets may be used under medical supervision when rapid weight loss is indicated. Total fasting is also an option, but carries increased risk. Surgical intervention may be used when dietary intervention fails.

Very-Low-Calorie Diets

For moderately to morbidly obese clients, especially those with serious complications such as diabetes mellitus, hypertension, and sleep apnea, traditional low-calorie diets may promote too slow a rate of weight loss. A more aggressive alternative for these clients is the use of a very-low-calorie diet (VLCD), otherwise known as a protein-sparing modified fast. It is designed to produce large and rapid weight loss in clients whose health is so jeopardized by obesity that the risk of a modified fast is less than the risk of maintaining obesity.

Liquid protein modified fast formulas were introduced and became popular during the late 1970s. They were composed of an incomplete protein of low biologic value and lacked adequate vitamins, minerals, and electrolytes; no recommendations regarding the use of supplements were made. Diuresis and extensive electrolyte losses that resulted from the use of these extremely low-calorie diets probably played a role in the numerous deaths attributed to the diet.[1]

Today's VLCD, of which Optifast and Health Management Resources (HMR) are the most popular, bear little resemblance to their predecessors. Although virtually a fasting diet, it provides 50 to 100 g of high biologic protein a day, or approximately 1.5 g/kg of IBW. The protein, provided either through small portions of meat, fish, or poultry, or as a

Table 4-10
Comparison of Currently Popular Diet Programs

	Programs				
Criteria	_Diet Workshop_	_Jenny Craig_	_Nutri-System_	_Slim Fast/ Ultra Slim Fast_	_Weight Watchers_
Does the diet have long-term possibilities?	Yes	No	No	Not really	Yes
What is the recommended rate of weekly weight loss?	1.5–3 lb	1–2 lb	1.5–2 lb	Up to the in-dividual	1–2 lb
How extensive is the education component: nutrition, behavior modification, and the importance of exercise?	1 hr/wk in group setting	14 1-hr video classes plus weekly individual sessions with a counselor	Weekly 30-min group mtgs plus 10-min indi-vidual sessions with a counselor	None	45-min weekly group mtg
What percentage of clients who reach their weight loss goal?	10%	10%	Not available	Unknown	Not available
Is a maintenance plan offered?	Yes	Yes	Yes	No	Yes
What is the cost?	$14 mem-bership plus $9/wk until mainte-nance phase reached	$185 mem-bership + $60–$70 per week for food	Not avilable	$8–$12 per week	$12–$20 for mem-bership plus $7–$9/week until maintenance

powdered protein supplement mixed with water, minimizes the loss of lean body tissue that occurs with complete fasting. Very-low-calorie diets also use critical amounts of supplemental vitamins and minerals based on laboratory data, especially serum electrolyte values. Small amounts of carbohydrates are provided.

A very-low-calorie diet can be safe if used under close medical supervision, and it produces rapid weight loss. During the first week of the fast, weight loss averages 0.78 kg/day, which falls to about 0.28 kg/day by the third week of the program.[1] Total weight loss during the 12-week program averages at least 45 pounds; the longer the program is used, the greater the weight loss. Some programs have used the diet for up to 12 months.

Other benefits include significant reductions in serum cholesterol and triglyceride

Table 4-11
Weight Loss Gimmicks of Questionable Reliability, Validity, and Safety

The Gimmick	The Effect
SAUNAS, STEAM BATHS, AND INFLATABLE CLOTHING	Induce a temporary loss of body water with no effect on body fat.
VIBRATING MACHINES	No weight control benefit; they merely jiggle body fat.
DIET PILLS Numerous prescription and over-the-counter drugs are used to aid weight reduction. When used as the only means of weight control, drugs are ineffective and inappropriate. Some drugs may be useful on a short-term basis when used in combination with a calorie-restricted diet, behavior modification, and exercise. Some commonly used drugs include:	
Diuretics	Temporary decrease in body weight due to the loss of fluid, not fat. Electrolyte imbalances and dehydration may occur with indiscriminate use.
Laxatives	Methyl cellulose and other bulk-producing agents have been used based on the idea that bulk increases the feeling of satiety and thus decreases the desire to eat. Their effectiveness and safety are unproven.
Benzocaine	Numbs the tongue and mucous membranes, and therefore decreases the desire to eat. Presently there appears to be no evidence of danger with overuse.
Amphetamines (dexedrine and benzedrine)	May be prescribed as appetite suppressants. Initially, these drugs do decrease appetite and produce an average weekly weight loss of about 0.5 lb to 1.0 lb. After a couple of months, their effectiveness is limited, and once discontinued, weight reduction stops and weight loss is poorly maintained. Possible side effects include nervousness, restlessness, irritability, euphoria, insomnia, hypertension, and drug dependence. It is recommended that anorectic drugs not be used continuously for more than 6 months because the long-term effects are unknown.
Thyroid hormones	Promote loss of lean body mass, not fat. Thyroid hormone is a powerful hormone that should be used only when a thyroid deficiency has been diagnosed.

levels, improved glucose tolerance, and improvements in hypertension, pulmonary problems, and surgical risks.

Unfortunately, loss of body protein and potassium remains a major concern with VLCD. Studies have shown that the degree of obesity is inversely related to the degree of protein depletion—lighter people tend to lose more protein than people with a higher percentage of body fat. Because of this, it is recommended that VLCD be used only in individuals who are at least 130% to 140% of ideal weight. Other contraindications include arrhythmias, unstable angina, protein-wasting diseases, major system failure, drug therapy causing protein wasting (*i.e.*, steroids), and pregnancy and lactation. Common side effects include moderate ketosis, decreased cold tolerance, hair loss, dry skin, fatigue, light-headedness, nervousness, constipation or diarrhea, and menstrual irregularities.[1] In addition, the drop-out rate is very high, and weight loss tends to be poorly maintained after the diet is discontinued. Researchers are hoping that behavior modification used in combination with VLCD will help clients maintain their weight loss.

Total Fasting

Because total fasting alters normal physiology and biochemistry of the gastrointestinal tract, it should be used only under complete medical supervision. Potassium, sodium, bicarbonate, and multivitamin–mineral supplements are necessary. Although total fasting does produce weight loss, loss of lean body tissue is extensive and weight loss is poorly maintained. Other potential complications include dehydration, hyperuricemia, nausea, dizziness, hepatic and renal impairment, mineral depletion, acidosis, severe postural hypotension, and muscle wasting.

Surgical Procedures

Surgical intervention may be considered as a last resort for morbidly obese clients who fail to lose weight by nonsurgical means and who are at increased risk of morbidity and mortality because of their obesity. Surgery should be contemplated only when the risk of remaining obese is greater than the risk of surgery. Unfortunately, surgery cannot guarantee that weight loss will be maintained, especially if eating attitudes and habits do not change. Follow-up care and behavior modification are vital to the long-term success of any surgical procedure.

The types of surgical procedures that may be performed include the following:

Jejunoileal Bypass: A procedure that disconnects a large portion of the small intestine so that the absorption of calories is greatly reduced; malabsorption causes weight loss even if eating behaviors do not change. Unfortunately, nutrients are also malabsorbed, and common complications include malnutrition, liver failure, severe diarrhea, urinary stones, and intestinal infections. Because of the 15% to 39% incident rate of serious complications and a mortality rate of up to 6%, jejunoileal bypasses have been replaced largely with gastric stapling.

Gastric Stapling (Gastroplasty): Introduced in 1977, gastroplasty is a relatively safe procedure that reduces the capacity of the stomach. A row of staples across the stomach creates a small pouch that may initially hold 1 to 2 oz of food; when more than 2 oz of food is consumed, pain and/or vomiting results. Over time, however, the pouch stretches to hold more food. Although the incidence of postsurgical complications is low, the staples may burst if too much food or liquids is consumed before the staple line heals.[15] In addition, overindulgence can cause the pouch to accommodate more food, reducing its effectiveness, and obstruction can occur if food is improperly chewed. Nutritional complications reported with this procedure include hypoalbuminemia and vitamin deficiencies, in addition to vomiting and nausea.[12] Clients need to understand the importance of eating small meals, eating slowly, chewing food thoroughly, and progressing the diet from liquids, to puréed foods, to soft foods accordingly.

Intragastric Balloon Insertion: By endoscopy, a cylindrical implant is placed in the stomach and then inflated for the purpose of reducing stomach capacity. Diet therapy and behavior modification are included in the treatment program. Although standards were previously lower, the FDA revised its criteria for eligibility to 100 pounds overweight in

1986 after complications of vomiting, ulcers, gastric perforations, and intestinal obstructions were reported. Few studies have been conducted on the dietary intake of balloon recipients. However, one study showed that weight loss ranged from 0% to 16% of original weight, which is comparable to weight loss achieved through diet and behavior modification alone.[12] The effects of the balloon on long-term weight maintenance are not known. Some critics argue that the balloons have marginal effects on reducing stomach capacity.[12]

Jaw Wiring: An approach that attempts to reduce intake by preventing the intake of solid foods. It is possible, however, to continue consuming a high-calorie diet, depending on the client's choice of liquids. At best, jaw wiring is a temporary solution.

Fat Suctioning (Lipectomy): Fat cells are suctioned by a vacuum through a hollow tube that is inserted through an incision. Used primarily around the hips, abdomen, buttocks, and thighs, the procedure is designed only for people under 40 with congenital fat bulges. It is not a cure for obesity for, at best, it addresses only a symptom of obesity rather than treating the underlying problem.

NURSING PROCESS

Before a plan of care can be devised, a thorough assessment is needed to determine who is likely to succeed in a weight control program. Even though all obese clients have the potential to benefit from weight loss, not all obese clients are motivated to lose weight and to keep it off once lost. In addition, there are dangers if clients are selected indiscriminately. For example:

- Weight loss followed by regain, commonly referred to as "yo-yo" dieting, may be more dangerous than static obesity.
- Failure can have devastating consequences that may preclude later attempts at dieting when the client may be more motivated and have a better chance at success.
- "Negative contagion" may spread to the rest of the participants in a group setting and hinder their progress.
- The health professional's morale may suffer.
- The health professional's time may be better spent on clients who are truly motivated to lose weight.

Assessment

Assess for the following factors:

Current weight, weight status: Compare actual weight to "ideal" standard.

Distribution and degree of body fatness, based on triceps skinfold measurements, waist : hip ratio, and measurements of bust/chest and thighs, if available.

Abnormal values with nutritional significance, such as serum cholesterol, triglycerides, albumin, and glucose.

Signs or symptoms of malnutrition (see Chap. 9).

Usual 24-hour intake, including the portion sizes, the frequency and pattern of eating, and the method of food preparation.

Usual intake of high-fat foods.

The use of "diet" foods.

Overeaters Anonymous

> Overeaters Anonymous is founded on the belief that compulsive overeating is a physical, emotional, and spiritual disease. It is designed to complement medical and nutritional treatment of obesity; its focus is limited to the compulsive nature of overeating. There are no dues or fees, nor is there any weight requirement for entering the program. Like Alcoholics Anonymous, OA regards compulsive overeating as an addiction that can be arrested but not cured. A self-administered questionnaire that focuses on eating behaviors (such as eating in the absence of hunger, secret binge eating, feelings of guilt following overeating) may be used to help identify a compulsive eating disorder.

Eating behaviors and attitudes that can be improved. Early record-keeping of the amounts and types of foods eaten, where the food was consumed, and the client's feelings about the meal or snack will help.

Previous history of dieting, especially "successes" followed by weight gain. Evaluate the types of diets followed, the length of dieting, and the reason for abandoning the diet to determine the client's level of motivation and determination.

Cultural, familial, religious, and ethnic influences on eating habits.

Emotional triggers that stimulate overeating, such as depression, boredom, anger, guilt, frustration, or self-hate. People identified as compulsive overeaters may benefit from Overeaters Anonymous, a self-help group that uses the 12-step program of Alcoholics Anonymous (see box, Overeaters Anonymous).

Nutritional knowledge, level of intelligence, and willingness to learn.

The duration of obesity, the age of onset, and whether a family history exists.

Presence of complications (*i.e.*, hypertension, diabetes, heart disease, etc.); determine their impact on nutritional status or whether dietary intervention is needed.

Usual activity patterns and the client's willingness to adopt an exercise program.

The client's sense of body image and self-esteem and the presence or lack of support systems.

Nursing Diagnosis

Altered Nutrition: More Than Body Requirements, related to imbalance of intake versus activity expenditures.

Planning and Implementation

It is rarely effective to preach about the hazards of obesity and the virtues of being thin to someone who must lose weight. A positive, supportive approach is needed to establish rapport with the client and develop the proper atmosphere conducive to weight control instruction. Set mutually agreeable realistic short- and long-term goals: Whereas a 100-lb weight loss in a year seems overwhelming and discouraging, a 6-lb weight loss per month may be within reach.

A balanced weight-reduction diet, like a normal diet, should provide approximately 50% to 55% of total calories from CHO, 30% or less from fat, and the remainder from protein. Stress the importance of consuming a nutritionally adequate diet even though calorie intake is reduced. Include all major food groups in the diet; avoid items from the "Fats, Sweets, and Alcohol" group that provide mostly calories with few nutrients.

Moderately restricted weight loss diets range from 1000 to 1200 calories for women and 1500 to 1800 calories for men. Although extremely low-calorie diets can speed weight loss, they also make compliance more difficult. Generally, multivitamins, and possibly mineral supplements, are indicated when intake falls below 1200 calories.

When a food is forbidden, it suddenly takes on mystical qualities and becomes all the more appealing. Keep forbidden foods to a minimum and emphasize portion control.

Weight loss plateaus are to be expected because of a temporary increase in body water resulting from the oxidation of fat tissue. Eventually, an increase in urine output rids the body of excess water and weight loss continues.

Client Goals

The client will
Increase physical activity.
Explain the relationship between diet, physical activity, and weight control.
Plan menus for _____ days that are low in calories and nutritionally adequate.
Practice behavior modification techniques to avoid eating behaviors that lead to weight
  gain.
Lose _____ pounds/week until _____ pounds total weight loss is achieved.
Maintain weight loss.

Nursing Interventions

Diet management

Decrease calorie intake by 500 to 1000 calories/day from calculated requirements to promote gradual weight loss.

Individualize the diet as much as possible to correspond with the client's likes, dislikes, and eating pattern, since standard diets rarely fit into a person's lifestyle and eating habits.

Limit fat intake to 30% of total calories/day or less; encourage an adequate protein intake and a liberal intake of complex carbohydrates.

Client teaching

Instruct the client
On the relationship between calorie intake, physical activity, and weight status.
That weight control can be achieved by reducing intake or increasing physical activity but
  is most effectively and easily achieved by combining the two.
That any amount and kind of exercise is better than no exercise at all. Encourage the client
  to participate in some kind of enjoyable activity; the intensity, duration, and frequency
  of exercising can be increased after the client gains confidence.

That food is used more efficiently when consumed in small quantities three to four times per day rather than at one large meal per day. Encourage the client to avoid meal skipping and hunger, which often leads to snacking and a higher calorie intake.

That occasional deviations from the diet should be expected. Encourage the client to accept these without feelings of failure and to resume "normal" dieting as soon as possible.

Not to get weighed too frequently; weight losses less than anticipated can be discouraging.

That fats in the diet provide the most concentrated source of calories—more than twice the calories in an equivalent amount of protein or CHO. Calorie intake can be reduced drastically by limiting fat intake, such as fatty meats, whole-milk dairy products, fried foods, butter, margarine, salad dressings, oils, nuts and peanut butter, and rich desserts and pastries.

To keep a food record to increase awareness of amounts and types of foods eaten and precipitating factors.

To practice behavior modification techniques designed to change food attitudes and habits (see box, Behavior Modification Techniques). Successful weight control is possible when the attitude of "always being on a diet" changes to an acceptance of eating lighter and less as a way of life.

That a dieter's friends are as follows:
- A scale and measuring utensils to control portion sizes
- Baked, broiled, steamed, and boiled foods
- Fresh fruits and vegetables prepared without added fat
- Lean meats, skinless poultry, and fish
- Starchy foods without added fat, such as bread, pasta, rice, potatoes, dried peas and beans, corn, peas, winter squash, and unsweetened cereals; whole-grain products and high-fiber foods are especially good at providing a feeling of fullness without a lot of excess calories
- Skim or low-fat milk and dairy products
- Herbs and spices, which impart flavor without any calories. The same is true of cooking with wine; as the food cooks, the calories evaporate, leaving only the flavor of wine

How to order from a menu while dining out:
- Estimate portion sizes of all foods
- Stick to plain foods rather than casseroles and stews
- Choose tomato juice, unsweetened fruit juice, clear broth, bouillon, or consommé as an appetizer instead of sweetened juices, fried vegetables, seafood cocktail, or cream or thick soups
- Choose fresh vegetable salads and use oil and vinegar or fresh lemon instead of regular salad dressings, or request that the dressing be served separately; avoid coleslaw and other salads with the dressing already added
- Order plain roasted, baked, or broiled meat, fish, or poultry; request a "doggy bag" if the portion size is too large
- Order steamed, boiled, or broiled vegetables
- Choose plain baked, mashed, boiled, or steamed potatoes, rice, or noodles
- Select fresh fruit for dessert
- Request milk for coffee and tea, if desired, instead of cream
- Most airlines will provide low-calorie meals if requested at the time that flight reservations are made.

On food preparation ideas:
- Food does not have to be prepared separately from the rest of the family's as long as extra sugar and fat are not added
- Nonstick sprays are effective and virtually calorie-free
- Trim all visible fat from meat after cooking, and remove the skin from poultry
- Use low-calorie or diabetic cookbooks for variety

On food purchasing and label reading:
- Avoid temptation by not buying problem foods
- Stick to a shopping list
- Do not shop while hungry
- Only buy the amount needed
- "Lite" foods do not necessarily have fewer calories than regular foods; for instance, one type of corn chip marketed as "lite" has only 1 calorie less than the regular variety
- "Low-calorie" foods cannot have more than 40 cal/serving or 0.4 cal/g
- "Reduced-calorie" items must be reduced in calories by one-third
- "Sugar-free" and "dietetic" do not necessarily mean low-calorie

Counsel overweight parents about the dangers of overfeeding infants and the inappropriate use of food to convey love, support, or acceptance. Advise parents to encourage their children to participate in regular physical activity.

Advise the client to consult his or her physician or dietitian if questions concerning the diet or weight loss arise.

Monitor

Monitor for the following signs or symptoms:
Compliance to diet, and the need for follow-up diet counseling
Effectiveness of the diet (*i.e.*, weight loss), and assess the need for further diet modification
Weight, weight changes
Lab values, when available

Evaluation

Evaluation is ongoing. Assuming the plan of care has not changed, the client will achieve the goals as stated above.

BIBLIOGRAPHY

1. American Dietetic Association: Position Paper of the American Dietetic Association: Very-Low-Calorie Weight Loss Diets. J Am Diet Assoc 90:722, 1990
2. American Dietetic Association: Position of The American Dietetic Association: Optimal Weight as a Health Promotion Strategy. J Am Diet Assoc 89:1814, 1989
3. Brownell KD: The psychology and physiology of obesity: Implications for screening and treatment. J Am Diet Assoc 84:406, 1984
4. Brownell KD: The Learn Program for Weight Control. Philadelphia: University of Pennsylvania School of Medicine, 1988
5. Frankle RT: Obesity, a family matter: Creating new behavior. J Am Diet Assoc 85:597, 1985

6. Gortmaker SL, Dietz WH, Cheung LWY: Inactivity, diet, and the fattening of America. J Am Diet Assoc 90:1247, 1990

7. Jacobson M (ed): Bulging bellies and breast cancer. Nutrition Action Health Letter 17(3):4, 1990

8. Kemnitz JW: Body weight set point theory. Contemporary Nutrition 10(2), 1985

9. Mayer J (ed): Some calories count more than others. Tufts University Diet and Nutrition Letter 6(9):2, 1988

10. Mayer J (ed): Smart losers' guide to choosing a weight-loss program. Tufts University Diet and Nutrition Letter 8(6):3, 1990

11. Mayer J (ed): When a dieter hits a stubborn plateau. Tufts University Diet and Nutrition Letter 8(3):1, 1990

12. Morrow SR, Mona LK: Effect of gastric balloons on nutrient intake and weight loss in obese subjects. J Am Diet Assoc 90:717, 1990

13. National Dairy Council: Weight Management: A Summary of Current Theory and Practice. Rosemont, IL: National Dairy Council, 1985

14. National Research Council: Recommended Dietary Allowances. 10th ed. Washington, DC: National Academy Press, 1989

15. Priddy MLB: Gastric reduction surgery: A dietitian's experience and perspective. Am J Diet Assoc 85:455, 1985

16. United States Department of Agriculture, and United States Department of Health and Human Services: Nutrition and Your Health: Dietary Guidelines for Americans. 3rd ed. Home and Garden Bulletin no. 232, 1990

17. Weigley ES: Average? Ideal? Desirable? A brief overview of height–weight tables in the United States. J Am Diet Assoc 84:417, 1984

2 *Regulatory Nutrients*

5 Vitamins

CHARACTERISTICS OF VITAMINS AS A GROUP

Vitamins are chemical compounds made of the elements carbon, hydrogen, oxygen, and sometimes nitrogen or other elements. The presence of carbon classifies vitamins as organic substances, which can be converted to other forms and are susceptible to oxidation and destruction. Vitamins are soluble in either water or fat. Solubility influences their absorption, movement through the blood, storage, and excretion.

The body needs vitamins in very small amounts to help regulate body processes, such as the synthesis of numerous body compounds like bones, skin, nerves, brain, and blood. Vitamins do not provide energy (calories), but are required for the metabolism of the energy-providing nutrients (CHO, protein, and fat). Most vitamins function by combining with a protein (apoenzyme) to form a coenzyme that promotes the action of enzymes. Without vitamins, thousands of chemical reactions cannot occur, and health and life are seriously threatened.

Vitamins are essential in the diet because either they cannot be synthesized by the body or they are produced in inadequate amounts (see Appendices 2 and 3). The body can

105

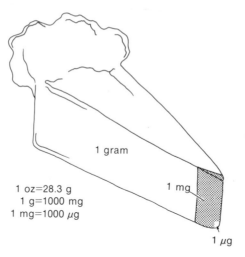

Figure 5-1
Comparative units of measure.

1 gram

1 oz=28.3 g
1 g=1000 mg
1 mg=1000 µg

1 mg

1 µg

make vitamin D, vitamin A, and niacin *if* the proper precursors are available. Microorganisms in the gastrointestinal (GI) tract can synthesize vitamin K and vitamin B_{12}, but not enough to meet the body's needs.

Vitamins are present in foods only in very small amounts; vitamins usually are measured in milligrams (mg), which are 1/1000 of a gram, or micrograms (µg), 1/1000 of a milligram (Fig. 5-1).

INDIVIDUAL VITAMINS

Individual vitamins vary greatly in how their elements are arranged, so that each is a distinct chemical individual. Each vitamin has one or more specific functions and cannot be converted to or substituted for another. Individual vitamins may exist in several different active forms; different forms perform different functions.

DEFINITIONS
Provitamins

Provitamins (or vitamin precursors) are vitamin-related compounds that can be converted to an active vitamin in the body under proper conditions. Examples include tryptophan (an amino acid), which can be converted to niacin; carotene, which can be converted to vitamin A; and cholesterol, which can be converted to vitamin D.

Antivitamins

Antivitamins (vitamin antagonist or antimetabolite) are substances that block the synthesis or metabolism of a vitamin. Some drugs, like methotrexate (a folic acid antagonist), antibiotics (because they interfere with vitamin K synthesis), and dicumarol (an antagonist of vitamin K), are common antivitamins.

Avitaminosis

Avitaminosis means literally "without vitamins." When followed by the letter of a vitamin, avitaminosis means that particular vitamin is deficient (*i.e.*, avitaminosis A)

Hypervitaminosis

When followed by the letter of a vitamin, hypervitaminosis means that an excess of that particular vitamin has accumulated in the body to toxic levels. Examples include hyper-vitaminosis A and hypervitaminosis D.

Megadose

A megadose is an amount at least 10 times greater than the RDA. Vitamins in megadoses have pharmacologic strength and act more like drugs than nutrients.[5]

VITAMIN SOURCES

Although the American Diabetic Association and American Dietetic Association exchange lists are useful for identifying the sources and amounts of CHO, protein, and fat contained in the diet, the exchange lists do not indicate sources of vitamins and minerals. Likewise, dietary recommendations made by leading health organizations focus mostly on avoiding excesses of macronutrients (CHO, protein, fats, and cholesterol), rather than on obtaining adequate amounts of vitamins and minerals. Despite the emphasis on avoiding too much, a "balanced diet" (*i.e.*, the food-group approach to meal planning) is still important to ensure nutritional adequacy.

The food-group approach, such as the USDA's Food Guide Pyramid discussed in Chapter 8, divides foods into six groups. Although nonspecific with regard to quantities of *nutrients* that must be consumed, daily amounts of foods are recommended from each group. It is assumed that the vitamin and mineral content of the diet will be adequate if appropriate amounts of a variety of foods from each food group are chosen.

However, a person may eat the recommended amount of servings from each of the food groups and still not have an adequate vitamin intake if food selections are not varied. Because not all foods within a group are nutritionally equivalent (*i.e.*, pork is rich in thiamine but other meats are not), actual vitamin intake varies considerably depending on actual food choices. Also, vitamin retention in foods, especially of water-soluble vitamins, depends on proper handling, storage, and preparation. The theoretical vitamin content of a food listed in a food composition table may greatly exceed the amount of vitamin actually eaten after that food has been prepared for consumption. And lastly, people with individual needs that are higher than normal due to metabolic disorders, inadequate absorption, the use of certain medications, substance abuse, or genetic background, may require additional vitamins, either through diet or supplements.

VITAMIN DEFICIENCIES

Before the 1940s, vitamin deficiencies were prevalent in the United States and throughout the world. As a result of an abundant food supply, selected fortification of certain foods, and better methods of determining and improving the nutrient content of foods, vitamin deficiency diseases have virtually been eliminated in developed countries. Today the emphasis of public health nutrition is not on consuming adequate amounts of nutrients, but on avoiding dietary excesses, like fat, cholesterol, and calories, that are associated with chronic diseases and are the leading causes of death in the United States.

Although severe vitamin deficiencies are rare in the United States, food consumption surveys indicate that some population groups consume less than the RDA for some vitamins. That does not necessarily mean a deficiency will result, because the RDAs are intended to exceed the needs of most healthy people. However, the potential exists for subclinical or marginal deficiencies, especially of vitamin B_6.[11] Groups especially at risk for developing vitamin deficiencies include those in certain age groups (infants, adolescents, pregnant and lactating women, and the elderly); smokers, alcoholics, and chronic users of certain medications; people of low socioeconomic status; people who are chronically ill; people with psychological disturbances; and poor or finicky eaters, such as dieters, strict vegetarians, and food faddists.

Although the actual biochemical and clinical findings vary depending on which vitamin is deficient, the progression of vitamin deficiencies is the same for all vitamins (Fig. 5-2).

VITAMIN SUPPLEMENTS

Vitamin supplements are a $2.7 billion-a-year business. Although estimates vary, 35% to 40% of American adults take vitamin supplements; the incidence may rise as high as 72% among people living on the West Coast or those aged 60 or older.[5] The use of vitamin supplements is greater among women than men, especially women who work full time, and also higher among college graduates than noncollege graduates. Professional, clerical, and sales people tend to use supplements more than manual laborers and unemployed people. Nonsmokers who exercise and diet tend to use supplements more than the general population.

Healthy adults who consume a variety of foods properly prepared from each of the

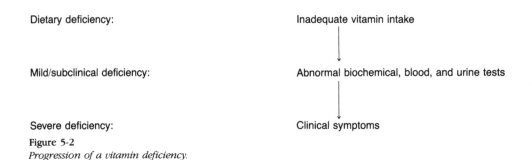

Dietary deficiency: Inadequate vitamin intake

Mild/subclinical deficiency: Abnormal biochemical, blood, and urine tests

Severe deficiency: Clinical symptoms

Figure 5-2
Progression of a vitamin deficiency.

food groups rarely require vitamin supplements. In the National Research Council's report entitled *Diet and Health*,[13] eating a variety of foods, not consuming supplements, was recommended as the desirable way for the general public to obtain adequate amounts of nutrients. However, many people self-prescribe vitamins based on widespread beliefs that the typical American diet is deficient in vitamins, that taking supplements will provide energy, increase endurance, and combat stress, and that vitamin supplements can prevent or cure a wide variety of ills like cancer, colds, and arthritis.[4] Many vitamin users are convinced that supplements help them cope better during times of stress or worry, and that supplements can make up for a "bad" diet.

A multivitamin supplement may be indicated when intake is marginal, unbalanced, or lacks variety, as in the case of people on very-low-calorie diets, strict vegans, and the elderly. Other population groups who may benefit from the use of supplements include people with increased vitamin requirements who may not be able to consume adequate amounts of vitamins through diet alone. Pregnant and lactating women, people with malabsorption disorders or certain other chronic diseases, and people who use specific medications that interfere with the absorption or metabolism of vitamins fall into this category. Severe physical stress, such as major surgery, second- and third-degree burns, large bone fractures, and multiple injuries, increases the need for vitamin C and certain other nutrients. Despite advertising claims, it has never been determined what, if any, effect psychological stress has on vitamin requirements.

People who need vitamin supplements should take them. People who do not need them are wasting their money and risk health problems if they take vitamins in excess of the RDA, especially high doses of single nutrients.[1] Certainly, food is the best and safest source of nutrients. But if someone chooses to take unprescribed supplements, they should take a balanced multivitamin instead of only one or two vitamins, because vitamins work best together and when they are in balanced proportions. Too much of one vitamin can alter the need for other nutrients. In addition, people who are deficient usually need more than one vitamin because singular vitamin deficiencies, especially of the B complex, are rare.

It is also best to take supplements that do not provide more than 100% of the RDA for established vitamins. Unless medically indicated, there is not only no benefit from taking more than 100% of the RDA for vitamins, but it is also potentially dangerous, especially for vitamins A, D, and B_6. Moreover, taking supplements of non-nutrients is economically wasteful and nutritionally worthless (see box, Food for Thought: Nonvitamin Vitamins).

Unlike drugs that must be tested to ensure potency and that they can be absorbed by the body, there are no such laws governing the sale of vitamins—there are no guarantees that supplements are either effective or in a form that the body can readily and easily absorb.[5] Marketing tactics that promote vitamins as "natural," "organic," "therapeutic," "high-potency," and "stress formula" are open to interpretation. Regardless of whether a vitamin is synthetically prepared in a laboratory or extracted from natural food sources, the chemical structure is the same. For instance, the body cannot distinguish between inexpensive synthetic vitamin C and vitamin C from rosehips that costs twice as much. Vitamin supplements do not necessarily follow the dictum of "you get what you pay for." However, freshness should be a consideration, because over time, supplements can decompose or become too hard to dissolve.[5] Prolonged storage, especially under hot, humid conditions like a bathroom, causes vitamins to lose their potency. Unfortunately, the FDA does not require expiration dates on vitamin supplements.

Nonvitamin Vitamins

Vitamin and food supplements are big business, with about 35% or more of the adult American population using vitamin supplements regularly at an annual tab of over $1.5 billion. Unfortunately, there may be no other single class of drugs that has fallen prey to as much quackery, misunderstanding, misrepresentation, and misuse as vitamins. Although the First Amendment to the United States' Constitution guarantees freedom of speech, it also gives everyone the right to make statements about food and nutrition—whether or not they are true. However, by law, consumers are protected against deceptive advertising. Thus, although health food faddists can *state* that a particular supplement or product is a miracle cure-all, they cannot *advertise* it as such.

Most experts believe healthy people do not benefit from taking nutrients in quantities greater than the RDA, and considering there are almost 4000 cases of vitamin poisoning a year (80% of them children), supplements can be very dangerous. In addition, taking supplements that contain non-nutrients is ineffective, costly, and potentially harmful.

Flavonoids or Bioflavonoids

As a group of over 200 biologically similar compounds, flavonoids were called vitamin P because they were shown to reduce capillary permeability. Rutin, hesperidin, and quiercetin are the only flavonoids purported to have therapeutic roles; however, they are broken down in the gastrointestinal tract so that little or no flavonoids are absorbed intact. Although essential for crickets and other insects, flavonoids have not been shown to be essential for humans and have been disqualified as a true vitamin. Despite numerous claims, there is no evidence that flavonoids are needed in the diet or are effective against hypertension, vascular disease, rheumatic fever, arthritis, or cancer.

Inositol

Inositol, which is a six-carbon sugar alcohol, is widespread in the diet and is made in the body from glucose. In the body, inositol is a component of phospholipids and is concentrated in cerebrospinal fluid, the brain, the heart, and other skeletal muscles. It is believed to play a role in nerve transmissions and regulating enzyme activity. Because of its anti-hair loss effect in mice, it was believed to be a vitamin. However, it has not been proven to be essential for humans. Claims that inositol can treat baldness and thinning hair, dissolve fat, and improve brain cell nutrition are unproven. It is doubtful that healthy people need inositol supplements, although supplements may be beneficial for people with diabetes, chronic renal failure, and multiple sclerosis who have altered inositol metabolism.

(continued)

Nonvitamin Vitamins

Laetrile (Amygdalin)

Laetrile, found in apricot pits and other stone fruits and nuts, contains 6% cyanide by weight. It has been falsely labeled as vitamin B_{17} and promoted as a cure for cancer, based on the idea that cancer cells have an enzyme that releases cyanide from laetrile, which kills cancer cells. Normal cells supposedly do not have the enzyme. In truth, normal cells may actually have more of the enzyme, and according to the National Cancer Institute, laetrile does not cure, improve, or even slow the progression of cancer, nor does it improve cancer-related symptoms or extend life span. In addition, laetrile is potentially toxic: There have been numerous reports of cyanide poisoning related to oral ingestion of laetrile.

Pangamic Acid

Because it increases the oxygen content of the blood and oxygen uptake by tissues, pangamic acid has been called vitamin B_{15} and promoted as the "feel good" pill. There is no evidence that pangamic acid is a vitamin, even though it supposedly cures fatigue, cancer, alcoholism, schizophrenia, heart disease, autism, gangrene, and allergies, as well as reverses the aging process and increases sexual fulfillment. The actual composition of pangamic acid varies with the manufacturer. Some compounds in pangamic acid are inert; others are potentially toxic, mutagenic, or carcinogenic.

Para-aminobenzoic Acid

Although para-aminobenzoic acid (PABA) is a component of folic acid and is often classified as a B vitamin, it cannot be substituted for folic acid and is not a vitamin. The only medically accepted use of PABA is as a sunscreen in suntan lotions.[5] Claims that PABA cures gray hair, infertility, and impotence are unproven. Although large amounts of PABA may be used to darken hair, it may produce nausea, vomiting, acidosis, and blood disorders.

Choline

Choline is an essential component of animal tissues but cannot be considered a vitamin since its need in the diet has not been established. Choline plays a role in the metabolism and transportation of fat, is a component of lecithin, and is a precursor of acetylcholine, a compound involved in the transmission of nerve impulses. In the diet, choline is found in egg yolk, liver, organ meats, lean meats, legumes, and wheat germ and is also synthesized in the body. A deficiency in humans has not been documented.

FAT-SOLUBLE VITAMINS

Vitamins A, D, E, and K are the four fat-soluble vitamins. A summary of the fat-soluble vitamins is outlined in Table 5-1.

Group Characteristics

As a group, fat-soluble vitamins have the following characteristics:
- They are absorbed into the lymphatic system with fat. Fat-soluble vitamin deficiencies

Table 5-1
Summary of Fat-Soluble Vitamins

Vitamin	Functions	Deficiency Signs and Symptoms
VITAMIN A		
Vitamin precursor: carotene	The formation of visual purple,	Night blindness, or the slow recovery
Vitamin: retinol	which enables the eye to	of vision after flashes of bright
Adult RDA	adapt to dim light	light at night
	Normal growth and develop-	Bone growth ceases; bone shape
Men: 1000 μg RE*	ment of bones and teeth	changes; enamel-forming cells in
Women: 800 μg RE	The formation and maintenance	the teeth malfunction, teeth crack
Pregnancy: 800 μg RE	of skin and mucous mem-	and tend to decay.
Lactation: 1300 μg RE	branes	Skin becomes dry, scaly, rough, and
		cracked; keratinization or hyper-
		keratosis develops; mucous mem-
		brane cells flatten and harden:
		Eyes become dry (xerosis); irre-
		versible drying and hardening of
		the cornea can result in blindness.
		Decreased saliva secretion → diffi-
		culty chewing, swallowing →
		anorexia
		Decreased mucous secretion of the
		stomach and intestines → im-
		paired digestion and absorption
		→ diarrhea, increased excretion
		of nutrients
		Susceptibility to respiratory, urinary
		tract, and vaginal infections
		increases.

Food Sources
Preformed retinol is found in liver, fish liver oils, whole + fortified milk and dairy products, fortified margarine, and fortified breakfast cereals. Carotenes are found in dark green and yellow vegetables, such as sweet potatoes, winter squash, carrots, broccoli, spinach, "greens," peaches, apricots, and cantaloupe

VITAMIN D		
Vitamin precursors: ergosterol,	Helps maintain optimal serum	Rickets (in infants and children)
7-dehydrocholesterol	levels of calcium and phos-	Retarded bone growth
Vitamins: D_2 (ergochole-	phorus for normal bone min-	Bone malformations (bowed
calciferol), D_3	eralization by	legs)
(cholecalciferol)	Stimulating the intestinal	Enlargement of ends of long

(continued)

Table 5-1 (*continued*)

Vitamin	Functions	Deficiency Signs and Symptoms
Adult RDA	absorption of calcium	bones (knock–knees)
19–24-year olds: 10 micrograms	Mobilizing calcium and	Deformities of the ribs
After age 24: 5 micrograms	phosphorus from the bone	(bowed, with beads or
Pregnancy or lactation: 10	Stimulating reabsorption of	knobs)
microgr ams	calcium by the kidney	Delayed closing of the fontanel →
	Increasing reabsorption of	rapid enlargement of the head
	phosphorus by the kidney	Decreased serum calcium and/
		or phosphorus
		Malformed teeth; decayed teeth
		Protrusion of the abdomen
		related to relaxation of the
		abdominal muscles
		Increased secretion of para-
		thyroid hormone
		Osteomalacia (in adults)
		Softening of the bones →
		deformities, pain, and easy
		fracture
		Decreased serum calcium and/or
		phosphorus, increased alkaline
		phosphatase
		Involuntary muscle twitching
		and spasms

Food Sources

Fortified milk, margarine, and breakfast cereals; small amounts are found in butter, egg yolk, liver, salmon, sardines, and tuna fish

---

VITAMIN E

Tocopherol	Acts as an antioxidant to protect	Increased RBC hemolysis
Adult RDA	vitamin A and PUFA from	In infants, causes anemia, edema, and
Men: 10 mg α–TE	being destroyed	skin lesions
Women: 8 mg α–TE	Protects cell membranes	
Pregnancy: 10 mg -TE		
Lactation: 12 mg α-TE		

Food Sources

Vegetable oils, wheat germ, leafy vegetables, soybeans, corn, peanuts, pecans, walnuts, margarine and salad dressings made with vegetable oils

---

VITAMIN K

Vitamin K_1 (phylloquinone)	Essential for the formation of 5	Delayed blood clotting →
Vitamin K_2 (menaquinone)	proteins necessary for nor-	hemorrhage
Adult RDA	mal blood clotting	Hemorrhagic disease of the newborn
Men: 80 micrograms		
Women: 65 micrograms		
Pregnancy or lactation:		
65 micrograms		

Food Sources

Green leafy vegetables, cabbage, cauliflower, spinach, cheese, egg yolk, and liver. Synthesized by GI flora.

---

* RE = retinol equivalents. 1 retinol equivalent = 1 μg retinol or 6 μg β-carotene

can occur secondary to any condition that interferes with fat absorption, such as malabsorption syndromes, and pancreatic and biliary diseases.

- They must be attached to protein carriers to be transported through the blood, because fat is not soluble in water (blood).
- They are not excreted when consumed in excess of need; rather, they are stored primarily in the liver and adipose tissue.
- Fat-soluble vitamin deficiency symptoms are slow to develop.
- Because of the body's storage reserve, they do not have to be consumed every day.
- They can be toxic when consumed in large doses over a prolonged period of time, particularly vitamin A and vitamin D.

Vitamin A

Vitamin A was recognized in 1913 as the first fat-soluble vitamin. Although relatively stable, vitamin A is destroyed gradually by exposure to air, light, and heat.

Preformed vitamin A exists as a group of compounds commonly known as retinoids, and incudes retinol, retinaldehyde, and retinoic acid. Actual vitamin A activity differs among retinoids. Preformed vitamin A is found only in animal sources such as any kind of liver (beef, veal, pork, lamb, chicken, and turkey), butter, cream, and egg yolk. Fish oils are rich in vitamin A but are not generally consumed as foods.

The precursors of vitamin A are carotenes or carotenoids, the yellow pigment in yellow fruits and yellow and dark-green vegetables (the green pigment, chlorophyll, masks the presence of carotenes in green vegetables). Although there are some 500 naturally occurring carotenoids in plants and some animal fats, only 50 actually are precursors of vitamin A, of which beta carotene is the most common. Because not all carotenes can be converted into vitamin A, the color intensity of a fruit or vegetable is not a reliable indicator of provitamin A content.[10] Excellent sources include sweet potatoes, winter squash, carrots, broccoli, spinach, green leafy vegetables, peaches, apricots, and cantaloupe. Significant amounts of vitamin A are supplied by foods fortified with vitamin A, such as milk, dairy products, and breakfast cereals. The RDA for vitamin A is measured in retinol equivalents.

Functions

Vitamin A is best known for its role in night vision, the normal growth of bones and teeth, and the formation and maintenance of skin and mucous membranes. The role of vitamin A is less well understood in reproduction, cell membrane stability, the synthesis of corticosterone (a hormone produced by the adrenal glands), the output of thyroxine (the hormone secreted by the thyroid gland), the development of the nervous system, red blood cell (RBC) production, and immune system functioning.

Clinical Applications

Vitamin A Deficiency

Even if the diet is devoid of vitamin A, it may take several years for a vitamin A deficiency to become apparent because (1) the body is capable of storing large amounts of vitamin A, and (2) deficiency symptoms do not appear until body stores are exhausted. Vitamin A deficiency is often associated with protein-calorie malnutrition.

Vitamin A deficiency may be caused by an inadequate intake (primary deficiency) or may occur secondary to malabsorption disorders, pancreatic and biliary diseases, disorders that interfere with vitamin A storage, or conditions that prevent the conversion of carotenes to vitamin A.

Severe vitamin A deficiency is rare in the United States, although mild vitamin A deficiency may be seen among low socioeconomic groups. In many developing nations, vitamin A deficiency is the major cause of blindness.

Clinical Findings

Vitamin A deficiency may produce the following clinical findings:
Night blindness or changes in the eyes, such as dryness, wrinkling, keratinization, ulceration, or softening and perforation of the cornea may occur.
Skin may appear dry, scaly, or bumpy.
Diarrhea may develop, and susceptibility to respiratory infections increases.
Teeth may appear cracked or decayed.
Fatigue and other symptoms of anemia may develop.

Treatment

Acute vitamin A deficiency is treated with large doses of oral supplements; the more severe the symptoms, the longer the response time to vitamin A therapy.

Vitamin A Toxicity

Vitamin A toxicity is not likely to occur from diet alone; toxicity is usually associated with megadoses of vitamin A supplements. Toxicity can develop in adults with sustained daily intakes exceeding 15,000 µg. Short of consuming liver or fish liver oils daily, this dose cannot be achieved from foods alone. Children can develop toxic reactions to vitamin A at lower doses. Individual tolerance to vitamin A varies considerably. However, toxicity occurs only from excessive intakes of preformed vitamin A, not from the vitamin A precursor carotene, which is not converted to vitamin A quickly enough to cause a toxicity. Instead, carotene is stored in adipose tissue and may accumulate under the skin to the extent that it causes the skin color to turn yellowish orange, a harmless condition known as hypercarotenemia.

Symptoms of vitamin A toxicity include anorexia, abnormal skin pigmentation, nausea, vomiting, abdominal pain, diarrhea, weight loss, irritability, fatigue, ascites and portal hypertension, brittle nails, loss of hair, dry skin, bone pain and fragility, hydrocephalus and vomiting (in infants and children), spleen enlargement, and extensive liver damage. Symptoms can be reversed if toxicity is detected early and vitamin supplementation is stopped, although complete recovery may take several weeks. Permanent damage can result if prompt action is not taken.

Pharmacologic Uses of Vitamin A

Large doses of vitamin A may be used pharmacologically not only to treat vitamin A deficiency, but also to treat severe, resistant forms of acne. By some unknown mechanism, the drug Accutane (a retinoid, 13-*cis*-retinoic acid or isotretinoin; Roche Laboratories, Nutley, NJ) can cause a complete and prolonged remission of acne. Although vitamin A toxicity can develop depending on the dose and duration of treatment, Accutane appears to be safer and more effective than other forms of vitamin A used in the past (*i.e.*, retinol). Because large doses of vitamin A can cause spontaneous abortion and fetal abnormalities, Accutane should not be used by women who are or may be pregnant.

Vitamin A has also been used experimentally to block the conversion of precancerous cells into cancerous cells. Studies have shown that the incidence of epithelial cancers, particularly lung, larynx, esophagus, and bladder cancers, is higher among people whose diets are low in vitamin A. Vitamin A does not seem to prevent the initiation of cancer but may prevent or retard tumor development. Research has also shown that animals injected with known carcinogens developed significantly fewer tumors when given doses of 13-*cis*-retinoic acid. This compound and other synthetic retinoids appear to be more effective and less toxic than natural vitamin A, at least in test animals. More testing and research are needed before vitamin A compounds are available for routine use. For now, the American Cancer Society recommends that Americans consume foods high in vitamin A to help protect against cancer.

Nutrient/Drug Interactions

Supplements of vitamin A may:
- Enhance hepatotoxicity of alcohol (if hypervitaminosis A exists)
- Increase the risk of vitamin A toxicity from the drug isotretinoin (13-*cis*-retinoic acid/Accutane)
- Enhance intracranial hypertension induced by tetracycline

Drugs that affect vitamin A are as follows:[6]
- Cholestyramine: decreases vitamin A and carotene absorption
- Clofibrate: decreases carotene absorption
- Colchicine: decreases carotene absorption
- Mineral oils: decrease vitamin A absorption
- Oral contraceptives: increase plasma vitamin A levels

Vitamin D (Calciferol)

Vitamin D was discovered in 1918 and isolated in 1930. It is very stable and is resistant to heat, aging, and storage.

7-Dehydrocholesterol, a precursor of vitamin D that is found in some animal sources, is converted to cholecalciferol (vitamin D_3) in the skin by ultraviolet light. D_2 (ergocalciferol) is the other major form of vitamin D. Its precursor is ergosterol, which is a plant sterol that is converted to vitamin D_2 when exposed to ultraviolet light. Ergocalciferol is produced commercially for use in vitamin supplements.

Both vitamin D_2 and vitamin D_3 must be converted to the active form of vitamin D. The liver converts vitamin D_3 to a more potent form of vitamin D (25-hydroxycholecalciferol), which the kidneys convert to calcitrol, the most potent and active form of vitamin D. Because calcitriol can be synthesized in the kidney and stimulates functional activity elsewhere in the body, vitamin D is considered by some to be a hormone, not a vitamin.

There are few food sources of vitamin D in the diet, except for liver, fish liver oils, and eggs. Fortified foods are the major source of vitamin D in the average American diet. Fortunately, the body can synthesize all the vitamin D it needs if enough sunlight is available. However, the amount of vitamin D synthesized in the skin depends on the area of skin exposed, the length of exposure, and the character of the skin. For instance, light skin synthesizes vitamin D more readily than dark skin, and aging reduces an 80-year-old's ability to about half that of a 20-year-old.[8]

Because the body is capable of synthesizing vitamin D, a dietary source is unnecessary if exposure to sunlight is regular and under optimal conditions. However, because few people meet those conditions, a dietary source of vitamin D is considered essential (see Table 5-1). Some studies have found that average daily consumption of vitamin D is below the RDA, and that because of a decreased ability to produce vitamin D with aging, the RDA may be set too low for certain age/sex groups.[8]

Functions

Through its role in calcium and phosphorus metabolism, vitamin D is essential for normal growth and development (see Table 5-1).

Clinical Applications

Vitamin D Deficiency

A deficiency of vitamin D results in the diseases rickets in children and osteomalacia in adults. Children at high risk for rickets are those who have malabsorption syndromes, are born prematurely, are given vitamin D-deficient formulas or breastfed by vegan mothers, and those who have received anticonvulsant therapy for a long time. The fortification of foods with vitamin D has almost eliminated rickets in the United States, though it continues to be a problem in underdeveloped countries.

Clinical osteomalacia is rare in the United States but may be observed in women who have had chronically low intakes of vitamin D and multiple pregnancies. Also at risk are house-bound or institutionalized elderly, because aging impairs the ability to synthesize vitamin D, and exposure to sunlight is limited. Pure vegans are at risk because they exclude milk and dairy products, which are fortified with vitamin D, from their diet. Secondary vitamin D deficiency can develop in people with liver or kidney diseases, because the conversion of previtamins to the active form of vitamin D is impaired, or from fat malabsorption syndromes that interfere with vitamin D absorption.

Vitamin D deficiency may also occur when exposure to sunlight is limited, such as in northern climates. Unfortunately, ultraviolet light cannot penetrate atmospheric pollution, fog, smoke, glass, or clothing; even dark pigment in the skin limits the synthesis of vitamin D.

Clinical Findings

Children with rickets may be observed to have the following:
Profuse sweating and restlessness, which may be the first sign of rickets
Tetany and convulsions
Growth retardation
Skeletal deformities, such as bowed legs or knock-knees; enlarged, malformed skull; beading on the ribs and pigeon chest; curvature of the spine; enlarged wrists and ankles
Delayed tooth eruption; defective enamel
In adults, signs and symptoms of osteomalacia may include the following:
Softening of the bones leading to bone deformities, especially of the limbs, chest, and pelvis
Muscular weakness and back pain
Development of a waddling gait

Treatment

Symptoms of rickets and osteomalacia are reversible with therapeutic doses of 2000 to 6000 IU of vitamin D daily; calcium supplements may also be prescribed and exposure to the sun is encouraged. Doses of up to 50,000 IU may be necessary in adults with malabsorption.

Vitamin D Toxicity

Vitamin D may be the most toxic fat-soluble vitamin. Although vitamin D toxicity generally occurs when large doses are consumed over time, toxic levels for some groups may be as low as five times the RDA. Individual tolerance varies significantly; however, young children are especially vulnerable. An excess of vitamin D produces hypercalcemia, which causes excessive calcification of the bones and soft tissues, formation of kidney stones and the potential for permanent kidney damage and irreversible cardiovascular damage. Symptoms include nausea, vomiting, headache, weakness, weight loss, constipation, polyuria, and polydipsia. Children may also experience mental and physical growth retardation, and failure to thrive. Drowsiness and coma may develop in severe cases.

Toxicity is treated by discontinuing the vitamin supplement, correcting fluid and electrolyte imbalances, reducing calcium intake, and administering a loop diuretic to increase renal calcium excretion. Glucocorticoid therapy may be used to lower serum calcium levels.

Pharmacologic Uses of Vitamin D

Vitamin D preparations may be used to treat hypocalcemic diseases such as vitamin D-dependent rickets, renal osteodystrophy, postoperative tetany, idiopathic tetany, and hypoparathyroidism. In healthy people, vitamin D in excess of the RDA offers no known benefit and the possibility of toxicity; therefore, intakes greater than the RDA are not recommended.

Nutrient/Drug Interactions

Supplements of vitamin D may
- Precipitate cardiac arrhythmias in patients receiving digoxin who have vitamin D-induced hypercalcemia.

Drugs that affect vitamin D are as follows:[6]
- Adrenal corticosteroids: antivitamin D activity inhibits intestinal absorption of calcium
- Anticonvulsants: increase inactivation of vitamin D
- Barbiturates: increase inactivation of vitamin D
- Cholestyramine: decreases intestinal absorption of vitamin D
- Mineral oil: prolonged use causes vitamin D malabsorption
- Thiazide diuretics: may potentiate vitamin D-induced hypercalcemia in hypoparathyroid patients

Vitamin E

Vitamin E was discovered in 1922 and first synthesized in 1937. Processing, storage, and preparation techniques may result in large losses of vitamin E in foods.

Compounds with vitamin E activity are known as tocopherols. Alpha-tocopherol is the most active form of vitamin E and the most abundant in food. Vitamin E is found in plant fat and is especially abundant in vegetable oils, products made with vegetable oils (like margarine and shortening), wheat germ, nuts, and to a lesser extent, green leafy vegetables. Animal fats are poor sources of vitamin E. The actual vitamin E content of the diet varies considerably depending on the type and amount of fat consumed. The RDA for vitamin E is expressed as tocopherol equivalents.

Functions

Although the mechanism by which it functions is not fully understood, vitamin E is the primary antioxidant in the body and serves to protect polyunsaturated fatty acids (PUFA) from oxidation. Correspondingly, the need for vitamin E increases as the intake of PUFA increases; fortunately, both are found in the same foods. Because cell membranes, especially RBC membranes, are rich in PUFA, vitamin E helps maintain cell membrane integrity and protects RBC against hemolysis.

Clinical Applications

Vitamin E Deficiency

Premature and very-low-birth-weight infants are at risk for vitamin E deficiency because they are born with low body reserves, their intestinal absorption is impaired, and accelerated growth rates increase vitamin E demand. Feeding these infants commercial formulas with high concentrations of PUFA and iron, which destroys vitamin E, compounds the problem.

The only other population group likely to develop vitamin E deficiency are people with chronic fat malabsorption related to celiac disease, cystic fibrosis, or pancreatic disorders. Vitamin E deficiency related to poor intake is not likely.

Clinical Findings

In infants, symptoms of hemolytic anemia, edema, and skin lesions may develop. In adults, neurologic symptoms do not appear until malabsorption has persisted for 5 to 10 years.

Treatment

Infants may be given formula with added vitamin E, vitamin E drops, or, in case of a severe deficiency, injections of vitamin E. Adults may be given supplements of vitamin E or a multivitamin containing vitamin E.

Vitamin E Toxicity

Compared to vitamin A and vitamin D, vitamin E appears to be relatively nontoxic. Although individual tolerance varies, it appears that oral doses of up to 100 to 800 mg/day are harmless and useless. At 900 mg/day, vitamin E has been shown to cause depression and fatigue. Diarrhea, cramps, blurred vision, headaches, and dizziness may occur with higher doses. Megadoses of vitamin E can also interfere with normal blood clotting and vitamin A metabolism.

Pharmacologic Uses of Vitamin E

The only established use of vitamin E is to treat or prevent vitamin E deficiency. Numerous claims that vitamin E can treat coronary heart disease, infertility, cancer, diabetes, ulcers, skin disorders, burns, shortness of breath, and muscular dystrophy, as well as increase physical performance and sexual potency, protect against heart disease and air pollution, reverse gray hair and wrinkles, and slow the aging process are unfounded. However, the use of vitamin E to reduce the toxic effects of oxygen therapy on lung parenchyma and the retina in premature infants is being investigated.

Nutrient/Drug Interactions

Vitamin E may enhance anticoagulant response to warfarin and can reduce the efficacy of oral iron supplements. Mineral oil can cause vitamin E malabsorption.

Vitamin K

Vitamin K was recognized as the antihemorrhagic factor in 1935. It is resistant to heat and air but is destroyed by light, strong acids and alkalis, and oxidizing agents. The body is able to store small amounts of vitamin K in the liver, heart, skin, muscles, and kidney.

Vitamin K occurs naturally in two forms: phylloquinone, which is found in dark-green leafy vegetables and members of the cabbage family, and menaquinones, which are synthesized in the intestinal tract by bacteria. Animals provide both forms of vitamin K. The RDA for vitamin K was established for the first time in 1989.

Functions

Vitamin K is essential for the synthesis of prothrombin and at least five other proteins required for normal blood clotting.

Clinical Applications

Vitamin K Deficiency

Because intestinal bacteria and a balanced diet provide ample amounts of vitamin K, a deficiency is not likely in a healthy person. However, recent research indicates that intestinal synthesis is not sufficient to meet total vitamin K needs, and alterations in clotting factors will result when dietary intake of vitamin K is restricted.

Newborns are prone to vitamin K deficiency because they have sterile GI tracts, thus, no bacteria results in no vitamin K synthesis. Although newborns are exposed to intestinal bacteria when they pass down the birth canal, it takes 1 to 2 days for the bacteria to become established in the GI tract. In addition, newborns may not have an immediate dietary source of vitamin K; initial feedings are often delayed for a number of hours, and breast milk is a poor source of vitamin K. Because of this, a single parenteral dose of vitamin K is usually given prophylactically at birth.

A secondary deficiency may occur from impaired intestinal synthesis related to prolonged use of antibiotics or vitamin K antagonists (see Nutrient/Drug Interactions) or from impaired vitamin K absorption related to chronic fat malabsorption, or chronic biliary obstruction. People on long-term total parenteral nutrition are also at risk.

Clinical Findings

Signs of hemorrhaging may be observed related to delayed blood clotting.

Treatment

Vitamin K deficiency in adults is treated with either oral or intramuscular administration of vitamin K.

Vitamin K Toxicity

Excessive doses of vitamin K over long periods of time have failed to produce toxic symptoms. However, menadione may cause hemolytic anemia and hyperbilirubinemia in the newborn.

Pharmacologic Uses of Vitamin K

Vitamin K is used pharmacologically to treat coagulation disorders related to impaired vitamin K synthesis or absorption and prophylactically to treat hemorrhagic disease of the newborn. Vitamin K also is given for oral anticoagulant-induced prothrombin deficiency.

Nutrient/Drug Interactions

Vitamin K in liquid food supplements may inhibit the hypoprothrombic effect of warfarin. Drugs that affect vitamin K are as follows:

- Coumarin and indanedione anticoagulants: interfere with hepatic synthesis of vitamin K-dependent clotting factors
- Cholestyramine: decreases vitamin K absorption
- Mineral oil: decreases vitamin K absorption
- Salicylates: antagonize vitamin K
- Tetracyclines: decrease intestinal synthesis of vitamin K

WATER-SOLUBLE VITAMINS

The water-soluble vitamins are vitamin C and the B-complex vitamins, all of which perform one or more functions in the body and must be supplied in the diet. Recommended dietary allowances have been established for vitamin C and six B vitamins: thiamine, riboflavin, niacin, vitamin B_6, folate, and vitamin B_{12}. Estimated safe and adequate intakes have been established for pantothenic acid and biotin. Table 5-2 is a summary of the water-soluble vitamins.

Group Characteristics

As a group, water-soluble vitamins have the following characteristics:

They are absorbed through the intestinal wall directly into the bloodstream, where they travel freely and without the aid of protein carriers.

Water-soluble vitamins are filtered through the kidneys and excreted in the urine when consumed in excess of need.

Although some tissues are able to hold limited amounts, water-soluble vitamins are generally considered nontoxic. However, that belief has come under scrutiny since

(*Text continued on page 124*)

Table 5-2
Summary of Water-Soluble Vitamins

Vitamin	Functions	Deficiency Signs and Symptoms
VITAMIN C (Ascorbic Acid)		
Adult RDA Men and women: 60 mg Pregnancy: 70 mg Lactation: 95 mg	Acts as an antioxidant Formation of collagen Enhances intestinal absorption of iron Converts folate to its active form Involved in the metabolism of certain amino acids	Bleeding gums, pinpoint hemorrhages under the skin Scurvy, characterized by Hemorrhaging Muscle degeneration Skin changes Delayed wound healing: reopening of old wounds Softening of the bones → malformations, pain, easy fractures Soft, loose teeth Anemia Increased susceptibility to infection Hysteria and depression

Food Sources

Guava, broccoli, brussels sprouts, green peppers, strawberries, "greens," citrus fruits, potatoes, tomatoes, and cabbage

Vitamin	Functions	Deficiency Signs and Symptoms
THIAMINE (Vitamin B$_2$)		
Adult RDA Men: 1.2–1.5 mg Women: 1.0–1.1 mg Pregnancy: 1.5 mg Lactation: 1.6 mg	Energy metabolism, especially the metabolism of CHO Normal nervous system functioning	Beriberi Mental confusion Fatigue Peripheral paralysis Muscle weakness and wasting Painful calf muscles Anorexia Edema Enlarged heart Sudden death from heart failure

Food Sources

Pork, liver, organ meats, whole grain and enriched grains, nuts, legumes, potatoes, eggs, and milk

Vitamin	Functions	Deficiency Signs and Symptoms
RIBOFLAVIN (Vitamin B$_2$)		
Adult RDA Men: 1.4–1.7 mg Women: 1.2–1.3 mg Pregnancy: 1.6 mg Lactation: 1.8 mg	CHO, protein, and fat metabolism Other metabolic roles	Ariboflavinosis Dermatitis Cheilosis Glossitis Photophobia Reddening of the cornea

Food Sources

Milk and dairy products, organ meats, eggs, enriched grains, and green leafy vegetables

Vitamin	Functions	Deficiency Signs and Symptoms
NIACIN (Vitamin B$_2$)		
Adult RDA Men: 15 to 19 mg NE Women: 13–15 mg NE	CHO, protein, and fat metabolism	Pellagra: (4 Ds) Dermatitis (bilateral and symmetrical) and glossitis Diarrhea

(continued)

Table 5-2 (*continued*)

Vitamin	Functions	Deficiency Signs and Symptoms
Pregnancy: 17 mg NE Lactation: 20 mg NE		Dementia, irritability, mental confusion → psychosis Death, if untreated

Food Sources

Kidney, liver, poultry, lean meat, fish, yeast, peanut butter, enriched and whole grains, dried peas and beans, and nuts

VITAMIN B$_6$ (Pyridoxine)

Adult RDA

Men: 2.0 mg
Women: 1.6 mg
Pregnancy: 2.2 mg
Lactation: 2.1 mg

Amino acid metabolism
Blood formation
Maintenance of nervous tissue
Conversion of tryptophan to niacin

Dermatitis, cheilosis, glossitis, abnormal brain wave pattern, convulsions, and anemia

Food Sources

Chicken, fish, peanuts, oats, yeast, wheat germ, pork, organ meats, egg yolk, whole grain cereals, corn, potatoes, and bananas

FOLATE

Adult RDA

Men: 200 μg
Women: 180 μg
Pregnancy: 400 μg
Lactation: 280 μg

Amino acid metabolism
DNA and RNA synthesis; proliferation of cells
Blood formation

Glossitis, diarrhea, macrocytic anemia

Food Sources

Green leafy vegetables, asparagus, broccoli, liver, organ meats, milk, eggs, yeast, wheat germ, and kidney beans

VITAMIN B$_{12}$ (Cobalamin)

Adult RDA

Men and Women: 2 μg
Pregnancy: 2.2 μg
Lactation: 2.6 μg

RNA and DNA synthesis
Blood formation
Maintenance of nervous tissue
CHO, protein, and fat metabolism
Folate metabolism

GI changes: glossitis, anorexia, indigestion, recurring diarrhea or constipation, and weight loss
Macrocytic anemia → pallor, dyspnea, weakness, fatigue, and palpitations
Neurologic changes: paresthesia of the hands and feet, decreased sense of position, poor muscle coordination, poor memory, irritability, depression, paranoia, delirium, and hallucinations

Food Sources

Liver, kidney, fresh shrimp and oysters, meats, milk, eggs, and cheese

PANTOTHENIC ACID

Adult RDA

Men and women: safe and adequate intake 4 mg to 7 mg

CHO, protein, and fat metabolism

Not observed in humans

(*continued*)

Table 5-2 (*continued*)

Vitamin	Functions	Deficiency Signs and Symptoms
Food Sources		
Animal tissues, whole grain cereals, legumes, milk, vegetables, fruit		
BIOTIN		
Adult RDA	Fat and CHO metabolism	Observed only under experimental conditions
Men and women: safe and adequate intake 30 μg to 100 μg	Glycogen formation	
Food Sources		
Liver, organ meats, egg yolk, milk, and yeast. Synthesized by GI flora.		

1983, when neurologic abnormalities were reported in people taking megadoses of vitamin B_6.

Because tissue reserves of water-soluble vitamins are minimal, deficiency symptoms often develop rapidly when intake is inadequate.

Water-soluble vitamins should be supplied in the diet daily.

Vitamin C (Ascorbic Acid)

Vitamin C was not isolated in its pure form until 1932. Although the association between citrus fruits and the prevention of scurvy has long been known, it was not until the 20th century that vitamin C was discovered as the anti-scurvy ingredient. Vitamin C is labile; that is, it is easily destroyed by heat, air, alkalis, drying, and aging.

Active vitamin C exists in two forms: ascorbic acid and dehydroascorbic acid. The richest sources of vitamin C are citrus fruits, green and red peppers, collard greens, broccoli, spinach, tomatoes, and strawberries. Although potatoes and root vegetables are low in vitamin C, they contribute substantial amounts of vitamin C to the diet because they are eaten in large quantities. Ascorbic acid is often added to processed foods for its antioxidant properties.[10]

The RDA for vitamin C is listed in Table 5-2. However, there is considerable controversy over how much vitamin C is actually needed for optimal health. Even among different nations, recommended allowances vary, from 30 mg/day in Canada to 60 mg/day in the United States and 75 mg/day in Germany. Vitamin C requirement does increase in response to fever, chronic illness, infection, burns, multiple wounds, and smoking; the National Research Council recommends that regular cigarette smokers consume at least 100 mg of vitamin C daily. Although many people habitually take 1000 mg or more of vitamin C without toxic side effects, the long-term risks of such large doses are not known. Routine use of megadoses is not recommended.[10]

In the absence of continuous intake, vitamin C is poorly retained in the body.[10] Vitamin C consumed in excess of need is excreted in the urine.

Functions

Vitamin C has many important functions in the body, although the mechanism by which it works is not clearly understood. Vitamin C is needed for the formation of collagen, the most abundant protein in fibrous tissue such as connective tissue, cartilage, bone matrix, tooth dentin, skin, and tendon. The integrity of this "intracellular cement" is important for maintaining capillary strength, promoting wound healing, and resisting infection.

Vitamin C also acts as an antioxidant to protect vitamin A, vitamin E, PUFA, and iron from destruction. It is involved in many metabolic reactions, including promoting the absorption of iron, converting folacin to its active form, the formation of some neurotransmitters, the synthesis of thyroxine, and the absorption of calcium and its deposition and withdrawal from teeth.

Clinical Applications

Vitamin C Deficiency

According to the Nationwide Food Consumption Survey of 1977–1978,[11] vitamin C intake exceeds the RDA for all sex/age groups. Groups most at risk for vitamin C deficiency are alcoholics, people who do not eat fruits and vegetables, people with increased vitamin C requirements, and people of low socioeconomic status.

Clinical Findings

When the body's supply of vitamin C is exhausted and intake is inadequate, symptoms of scurvy appear. Defects in collagen synthesis are evidenced by swollen, inflamed gums that bleed easily, and pinpoint hemorrhages under the skin related to capillary fragility. Hemorrhaging worsens as the disease progresses. Softening of the ends of the long bones can lead to painful malformations and fractures, and ankle and wrist joints may appear swollen. Wound healing is delayed and previous wounds may reopen. Secondary infections are more likely. Changes in skin and teeth may become apparent.[10] In addition, psychological symptoms of hysteria and depression may develop. Internal hemorrhage may lead to heart failure and sudden death.

Treatment

Scurvy can be cured as quickly as 5 days after moderate doses of vitamin C are administered (100 mg).

Vitamin C Toxicity

Although large doses of vitamin C generally are considered nontoxic, it is possible that megadoses may cause undesirable side effects such as nausea, abdominal cramps, and diarrhea, and iron absorption may become excessive. Large doses of vitamin C also can cause a false-positive test for glucose in the urine. An increase in oxalic acid excretion (excess vitamin C may be excreted as vitamin C or oxalic acid, a waste product of vitamin C metabolism) theoretically increases the risk for oxalate renal stone formation. Certain population groups, including some black Americans, Sephardic Jews, and Orientals, may develop hemolytic anemia because they lack an enzyme that normally protects against the effects of large amounts of vitamin C and other strong reducing agents. Because the body becomes conditioned to catabolizing and excreting large amounts of vitamin C, rebound scurvy may develop between the time megadoses are stopped and normal vitamin C metabolism is restored.

Pharmacologic Uses of Vitamin C

The only proven effective therapeutic use of vitamin C is to prevent or treat scurvy. In large doses, vitamin C may have pharmacologic or drug-like effects. For instance, vitamin C may be used as adjunctive therapy to promote wound healing, as in the case of severe burns, multiple or serious pressure ulcers, and postoperative periods.[6]

Vitamin C and the Common Cold,[12] a book written by Nobel Prize winner Linus Pauling in 1970, claims that taking 1 g of vitamin C daily can reduce the incidence of colds by 45% and that during a cold, doses of 500 to 1000 mg of vitamin C every hour will alleviate symptoms. However, most studies conclude that megadoses of vitamin C do not prevent colds. Whereas large amounts of vitamin C may lessen the duration and severity of colds, the benefit is so small that supplements are not recommended.

Researchers are also investigating the role of vitamin C in cancer prevention. Studies indicate that foods high in vitamin C may protect against certain kinds of cancer, such as cancer of the stomach and esophagus. However, it has not been determined whether vitamin C alone, or vitamin C together with some other components in those foods, is to be credited for the reduced risk. It is known that vitamin C may help prevent cancer by blocking the conversion of nitrites and amines (both present in food) to nitrosamines, which are potent animal carcinogens. Although vitamin C may reduce the risk of cancer from nitrosamines, that is not the same as saying vitamin C prevents cancer. Most experts agree that the recommendation to take megadoses of vitamin C to prevent cancer is premature and unsupported by current evidence. However, the American Cancer Society does recommend that Americans choose foods rich in vitamin C to reduce their risk of cancer.

Linus Pauling and Ewan Cameron[14] claim that high doses of vitamin C are beneficial in the treatment of patients with advanced cancer, especially patients who have not had chemotherapy. However, in a recent study conducted at the Mayo Clinic, two groups of advanced colon and rectal cancer patients who had not previously been treated with chemotherapy were treated with either 10 g of vitamin C daily or a placebo. Their results indicated that vitamin C showed no advantage over the placebo with regard to the progression of the disease or survival of the patient.

In some hypercholesterolemic people, large doses of vitamin C have lowered serum cholesterol levels; however, these results have not been confirmed by others.

Although vitamin C has been shown to relieve infertility caused by nonspecific sperm agglutination, the men who were successfully treated tended to be deficient in vitamin C. Evidence that vitamin C cures infertility in well-nourished people is lacking.

Nutrient/Drug Interactions

Supplements of vitamin C may
- Interfere with the absorption of fluphenazine, an antipsychotic agent.
- Decrease prothrombin time in clients receiving oral anticoagulants.
- Increase the excretion of acidic drugs (salicylates, barbiturates) and increase excretion of basic drugs (quinidine, atropine, amphetamines, tricyclic antidepressants, phenothiazines).

- Increase the risk of crystalluria with sulfonamides.
- Enhance absorption of oral iron supplements.

Drugs that affect vitamin C are as follows:
- Adrenal corticosteroids: increase urinary excretion of vitamin C
- Barbiturates: increase urinary excretion of vitamin C
- Indomethacin: decreases plasma and platelet ascorbic acid levels
- Levodopa: increases the need for vitamin C
- Oral contraceptives: decrease serum, leukocyte, and platelet levels of vitamin C
- Phenacetin: increases urinary excretion of vitamin C
- Salicylates: increase urinary excretion of vitamin C
- Sulfonamides: increase urinary excretion of vitamin C

Thiamine (Vitamin B₁)

Thiamine was discovered in 1921 and synthesized in 1936. Thiamine is lost in cooking, especially when cooking is prolonged or at high temperatures. Alkalis also destroy thiamine.

Rich sources of thiamine include unrefined and enriched grains, pork, and organ meats, legumes, seeds, and nuts. Enriched and fortified grains and cereals contribute substantial amounts of thiamine to the diet.

Thiamine requirements are based on the calorie content of the diet—a high CHO diet increases the need for thiamine. The heart and brain are the tissues that store, or become saturated with, thiamine when intake exceeds requirement; thiamine remaining after tissues are saturated is excreted in the urine.

Functions

Thiamine is an important component in the coenzyme thiamine pyrophosphate (TPP), which is involved in converting CHO (glucose) to energy. Thiamine is also necessary for protein and fat metabolism and normal nervous system functioning.

Clinical Applications

Thiamine Deficiency

Significant thiamine depletion can develop within 3 weeks on a diet devoid of thiamine. In the United States, thiamine deficiency is most commonly related to alcohol abuse, which alters thiamine intake, absorption, and metabolism. Other high-risk groups include renal patients undergoing long-term dialysis, patients receiving long-term parenteral nutrition, people with chronic fever, and the relatively few people with thiamine-responsive inborn errors of metabolism.[10]

Severe thiamine deficiency, known as *beriberi*, is rare in the United States, although subclinical deficiencies may be seen. Throughout history, countries in the Orient, which rely heavily on milled rice (refining rice removes much of the thiamine content) and foods with antithiamine activity, have had a high incidence of beriberi. However, food enrichment programs have virtually eradicated beriberi in Japan and the Philippines.

Clinical Findings

Beriberi, which translates literally to "I can't, I can't," is an accurate description of the weakening disease that primarily affects the nervous and cardiovascular systems. Adult beriberi produces symptoms of anorexia, fatigue, nausea, vomiting, irritability, mental confusion, muscular weakness, peripheral paralysis, emotional instability, depression, and general lethargy.

Beriberi may be classified as "mixed," which is characterized by neuritis and heart failure, "dry," of which polyneuritis is the major finding, or "wet," which is identified by edema and heart failure. Without treatment, most patients die from sudden heart failure.

Infantile beriberi is common in breastfed infants living in underdeveloped countries. Symptoms include restlessness, pallor, inability to sleep, edema, diarrhea, muscle wasting, and breathing difficulties. Death caused by acute heart failure may occur 1 to 2 days after the onset of symptoms.

Treatment

Large oral doses of thiamine or a thiamine derivative are administered. Wet beriberi responds within a few hours after treatment is initiated if the nervous system is not badly damaged; recovery from dry beriberi is slower. Infantile beriberi is treated by giving thiamine to both the lactating mother and to the infant. Because thiamine deficiency rarely occurs alone, a B-complex multivitamin preparation frequently is given.

Thiamine Toxicity

Thiamine consumed orally produces no known toxic effects; large parenteral doses may produce evidence of toxicity.

Pharmacologic Uses of Thiamine

The only pharmacologic use of thiamine is to treat thiamine deficiency.

Nutrient/Drug Interactions

Supplements of thiamine can enhance the response to peripherally acting muscle relaxants.[6]

Drugs that affect thiamine are as follows:
- Antacids: destroy thiamine
- Barbiturates: decrease thiamine absorption
- Diuretics, mercurial: increase urinary excretion of thiamine

Riboflavin (Vitamin B₂)

Riboflavin was discovered in 1932 and synthesized in 1935. Although resistant to heat, acid, and oxidation, riboflavin is quickly destroyed by light.

Riboflavin is widely distributed in foods but only in small amounts. Good sources include milk and dairy products, followed by meats, poultry, and fish. Enriched and fortified grains and cereals contribute large amounts of riboflavin to the diet.

The RDA listed for riboflavin is a recommended minimum daily intake. Actual riboflavin requirements are based on calorie intake: As calorie intake increases, the amount of riboflavin needed also increases. Because only small amounts of riboflavin are "stored" in the liver and kidney, a daily intake is necessary. However, riboflavin consumed in excess of need is excreted in the urine; protein-wasting conditions increase riboflavin excretion.

Functions

Riboflavin is part of the coenzymes FAD (flavin adenine dinucleotide) and FMN (flavin mononucleotide), which have vital metabolic roles in energy metabolism, DNA and protein synthesis, and gluconeogenesis. Riboflavin is also involved in the activation of vitamin B_6, the conversion of folacin to its coenzyme, corticosteroid synthesis, RBC production, and thyroid enzyme activity.

Clinical Applications

Riboflavin Deficiency

Riboflavin deficiency is uncommon in the United States. However, people with marginal calorie intakes, such as adolescent women, alcoholics, and the elderly, are at risk for riboflavin deficiency, as are people with malabsorption syndromes and those using certain drugs (see Nutrient/Drug Interactions).

Clinical Findings

Signs of riboflavin deficiency may not appear for several months on a riboflavin-deficient diet. Early symptoms include oral lesions, dermatitis, normocytic anemia, and scrotal and vulval skin changes.[10]

Cheilosis (fissuring of the lips), angular stomatitis (cracks in the skin at the corners of the mouth), a purplish swollen tongue, and reddening of the cornea are characteristics of a severe riboflavin deficiency (ariboflavinosis).

Treatment

Riboflavin deficiency is treated with large oral doses of riboflavin or B-complex vitamins; severe deficiency may require parenteral administration. Lesions may heal within a few days or weeks.

Riboflavin Toxicity

Riboflavin produces no known toxic effects.

Pharmacologic Uses of Riboflavin

Riboflavin is used pharmacologically only to treat riboflavin deficiency.

Nutrient/Drug Interactions

Drugs that affect riboflavin are as follows:
- Amitriptyline: interferes with riboflavin metabolism
- Chloramphenicol: may increase the need for riboflavin
- Chlorpromazine: may interfere with riboflavin metabolism
- Imipramine: may interfere with riboflavin metabolism
- Probenecid: increases urinary excretion of riboflavin

Niacin or Nicotinic Acid

Although known since 1867, niacin was not recognized as a vitamin until 1936. Niacin is relatively stable to heat, oxidation, light, acid, and alkalis; therefore, little is lost through food preparation, cooking, or storage. However, bioavailability of niacin may be low in some foods.

Lean meats, kidney, liver, poultry, fish, yeasts, and peanut butter are excellent sources of niacin. Enriched and whole grain products, dried peas and beans, and nuts contain lesser amounts of niacin.

The body is able to synthesize niacin from its precursor tryptophan, an amino acid abundant in milk, eggs, and other foods rich in protein. At least 1% of the total protein intake is in the form of tryptophan, and 60 mg of tryptophan are needed to synthesize 1 mg of niacin (*i.e.*, 60 g of protein = 0.6 g [or 600 mg] tryptophan, which may be converted to 10 mg of niacin).

The RDA for niacin represents the minimum total milligrams of niacin equivalents required daily; as with riboflavin, actual need is based on total calorie intake, which increases niacin requirements. "Niacin equivalents" is the total amount of niacin available in the diet from preformed niacin and the precursor tryptophan. Little niacin accumulates in the body, and amounts consumed in excess of need are excreted in the urine.

Functions

As part of the coenzymes NAD (nicotinamide adenine dinucleotide) and NADP (nicotinamide adenine dinucleotide phosphate), niacin (nicotinamide is its active form) is required by all living cells for oxidation and the release of energy from CHO, protein, and fat. Nicotinamide adenine dinucleotide also plays a role in glycogenesis. Reduced NADP is required for the synthesis of fatty acids, cholesterol, and steroid hormones.

Clinical Applications

Niacin Deficiency

A severe deficiency of niacin leads to pellagra, which literally means "rough skin." In the United States, pellagra is uncommon and most often associated with alcohol abuse or clinical stresses. Pellagra is widespread in areas that rely on corn as a staple, such as parts of Africa and Asia, and was common in the southern United States before grain products were enriched.

Clinical Findings

The symptoms of niacin deficiency are similar to those of a deficiency of riboflavin. Early symptoms include anorexia, apathy, weakness, indigestion, and skin lesions. Classic symptoms of pellagra are the "four Ds":
- Dermatitis, which occurs bilaterally and symmetrically—especially on skin exposed to the sun; the tongue also becomes smooth, sore, and "beefy"
- Diarrhea
- Dementia; also irritability, depression, confusion, psychosis, and tremors
- Death if untreated

Treatment

Niacin deficiency may be treated with niacin and/or tryptophan. However, because a deficiency of niacin rarely occurs alone, treatment is most effective when other B-complex vitamins are administered, especially thiamine and riboflavin.

Severe pellagra may be treated with oral doses of 150 to 600 mg of nicotinic acid or nicotinamide several times daily (nicotinamide is preferred because it produces fewer side effects). Response may begin within the first 24 hours of treatment and be complete within a few weeks; some mental disturbances may be permanent if related to chronic malnutrition.

Niacin Toxicity

Large doses of nicotinic acid may produce flushing and itching. Doses of 3 to 9 g of nicotinic acid daily decrease serum lipids and mobilization of fatty acids from adipose during exercise. Other reported side effects include nausea, vomiting, diarrhea, hypotension, tachycardia, fainting, hypoglycemia, and liver damage.

Pharmacologic Uses of Niacin

Niacin is used pharmacologically to treat niacin deficiency and pellagra. Megadoses of nicotinic acid (3 to 6 g/day) may be used as adjunctive therapy to lower serum cholesterol in people who do not respond adequately to diet and weight loss. However, it is not clear whether niacin has a positive, negative, or neutral effect on morbidity or mortality related to atherosclerosis or coronary heart disease. Adverse reactions include nausea, vomiting, abdominal pain, diarrhea, GI disorders, generalized flushing, sensation of warmth, and dry, itchy, tingling skin.

Although "orthomolecular therapists" use megadoses of niacin alone or in combination with large doses of other vitamins and minerals, enzymes, hormones, diets, and electroconvulsant therapy to treat schizophrenia, its efficacy and safety are unproven. According to a Task Force on Vitamin Therapy in Psychiatry of the American Psychiatric Association, orthomolecular therapy is based on uncontrolled studies, casual observations, and questionable diagnostic procedures.[2]

Nutrient/Drug Interactions

Large doses of niacin can potentiate the vasodilating effect of sympathomimetic blocking-type antihypertensive drugs and cause postural hypotension.

Niacin can reduce the effectiveness of oral hypoglycemic agents by elevating blood glucose levels.[6]

Drug that affects niacin is as follows:

- Isoniazid: causes pyridoxine depletion; pyridoxine is necessary for the conversion of tryptophan to niacin

Vitamin B6

Vitamin B_6 was identified in 1934 and isolated in 1939. Food processing can cause considerable losses of vitamin B_6.

Vitamin B_6, sometimes referred to as pyridoxine, is actually a group of three active compounds: pyridoxine (plant sources), pyridoxal, and pyridoxamine (animal sources). Chicken, fish, kidney, liver, pork, and eggs are rich sources of vitamin B_6. Whole-wheat products, peanuts, walnuts, oats, and unmilled rice are also good sources.

Vitamin B_6 requirement is related directly to protein intake: As protein intake increases, so does the need for vitamin B_6. Very little vitamin B_6 is stored in the body. The most recent edition of the RDAs lowered the recommendations for vitamin B_6 because metabolic maintenance is observed with lower intakes than previously suggested. Approximately 40 drugs are known to affect vitamin B_6 metabolism or bioavailability (see Nutrient/Drug Interactions).

Functions

As part of the coenzyme pyridoxal phosphate (PLP) or pyridoxamine phosphate, vitamin B_6 is involved in more than 60 biochemical reactions, especially in protein and amino acid metabolism. Vitamin B_6 is also important for the synthesis and conversion of tryptophan to niacin, the synthesis of gamma-aminobutyric acid (GABA, a compound that inhibits neurotransmitters in the brain), the formation of heme for hemoglobin, fatty acid metabolism, myelin sheath synthesis, and maintaining cellular immunity.

Clinical Applications

Vitamin B_6 Deficiency

Because vitamin B_6 is so widespread in foods and the daily requirement is small, a dietary deficiency of vitamin B_6 is uncommon. When a dietary deficiency does develop, it most often occurs in people with multiple B vitamin deficiencies.

A primary deficiency of vitamin B_6 occurs in people with an inborn error of vitamin B_6 metabolism, which prevents the synthesis of GABA. Infants born with the disorder become mentally retarded and develop uncontrollable convulsions unless treated early in the neonatal period with large daily doses of vitamin B_6.

A secondary deficiency may result from malabsorption syndromes, alcohol abuse, or certain drug therapies.

Clinical Findings

Deficiency symptoms include depression, nausea, vomiting, irritability, drowsiness, dermatitis, weight loss, increased susceptibility to infection, cheilosis, glossitis, anemia, abnormal brain wave pattern, and convulsions. A high protein intake increases the severity and speeds the onset of vitamin B_6 deficiency symptoms.

Treatment

Deficiency is treated with oral doses of vitamin B_6; parenteral injections are used if oral intake is contraindicated or absorption is impaired. Patients with vitamin B_6 dependency syndromes require large doses for life.

Vitamin B_6 Toxicity

Although acute toxicity is low, high doses of vitamin B_6 (*i.e.*, gram quantities) used for months or years have been blamed for neurologic problems, such as difficulty in walking, numbness of the feet and hands, clumsiness, and nerve degeneration.[3] Damage is not permanent, and symptoms improve gradually when the vitamin is discontinued.

Pharmacologic Uses of Vitamin B₆

In pharmacologic doses, vitamin B₆ is used to treat vitamin B₆ deficiency related to poor intake, malabsorption, secondary to drug therapy, or inborn errors of metabolism.

Vitamin B₆ has also been used experimentally in doses of 10 to 15 mg to relieve malaise and depression in women using oral contraceptives and to relieve symptoms of premenstrual syndrome, even though its efficacy has not been proven in controlled, double-blind studies. Vitamin B₆ has also been used with some success to relieve nausea and vomiting during pregnancy and after radiation therapy.

New research has found that victims of sickle cell anemia have low plasma levels of B₆. When given 50 mg of the vitamin twice a day for 2 months, the sickest patient had much shorter, much less severe crises.[3] Further studies need to be conducted to determine the relationship between sickle cell disease and vitamin B₆. By happenstance, during this study, it was discovered that all healthy "controls" (participants without sickle cell anemia) who had low vitamin B₆ levels also had bronchial asthma. An earlier study done with asthmatic children found that 200-mg supplements of vitamin B₆ given for 1 month decreased asthmatic symptoms. Like sickle cell, this is an area for future investigation.

Nutrient/Drug Interactions

Supplements of vitamin B₆ may
- Reverse the antiparkinsonism of the drug levodopa.
- May reduce phenytoin levels.
- May correct drug-induced peripheral neuropathy caused by hydralazine, isoniazid, and penicillamine.

Drugs that affect vitamin B₆ are as follows:
- Adrenal corticosteroids: increase the need for vitamin B₆
- Chloramphenicol: may increase the need for vitamin B₆
- Cycloserine: decreases serum vitamin B₆
- Diuretics: increase urinary excretion of vitamin B₆
- Hydralazine: inactivates vitamin B₆ and increases its urinary excretion
- Isoniazid: increases urinary excretion of vitamin B₆; causes vitamin B₆ depletion
- Levodopa: vitamin B₆ antagonist; depletes vitamin B₆
- Oral contraceptives (estrogen-containing): increases vitamin B₆ requirement
- Penicillamine: inhibits pyroxidal-dependent enzymes

Folic Acid (Folate, Folacin)

Folate was synthesized in 1946. Unfortunately, up to 50% of folate in foods may be lost during preparation, processing, and storage.

Folate is widespread in the diet. Excellent sources of folate include green leafy vegetables, asparagus, broccoli, liver, organ meats, milk, eggs, yeast, wheat germ, and kidney beans; beef, potatoes, dried peas and beans, whole grain cereal, nuts, bananas, cantaloupe, lemons, and strawberries are good sources.

In its most recent edition, the RDA for folate was lowered by one-half the previous recommendation because adult diets providing only 200 μg adequately maintained folate status and liver stores.[10] Folate requirements increase in response to pregnancy, lactation, alcohol abuse, malabsorption syndromes, certain medications, and other stresses.

Functions

The conversion of folate to the coenzyme tetrahydrofolic acid may depend on an adequate supply of vitamin B_{12}. As a coenzyme, folate plays a role in the synthesis of RNA (ribonucleic acid) and DNA (deoxyribonucleic acid) and is therefore necessary for the proliferation of cells and the transmission of inherited characteristics. Other functions of folic acid include the formation and maturation of RBC and white blood cells, amino acid metabolism, and the synthesis of enzymes.

Clinical Applications

Folate Deficiency

Folate deficiency is widespread in all parts of the world. In developing nations, folate deficiency commonly is caused by parasitic infections. Americans typically consume less than the previous RDA for folate without becoming deficient; the incidence of folate deficiency related to inadequate intake alone is difficult to estimate. Americans most at risk for folate deficiency are alcoholics because of poor folate intakes, impaired folate absorption, and altered folate metabolism. At risk for deficiency related to poor intake are the elderly, fad dieters, and the poor. Because growth increases folate requirements, infants, adolescents and pregnant women may have difficulty consuming adequate amounts. Lastly, risk is increased when absorption is altered, which may occur secondary to certain medications (see Nutrient/Drug Interactions), malabsorption syndromes, and general effects of aging. Absorption can be improved by eating a rich source of vitamin C with folate-containing foods.

Clinical Findings

Folate deficiency results in macrocytic or megaloblastic anemia characterized by large, immature RBC; anemia leads to fatigue, weakness, and pallor.

Other symptoms that may be observed include diarrhea, weight loss, and glossitis.

Treatment

Large oral doses result in rapid improvement of most symptoms; however, anemia is gradually reversed.

Folic Acid Toxicity

Folic acid produces no known toxic effects, although large doses may interfere with anticonvulsant therapy and precipitate convulsions in epileptics controlled by phenytoin.[10] Large parenteral doses of folic acid given to animals can produce kidney damage and hypertrophy.

Pharmacologic Uses of Folic Acid

Pharmacologic doses of folic acid are used to treat megaloblastic anemia related to inadequate folic acid intake, impaired absorption, altered requirements, or altered metabolism.

Folic acid may be used prophylactically during pregnancy to prevent anemia.

Nutrient/Drug Interactions

Supplements of folic acid may
- Alter the response to the drug methotrexate.

- Decrease the anticonvulsant action of the drug phenytoin.

Drugs that affect folic acid are as follows:

- Adrenal corticosteroids: increase the need for folic acid
- Alcohol: decreases folic acid absorption
- p-Aminosalicylic acid: decreases folic acid absorption
- Anticonvulsants: may decrease serum folate levels
- Azathioprine: folic acid antagonist
- Barbiturates: increase the need for folic acid
- Chloramphenicol: can antagonize response to folic acid
- Cycloserine: may decrease serum folate
- Isoniazid: may decrease serum folate
- Methotrexate: folic acid antagonist
- Nitrofurantoin: decreases serum folate
- Oral contraceptives: may impair folic acid metabolism and produce folate depletion
- Pyrimethamine: decreases serum folate
- Salicylates: decrease serum folate in patients with rheumatoid arthritis
- Sulfasalazine (salicylazosulfapyridine): decreases folic acid absorption
- Triamterene: folic acid antagonist
- Trimethadione: may lower serum folate levels when used on a long-term basis
- Trimethoprim: may decrease folic acid absorption

Vitamin B_{12} (Cobalamin)

Vitamin B_{12} was discovered in 1948 and synthesized in 1974. It is stable during normal cooking.

Vitamin B_{12} is found only in animal products and is especially abundant in kidney, liver, fresh shrimp and oysters, milk, eggs, fish, cheese, and muscle meats. Although GI flora synthesize small amounts of vitamin B_{12}, it is not absorbed because it is synthesized beyond the terminal ileum.

Vitamin B_{12} equilibrium can be maintained over a wide range of intakes. Excess vitamin B_{12} is stored in the liver in amounts sufficient to last 5 to 6 years or longer. Actual RDA for vitamin B_{12} is set high enough to maintain stores at substantial levels in view of the increasing evidence that vitamin B_{12} absorption appears to decrease in the elderly.[10]

Functions

Vitamin B_{12} is essential for the normal function of all cells, especially those of the GI tract, bone marrow, and the nervous system. Vitamin B_{12} plays a role in the synthesis of RNA and DNA and is therefore required for growth and RBC maturation. Myelin formation, CHO, protein, and fat metabolism, and folic acid metabolism are additional functions of vitamin B_{12}.

Clinical Applications

Vitamin B_{12} Deficiency

Vitamin B_{12} deficiency may develop from impaired absorption related to aging, iron deficiency, hypothyroidism, malabsorption syndromes, intestinal infestations, or intestinal resections that bypass the ileum. Impaired absorption accounts for more than 95% of the cases of vitamin B_{12} deficiency in the United States.

The absorption of vitamin B_{12} from the lower ileum requires the presence of intrinsic factor (IF), a glycoprotein secreted in the stomach. Conditions that alter IF secretion, such as gastric surgery or gastric cancer, lead to vitamin B_{12} malabsorption and a megaloblastic anemia called *pernicious anemia* (see Chap. 16).

A dietary deficiency of vitamin B_{12} is rare, except among pure vegetarians who consume no animal products and who do not supplement their diet. Even then, symptoms may not develop for 5 to 10 years.

Clinical Findings

Symptoms related to anemia that may be observed include pallor, dyspnea, weakness, and fatigue. Gastrointestinal changes may become apparent, including glossitis, anorexia, indigestion, recurring diarrhea or constipation, and weight loss.

Observe for neurologic changes, including paresthesia of the hands and feet, decreased sense of position, poor muscle coordination, poor memory, irritability, depression, paranoia, delirium, and hallucinations.

Treatment

Vitamin B_{12} deficiency caused by an inadequate intake can be reversed with oral vitamin B_{12} supplements. When vitamin B_{12} deficiency is related to impaired absorption, intramuscular injections are necessary.

Correct diagnosis and early treatment are necessary to prevent irreversible nervous system damage. Folic acid supplements will relieve vitamin B_{12} deficiency symptoms of anemia and GI changes, but do not halt the progressive nervous system damage that only vitamin B_{12} can treat.

Vitamin B_{12} Toxicity

Large oral doses of vitamin B_{12} produce no known toxic effects, nor do they offer any benefit.

Pharmacologic Uses of Vitamin B_{12}

Pharmacologic doses of vitamin B_{12} are used only to treat vitamin B_{12} deficiency.

No evidence exists to support claims that vitamin B_{12} relieves infectious hepatitis, multiple sclerosis, poor appetite, poor growth, aging, or fatigue.[5]

Nutrient/Drug Interactions

Drugs that affect vitamin B_{12} are as follows:
- Alcohol: decreases vitamin B_{12} absorption
- p-Aminosalicylic acid: decreases vitamin B_{12} absorption; causes a depletion in serum levels
- Anticonvulsants: may decrease serum levels of vitamin B_{12}
- Barbiturates: decrease serum vitamin B_{12} levels
- Chloramphenicol: may increase the need for vitamin B_{12}
- Cholestyramine: may decrease absorption of vitamin B_{12}; decreases serum levels
- Clofibrate: decreases vitamin B_{12} absorption
- Colchicine: decreases vitamin B_{12} absorption; decreases serum levels

- Cycloserine: may decrease serum vitamin B_{12} levels
- Metformin: decreases vitamin B_{12} absorption; decreases serum levels
- Methotrexate: decreases vitamin B_{12} absorption; decreases serum levels
- Neomycin: decreases vitamin B_{12} absorption; decreases serum levels
- Oral contraceptives: may alter tissue distribution of vitamin B_{12}
- Phenformin: decreases vitamin B_{12} absorption
- Phenobarbital: decreases serum and cerebrospinal fluid levels of vitamin B_{12}
- Potassium chloride: decreases vitamin B_{12} absorption
- Pyrimethamine: decreases serum levels of vitamin B_{12}
- Sodium nitroprusside: depletes plasma vitamin B_{12} by increasing urinary vitamin B_{12} excretion

Pantothenic Acid

Pantothenic acid was discovered in 1933 and synthesized in 1940. It is stable in moist heat, but destroyed by dry heat, acid, alkalis, and certain salts.

Pantothenic acid is found to some degree in all plants and animals. The richest sources of pantothenic acid are animal tissues, whole-grain cereals, and legumes; milk, vegetables, and fruit are good sources. Pantothenic acid may be synthesized by GI flora.

An RDA has not been established for pantothenic acid because of a lack of conclusive evidence regarding dietary requirements. An estimated safe and adequate intake of 4 to 7 mg is probably adequate for adults, most of whom consume 5 to 10 mg/day. Pantothenic acid consumed in excess of need is excreted in the urine.

Functions

As part of coenzyme A, pantothenic acid is important in the metabolism of CHO, protein, and fat; it is essential to most living things.

Clinical Applications

Pantothenic Acid Deficiency

No cases of pantothenic deficiency from natural causes have been reported. Laboratory-induced pantothenic deficiency produces dermatitis, burning sensations of the feet, fatigue, insomnia, nausea, intestinal disturbances, irritability, depression, and increased susceptibility to infections.

Pantothenic Toxicity

Pantothenic acid produces no known toxic effects, although large amounts may cause diarrhea.

Pharmacologic Uses of Pantothenic Acid

Although a natural dietary deficiency of pantothenic acid has not been documented and exact requirements are unknown, symptoms of weakness, fatigue, mood changes, dizziness, psychoses, unsteady gait, and torpor develop in people on low pantothenic acid diets who are also receiving drugs that may act as pantothenic antagonists. Pantothenic supplements have been credited with improving the burning-foot syndrome. Oral doses of 20 to 100 mg have been used for experimental and therapeutic purposes.

Nutrient/Drug Interactions

Drugs that affect pantothenic acid are as follows:
- Mercaptopurine: may antagonize pantothenic acid
- Probenecid: decreases urinary excretion of pantothenic acid

Biotin

Biotin was discovered in 1935 and synthesized in 1942. It is resistant to heat, but is unstable to alkali and oxidation, and may be leached from food by water.

Biotin is widely distributed in nature. Biotin bound to protein is fat-soluble and found in animal tissues. The richest sources are liver, organ meats, egg yolk, milk, and yeast. Biotin found freely in nature is water-soluble and is found mostly in plants and plant products: legumes, nuts, soy flour, and cereals. Gastrointestinal flora synthesize significant amounts of biotin, but it is not known how much is available for absorption.

Although an RDA for biotin cannot be established on the information currently available, it is assumed that the average American diet contains amounts adequate to meet the needs of most healthy adults. The newest estimated safe and adequate daily dietary intake is lower than those that appeared in previous editions of the RDA.

Functions

As a coenzyme, biotin plays a role in the metabolism of fats and CHO, the conversion of tryptophan to niacin, glycogen formation, and chemical reactions that add or remove carbon dioxide from other compounds.

Clinical Applications

Biotin Deficiency

Biotin deficiency symptoms have been induced in humans only by adding the equivalent of 24 raw egg whites to a biotin-deficient diet. Avidin, a chemical in raw egg white, prevents the absorption of biotin from the intestinal tract and leads to a dry, scaly dermatitis, anorexia, nausea, vomiting, glossitis, pallor, and mental depression. A biotin deficiency may also result from long-term use of biotin-free total parenteral nutrition. Biotin supplements reverse most deficiency symptoms within 2 to 3 days; all symptoms are alleviated after 3 months of biotin therapy.

Biotin Toxicity

Biotin produces no known toxic effects.

Pharmacologic Uses of Biotin

None known.

Nutrient/Drug Interactions

None known.

BIBLIOGRAPHY

1. American Dietetic Association: Recommendations concerning supplement usage: ADA statement. J Am Diet Assoc 87:1342, 1987
2. Gershoff SN: More on B_6 supplements. Tufts University Diet and Nutrition Letter 3:8(2), 1985
3. Liebman BF: Vitamin and drug? Nutrition Action Health Letter 13(9):1, 1986
4. Liebman BF: Stress pills: Burning the consumer at both ends. Nutrition Action Health Letter 12(3):1, 1985
5. Liebman BF: Getting your vitamins? Nutrition Action Health Letter 17(5):1, 1990
6. Malseed RT: Pharmacology Drug Therapy and Nursing Considerations. 3rd ed. Philadelphia: JB Lippincott, 1990
7. Mayer J (ed): The do's and don'ts of taking supplements. Environmental Nutrition 10(11):1, 1987
8. Mayer J (ed): Over 50? Chances are you need more vitamin D. Tufts University Diet and Nutrition Letter 8(4):1, 1990
9. Mayer J (ed): No supplements for anyone at all? Tufts University Diet and Nutrition Letter 7(4):1, 1989
10. National Research Council: Recommended Dietary Allowances. 10th ed. Washington, DC: National Academy Press, 1989
11. United States Department of Agriculture, Human Nutrition Information Service Consumer Nutrition Division: Nutrient Intakes: Individuals in 48 States, Year 1977–78. Nationwide Food Consumption Survey 1977–78, Report no. 1-2, 1984
12. Pauling L: Vitamin C and the Common Cold. San Francisco: WH Freeman, 1970
13. Committee on Diet and Health, National Research Council. Diet and Health: Implications for reducing chronic disease risk (executive summary). Washington, DC: National Academy Press, 1989
14. Gentry M (ed): From the editor. American Institute of Cancer Research Newsletter 8:4, 1985

6 Minerals

GROUP CHARACTERISTICS

Minerals are *inorganic elements*, unlike the energy nutrients and vitamins, which are *organic compounds* made of elements. As such, minerals are not metabolized; that is, they are not broken down and rearranged in the body, nor are they destroyed during food preparation. However, some minerals in food may be lost through excessive soaking and cooking in water. Minerals are contained in the ash that remains after food has been digested.

Although minerals comprise only about 4% of the body's total weight, they are found in all body fluids and tissues either in the form of salts (*e.g.*, sodium chloride) or combined with organic compounds (*e.g.*, iron in hemoglobin). In their ionic form, minerals are water-soluble. Minerals function as structural components in the body and serve to regulate body processes (Table 6-1).

Although they have several common group characteristics, there are distinct differences between individual minerals. For instance, some minerals are excreted in the urine, whereas others are excreted in the feces. Minerals that are easily excreted do not accumulate to toxic levels in the body; others are stored and can produce toxicity symptoms when consumed in excess of need. Toxicities are not likely to occur from eating a balanced diet; rather, they are most often related to excessive use of mineral supplements, environmental or industrial exposure, human errors in commercial food processing, or alterations in metabolism (*e.g.*, a genetic defect in iron absorption causes hemosiderosis, an excessive accumulation of iron in the liver).

Three minerals discussed in this chapter, calcium, phosphorus, and magnesium, are classified as macrominerals because they are found in the body in amounts greater than 5 g and are needed by the body in relatively large amounts (100 mg/day or more) (Fig. 6-1). Nine minerals discussed in this chapter are considered microminerals, or trace elements,

Table 6-1
General Functions of Minerals

Mineral	Regulating Function	Structural Function
Calcium	Nerve cell transmissions Muscle contractions Blood clotting	Bones and teeth
Phosphorus	Acid-base balance	Bones and teeth Soft tissues
Magnesium	Nerve cell transmission Muscle contractions	Bones and teeth
Fluorine		Bones and teeth
Sulfur	Vitamin, enzyme, and hormonal activity	Skin Hair Nails Soft tissues
Iron		Blood (hemoglobin) Soft tissues
Potassium	Fluid balance	Soft tissues
Sodium	Acid-base balance	
Chlorine	Fluid balance	
Zinc	Vitamin, enzyme, and hormonal activity	
Manganese		
Cobalt		
Copper		
Chromium		
Iodine		
Selenium		

because they are found in the body in amounts less than 5 g and are needed in only very small amounts (15 mg/day or less) (Table 6-2). Other elements, such as cobalt, nickel, and vanadium, may prove essential to human nutrition in the future. At present, their functions and requirements have not been established.

MAINTENANCE OF MINERAL BALANCE IN THE BODY

The body has several mechanisms by which it maintains mineral balance, or homeostasis, depending on the mineral involved. Some minerals can be released from storage and redistributed as needed, which is what happens when calcium is released from the bones to restore normal serum calcium levels. The body can also compensate for low or high levels of some minerals by increasing or decreasing the amount of mineral absorbed. For example, the normal absorption rate of iron from a mixed diet is only 10%, but the rate may increase up to 50% during iron deficiency. Finally, the excretion rate of some minerals can be adjusted as needed, as in the case of sodium. Virtually all the sodium consumed in the diet is absorbed, and the only way the body can get rid of it is by excreting it in the urine. Hence, for healthy individuals, the higher the sodium intake, the greater the urinary sodium excretion.

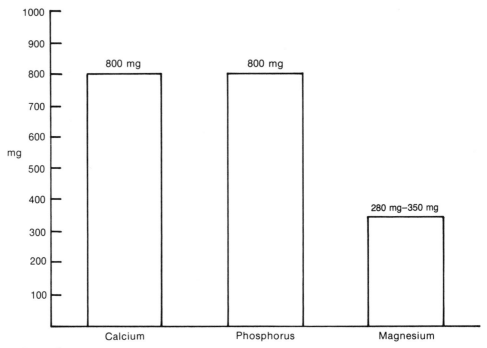

Figure 6-1
The RDAs of macrominerals for adults.

MACROMINERALS

Calcium, phosphorus, and magnesium are macrominerals. A summary of each appears in Table 6-3. Although sodium, potassium, and chlorine are also macrominerals, they function primarily as electrolytes and are discussed in Chapter 7.

Calcium

Calcium is the most abundant mineral in the body, comprising about half of the body's total mineral content. Almost all of the body's calcium (99%) is combined with phosphorus, magnesium, and other elements to give rigidity and structure to bones and teeth. As a large, dynamic reservoir of calcium, bones continually take up and release calcium to keep serum calcium levels within a narrow range. The remaining 1% of calcium in the body is found in plasma and other body fluids. It plays important roles in blood clotting, nerve transmission, muscle contraction and relaxation, cell membrane permeability, and the activation of certain enzymes.

Milk and milk products are the richest sources of calcium in the diet, so much so that an inadequate intake of calcium is likely if dairy products are omitted from the diet. It is estimated that dairy products contribute more than 55% of calcium intake in the average American diet.[3] Canned fish with bones may also be an excellent source of calcium. Although green leafy vegetables, whole grains, nuts, and legumes are good sources of

Table 6-2
The RDA and Estimated Safe and Adequate Dietary Intakes of Trace Elements for Adults

Micromineral	RDA
Chromium	50–200 μg
Selenium	55–70 μg
Molybdenum	75–250 μg
Iodine	150 μg
Copper	1.5–3.0 mg
Fluoride	1.5–4 mg
Manganese	2.0–5.0 mg
Iron	10–15 mg
Zinc	12–15 mg

calcium, fiber and other binding agents decrease the amount of calcium available for absorption. See Appendix 13 for the calcium content of selected foods.

Absorption and Excretion

Normally, only 30% to 40% of the calcium consumed in the average mixed diet is absorbed. The percentage of calcium absorbed is known to increase in response to body need, such as during pregnancy, lactation, growth, and recovery from bone fractures. Lactose, the CHO in milk and dairy products, and vitamin D both promote calcium absorption. At normal and below-normal intakes of protein, calcium absorption is enhanced; however, protein intakes in excess of the RDA do not offer any additional benefit. Phosphorus, in all forms except phytate phosphorus, has little if any negative effect on calcium absorption.[3] The ratio of calcium to phosphorus in the diet probably does not play an important role in the utilization of calcium.[6]

Calcium absorption is impaired when gastrointestinal (GI) motility is increased, because of reduced transit time. Likewise, excessive fat intake or fat malabsorption syndromes cause calcium to precipitate into insoluble calcium soaps, which are excreted in the feces. Phytates and oxalates, chemicals present in whole wheat and green, leafy vegetables, respectively, also combine with calcium to prevent its absorption. Excessive intakes of certain fibers may impair calcium absorption, as can excessive intakes of magnesium or iron. Because of changes in the levels of circulating vitamin D metabolites, the efficiency of calcium absorption decreases with age. Calcium that is not absorbed is excreted in the feces.

The kidneys help maintain serum calcium levels by increasing urinary excretion when serum levels rise. Calcium excretion is also influenced by other factors. Studies using purified proteins showed that a high protein intake increases urinary calcium excretion. However, when red meat was used as the protein source, there was no effect on urinary calcium, nor on fecal calcium, calcium balance, or intestinal absorption.[6] An increase in phosphorus intake decreases calcium excretion. Because many sources of protein are also high in phosphorus (milk, eggs, and meat), an increase in the intake of one is usually accompanied by an increase in the other. The net effect on calcium balance is negligible at recommended levels of calcium intake.[3]

Table 6-3
Summary of Macrominerals

Mineral and Sources	RDA	Estimated Average Adult Intake in the U.S.	Functions
CALCIUM			
Milk and dairy products	18–24 yo: 1200 mg	Men: 854 mg	Bone and teeth formation and maintenance
Green leafy vegetables	25 and older: 800 mg	Women: 574 mg	Blood clotting
Whole grains			Nerve transmission
Nuts			Muscle function
Legumes			Cell membrane permeability
PHOSPHORUS			
Meat	18–24 yo: 1200 mg	1000–1500 mg	Bone and teeth formation and maintenance
Poultry	25 and older: 800 mg		Acid-base balance
Fish			Energy metabolism
Eggs			Cell membrane structure
Legumes			Regulate hormone and coenzyme activity
Milk and dairy products			
Soft drinks			
MAGNESIUM			
Green leafy vegetables	Men: 350 mg	207–329 mg	Bone formation
Nuts	Women: 280 mg		Smooth muscle relaxation
Legumes			Protein synthesis
Whole grains			CHO metabolism
Seafood			

In the past, it was believed that high intakes of phosphorus combined with low calcium consumption led to secondary hyperparathyroidism, and the loss of calcium from the bones. However, studies on humans have failed to establish a negative effect of phosphorus intake on calcium balance when calcium intake is adequate.[3]

Maintenance of Serum Calcium Levels

Normal serum calcium = 4.5–5.3 mEq/liter or 9–11 mg/dl

Serum calcium levels, and the ratio of serum calcium to phosphorus, are held relatively constant at the expense of bone when dietary intake of calcium is inadequate. By the action of hormones, the body can correct deviations in calcium levels by increasing the amount of calcium absorbed, by depositing or withdrawing calcium from the bones, or by increasing urinary excretion.

Low serum calcium levels are raised by *vitamin D*, which increases calcium absorption, mobilizes calcium from the bone, and, to a small extent, increases renal reabsorption of calcium. *Parathyroid hormone* also functions to raise serum calcium by increasing calcium absorption, mobilizing calcium from the bone, and increasing renal reabsorption of calcium. High serum calcium levels are corrected by *calcitonin*, which prevents further bone resorption. Altered serum calcium levels are not related to dietary intake, but rather are the result of hormonal abnormalities or occur secondary to other clinical conditions. Hypocalcemia (low serum calcium levels) is caused by an inadequate secretion of parathyroid hormone related to idiopathic or surgically induced hypoparathyroidism (thyroidectomy, parathyroidectomy, or neck dissections). Tetany, a symptom of hypocalcemia, is characterized by severe, intermittent, tonic contractions of the extremities, muscular cramps, uncontrolled seizures, and possible convulsions. Tetany occurs when serum calcium levels fall in response to an increase in serum phosphorus levels, possibly due to an excessive phosphorus intake or a decrease in parathyroid hormone secretion.

Hypercalcemia (elevated serum calcium levels) can cause nausea, vomiting, anorexia, abdominal pain, constipation, polyuria, polydipsia, mental changes, calcium renal stones, and excessive calcification of the bones and soft tissues. Coma and death may result if not treated. Hypercalcemia may be caused by cancer, excessive combined intakes of vitamin D and calcium, hyperparathyroidism (increased secretion of parathyroid hormone), thyroid disorders, and hypophosphatemia.

Resorptive hypercalciuria is a condition that occurs during periods of prolonged immobility when an excessive amount of calcium is withdrawn from the bone and excreted in the urine, which increases the risk of calcium renal stones.

See Chapter 17 for more on alterations in calcium metabolism.

Recommended Dietary Allowance and Average Intake

The RDA for calcium is 800 mg/day for both women and men aged 25 and older. The newest edition of the RDA raised the RDA for men and women aged 18 to 24 years to 1200 mg/day, in view of the evidence that peak bone mass is not attained before age 25, and that an apparent protective measure against osteoporosis later in life is to maximize genetically programmed peak bone mass by consuming an adequate calcium intake during early adulthood. The average daily adult intake of calcium is reported to be 854 mg for men and 574 mg for women.

Because the body has the ability to adapt during times of inadequate calcium intake, and because evidence of inadequate intake is slow to develop, there is considerable controversy regarding how much calcium is actually needed to maintain calcium balance. Some studies have shown that at intakes of 800 mg/day, a substantial percentage of ambulatory people are in negative calcium balance. Increasing calcium intake to 1200 mg caused a significant increase in calcium balance; however, intakes of 2000 mg and higher did not offer any real improvement in calcium balance.[6] Because 800 mg does not appear adequate to maintain calcium balance and because calcium losses increase with aging, many researchers believe the RDA should be higher, especially for women. In fact, it has been recommended that postmenopausal women may need 1500 mg of calcium per day to maintain calcium balance.

Clinical Applications

Calcium Deficiency

Calcium deficiency may be related to an inadequate calcium intake or may occur secondary to malabsorption syndromes, vitamin D deficiency, or endocrine disorders. A long-standing deficiency of calcium, which causes loss of calcium from the bones in order to maintain serum calcium levels, can result in osteoporosis, a prevalent condition among middle-aged and elderly women that is characterized by a negative calcium balance and a loss of total bone mass. Although all people lose bone with age, the rate of bone loss appears to be accelerated by a calcium deficiency (see Chap. 19 for more on osteoporosis).

Calcium Excess

Although intakes up to 2500 mg/day have not produced adverse effects in healthy people, high intakes may cause constipation and increase the risk of calcium urinary stones in men with hypercalciuria. In addition, absorption of iron, zinc, and other minerals may be inhibited, and the potential for hypercalciuria, hypercalcemia, and renal function deterioration exists.[3]

Future Directions

Some studies have shown that high calcium intakes protect against high blood pressure; other studies have failed to establish a relationship. Another area of future research is the role calcium plays in the prevention of colon cancer promoted by fat and bile acids.[3]

Nutrient/Drug Interactions

When taken together, calcium decreases the absorption of tetracycline, phenytoin, and iron salts[1] and may antagonize the action of calcium channel blocking drugs.

Drugs that affect calcium are as follows:

- Acetazolamide: increases urinary calcium excretion
- Adrenal corticosteroids: decrease calcium absorption
- Anticonvulsants: may decrease serum levels of vitamin D and calcium
- Capreomycin: decreases serum calcium
- Cholestyramine: decreases calcium absorption with long-term use; decreases serum calcium; increases urinary calcium excretion
- Cycloserine: may decrease calcium absorption
- Dactinomycin: decreases calcium absorption
- Digitalis glycosides: may increase urinary calcium excretion
- Ethacrynic acid: increases urinary calcium excretion
- Furosemide: increases urinary calcium excretion; decreases serum calcium in hypercalcemia
- Glutethimide: may alter calcium need; long-term use may cause osteomalacia
- Lithium: increases urinary calcium excretion, decreases calcium uptake by bone
- Mercurial diuretics: increase urinary calcium excretion
- Neomycin: decreases calcium absorption
- Petrolatum, liquid: decreases calcium absorption
- Phenolphthalein: decreases vitamin D and calcium absorption
- Probenecid: increases urinary calcium excretion
- Spironolactone: increases urinary calcium excretion
- Tetracyclines: decrease absorption of calcium
- Thiazide diuretics: single dose increases calcium excretion, long-term use tends to decrease calcium excretion and increase serum calcium
- Triamterene: may increase urinary calcium excretion
- Viomycin: can cause hypocalcemia; causes excessive urinary excretion of calcium, which persists after the drug is discontinued

Phosphorus

Next to calcium, phosphorus is the second most abundant mineral in the body. Approximately 85% of the body's phosphorus is found in bones; with calcium, it is essential for their formation and maintenance. The rest of the body's phosphorus is metabolically active and is found in every body cell. It performs numerous functions, such as regulating acid–base balance, metabolizing energy, providing structure to cell membranes, serving as an essential component of nucleic acids, regulating the activity of hormones and coenzymes, aiding in the absorption and transportation of fats, and facilitating the absorption of glucose.

Almost all foods contain phosphorus. Foods rich in protein (meat, poultry, fish, eggs, legumes, and nuts), and calcium (milk and milk products) are also high in phosphorus. In the average adult American diet, soft drinks and processed foods supply a significant amount of phosphorus. Grains, eggs, nuts, and legumes are also good sources. See Appendix 13 for the phosphorus content of selected foods.

Absorption, Excretion, and Maintenance

Normally, about 50% to 70% of the phosphorus in the adult diet is absorbed. Like calcium, the absorption of phosphorus is enhanced by the presence of vitamin D and is regulated by parathyroid hormone. The major route of phosphorus excretion is the urine.

Normal serum inorganic phosphorus is maintained at 2.5 to 4.8 mg/dl. Hyperphosphatemia (high serum phosphorus level), which may be related to renal insufficiency or hypoparathyroidism, is characterized by symptoms of hypocalcemic tetany. Hypophosphatemia (low serum phosphorus levels) may occur as a result of administering long-term, phosphorus-free total parenteral nutrition, excessive use of phosphate-binding antacids, malabsorption syndromes, vitamin D deficiency leading to rickets or osteomalacia, hyperparathyroidism, treatment of diabetic acidosis, or alcoholism. Clinical findings include anorexia, weakness, circumoral paresthesia, and hyperventilation.

Recommended Dietary Allowance and Average Intake

With the exception of young infants, who need less phosphorus in relation to calcium, the RDA for phosphorus equals the RDA for calcium for all age/sex groups. The typical adult American diet supplies 1000 to 1500 mg/day, well above the RDA of 800 mg, and those figures may even be underestimated by 15% to 20% because of the prevalence of phosphorus-containing additives in the diet.

Clinical Applications

Phosphorus Deficiency

Because phosphorus is pervasive in the diet, a dietary deficiency is rare. However, premature infants fed only breast milk may develop hypophosphatemic rickets from a low phosphorus intake during a period when need is increased because of rapid bone mineralization.

Phosphorus deficiency may be induced in people on long-term aluminum hydroxide (antacid) therapy, since aluminum hydroxide binds with phosphorus, making it unavailable for absorption. Weakness, anorexia, malaise, and pain characterize the loss of bone.

Phosphorus Excess

In animals, an excessive phosphorus intake has been shown to lower serum calcium levels and to cause secondary hyperparathyroidism and loss of bone. In humans, only lowered serum calcium levels have been observed. An intake of phosphorus excessive enough to cause adverse effects is not likely from normal diets.[3]

Nutrient/Drug Interactions

Drugs that affect phosphorus are as follows:
- Aluminum hydroxide: decreases phosphorus absorption; may cause hypophosphatemia if used frequently and on a long-term basis
- Magnesium hydroxide: may decrease phosphorus absorption
- Petrolatum, liquid: decreases phosphorus absorption

Magnesium

Of the 20 to 28 g of magnesium in the adult body, approximately 60% is deposited in the bone with calcium and phosphorus. The rest of the body's magnesium is distributed in various soft tissues, muscles, and body fluids. Magnesium plays a role in smooth muscle relaxation, protein synthesis, CHO metabolism, cellular growth and reproduction, and hormonal activity. Serum magnesium concentration is held constant in healthy individuals by poorly understood homeostatic mechanisms[3] and does not appear to be controlled by hormones.

Magnesium is abundant in the diet, especially in green, leafy vegetables as a component of chlorophyll (green pigment). Other sources include whole grains, nuts, legumes, seafood, cocoa, and chocolate.

Absorption and Excretion

Average magnesium absorption averages from 40% to 60% of intake. An inverse relationship exists between magnesium intake and absorption—as intake increases, absorption decreases. In animal studies, the absorption of calcium and magnesium is competitive and mutually exclusive. The higher the intake of calcium, the lower the absorption of magnesium. However, studies with humans have not shown magnesium absorption or balance altered by calcium intakes of up to 2000 mg/day.[6] Other factors that decrease the absorption of magnesium include phytates and oxalates, and the presence of fat. Because the kidneys efficiently conserve magnesium, urinary excretion is very low.

Recommended Dietary Allowance and Average Intake

It is reported that the average American man consumes 329 mg of magnesium per day and the average adult woman 207 mg,[3] figures that fall below the current RDA of 350 mg and

280 mg for men and women, respectively. However, there is no evidence that magnesium deficiency is common among healthy American adults.

Factors that may increase the need for magnesium include diets high in calcium, protein, vitamin D, or alcohol, as well as psychological or physical stress, including athletic training.

Clinical Applications

Magnesium Deficiency

A dietary deficiency of magnesium has not been reported in people consuming a normal mixed diet.[3] However, magnesium deficiency may occur secondary to malabsorption syndromes, renal dysfunction, general malnutrition and alcoholism, and iatrogenic causes such as nasogastric suctioning, parenteral or enteral feedings deficient in magnesium, or as a side effect of certain medications.

Hypomagnesemia (low serum magnesium level of less than 1.8 mg/dl) is uncommon because of the supply of magnesium available on the surface of bones, coupled with the kidneys' ability to conserve magnesium. However, hypomagnesemia may occur secondary to numerous clinical conditions, including GI disorders such as malabsorption, vomiting, and diarrhea; as a side effect of certain medications (see Nutrient/Drug Interactions); alcoholism; kwashiorkor; hyperthyroidism and parathyroid disorders; diabetic acidosis; the administration of magnesium-free parenteral fluids after surgery; postsurgical stress; renal disease; and rickets in patients who are receiving massive doses of vitamin D.

Signs and symptoms of hypomagnesemia include increased neuromuscular and central nervous system irritability, progressing to loss of muscular control, tremors, disorientation, tetany, positive Trousseau's signs, positive Chvostek's signs, and convulsions.

Magnesium Excess

Large oral intakes of magnesium appear to be safe when renal function is normal. However, hypermagnesemia (high serum magnesium level greater than 3.0 mg/dl) may occur in people with impaired renal function who take therapeutic doses of magnesium. Central nervous system depression, coma, and hypotension may occur.

Nutrient/Drug Interactions

When they are taken together, magnesium decreases the absorption of tetracycline. Drugs that affect magnesium are as follows:
- Alcohol: increases urinary excretion of magnesium
- Amphotericin B: decreases serum magnesium
- Capreomycin: decreases serum magnesium
- Cycloserine: may decrease magnesium absorption
- Digitalis glycosides: may increase urinary excretion of magnesium
- Ethacrynic acid: increases urinary excretion of magnesium; can cause hypomagnesemia
- Furosemide: increases urinary excretion of magnesium
- Gentamicin: increases urinary excretion of magnesium
- Lithium: increases plasma magnesium
- Mercurial diuretics: increase urinary excretion of magnesium; may induce magnesium depletion

- Phenobarbital: decreases serum magnesium levels
- Phenytoin: decreases serum magnesium levels
- Probenecid: increases urinary excretion of magnesium
- Spironolactone: increases urinary excretion of magnesium
- Tetracyclines: may decrease magnesium absorption, but is not clinically significant
- Thiazides: increase urinary excretion of magnesium; can cause magnesium depletion
- Viomycin: can cause hypomagnesemia; excessive urinary excretion of magnesium persists after the drug is discontinued

TRACE ELEMENTS

Iron, iodine, and zinc are the best-known trace elements. Iron has always been listed in the RDA tables; iodine first appeared in 1968, and zinc was added in 1974. In 1980, estimated safe and adequate daily intakes for copper, manganese, fluoride, chromium, and molybdenum were listed separately from the RDA table. Selenium was included on that table, but was upgraded to RDA status for the first time in 1989. A summary of trace elements with defined RDA appears in Table 6-4. Although research shows that arsenic, nickel, silicon, and boron are essential in animals, human requirement has not been proven. Lead and mercury are toxic, nonessential trace elements (see Food for Thought: Other Trace Elements—Future RDA Candidates?).

Group Characteristics

Because trace elements are required in such infinitesimal amounts, measuring their presence in food and the body is difficult. With the exception of iron, manganese, and copper, food composition tables generally do not provide data on trace elements. Compounding the problem of not knowing how much of trace elements are provided in the diet is the variable of bioavailability. The metabolism of individual trace elements is strongly influenced by other dietary factors, so that absorption and utilization of an element can vary depending on the source of the nutrient and the presence of other dietary factors consumed at the same time. Assessing dietary intake is extremely difficult.

In the body, reliable and valid indicators of trace element status (*i.e.*, measuring serum levels, conducting balance studies, determining enzyme activity) are not available for all microminerals, so assessing trace element status is not always possible.

It appears that each trace element has its own curve or range of safe and adequate intakes over which the body can maintain homeostasis. The margin of safety may be narrower for some minerals than others. Extremely excessive or deficient intakes of any element have the potential to cause death. Somewhere in between optimal function and obvious alteration in function lies a gray area of marginal deficiency/marginal toxicity—an area that generates much controversy and interest. People consuming an adequate diet derive no further benefit from using supplements, and because a delicate balance exists among minerals, a large intake of one element may induce a deficiency of another. However, people with marginally deficient intakes may experience improved health by the judicious use of supplements.

Table 6-4
Summary of Essential Trace Elements with Defined RDAs

Trace Element	RDA	Estimated Average Adult Intake in the United States	Major Sources	Function	Signs of Deficiency	Signs of Toxicity
Iron (Fe)	Men: 10 mg Women: 15 mg	Men: >10 mg Women: 10–11 mg	Liver, lean meat, dried beans, fortified cereals	Oxygen transport via hemoglobin and myoglobin; constituent of enzyme systems	Depletion of iron stores, anemia (microcytic, hypochromic), pallor, decreased work capacity	Hemochromatosis, hemosiderosis Acute poisoning → GI cramping, nausea, vomiting, possible shock, convulsions, and coma
Iodine (I)	150 µg	170 µg–250 µg	Iodized salt, seafood, milk, eggs, bread	Constituent of thyroid hormones that regulate BMR	Goiter (not a problem in the United States)	Acne-like skin lesions, "iodine goiter"
Zinc (Zn)	Men: 15 mg Women: 12 mg	10 mg to 15 mg	Meat, oysters, seafood, milk, egg yolks, legumes, whole grains	Tissue growth, development, and healing; sexual maturation and reproduction; constituent of many enzymes in energy and nucleic acid metabolism	Impaired growth, sexual maturation, and immune system functioning; skin lesions; acrodermatitis enteropathica; decreased sense of taste and smell	Excess use of supplements may cause anorexia, vomiting, nausea, diarrhea, muscle pain, lethargy, drowsiness, and bleeding gastric ulcers; may also interfere with copper metabolism and decrease serum levels of high-density lipoproteins (HDL, the "good" form of cholesterol)
Selenium (Se)	Men: 70 µg Women: 55 µg	108 µg	Seafood, kidney, liver, meat, some grains	Protects against oxygen damage and heavy metals; constituent of an enzyme that acts as an antioxidant	Usually occurs in combination with protein-energy malnutrition or other nutrient deficiency; may produce cardiomyopathy	Loss of hair, brittle fingernails, and fatigue

Trace element deficiencies may be related more to geographic location than "bad" eating habits. Because plants, and ultimately animals and humans, depend on the soil for trace elements, some mineral deficiencies (*e.g.*, goiter) are related to living in areas with soil poor in minerals (*e.g.*, the "goiter belt" area around the Great Lakes). So even foods that have been evaluated for their trace element content may not represent the actual amount of a trace element a person consumes, depending on where the food was harvested.

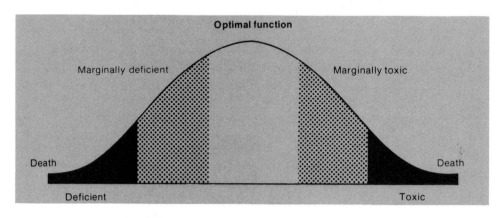

Iron

Of the 3 to 5 g of iron in the body, a small amount is found in the plasma bound to the protein transferrin, the transport carrier of iron. Seventy percent is in the heme portion of hemoglobin and 5% in myoglobin, the molecules that function to carry oxygen and carbon dioxide to and from the cells. About 20% is stored as ferritin in the liver, bone marrow, and spleen, and the remaining 5% is distributed throughout cells as part of enzyme systems active in the production of energy.

Iron in the diet comes in two forms: heme iron, which constitutes about half of the iron in animal sources such as meat, fish, and poultry, and nonheme iron, which comprises the remaining half of the iron found in animal sources and all of the iron found in plants such as grains, vegetables, legumes, and nuts. Although heme iron is much better absorbed than nonheme, nonheme iron accounts for a larger percentage of total iron intake. Table 16-8 lists heme and nonheme sources of iron.

Absorption and Excretion

Although the average rate of iron absorption is about 10% of the total consumed, the rate varies significantly during times of need. When iron requirements are increased, such as during growth, pregnancy, and iron deficiency, as much as 50% of the iron consumed may be absorbed, and iron absorption becomes more efficient for both forms of iron.

Heme and nonheme iron are absorbed by different mechanisms.[3] Heme iron generally is absorbed at a rate of about 15% to 35% of the amount consumed; the rate is influenced only by body need. Nonheme iron is less well absorbed, with a rate of only 3% to 8% of that consumed. In addition to need, its absorption rate is influenced by the presence of absorption enhancers and inhibitors. Factors that increase the absorption of nonheme iron include vitamin C, when consumed at the same meal; certain animal proteins, such as meat, fish, and poultry; alcohol; and gastric acidity, which increases iron solubility. Nonheme iron absorption decreases in the presence of tea, coffee, binding agents like bran, phosphates, oxalates, phytates, phosvitin, and EDTA (a metal-sequestering food additive), alkalinity (*e.g.*, from the use of antacids), diarrhea, and steatorrhea.

Iron absorption from supplements and enriched and fortified foods also varies with the particular form of iron used. Ferrous sulfate, lactate, fumarate, succinate, glycine sulfate, and glutamate are well absorbed; ferrous citrate, tartrate, and pyrophosphate are poorly absorbed (see Chap. 16 for more on iron).

Because the body maintains iron balance primarily by adjusting the rate of absorption, little or no iron is excreted in the urine. Even iron contained in hemoglobin and other body substances is recycled as the cells are replaced. However, a small amount of iron is lost daily through the skin, hair, feces, nails, sweat, and GI cells. Menstrual blood loss accounts for additional lost iron.

Recommended Dietary Allowance and Average Intake

To compensate for an average absorption rate of 10% and the daily (and monthly) iron losses, the RDA for iron is set at 10 mg/day for men and postmenopausal women and 15 mg/day for women of childbearing age. The previous RDA for women of childbearing age was 18 mg/day. The average iron intake from a typical American diet is 10 to 11 mg/day.

Iron requirements increase during periods of growth (infancy, adolescence, pregnancy) and in response to heavy or chronic blood loss related to menstruation, surgery, injury, childbirth, GI bleeding, and aspirin abuse. Iron needs may also increase secondary to the use of medications that alter iron absorption (see Nutrient/Drug Interactions).

Clinical Applications

Iron Deficiency

Iron may be the most common nutritional deficiency in the United States, especially among infants, adolescents, menstruating women, and pregnant women. Daily supplements of 30 to 60 mg are often prescribed for pregnant women. Because menstruating women, infants, and adolescents may not eat enough iron to meet their needs, iron supplements may be indicated (see Chap. 16 for more on iron deficiency).

Iron Toxicity

Iron toxicity is uncommon, because the body normally decreases the rate of iron absorption when its iron status is adequate. However, a rare genetic defect in iron metabolism, known as hemochromatosis, causes iron to accumulate in excessive amounts, which can eventually saturate the body's tissues, especially the skin, liver, and pancreas, and end in multiple systems organ failure.

Because alcohol enhances iron absorption, alcoholics and even people with a history of alcoholism absorb iron at rates much higher than average. One report found iron absorption rates as high as 50% among alcoholics who had abstained from alcohol for 4 weeks before the study, a rate similar to that in hemochromatosis.[6] The result may be toxic overload.

In the absence of genetic defects or alcohol abuse, excessive iron storage from diet alone is unlikely. However, iron supplements or vitamin pills with iron is a leading cause of accidental poisoning in young children, who have a much lower tolerance for iron loads than adults. Signs and symptoms of acute iron poisoning include GI cramping and pain, vomiting, and nausea, which may lead to shock, convulsions, and coma.

Nutrient/Drug Interactions

When they are taken together, iron may decrease the absorption of tetracycline.
Drugs that affect iron are as follows:
- Alcohol: increases absorption of ferric iron
- Antacids (carbonate): decrease iron absorption
- Chloramphenicol: increases serum iron, total iron binding capacity
- Cholestyramine: can decrease iron absorption; decreases iron reserves (high dose in animal studies)
- Clofibrate: decreases iron absorption
- Dactinomycin: decreases iron absorption
- Indomethacin: may cause anemia
- Neomycin: decreases iron absorption
- Oral contraceptives: may increase serum levels of iron
- Salicylates: may cause iron-deficiency anemia with long-term or overuse

Iodine

The average adult body has 20 to 50 mg of iodine, which is found in muscles, the thyroid gland, skin, skeleton, endocrine tissues, central nervous system, and bloodstream. It is an essential component of thyroxine and triiodothyronine (T_3), the thyroid hormones responsible for regulating basal metabolic rate.

The major source of iodine in the American diet is iodized salt, even though about half of the salt sold in the United States is not iodized. Because iodine is abundant in ocean water, seafood is an excellent source of iodine. Plants grown in iodine-rich soil, which includes most areas of the United States except the Rocky Mountain states and the Great Lakes areas, are also good sources of iodine. Although a naturally poor source of iodine, milk now provides a significant amount of iodine in the diet because of the iodized salt licks given to cows and the use of iodine chemicals to sanitize and disinfect udders, milking machines, and milk tanks. Iodates used as bread dough conditioners also contribute to iodine intake.

Absorption and Excretion

Dietary iodine is rapidly and almost completely absorbed from the small intestine in the form of iodides. Approximately two thirds of the amount absorbed is excreted in the urine; the small amount of iodine in the feces is from bile.

Recommended Dietary Allowance and Average Intake

The RDA for both men and women is set at 150 μg/day, which includes a measure of safety for the as-yet unquantified effect of goitrogens (thyroid antagonists found in members of the cabbage family) on iodine requirements. The average iodine intake is estimated at 250 μg for men and 170 μg for women, excluding the intake from iodized salt. This figure represents a gradual decline in iodine intake over the last decade, most probably due to the reduction in the use of the iodine-containing red dye erythrosine (FD&C Red No. 3) in ready-to-eat cereals.[4] Still, it is recommended that no new sources of iodine be added to the U.S. food supply.[3]

Clinical Applications

Iodine Deficiency

A deficiency of iodine leads to a decrease in the production of thyroid hormones. Over time, the thyroid hypertrophies, or develops endemic goiter. Severe and prolonged iodine deficiency may result in hypothyroidism, an endocrine disorder that affects the uptake of iodine by the thyroid gland (see Chap. 17).

Before the introduction of iodized salt, goiter was prevalent in the United States. Now, the problem of goiter is limited to developing countries.

Iodine Toxicity

Most people are unaffected by excess iodine; for those who are affected, the amount of iodine required to cause adverse effects is highly individualized.[4] Iodine toxicity may manifest itself as thyroiditis (inflammation of the thyroid gland), goiter, hypothyroidism (excess iodine may inhibit synthesis of the thyroid hormone), hyperthyroidism, sensitivity reactions (*i.e.*, allergic and anaphylactic responses), and acute responses with large doses (cardiovascular collapse, convulsions, asthma attacks).[4] Iodine is fatal in large amounts.

Nutrient/Drug Interactions

None known.

Zinc

Although zinc is present in the body in only a small quantity (about 2 g), it is found in many tissues, including the eye, bones, skin, hair, muscles, pancreas, liver, kidney, and male reproductive organs. It is a component of DNA, RNA, insulin, and numerous enzyme systems that function in tissue growth, maintenance, and healing; the metabolism of CHO, protein, fat, and nucleic acids; sexual maturation and reproduction; the senses of taste and smell; and immune reactions.

Generally, animal products are good sources of zinc, especially meats, oysters and other seafood, milk, and egg yolks. Legumes and whole grains are good sources of zinc but are less well absorbed.

Absorption and Excretion

On the average, only 15% to 35% of ingested zinc is absorbed; however, people with low zinc status absorb zinc more efficiently than people with good status, and small doses of zinc are absorbed more efficiently than large doses. The bioavailability of zinc varies significantly depending on the source. Whereas fiber and phytates interfere with zinc availability, the effect may be negligible in the average U.S. diet.[6] Protein, phosphorus, and iron may have greater impact on zinc status, but results from studies are inconsistent and contradictory.

Zinc homeostasis is strongly regulated, and its excretion, primarily through the feces, is directly proportional to zinc status.[3] Fecal excretion includes unabsorbed dietary zinc and zinc from enteropancreatic circulation. Small amounts of zinc are excreted in bile; under normal conditions, there is no urinary excretion of zinc.

Recommended Dietary Allowance and Average Intake

For the first time, sex-specific recommendations were made for zinc in the 10th edition of the RDA. Research shows that men need more zinc than women, as reflected in the RDA, which recommend 15 mg/day for men and 12 mg/day for women.

Zinc intake is related to total calorie intake: As calorie content increases, zinc content increases. It is estimated that men consume 90% or more of the RDA for zinc and women select diets that provide less than 81% of the RDA for zinc. The difference in zinc intake between men and women appears to be related solely to calorie intake, not the zinc density of foods chosen.[2]

Clinical Applications

Zinc Deficiency

Although clear evidence that zinc deficiency is prevalent in the general population is lacking, average intake among Americans may be marginal. Vegetarians consuming a high-fiber diet, as well as children, adolescents, and pregnant women may be especially at risk for zinc deficiency. Zinc deficiency can also occur secondary to malabsorption syndromes because zinc absorption is decreased while excretion is increased. Sickle cell anemia, long-term use of total parenteral nutrition, and a rare inborn error of metabolism that interferes with zinc absorption also can lead to zinc deficiency.

Growth retardation, hypogonadism, mild anemia, hypogeusia (decreased taste acuity), delayed wound healing, alopecia, and a dermatitis called acrodermatitis enteropathica characterize zinc deficiency. Symptoms are dramatically reversed with zinc supplements.

Zinc Toxicity

Muscle incoordination, GI irritation, vomiting, diarrhea, dizziness, drowsiness, lethargy, renal failure, and anemia may be caused by large supplemental doses of zinc. Zinc toxicity may also impair copper metabolism and decrease serum HDL (high-density lipoproteins, the "good" cholesterol).

Nutrient/Drug Interactions

When they are taken together, zinc may decrease the absorption of tetracycline. Drugs that affect zinc are as follows:

- Adrenal corticosteroids: increase urinary zinc excretion
- Alcohol: increases urinary zinc excretion
- Chlorthalidone: increases urinary zinc excretion
- Dimercaprol: binds zinc; alters taste acuity
- Mercaptopurine: may cause zinc deficiency
- Methotrexate: may cause zinc deficiency
- Oral contraceptives: high estrogen preparations increase erythrocyte zinc
- Penicillamine: binds zinc; increases urinary zinc excretion; decreases taste acuity
- Tetracyclines: may decrease zinc absorption, although not clinically significant
- Thiazide diuretics: increase urinary zinc excretion

Selenium

Selenium is a component of the enzyme glutathione peroxidase, which acts as an antioxidant. As such, selenium has a close metabolic relationship with vitamin E, the body's primary antioxidant.[3] Selenium deficiency has been postulated to be a predisposing condition to a cardiomyopathy disorder known as Keshan disease. Other functions of selenium are being explored.

Good sources of selenium include seafoods, kidney, liver, and other meats. The selenium content of grains and seeds depends on the selenium content of the soil in which they are grown. Grains, vegetables, and meat raised in South Dakota, Wyoming, New Mexico, and Utah are high in selenium; selenium content of the soil in the southern states and on both coasts of the United States is considerably lower.

Recommended Dietary Allowance and Average Intake

The RDA for selenium was established for the first time in 1989. Based on studies of Chinese men, the RDA has been set at 70 μg for men and 55 μg for women. Previously, the estimated safe and adequate daily intake was 50 to 200 μg. Average daily adult intake in the United States is 108 μg.

Clinical Applications

Selenium Deficiency

In animals, simultaneous deficiencies of vitamin E and selenium cause many diseases that can be prevented or cured by supplements of either nutrient alone.[3] Muscular discomfort or weakness that develops in humans receiving long-term total parenteral nutrition devoid of selenium responds to selenium supplementation. Cardiomyopathy may also develop.

Other Trace Elements—Future RDA Candidates?

Although definitive evidence is lacking, future research may reveal that other trace elements are essential for human nutrition. Unfortunately, evidence is difficult to obtain, and quantifying human need is even more formidable. And, as in the case of all trace elements, the potential for toxicity exists.

Arsenic, Nickel, Silicon, and Boron

Although "poison," "plastic," or cleaning solutions may come to mind, these trace elements are recognized as essential nutrients for animals. However, a deficiency in humans has not been identified, and therefore it is impossible to estimate human requirement.

Cadmium, Lead, Lithium, Tin, and Vanadium

They sound like pollutants, and in some cases they are. Yet it is remotely possible that humans need them in minute amounts, amounts easily met by levels naturally occurring in food, water, and air.

Cobalt

Cobalt is an essential component of vitamin B_{12}; however, there is no evidence that cobalt intake is limiting in the diet, and no RDA is necessary.[9]

Selenium Toxicity

It is not known exactly how much selenium is toxic. The residents of one particular county in China developed toxicity after consuming 50,000 μg a day. Symptoms included itchy scalp, dry brittle hair, cracked fingernails, mottled teeth, and blistering lesions over the limbs. Some people had nervous system alterations, such as numbness, convulsions, paralysis, and even death. In the United States, people who took an improperly manufactured supplement that contained 27.3 mg of selenium per tablet developed nausea, abdominal pain, diarrhea, nail and hair changes, peripheral neuropathy, fatigue, and irritability.[3] The margin of error between the present RDA and toxicity dose appears to be at least 500 μg.

Future Directions

Both laboratory and epidemiologic studies suggest that selenium may be protective against cancer. However, the evidence is not complete, and other contradictory studies have shown that large doses of vitamin C and selenium actually increase tumor growth. Because the long-term safety of selenium supplements and the possible interactions with other nutrients is not known, researchers refuse to endorse supplements.

Nutrient/Drug Interactions

None known.

Table 6-5
Summary of Trace Elements With Estimated Safe and Adequate Daily Dietary Intakes

Newer Trace Element	Adult Estimated Safe and Adequate Daily Intakes	Average Estimated Intake in the United States	Major Sources	Function	Signs of Deficiency	Signs of Toxicity
Copper (Cu)	1.5 mg–3.0 mg	0.9–1.2 mg	Organ meats, seafood, nuts, seeds	Integrity of heart and large arteries; bone and blood formation	Anemia, altered bone formation, impairment of cardiovascular system, hypercholesterolemia	None known
Manganese (Mn)	2.0 mg–5 mg	2.2 mg–2.7 mg	Whole grains and cereals, fruits, vegetables	Constituent of enzymes in mucopolysaccharide metabolism and in fat synthesis; also needed for growth, reproduction, and blood clotting	Deficiency in humans is unknown.	Dietary excess unlikely
Fluorine (Fl)	1.5 mg to 4 mg	0.9 mg–1.7 mg	Fluoridated water, tea	Structure of enamel of teeth; role in bone formation and integrity	Dental caries; may increase the risk of osteoporosis	2 mg/day to 8 mg/day may cause mottling of the teeth; doses of 20 mg to 80 mg may induce bone changes years later
Chromium (Cr)	50 µg–200 µg	25 µg–33 µg	Brewers yeast, whole grains, eggs, vegetable oil, nuts, meats	Cofactor for insulin	Insulin resistance; impaired glucose tolerance; low serum chromium is correlated with coronary heart disease in humans.	Dietary toxicity unlikely; occupational exposure to chromium dusts correlated to increase in bronchial cancer
Molybdenum (Mo)	75 µg–250 µg	76 µg–109 µg	Milk, beans, breads, cereals	Component of enzymes and flavoprotein, and therefore important for normal body metabolism	Sulfur amino acid toxicity; decreased production of uric acid (dietary deficiency unlikely)	Interferes with copper metabolism

"NEWER" TRACE ELEMENTS

Five other trace elements, copper, manganese, fluorine, chromium, and molybdenum, are considered essential for human nutrition. However, because not enough is known to firmly establish their RDA, they have been assigned estimated safe and adequate daily dietary intake ranges (Table 6-5).

BIBLIOGRAPHY

1. Malseed RT: Pharmacology: Drug Therapy and Nursing Considerations. 3rd ed. Philadelphia: JB Lippincott, 1990
2. Moser-Veillon PB: Zinc: Consumption patterns and dietary recommendations. J Am Diet Assoc 90:1089, 1990
3. National Research Council: Recommended Dietary Allowances. 10th ed. Washington, DC: National Academy Press, 1989
4. Pennington JAT: A review of iodine toxicity reports. J Am Diet Assoc 90:1571, 1990
5. Pennington JAT, Young BE, Wilson DB: Nutritional elements in US diets: Results from the Total Diet Study, 1982 to 1986. J Am Diet Assoc 89:659, 1989
6. Spencer H: Minerals and mineral interactions in human beings. J Am Diet Assoc 86:864, 1986

7 Fluid and Electrolytes

Body fluids are composed of water and electrolytes. Water is more vital to life than food because it is required for numerous functions, cannot be stored in the body, and is excreted daily. It is estimated that adults of normal weight can live about 70 days without food, but in a moderate climate, they die within 10 days without water.

Electrolytes are chemical compounds that dissociate into charged ions when dissolved in water. Together, water and electrolytes regulate the body's fluid balance and acid–base balance. The three major electrolytes are sodium, potassium, and chloride.

WATER

Water is absorbed rapidly into the blood and lymph by diffusion; it passes easily between body compartments, primarily by osmosis, depending on the concentration of electrolytes.

As the major body constituent present in every cell, water accounts for 50% to 60% of adult body weight. Muscle and viscera cells have the highest concentration of water; skeletal cells are low in water, and fat is practically water-free. Therefore, the higher the muscle mass, the greater the proportion of body water.

About two thirds of the body's water is within the cells (intracellular fluid or ICF); the rest of the body's fluid is called extracellular fluid (ECF) and includes plasma fluid, interstitial fluid, and all other body fluids such as lymph, cerebrospinal fluid, and gastrointestinal (GI)-tract fluids. Total body water and ECF decrease with age; ICF increases with an increase in body mass.

Water is involved in virtually every body function. Approximately 7 to 9 liters of water are secreted into the GI tract daily to aid in digestion and absorption. With the exception of 100 ml of water lost in the feces, almost all of the water contained in these secretions (saliva, gastric secretions, bile, pancreatic secretions, and intestinal mucosa secretions) is reabsorbed in the ileum and colon.

Water is the medium for all chemical reactions and a participant in many. Water is a solvent that dissolves many solutes, and as a component of blood, it helps transport nutrients to and carry wastes away from cells. By evaporating from the skin, water helps regulate body temperature. Water also acts as a lubricant along mucous membranes and between moving parts.

Water Balance

A state of water balance exists when the total fluid volume in the body is adequate and appropriately distributed among the body compartments. Normally, water intake equals water output to maintain water balance (Fig. 7-1).

Water Intake

For most healthy people, thirst is a reliable indicator of the body's need for water: A decrease in the ECF volume or an increase in the osmotic pressure of the blood stimulates the sensation of thirst by way of thirst receptors in the hypothalamus. However, thirst may not be a reliable indicator of need during illness and among infants and the elderly. Intense, sustained physical activity may also inactivate normal thirst mechanisms.

Most of the water consumed in the average American diet does not come from water, but from other beverages. Mean intake of water is estimated at 2.8 cups; the total amount of other beverages consumed (milk, coffee, tea, and soft drinks) is approximately 4.5 cups/

Water Intake		Water Output	
Fluids	500 ml-1700 ml	Urine	600 ml-1600 ml
Water in food	800 ml-1000 ml	Water in feces	50 ml-200 ml
Metabolic water	200 ml-300 ml	Water in expired air and perspiration	850 ml-1200 ml
Total=1500 ml-3000 ml		Total=1500 ml-3000 ml	

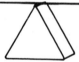

Figure 7-1
Water balance: Intake vs. output.

Table 7-1
Approximate Percentage of Water in Selected Foods

Food	% Water
Vegetables	70–95
Fruit	75–90
Whole milk	87
Eggs	75
Ice cream	60
Meats	40–75
White bread	36
Butter	15
Gelatin	13
All-purpose flour	12
Dried beans	11
Dry cereals	5
White sugar	0.5

capita/day.[5] Many solid foods provide water, with fruits and vegetables as the best sources (Table 7-1). Another source of water is metabolic water, which is produced from the oxidation of food. Every 100 g of CHO, protein, and fat oxidized yields 55, 41, and 107 g of water, respectively.

When oral intake is contraindicated, fluid can be given intravenously as glucose solutions, blood, plasma, or protein hydrolysate mixtures. Water may also be administered rectally in the form of isotonic saline solutions or given subcutaneously.

Water Output

Measurable water loss (sensible) occurs through the urine and feces. Water lost through expired air and perspiration is continuous, largely unconscious, and unmeasureable (insensible).

Urine

By far the largest output of water is through the urine. The amount of urine excreted daily varies with the amount of water consumed in the diet; normal adult urine output ranges from 600 to 1600 ml/day; the minimum or obligatory urine output needed to excrete nitrogenous and other wastes is about 600 ml.

When water intake is inadequate, the kidneys, under the influence of antidiuretic hormone (ADH), compensate by concentrating the urine to conserve water. Kidney diseases have a profound impact on water balance.

Feces

Normally, only a small amount of water (50 to 200 ml) is excreted daily in the feces. Conditions that interfere with intestinal reabsorption of water (*e.g.*, diarrhea and malabsorption syndromes) greatly increase water excretion and seriously affect the body's water balance.

Troubled Water

Bottled water sales exceed $2 billion a year and are increasing faster than any other beverage in the United States.[3,4] Taste and safety are the most common reasons why Americans choose bottled over tap water. However, despite the fact that bottled water can cost 300 to 1200 times more per gallon than tap water, there are no assurances of greater safety. In fact, the FDA has yet to adopt standards for contaminants that are as strict as those set for public water supplies, which are regulated by the Environmental Protection Agency. The bottom line is that bottled water can legally contain more toxins than tap water. The FDA has also been charged with not overseeing water bottling facilities closely enough to ensure that standards which do exist are being followed.

While it *may* be more dangerous than public water, bottled water appears to have a low potential for contamination or health hazards. Fortunately, 85% of American-sold water comes from bottlers who belong to a trade group called the International Bottled Water Association. Its members voluntarily permit unannounced annual inspections by the National Sanitation Foundation, a nonprofit testing and certification organization that makes sure bottlers are complying with standards as strict as those set for public water supplies. The International Bottled Water Association itself recommends more comprehensive regulation than is currently in place.

But let the buyer beware: About 25% of bottled water is virtually tap water in a pretty package, and bottled water may or may not contain sufficient quantities of fluoride to protect against cavities. So although bottled water may not be "bad," it may not be "good" either.

Natural water is water that is not from a public water system and has not been modified by the addition or removal of any minerals.

Spring water flows out of the ground on its own and is bottled at or near its source. If bottled by a member of the International Bottled Water Association, it is not modified by the addition or removal of minerals.

Purified water, also known as distilled water, tastes flat because it has had all of the minerals removed.

Mineral water, according to the International Bottled Water Association, contains not less than 500 parts per million total dissolved solids. Loosely defined, mineral water is any water that is not distilled. The greater the mineral content, the stronger the taste.

Seltzer water is water that is injected with carbon dioxide.

Expired Air

Expired air accounts for about 350 ml of water loss daily.

Perspiration

The amount of water lost through perspiration varies with activity and climate. As the amount of water excreted through perspiration increases, the volume of urine decreases.

Recommended Dietary Allowance

The requirement for water is highly variable and impossible to determine because actual need varies in response to other factors. The amount of water required is that needed to replace insensible losses, which vary considerably, and maintain a normal solute load, which can vary with diet and other factors. For practical purposes, adults need 1 ml/cal of energy expenditure, under average conditions of energy expenditure and environmental exposure.[5] Because the risk of water intoxication is rare, 1.5 ml/cal is often recommended to compensate for any variations in activity level, perspiration, and solute load.[5] The recommendation for infants is 1.5 ml/cal of energy expenditure because they have proportionately higher needs, are unable to express thirst, and have limited ability to concentrate the urine.

Clinical Applications

Dehydration

Dehydration, or fluid volume deficit, occurs when water output exceeds water intake, and may result from water deprivation, injection of hypertonic solutions, a reduction in the total quantity of electrolytes, or from excessive fluid loss. Conditions that increase fluid losses include fever; profuse perspiration caused by intense physical activity, especially during hot environmental temperatures accompanied by high humidity; and a variety of clinical conditions such as diarrhea, vomiting, fistulas, excessive urination (*e.g.*, uncontrolled diabetes), drainage tubes, hemorrhage, and severe burns. Signs and symptoms of dehydration vary in severity. Dry mucous membranes, decreased urinary output, concentrated urine, weak pulse, orthostatic hypotension, and decreased body temperature are early signs; stupor, coma, oliguria, and hypotension develop in the later stages. Dehydration is life-threatening when more than 10% of body weight is lost.[5] Oral or intravenous fluid and electrolytes are given, depending on the degree of depletion.

Fluid Intoxication

Fluid intoxication resulting from excessive water intake is rarely observed in healthy adults. Fluid volume excess, however, can occur secondary to impaired fluid output or altered sodium balance, as in the case of renal failure, congestive heart failure, excessive sodium intake, corticosteroid therapy, cirrhosis, or Cushing's syndrome. Depending on the severity, fluid volume excess may be treated by withholding fluid and electrolytes until the condition is resolved, or by administering diuretics.

ELECTROLYTES

By definition, electrolytes carry electrical charges when dissolved in solution. Cations, such as sodium and potassium, are positively charged ions; anions, like chloride, are negatively charged ions. In an electrolyte solution, the total number of cations and the total number of anions are exactly equal.

Within the body, the concentration of electrolyte ions or number of electrical charges in a liter of solution is expressed in milliequivalents per liter (mEq/liter). The concentration of electrolytes is maintained within a narrow range in both the ECF and ICF. Normally, serum contains about 150 mEq of cations/liter and 150 mEq of anions/liter, for a total serum osmolarity of about 300 mEq/liter. A summary of the electrolytes sodium, potassium, and chloride appears in Table 7-2.

EXAMPLE

$$\text{Milliequivalents} = \frac{\text{milligrams}}{\text{atomic weight}}$$

$$\frac{2000 \text{ mg of sodium}}{23 \text{ (atomic weight of sodium)}} = 86.96 \text{ mEq of sodium}$$

$$\frac{2000 \text{ mg of potassium}}{39 \text{ (atomic weight of potassium)}} = 51.3 \text{ mEq of potassium}$$

Sodium

Approximately 30% of the 120 mg of sodium in the body is located on the surface of the bone crystals; it is available to maintain serum sodium levels if hyponatremia develops. The rest of the body's sodium is in the ECF, mostly in plasma and in nerve and muscle tissue. It

Table 7-2
Summary of Sodium, Potassium, and Chloride

Electrolyte	Adult Estimated Minimum Requirement	Sources	Functions
Sodium	500 mg	Sodium chloride, processed foods like canned soups, meats, vegetables, pickled foods, snack items, convenience foods, soft water, milk, meats	Fluid balance, acid–base balance, muscle irritability, regulate cell membrane permeability and nerve impulse transmission
Potassium	2000 mg	Fruits and vegetables, legumes, whole grains, milk, meats	Fluid balance, acid–base balance, nerve impulse transmission, catalyst for many metabolic reactions, involved in skeletal and cardiac muscle activity
Chloride	750 mg	Sodium chloride, same sources as sodium	Fluid balance, acid–base balance, essential component of HCl

functions to maintain fluid balance, maintain acid–base balance, maintain muscular irritability, and to regulate cell permeability and nerve impulse transmission.

Sodium comprises 39% of salt, or sodium chloride, by weight. Because salt is used extensively in food processing and manufacturing, it is estimated that processed foods account for 75% of total sodium consumed. Canned meats and soups, condiments, pickled foods, foods prepared in brine solutions, and traditional snack items are high in added sodium. Naturally occurring sources of sodium, like milk, meats, egg, carrots, beets, spinach, celery, artichokes, and asparagus, provide only about 10% of sodium consumed. Salt added during cooking and at the table provides 15% of total sodium, and water supplies less than 10% (see Chap. 16 for high- and low-sodium foods).

Absorption and Excretion

About 95% of ingested sodium is absorbed, with the remaining 5% excreted in the feces. Sodium absorbed in excess of need is excreted by the kidneys. The hormone aldosterone acts to increase the reabsorption of sodium when blood volume, cardiac output, or extracellular sodium are low, or when extracellular potassium is high.

Normally, the amount of sodium ingested equals the amount of sodium excreted. When a salty meal is consumed, thirst is stimulated so that the transitory increase in sodium in the body can be diluted to normal concentration. With the increase in both sodium and fluid in the body, kidneys excrete more sodium and fluid to normalize blood volume. When sodium and fluid are both depleted, as in the case of profuse sweating, vomiting, or diarrhea, and only water is taken in, hyponatremia develops and water intoxication results. Symptoms of muscle weakness, apathy, nausea, and anorexia are alleviated with corrections of fluid and electrolyte balance.

Recommendations and Average Intake

The minimum amount of sodium needed by a healthy adult to replace obligatory losses and to provide for growth is probably only 115 mg/day. To compensate for wide variations in physical activity and climatic exposure, 500 mg has been set as the estimated minimum requirement for healthy adults. The previous edition of the RDA suggested 1100 to 3300 mg/day of sodium as a safe and adequate intake.

Calculating average sodium intake is extremely difficult, especially because "average" can vary considerably from day to day, depending on the amount of processed foods consumed. Also, the discretionary use of salt, which tends to be highly variable and can be considerable in amount, is practically impossible to estimate from dietary surveys. Depending on the method of assessment used, estimates of sodium intake range from 1800 to 5000 mg/day.[5] The Surgeon General estimates that average sodium intake for adults is 4000 to 6000 mg/day.[7]

The *Dietary Guidelines for Americans* suggests that Americans use salt and sodium only in moderation because current average intake greatly exceeds actual need, and because lower sodium intakes reduce high blood pressure in people who are sodium-sensitive.[8] Even people who are normotensive are urged to reduce sodium intake to help protect against hypertension and cardiovascular diseases in the future.

Clinical Applications

Normal serum sodium equals 132 to 145 mEq/liter.

Sodium Deficiency

Hyponatremia may occur as a result of severe vomiting, diarrhea, or profuse sweating in high temperatures; cystic fibrosis; adrenal insufficiency (Addison's disease); sodium-wasting renal disorders; and from excessive diuresis or excessive salt restriction. Clinical findings include cold, clammy skin, decreased skin turgor, apprehension, confusion, irritability, anxiety, hypotension, tachycardia, headache, tremors, convulsions, abdominal cramps, nausea, vomiting, and diarrhea.

Sodium Excess

Even on a diet high in sodium, sodium retention is not likely to occur. Most people can tolerate a wide range of sodium intakes because the kidneys are able to compensate by excreting more or less sodium in the urine. However, sodium excretion may be impaired by congestive heart failure, circulatory failure, or renal failure. Signs and symptoms of sodium retention include edema, weight gain; hot, flushed, dry skin; dry, red tongue; intense thirst, restless agitation, and oliguria or anuria. In the approximately 10% of the population who may be sodium-sensitive, a high sodium intake promotes high blood pressure.

Nutrient/Drug Interactions

Drugs that affect sodium are as follows:
- Castor oil: inhibits sodium absorption
- Captopril: may cause hyponatremia
- Colchicine: decreases sodium absorption
- Corticosteroids: cause sodium retention
- Diuretics: increase sodium excretion
- Levodopa: increases urinary sodium excretion
- Neomycin: decreases sodium absorption
- Probenecid: increases urinary excretion of sodium

Potassium

Most of the body's approximately 270 mg of potassium is located inside the cells as the major ICF cation; the remainder is in the ECF, where it serves to maintain fluid balance, maintain acid–base balance, transmit nerve impulses, catalyze metabolic reactions in the body, aid in CHO metabolism and protein synthesis, and control skeletal muscle contractility.

Potassium is widespread in the diet and is especially abundant in unprocessed foods, fruits, many vegetables, and fresh meats. Many salt substitutes contain significant amounts of potassium in place of sodium, which may convey both potential health risks and benefits.[1] Sources of potassium are listed in Appendix 9.

Absorption and Excretion

Potassium is absorbed readily from the small intestine at an efficiency rate of more than 90%. Only small amounts are excreted through the feces. Like sodium, an excess intake of potassium does not lead to an increase in serum concentration, due to the action of hormones. Aldosterone increases the urinary excretion of potassium when serum levels rise. Unfortunately, the kidneys cannot conserve potassium as efficiently as sodium, and urinary losses may be 200 to 400 mg/day even when the body is depleted in potassium.

Recommendations and Average Intake

In the 10th edition of the RDA, an estimated minimum requirement for potassium for healthy adults was set at 2000 mg/day. Previously, a daily intake of 1875 to 5625 mg/day for adults was recommended as safe and adequate.

Potassium intakes vary widely, depending on actual food selections. Diets high in fruits and vegetables may provide as much as 8 to 11 g/day.[5] It is estimated that the average adult consumes 800 to 11,000 mg/day.[6]

Clinical Applications

Normal serum potassium equals 3.5 to 5.0 mEq/liter.

Potassium Deficiency

Hypokalemia may occur from prolonged malnutrition and loss of protein tissue; prolonged GI loss related to vomiting, diarrhea, or gastric suctioning; kidney disease; diabetic acidosis; and the use of potassium-wasting diuretics. Signs and symptoms are muscle cramps and weakness, including cardiac muscle weakness; anorexia, nausea, vomiting, mental depression, confusion, drowsiness, abdominal distention, increased urine output, shallow respirations, and irregular pulse. Severe hypokalemia can result in cardiac dysrhythmias, which may be fatal.

Potassium Excess

Hyperkalemia, which may result from renal failure, or a too-rapid infusion of intravenous potassium, is characterized by irritability, anxiety, listlessness, mental confusion, nausea, diarrhea, poor respiration, GI hyperactivity, muscular weakness, numbness of the extremities, hypotension, cardiac arrhythmia, heart block, and cardiac arrest.

Future Directions

Numerous studies have shown that high intakes of potassium may be of benefit in preventing or treating hypertension.

Nutrient/Drug Interactions

Supplements of potassium may
Cause hyperkalemia when used concurrently with potassium-sparing diuretics.
Cause hyperkalemia when used concurrently with salt substitutes that contain potassium.

Increased serum potassium decreases both the toxicity and effectiveness of digitalis drugs.

Drugs that affect potassium are as follows:
- Adrenal corticosteroids: increase urinary potassium excretion
- p-Aminosalicylic acid: can cause hypokalemia
- Amphotericin B: increases urinary potassium excretion
- Capreomycin: decreases serum potassium
- Captopril: causes potassium retention, leading to hyperkalemia

- Colchicine: decreases potassium absorption
- Diuretics (except spironolactone, triamterene): increase urinary excretion of potassium; may cause hypokalemia
- Gentamicin: increases urinary potassium excretion
- Levodopa: increases urinary excretion of potassium
- Neomycin: decreases potassium absorption
- Penicillin: can cause hypokalemia, renal potassium wasting
- Phenolphthalein: causes hypokalemia in laxative abusers
- Probenecid: increases urinary excretion of potassium
- Salicylates: increase urinary excretion of potassium
- Viomycin: can cause hypokalemia; excessive urinary excretion of potassium persists after drug is discontinued

Chloride

Chloride is the major inorganic anion in the ECF; a relatively large amount is found as an essential component of hydrochloric acid (HCl) in the stomach. Its functions include fluid balance and acid–base balance. Its concentration in most cells is low.[5]

Almost all the chloride in the diet comes from salt (sodium chloride); therefore, rich sources of sodium are also rich sources of chloride.

Absorption and Excretion

Chloride is almost completely absorbed in the small intestine; the kidneys excrete chloride absorbed in excess of need. Diarrhea and vomiting increase chlorine losses.

Recommendations and Average Intake

An RDA for chlorine has not been established. Because both the sources of chloride and its normal losses from the body correspond to those of sodium, the estimated minimum requirements listed for all age and sex groups except infants equal those of sodium on a milliequivalent basis. For healthy adults, the estimated minimum requirement of 750 mg/day is easily exceeded considering the amount of salt in the average American diet. It is estimated that added salt provides approximately 6000 mg of chloride daily.[5]

Clinical Applications

Chloride Deficiency

Hypochloremia may be caused by prolonged vomiting, diarrhea, dehydration, the use of certain diuretics, fistual and tube drainage, cystic fibrosis, dehydration, and excessive perspiration. Clinical findings include muscle spasms, alkalosis, depressed respirations, and possible coma.

Chloride Excess

The only known cause of hyperchloremia is water-deficiency dehydration.[5] Excessive intakes of chloride (in the form of salt) are associated with an increased risk of hypertension in salt-sensitive people.

Nutrient/Drug Interactions

Drug that affects chloride is as follows:

- Probenecid: increases urinary excretion of chloride

FLUID AND ELECTROLYTE BALANCE AND IMBALANCES

Normal Fluid Balance

The volume of water in the body and how it is distributed among body compartments is determined largely by the concentration of solutes in solution, namely sodium and potassium. Sodium in the ECF draws water from the ICF (water follows salt); potassium inside the cell attracts water from the ECF. Water moves easily and reversibly between the ECF and the ICF from areas of low-solute concentration to areas of high-solute concentration to equalize the solute concentration on both sides of the semipermeable membrane (Fig. 7-2). For instance, a slight increase in the sodium concentration of the ECF causes water to move from the ICF to the ECF to equalize the solute concentration in both compartments.

The movement of water across cell membranes is caused by a force known as *osmotic pressure*, which is directly proportional to the total number of dissolved particles in solution. *Oncotic pressure*, the pressure at the capillary membrane caused by dissolved protein in the plasma and interstitial fluid, contributes to osmotic pressure. Protein acts to prevent plasma fluid in the blood vessels from leaking into the interstitial fluid. However, changes in the concentration of water, water and solutes, or serum protein can result in dehydration or edema.

Alterations in Fluid Balance

Hypertonic Dehydration

Hypertonic dehydration occurs when the ECF water loss exceeds the electrolyte loss, which causes water to move from the ICF to the ECF to compensate for the change in osmotic pressure. Excessive fluid losses or inadequate fluid intake can cause hypertonic dehydration. Symptoms include intense thirst; hot, flushed skin; vomiting; confusion; and oliguria or anuria.

Hypotonic Dehydration

Hypotonic dehydration occurs when the ECF becomes hypotonic to the ICF, resulting in the movement of water from the ECF to the ICF and a resultant decrease in blood volume. Giving fluid without electrolytes or giving only plain water when both fluid and electrolytes have been lost may bring about hypotonic dehydration, which is characterized by weakness, decreased urine output, and an increase in hematocrit related to the decrease in blood volume.

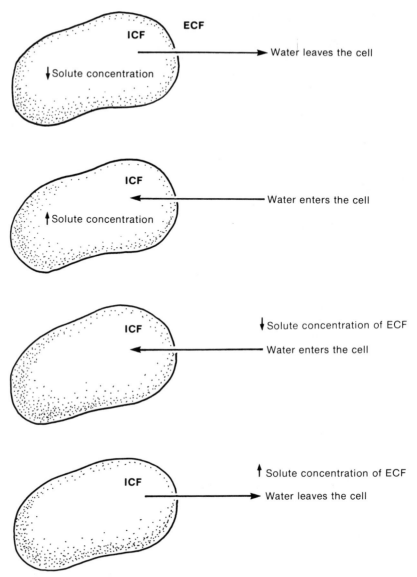

Figure 7-2
The movement of water across cell membranes.

Edema

Edema is the accumulation of fluid in the body that occurs when the body retains sodium, as in the case of some renal diseases and circulatory disorders. Edema also occurs when oncotic pressure falls due to a decrease in serum albumin levels, like during protein malnutrition.

ACID–BASE BALANCE

Acids and Their Sources

Acids are substances that donate hydrogen ions (H^+) to neutralize bases; bases are H^+ acceptors that neutralize acids. Acid–base balance refers to maintaining the body's concentration of H^+. Most of the body's hydrogen ion concentration is produced through the metabolism of food: The oxidation of CHO, protein, and fat for energy yields carbon dioxide and water, which combine to form carbonic acid, the most abundant acid in the body.

pH

The degree of acidity of a solution, or the concentration of hydrogen ions, is expressed in terms of pH, which ranges from 0 to 14. Normal blood pH is maintained between 7.35 and 7.45; other body fluids vary in pH from 1.2 to 8.6 (Fig. 7-3). A pH of 7 indicates the solution is neutral; that is, it contains an equal number of hydrogen and hydroxide ions.

A pH lower than 7 indicates the solution is acidic; the lower the number, the more acidic the solution. Acidic solutions have more hydrogen ions than hydroxide ions. Alkaline solutions have a pH greater than 7; the higher the number, the more alkaline the solution and the fewer the number of hydrogen ions.

REGULATION OF ACID–BASE BALANCE

Buffer systems, respirations, and the kidneys help regulate normal pH.

Buffer Systems

Buffers are substances that prevent drastic changes in pH by accepting or donating hydrogen ions to neutralize acids or bases. Most of the body's buffer systems are composed of a weak acid and a weak base, which can weaken strong acids and bases within a fraction of a second. There are three major buffer systems in the body.

The carbonic acid–bicarbonate system functions to regulate the pH of the blood. Carbonic acid (a weak acid) buffers strong bases like sodium hydroxide, and sodium bicarbonate (a weak base) buffers strong acids like hydrochloric acid.

The phosphate buffer system acts to regulate the pH of red blood cells and the kidney tubular fluids. Dihydrogen phosphate (a weak acid) buffers strong bases like sodium hydroxide, and monohydrogen phosphate (a weak base) buffers strong acids like hydrochloric acid.

The pH of body cells and plasma is regulated by the protein system. Amino acids are amphoteric—that is, they can act as either acids or bases because they have at least one carboxyl group that acts like an acid to buffer bases, and at least one amine group that acts like a base to buffer acids.

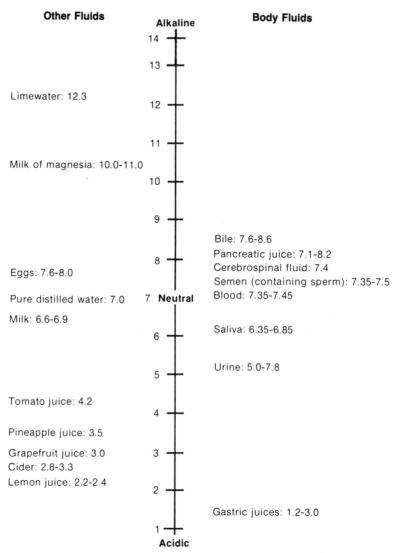

Figure 7-3
The pH of various body fluids and other fluids.

Respirations

The pH of body fluids can be changed within a matter of minutes by adjusting the rate of breathing. Carbonic acid, the most abundant acid produced from metabolism, is converted to carbon dioxide and is exhaled through the lungs. Changes in the carbon dioxide content of the blood can cause a change in the rate of breathing; likewise, a change in the rate of breathing causes a change in blood pH. For instance, a decrease in blood CO_2 causes an increase in pH. As a compensatory mechanism, breathing rate slows to retain CO_2 and lower pH. Conversely, an increase in blood CO_2 followed by a decrease in pH stimulates an increase in breathing rate so that CO_2 exhalation is increased and pH is ultimately increased.

The Kidneys

Although it may take as long as several hours to a few days, the kidneys are the most potent regulators of pH through their ability to excrete hydrogen ions in the form of ammonium ions, weak acids, and small amounts of free hydrogen ions. The kidneys also regulate the excretion of electrolytes and bicarbonate. A decrease in the pH of body fluids (becomes more acidic) causes the kidneys to excrete more hydrogen ions. When the pH of body fluids increases (becomes more alkaline), the kidneys excrete more bicarbonate and retain hydrogen ions to lower pH.

ACID–BASE IMBALANCES

Acidosis

Acidosis is a condition that occurs when the hydrogen ion concentration of the blood increases, resulting in a pH of 7.35 to 6.8. Acidosis depresses the central nervous system (CNS), which may result in confusion, coma, and death.

Respiratory Acidosis

Respiratory acidosis is caused by a decrease in respirations, which leads to an increase in the CO_2 content of the blood. Emphysema, pulmonary edema, pneumonia, and asphyxia can cause respiratory acidosis.

Metabolic Acidosis

Metabolic acidosis is caused by an increase in metabolic acids, like ketones or lactic acid, due to conditions such as diabetic acidosis and starvation. Diarrhea and renal tubular disorders that cause an increase in the excretion of bicarbonate ions can also lead to metabolic acidosis.

Alkalosis

Alkalosis, characterized by a pH of 7.45 to 7.8, occurs when the hydrogen ion concentration of the blood is abnormally low. Nervousness, muscle spasms, and convulsions may develop as the nerves of both the CNS and peripheral nervous system become overexcited and conduct impulses in the absence of stimulation.

Respiratory Alkalosis

Respiratory alkalosis is caused by hyperventilation, which decreases the concentration of CO_2 in the blood. Salicylate poisoning, acute anxiety, fevers, infections, and high altitudes can cause respiratory alkalosis.

Metabolic Alkalosis

Metabolic alkalosis occurs when the hydrogen ion concentration decreases in response to an increase in bicarbonate. Vomiting, which causes the loss of hydrogen ions in hydrochloric acid, potassium depletion, and the excessive use of alkaline drugs may cause metabolic alkalosis.

ACID AND BASE FORMERS

Because minerals are not broken down during metabolism, they leave an acid or alkaline ash in the body depending on their chemical composition. Calcium, sodium, potassium, and magnesium are bases; foods containing large amounts of these cations are said to be alkaline-forming or alkaline-producing (see Table 18-6). Foods containing predominately chloride, sulfur, and phosphorus are acid-formers (see Table 18-6). Because they contain no minerals and, therefore, do not leave an ash, pure fats and pure CHO are considered neutral foods.

Even if the diet contains predominately acid-forming or alkaline-forming foods, the pH of the blood is maintained by renal excretion of electrolytes. For instance, the higher the intake of sodium or potassium, the higher the amount of these electrolytes in the urine. Although it is possible to treat renal stones by manipulating the diet to alter urinary pH, drug therapy is a much more effective and consistent method of treatment (see Chap. 18).

BIBLIOGRAPHY

1. Ahern DA: Electrolyte content of salt-replacement seasonings. J Am Diet Assoc 89:935, 1989
2. Malseed RT: Pharmacology: Drug Therapy and Nursing Considerations. 3rd ed. Philadelphia: JB Lippincott, 1990
3. Mayer J (ed): Bottled water's image muddied. Tufts University Diet and Nutrition Letter 9(5):1, 1991
4. Mayer J (ed): Water, water everywhere, but is it fit to drink? Tufts University Diet and Nutrition Letter 9(1):1, 1991
5. National Research Council: Recommended Dietary Allowances. 10th ed. Washington, DC: National Academy Press, 1989
6. Pennington JA, Young B: Total Diet Study nutritional elements, 1982–1989. J Am Diet Assoc 91:179, 1991
7. Public Health Service, United States Department of Health and Human Services: The Surgeon General's Report on Nutrition and Health: Summary and Recommendations. DHHS (PHS) Publication no. 88-50211. Washington, DC: Government Printing Office, 1988
8. United States Department of Agriculture, United States Department of Health and Human Services: Nutrition and Your Health: Dietary Guidelines for Americans. 3rd ed. Home and Garden Bulletin no. 232, 1990

II
Nutrition in Health Promotion

8 Planning an Adequate Diet

An adequate diet obviously provides a balanced intake of sufficient amounts of all nutrients required for growth and development and for maintenance or restoration of health. Exactly what constitutes an adequate diet, and for whom, is less obvious. Nutritional deficiency diseases are now uncommon in the United States except among the poor, the elderly, alcoholics, fad dieters, and, ironically, hospitalized clients. In fact, public health concern has shifted away from undernutrition to overnutrition: of the 10 leading causes of death in the United States today, 5 are associated with dietary excesses and another 3 with excessive alcohol consumption.[15]

A "good" diet contains mostly "good" foods, but "good" can mean different things to different people. Fortunately, most leading government and health organizations agree on what constitutes a healthy diet. With their guidelines as a foundation, the food group approach to meal planning can be used to make actual food choices, or implement the guidelines. Recommended Dietary Allowances can be used to plan a diet or to evaluate the nutritional adequacy of a diet. However, they deal with individual nutrients, not food groups, and are too complex for use by the general public. Both the USRDA and Nutrient Density approach can be used to evaluate a food's or diet's relative nutritional quality.

Because eating supplies food for the body and the soul, diet planning is an art as well as a science. Personal food preferences and aversions, as influenced by culture, geography, and religion, have a greater impact on most people's actual food choices than do nutritional considerations: Ignoring their significance can undermine diet planning. Other factors to consider while planning a diet include food quality, safety considerations, and economic feasibility.

NUTRITIONAL CONSIDERATIONS

Dietary Guidelines

In the past, the purpose of dietary guidelines was to help prevent nutrient deficiencies. Today, numerous governmental and health agencies publish dietary guidelines whose focus is not on getting enough, but on avoiding excesses for the possible prevention of chronic diet-related diseases, as identified in Table 8-1. Just how much of an impact diet actually has on these disorders is unknown, because diet is difficult to separate from genetic, behavioral, and environmental factors. However, it is certain that diet contributes to the development of these diseases and that dietary change can contribute to their prevention.[15] Guidelines are suggestions for dietary change for the general population, not individuals. As such, they should be used as a starting point from which to develop an adequate diet for an individual.

Although specific recommendations vary somewhat in wording and phrasing (Table 8-2), most experts agree that Americans should adhere to the following dietary suggestions:

- Eat less cholesterol and fat, especially saturated fat. Diets high in fat increase the risk of obesity and certain types of cancer, and high intakes of saturated fat and cholesterol increase the risk of heart disease. Most recommendations suggest that total fat intake not exceed 30% of calories and that saturated fat contribute less than 10% of total calories. In his report entitled *Nutrition and Health*, the Surgeon General states that reducing fat intake is "clearly emerging as the primary priority for dietary change."[15]
- Eat a variety of foods, because no single food supplies all 40-plus essential nutrients. In

Table 8-1
Disorders Associated with Dietary Excesses

Disorder	Associated Dietary Excess
Coronary heart disease, cerebrovascular disease, and atherosclerosis	Total fat, saturated fat, and cholesterol
Cancer (bowel and breast)	Fat
Hypertension	Sodium, calories
Obesity	Calories, fat
Diabetes (type II)	Calories
Cirrhosis of the liver	Alcohol
Dental caries	Sugar

Table 8-2
Comparison of Selected Dietary Recommendations*

	Step One Diet (American Heart Association)	Nutrition, Common Sense and Cancer (American Cancer Society)	Dietary Guidelines for Americans (USDA and USDHHS)
Eat a variety of foods	x		x
Avoid obesity	x	x	x
Increase intake of complex CHO	x		x
Include foods rich in vitamins A and C in your daily diet		x	
Include cruciferous vegetables in your diet		x	
Increase fiber intake		x	x
Decrease intake of sugar			x
Decrease fat intake	x	x	x
Decrease intake of cholesterol	x		x
Avoid salt-cured, smoked, or charcoal-broiled foods		x	
Limit sodium intake	x		x
Drink alcohol only in moderation	x	x	x

* "x" indicates specifically recommended.

addition, variety helps reduce the risk of nutrient toxicity and accidental contamination. The Guide to Daily Food Choices appears in Table 8-3.

- Maintain healthy body weight. The risk of health problems is higher among both underweight and overweight people. However, "healthy" weight is not precisely defined because it is relative to other health status indicators, like serum cholesterol levels and blood pressure. A change in terminology to "healthy" weight from "desirable" weight emphasizes the shift in focus away from appearance and toward health.
- Eat more starch from vegetables, fruits, and grains because they are generally low in fat and high in fiber.
- Eat less sugar and sodium. High intakes of sugars and frequent sugary snacks contribute to tooth decay. Sodium can aggravate or increase the risk of hypertension in sodium-sensitive individuals.
- Use alcohol only in moderation. Alcohol provides little or no nutrients, no overall health benefits, increases the risk of health problems, causes many accidents, and can lead to addiction.

These suggestions are presented formally in *Dietary Guidelines for Americans*,[18] which represents the current Federal nutrition policy. Its predecessor, *Dietary Goals for the United States*, was published in 1977 by the Select Committee on Nutrition and Human Needs of the United States Senate. It recommended that Americans consume 30% of their total calories from fat, 12% from protein, and the remainder from carbohydrates, mostly in the form of starch and fiber. Because the goals generated a lot of controversy and criticism, the committee was disbanded and its responsibilities were delegated to the United States Department of Agriculture (USDA) and the United States Department of Health, Education,

Table 8-3
Guide to Daily Food Choices

Food Group	Nutritional Attributes	Suggested Daily Servings and Serving Sizes	Selection Tips
Bread, Cereal, Rice, and Pasta Group	Provide complex CHO, vitamins, minerals, and fiber	6–11 servings 1 serving is: 1 slice bread 1 oz ready-to-eat cereal ½ cup cooked cereal, rice, or pasta	Choose whole grain items often for fiber. Choose items made with little fat and sugar: bread, English muffins, rice, pasta. Avoid baked products high in fat and sugar: cakes, cookies, croissants, pastries. Limit fats and sugars used as toppings and spreads. When preparing package mixes, use less fat than directed and if milk is called for, use lowfat.
Vegetable Group	Provide vitamins A, C, and folate; iron, magnesium and fiber. Naturally low in fat	3–5 servings 1 serving is: 1 cup raw leafy vegetables ½ cup other vegetables, cooked or chopped raw ¾ cup vegetable juice	Because different vegetables provide different nutrients, be sure to eat: • dark green leafy vegetables several times a week (broccoli, spinach) • deep yellow vegetables (carrots, sweet potatoes) • starchy vegetables (potatoes, corn, peas) • legumes several times a week (navy, pinto, and kidney beans) Limit fat added to vegetables. Use low-fat salad dressing.
Fruit Group	Provide vitamins A and C and potassium Naturally low in fat and sodium	2–4 servings 1 serving is: 1 medium apple, banana, or orange ½ cup chopped, cooked, or canned fruit ¾ cup fruit juice	Choose fresh, frozen, canned or dried fruit. Eat whole fruits often. Eat fruits high in vitamin C regularly: citrus fruits, melons, berries. Choose 100% fruit juice instead of punches, ades, and drinks.
Meat, Poultry, Fish, Dry Beans, Eggs, and Nuts	Provide protein, B vitamins, iron, and zinc.	2–3 servings, the equivalent of 5–7 ounces of cooked lean meat, poultry, or fish 1 serving is: 2–3 ounces of cooked lean	Choose lean meat, poultry without skin, fish, and dried peas and beans. Often, they are lowest in fat. Use low-fat preparation techniques: trim away visible fat, don't add fat

(*continued*)

Table 8-3 (*continued*)

Food Group	Nutritional Attributes	Suggested Daily Servings and Serving Sizes	Selection Tips
		meat, poultry, or fish For the other items in this group, 1 ounce of meat equals: ½ cup cooked, dry beans 1 egg 2 tablespoons peanut butter	during cooking. Limit egg yolks; use egg whites freely. Because nuts and seeds are high in fat, use them in moderation.
Milk, Yogurt, and Cheese Group	Provide protein, vitamins, calcium, and other minerals	2–3 servings 1 serving is (based on calcium content): 1 cup milk or yogurt 1½ ounces natural cheese 2 ounces process cheese	Choose skim milk and non-fat yogurt often; they are lowest in fat. Cottage cheese is lower in calcium than most cheeses; 1 cup cottage cheese = ½ cup milk. Limit high fat cheese and ice cream. Choose lowfat cheeses and milk desserts (ice milk, frozen yogurt).
Fats, Oils, and Sweets	Provide calories with little else nutritionally	Use sparingly	

Source: USDA (prepared by Human Nutrition Information Service), USDA's Food Guide Pyramid. Home and Garden Bulletin Number 249 Hyattsville, MD, 1992

and Welfare (USDHEW), which later became the United States Department of Health and Human Services. Together these agencies published the first edition of *Dietary Guidelines for Americans*, which proved to be a less controversial, watered-down version of *Dietary Goals*. The guidelines have evolved into the current (third) edition, which was published in 1990. They provide more direction and have replaced negative suggestions ("avoid") to positive ones ("use in moderation") (see box, Dietary Guidelines for Americans and Suggestions for Food Choices).

Unfortunately, the guidelines are difficult for most consumers to use on a daily basis and they lack specificity regarding actual food choices.

The Food Guide Pyramid

In 1992, the USDA replaced the classic Basic 4 food wheel with a new graphic entitled the Food Guide Pyramid (Fig. 8-1). Based on recommendations set forth in the 3rd edition of the Dietary Guidelines for Americans, the Pyramid seeks to emphasize not only variety, but also proportion and moderation, two concepts previously unaddressed.

Dietary Guidelines for Americans and Suggestions for Food Choices

Eat a variety of foods. Eat a variety of foods daily, choosing different foods from each group, including selections of: fruits, vegetables; whole-grain and enriched breads, cereals, and other products made from grains; milk, cheese, yogurt, and other products made from milk; meats, poultry, fish, eggs, and dry beans and peas.

Maintain healthy weight. To help control overeating, eat slowly, take smaller portions, and avoid "seconds." To lose weight, eat a variety of foods that are low in calories and high in nutrients. Eat more fruits, vegetables, and whole grains prepared without added fats or sugar; eat less fat and fatty foods; eat less sugar and sweets; drink little or no alcoholic beverages; increase your physical activity.

Choose a diet low in fat, saturated fat, and cholesterol. Choose lean meat, fish, poultry, and dry beans and peas as protein sources; use skim or low-fat milk and milk products; moderate your use of egg yolks and organ meats; use fats and oils sparingly, especially those high in saturated fat, such as butter, cream, lard, heavily hydrogenated fats (some margarines), shortenings, and foods containing palm and coconut oils; choose liquid vegetable oils most often because they are lower in saturated fat; trim fat off meats; remove skin from poultry; have meatless meals occasionally; broil, bake, or boil rather than fry; read labels carefully to determine both amount and type of fat present in foods.

Choose a diet with plenty of vegetables, fruits, and grain products. Choose three or more servings of various vegetables, two or more servings of various fruits, and six or more servings of grain products. Increase fiber intake by eating more of a variety of foods that are natural sources of fiber.

Use sugars only in moderation. Use sugars in moderate amounts—sparingly if your calorie needs are low. Avoid excessive snacking and brush and floss your teeth regularly.

Use salt and sodium only in moderation. Use salt sparingly, if at all, in cooking and at the table. Choose foods lower in sodium instead of high-sodium foods. Use salted snacks, such as chips, crackers, pretzels, and nuts, sparingly. Read food labels carefully to determine the amounts of sodium. Use lower-sodium products, when available, to replace those you use that have higher sodium content.

If you drink alcoholic beverages, do so in moderation. If you drink, be moderate in your intake: Women should drink no more than one drink a day, men should not drink more than two drinks a day. Alcohol should not be consumed by women who are pregnant or trying to conceive, individuals who plan to drive or engage in other activities that require attention or skill, individuals using medicines, even over-the-counter kinds, individuals who cannot keep their drinking moderate, and children and adolescents.

*U.S. Department of Agriculture, and U.S. Department of Health and Human Services: Nutrition and Your Health: Dietary Guidelines for Americans. 3rd ed. Home and Garden Bull. no. 232, 1990.

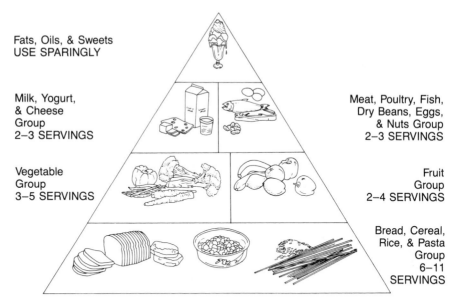

Figure 8-1
The Food Guide Pyramid: A Guide to Good Eating.

At the broad base of the pyramid, symbolizing the mainstay of the diet, is the Bread, Cereal, Rice, and Pasta group. Moving up the pyramid, next is a layer comprised of the Fruit group and Vegetable group, which is topped by a layer of the Milk group and Meat group. The apex of the pyramid is occupied by Fats, Oils, and Sweets. Because items in this group are high in calories and low in nutritional value, they should be used sparingly.

Simple and easy to use, the food group approach has long been used to teach basic principles of nutrition to the general public and to assist individuals in choosing balanced diets. Unlike previous Basic 4 guidelines, the Food Guide Pyramid suggests *average* amounts from each major food group, instead of *minimum* recommendations (see Table 8-3).

Although the pyramid is intended to help Americans choose diets lower in fat, the actual fat content of items within a group are not addressed for the sake of simplicity. For instance, no distinction is made between skim milk and whole milk or high-fat meats and low-fat meats nor are total calories addressed. For instance, two servings from the milk group could mean 2 cups of skim milk (180 calories) or 2 cups of flavored whole-milk yogurt (570 calories).

Recommended Dietary Allowances

The RDA were initially developed as a guide for planning and procuring food supplies for a wartime nutrition program in 1943. Today, they are used primarily by professionals not only to plan, but also to evaluate the nutritional quality of diets, the adequacy of food supplies in meeting nutritional needs, and the adequacy of government feeding programs. The RDA also are useful in developing new food products, developing guidelines for nutrition labeling, and developing nutrition education programs.

Recommended Dietary Allowances

Definition*	Comments
The levels of intake of essential nutrients that, on the basis of scientific knowledge, are judged by the Food and Nutrition Board to be adequate to meet the known nutritional needs of practically all healthy persons.	Recommended dietary allowances (RDA) have not been established for all the essential nutrients; therefore, a variety of foods should be consumed. RDA are revised periodically (about every 5 years) as more information becomes available. Does not guarantee to meet the needs of *all* healthy people: Some people consuming the RDA may not be meeting their individual needs for certain nutrients. The RDA are not appropriate for people who have acute or chronic illnesses, genetic disorders, or those using medications that alter nutritional requirements. The RDA also do not cover nutritional needs of low birthweight infants.
RDA are recommendations for the average daily amounts of nutrients that population groups should consume over a period of time.	Designed for a reference population of Americans who live in a temperate climate and are moderately active. Separate categories have been established for age, sex, pregnancy, and lactation (Appendix 2). Estimated safe and adequate daily dietary intakes of additional selected vitamins and minerals supplement the 1980 edition of the RDA (Appendix 3). Estimated sodium, chloride, and potassium Minimum Requirements of Healthy Persons was added to the 1989 edition of the RDA. Because the body has adaptive mechanisms and the ability to store many nutrients, the RDA are more meaningful over a 5- to 8-day period than on any given day.
RDA should not be confused with requirements for a specific individual.	The definition of requirement is the amount of a nutrient needed to pre-

(continued)

Recommended Dietary Allowances (*continued*)

Definition*	Comments
Differences in the nutrient requirements of individuals are usually unknown. Therefore, RDA (except for energy) are estimated to exceed the requirements of most individuals and thereby to ensure that the needs of nearly all in the population are met. Intakes below the recommended allowance for a nutrient are not necessarily inadequate, but the risk of having an inadequate intake increases to the extent that intake is less than the levels recommended as safe.	vent a deficiency; the definition of allowance is requirement plus a safety factor to account for individual variations. To accurately assess an individual's nutritional status and dietary adequacy, dietary factors, as well as anthropometric measurements, medical-socioeconomic data, biochemical findings, and clinical observations, should be evaluated (see Chap. 9).

* Data from National Research Council: Recommended Dietary Allowances, 10th ed. Washington, DC: National Academy Press, 1989.

In order to evaluate a person's intake according to the RDA, the nutritional composition of the diet must be calculated. This can be done most effectively by using food composition tables, such as the 14th edition of Pennington's *Food Values of Portions Commonly Used*,[13] that list the average nutrient content for a given amount of food based on the chemical analysis of a number of samples (see Appendix 1). They are intended to be used as a standard reference for the nutritional value of foods consumed throughout the country on a year-round basis. Besides being used to calculate the nutrient intake of individuals or groups, food composition tables also can aid in planning therapeutic diets with restricted or increased amounts of one or more nutrients, in developing food guides and nutrition education teaching materials, and in selecting nutritionally comparable alternatives among foods to control costs.

Food composition tables are widely available, easy to use, and inexpensive. However, there may be wide variations in nutrient composition among different samples of the same food related to the ripeness or maturity of the food, the portion of the food analyzed (*e.g.*, outer or inner leaves), the variety of a food, the length of time the food has been stored, the degree of processing and cooking used in preparation, the soil content where the food is grown, and the time of year the food is harvested. Also, not all foods have been analyzed for their nutrient content (*e.g.*, food fads and convenience items), and not all nutrients are listed in food composition tables (*e.g.*, trace elements like selenium). Likewise, even if the nutrient composition of a food is known, the bioavailability of the nutrients present in that food may be altered by other foods or nutrients consumed in a mixed diet. For instance, although iron-fortified cereals are high in iron, little iron may be absorbed if tea is consumed with the cereal. Conversely, orange juice can significantly increase the amount of iron absorbed from iron-fortified cereal.

Despite the shortcomings inherent with the use of food composition tables, the RDA is still the only method available that gives specific nutrient and calorie recommendations based on age and sex, and offers the advantage of providing close evaluation of actual intake. In addition, the RDA is revised periodically to reflect current data. The most recent edition of the RDA was published in 1989 and appears in Appendices 2, 3, and 4.

Unfortunately, the RDA are too complex for use by the general public and are established for healthy people only. Another disadvantage is that the RDA are appropriate for populations, but not necessarily for individuals. Ten percent of the population may be consuming a deficient diet even if they meet 100% of the RDA. Conversely, some people may habitually consume less than the RDA for some nutrients and may not necessarily have an inadequate intake of those nutrients.

Due to the lack of sufficient studies on the nutritional requirements of the elderly, the RDA for people aged 51 years and older has been extrapolated from studies on younger adults and may not be valid. In addition, there is no distinction made between the nutritional requirements of a 51-year-old and the requirements of a 90-year-old, although one can surmise they may be different.

In some cases, it may be necessary to exceed the RDA for some nutrients (*e.g.*, protein) in order to meet the RDA for others (*e.g.*, trace minerals such as iron and zinc), and the RDA do not consider nutrient losses incurred during food storage and preparation.

United States Recommended Dietary Allowance

The USRDA is the reference standard used in nutrition labeling that provides information on the approximate percentage, in relation to total daily need, of certain essential vitamins and minerals contained in a single serving. The USRDA apply to four general population groups.[19] For most foods, the allowances are for people aged 4 years and older. Other USRDA on labels may be found on products for infants up to 1 year (infant foods), for children under 4 (junior foods), and for women who are pregnant or breastfeeding (used for vitamin and mineral supplements).[19]

The USRDA generally represent the highest RDA for each nutrient for any age or sex within the four major categories. For instance, for all foods except infant and junior foods, the USRDA for thiamine is 1.5 mg (the RDA for men), even though the RDA for adult women is only 1.0 mg. Thus, a serving of cereal that supplies 100% of the USRDA for thiamine provides 1.5 mg of thiamine. The FDA has suggested definitions for fair, good, and excellent sources of nutrients according to the percentage of USRDA provided in a serving (Table 8-4; see Food for Thought: Labeling Lingo, for more on nutrition labeling.)

If all foods eaten in a day are labeled with the USRDA, the day's total nutrient intake can be determined by adding the percentages of USRDA for each nutrient. However, fresh fruits and vegetables, most meats, and many other items are not yet required to provide USRDA information, so it is extremely difficult to tally a whole day's intake. The USRDA is not specific for age or sex, and therefore may not accurately reflect an individual's actual requirements. Similarly, because the highest RDA for each nutrient is used for the USRDA, a

Table 8-4
FDA Guidelines for Descriptions
of Nutrients with USRDAs

(Fair) source	10% or more USRDA
Good source	25% or more USRDA
Excellent source	40% or more USRDA

(Pennington JAT, Wilkening VL, Vanderveen JE: Descriptive terms for food labeling. Journal of Nutrition Education 22(1): 51, 1990)

margin of safety is built in. A person's intake is not necessarily deficient if the USRDA is not met.

Nutrient Density

Nutrient density is another method of evaluating the relative quality of individual food items by comparing the ratio of nutrients to calories (Fig. 8-2). Nutrient-dense foods, or "protective" foods such as milk, liver, citrus fruit, dark-green and yellow fruits and vegetables, and whole-grain breads and cereals, provide the most nutrients for the fewest calories. Foods with low nutrient density, such as soft drinks, cakes, pies, candy, other sweets, and snack foods, provide large amounts of calories with few nutrients.

The index of nutritional quality (INQ) is an approach to diet planning based on nutrient density.[8] By comparing the amount of a particular nutrient in 1000 calories of a food to the RDA for that nutrient per 1000-calorie intake, a food's nutrient density for individual nutrients can be determined. An INQ value greater than 1.0 indicates that the food is a good source of that nutrient. The nutrient density approach is a particularly useful tool for anyone on a calorie-controlled diet or limited food budget: It shows which foods within each group are the best caloric and economic "buys" for the amount of nutrients provided.

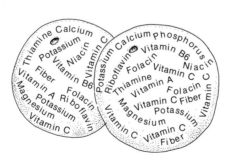

2 Medium Navel Oranges =130 Calories

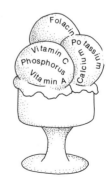

1/2 Cup Orange Sherbert=135 Calories

Figure 8-2
Nutrient density.

Labeling Lingo

The FDA, the U.S. Department of Agriculture, and the Federal Trade Commission share responsibility for food labeling, which currently is undergoing a major overhaul in both content and format. Over the last 85 years, the focus of food-labeling regulations has shifted from protecting the consumer from economic risk to protecting the consumer from health risk.[7] Surveys reveal that consumers want additional and revised information from what is currently available on labels, and want more products to be labeled. However, change is slow: Initial nutrition labeling regulations were proposed by the USDA in 1974 but were never finalized.[7]

In November 1990, the Nutritional Labeling and Education Act was signed to ultimately make labels more "user friendly."[15] The act requires the FDA to issue proposed regulations to implement the act within 12 months and to issue final regulations within 24 months.[7] If the FDA does not announce final regulations by the 24-month deadline, the proposed regulations will be considered final.

The act provides for mandatory nutritional labeling of most foods under FDA jurisdiction and allows voluntary labeling on fresh produce, seafood, meats, and poultry. However, if these items are not directly labeled, nutritional information must be displayed at the point of purchase. Serving sizes will be expressed in an appropriate common household measure. It also provides for labeling of total calories from fat, total fat, saturated fat, cholesterol, sodium, total carbohydrates, complex carbohydrates, sugars, dietary fiber, and total protein per serving, which should prove to be useful for consumers concerned with nutrition and health. Potentially misleading descriptions such as "light" or "lite," "diabetic," "reduced fat," and "imitation" will be prohibited. Health claims are forbidden unless they are consistent with FDA final regulations. And finally, the act provides for consumer education.

Labels can provide a wealth of information, provided the consumer knows what he is looking for and how to interpret what he finds. In the future, label information should be more abundant, clearer, and ultimately more helpful. Until then, consider the following when comparison shopping . . . and let the buyer beware!

Ingredient List

All packaged foods, except those with standardized ingredients such as ice cream and peanut butter, must be labeled with a list of ingredients written in order of descending weight. Items appearing at the beginning of the list are contained in greater concentration than those at the end. For instance, ingredient lists of fruit-ades reveal that they contain more sugar than fruit.

(continued)

Labeling Lingo

Serving Size

Unfortunately, serving sizes are not yet uniform among comparable items, and inaccurate comparisons regarding nutritional value and cost can easily be made. The sugar content of cereals can vary from 0 to 15 g, but portion sizes also vary from ⅓ to 1¼ cup.

Nutrient Claims

Claims of "No Cholesterol" on a container of hydrogenated vegetable shortening are misleading: Vegetable oils never contained cholesterol, but their saturated fat content may render the product unacceptable for people trying to eat a heart-healthy diet. Likewise, claims that a product is, for instance, "80% fat free" (therefore 20% fat) mislead the consumer into thinking that the product is within the recommended 30% level for fat. The product actually contains 20% fat by *weight*, not by calories, as recommended by the Dietary Guidelines. For instance, 2% milk contains 2% fat by weight. Unfortunately, that 2% fat weight translates into 37.5% fat calories: 5 g of fat contained in a cup of 2% milk provides 45 fat calories (5 g × 9 cal/g), or 37.5% of the 120 total calories provided.

Vegetable Oils

For the convenience of food manufacturers who vary the type of oils in their products based on availability and price, the disclaimer "may contain one or more of the following partially hydrogenated oils..." can be used on ingredient lists. However, it leaves consumers in the dark as to the actual oil used in that particular batch of product. If the disclaimer is used near the end of the ingredient list, or if the fat content per serving is small, it may not matter that the specific type of oil used is not known. But if it is a high-fat item, it may be wise to shop for a comparable item made with a known, and accepted, type of fat.

The following descriptive terms regarding calories and sodium are established; the cholesterol definitions are awaiting completion of the regulatory process.

Established Terms	*Definition and Requirement*
Low calorie	Less than or equal to 40 calories per serving and less than or equal to 0.4 calories per gram
Reduced calorie	At least ⅓ fewer calories, but otherwise nutritionally equivalent to the food it replaces; requires a statement of comparison

(continued)

Food for Thought
(continued)

Labeling Lingo

Sodium-free	Less than 5 mg of sodium per serving
Very low sodium	35 mg of sodium or less in a serving
Reduced sodium	For foods in which the usual level of sodium is reduced by at least 75%
Unsalted or no salt added, or some equivalent	For foods once processed with salt but now produced without it. However, the food may contain other forms of sodium

Proposed terms:

Cholesterol-free	Less than 2 mg of cholesterol per serving
Low cholesterol	Less than 20 mg of cholesterol per serving
Cholesterol reduced	For products reformulated or processed to reduce cholesterol by 50% or more

Guidelines only
(proposed regulations are under development):

Low fat	Less than or equal to 3 gm of fat per serving and less than or equal to 10% fat dry weight basis
Reduced fat	At least 50% reduction of fat compared to food it replaces; requires a statement of comparison

(Adapted from Pennington JAT, Wilkening VL, Vanderveen JE: Descriptive terms for food labeling. Journal of Nutrition Education 22(1): 51, 1990)

EXAMPLE

Nutrient	Amount/1000 Calories of Braised Beef Kidney*	Nutrient Allowances/ 1000 Calories†	INQ
Iron	41.6 mg	8 mg	41.6/8 = 5.2
Calcium	43.4 mg	450 mg	43.4/450 = 0.096

Conclusion: Braised beef liver is an excellent source of iron and a poor source of calcium.

* *Information from Pennington JAT, Church HN: Food Values of Portions Commonly Used, 15th ed. Philadelphia, JB Lippincott, 1989*

† *Information from Hansen RG, Wyse BW: Expression of nutrient allowances per 100 kilocalories. J Am Diet Assoc 76:223, 1980*

Unfortunately, the nutrient density approach is a complex plan that requires mathematical calculation or the use of tables. Also, there is limited information currently available on the amounts of nutrients per 1000 calories of food or the RDA for nutrients per 1000 calories of intake, and it does not provide data on whether total nutrient needs are met.

PERSONAL CONSIDERATIONS

A person's food preferences, choices, and aversions are continuously shaped by evolving physical, physiologic, and psychosocial factors (Table 8-5). Before planning a diet, factors influencing food habits and their relative importance to the person must be assessed. Positive aspects of an individual's food habits should be maintained and encouraged; diet changes should be implemented prudently within the context of the person's normal diet.

Although not static, conservative traditional influences like culture, geographic region, and religion have a stabilizing effect on food habits. Even though these influences do not have an equal impact on all people within a group, generalizations can be made about their characteristic food patterns and habits.

Culture

Culture encompasses the total way of life of a particular population or community at a given time. Culture, as such, defines what food is, which foods are appropriate for particular groups within the culture, how food should be handled, prepared, and stored, eating behaviors, the meaning of food and eating, attitudes towards obesity and body size, and the relationship between diet and health. However, culture is not a static influence, and at any given time culture may change to reflect ongoing changes in lifestyle, attitudes, technology, and environment.

As people of various ethnic backgrounds and nationalities settled in the United States, different cultural food patterns blended and adapted to American culture. First-generation Americans usually adhere more closely to cultural food patterns than subsequent generations, who may follow cultural patterns only on holidays and family gatherings. Even within a cultural group, food habits vary significantly among individuals and families.

Black American or "soul food" is based on foods abundant in the South; Blacks living in the North may be unfamiliar with the following "soul foods":

- Meat from all parts of the pig: ears, tails, feet, chin bone, pork chops, ham hocks, bacon, salt pork, spareribs, and chitterlings (intestines)
- Poultry, fried fish, wild game when available (rabbit, woodchuck, pheasant, possum, beaver, squirrel)
- Stewed okra, corn, tomatoes
- Greens cooked in fatback or salt pork served with cornbread
- Sweet potatoes, sweet potato pie, rice, grits
- Black-eyed peas and other dried beans
- Sweets, sweetened flavored drinks

Frying, barbecuing, and stewing are the most popular methods of preparation; milk and dairy products are not often used.

Mexican staples are corn, pinto or calico beans, rice, and chili peppers. Tomatoes are used frequently; meat, eggs, and milk infrequently. Most foods are fried and liberally seasoned with red chili powder, garlic, onion, and spices. Popular foods include the following:

- Chili con carne: a seasoned mixed dish made with beans and meat
- Tamales: seasoned mixture of corn meal and ground pork rolled in corn husks and steamed

Table 8-5
Factors Influencing Food Habits

Factors	Comments
PHYSICAL FACTORS	
Geographic location and climate	Food supply and price are influenced by location and climate.
Food technology	Food technology has greatly increased the variety and amount of foods available.
Income	Generally as income rises protein intake increases and carbohydrate intake decreases.
Storage and cooking facilities	Inadequate storage and cooking facilities limit the type and variety of food consumed.
PHYSIOLOGIC FACTORS	
Stage of development	Foods are often associated with certain age groups: milk with infancy, peanut butter and jelly with childhood, hamburgers and fries with adolescence, and tea and toast with the elderly.
State of health	People often revert to childhood eating behaviors and food preferences when recovering from an illness. They may, for example, request chicken noodle soup and ice cream because these items are associated with recovery from childhood illnesses.
Sense of taste and smell	Sense of taste and smell, and therefore food preferences, vary widely among individuals. The ability to taste and smell decreases in the elderly.
Hunger	Hunger is the least common reason why Americans eat.
PSYCHOSOCIAL FACTORS	
Culture	See section on Culture.
Religion	See section on Religion.
Advertising	Food companies spend millions of dollars annually promoting their products. Advertising tends to have the greatest impact on school-aged children.
Family tradition	Parents are the primary gatekeepers of young children's food intake, and young children tend to imitate their parents' food preferences, aversions, and habits.
Education	Generally, the more education that an individual has, the greater his variety of food choices.
Politics	May influence the availability, price, and quality of the food supply.
Social status	Certain foods are associated with poverty or low social status (macaroni, nonfat dry milk); others with wealth and social position (wild rice, caviar)
Food ideology	People may assign meanings to foods; for example, red meat and potatoes may be viewed as "masculine," salads and quiche as "feminine."
Learned aversions	Foods associated with a previous illness may be avoided, whether or not the food actually caused the illness.

- Tortillas: thin baked or fried "bread" made from lime-treated wheat flour or whole corn
- Frijoles refritas: refried pinto or calico beans
- Enchiladas: tortillas filled with cheese, onion, and lettuce
- Tacos: fried tortillas filled with meat or beans, onion, lettuce, and hot sauce

- Chorizo: Mexican sausage
- Sopapillas: fried bread dough

Puerto Rican staples are rice, beans, and viandas (starchy root vegetables such as sweet potatoes, cassava, and plantains). Other commonly used foods are as follows:

- Salted codfish, chicken, pork, and beef
- Dried peas and beans cooked with tomatoes, peppers, onions, garlic, salt pork, and seasonings
- Fruits abundant in Puerto Rico, such as bananas, oranges, pineapple, mango, papaya, and acerola
- Cafe con lèche (coffee and hot milk)

Italian staples are pasta served with a variety of sauces and crusty Italian bread. Eggs, cheese, tomatoes, and green vegetables are used liberally. Only small amounts of meat are used in many dishes. Popular foods include

- Pepperoni: highly seasoned sausage
- Minestrone: soup made with dried peas and beans
- Polenta: thickened cornmeal mush served plain or with tomato sauce and cheese
- Pizza: dough topped with vegetables, meat, cheese, and spices
- Ravioli: pockets of noodles filled with cheese and topped with sauce

Middle Eastern staples are rice and bulgur (cracked whole wheat), served alone or with vegetables and meat. Lamb, mutton, poultry, and chickpeas are commonly used, as is fermented milk (yogurt, matzoon, and leben). Fresh fruits are used liberally; eggplant, tomatoes, okra, beets, and spinach are favorite vegetables. Dates, olives, and figs are native to the area. Popular dishes include

- Shashlik: ground meat baked in cabbage leaves, and pieces of cut lamb skewered with tomato and onion
- Tabouli: salad made with bulgur, vegetables, and mint
- Hummus: seasoned chickpea spread
- Kibee: fresh raw ground lamb, seasoned and eaten uncooked

Oriental staples are rice, wheat, and millet. Soybean sprouts and soybean paste (miso) are used extensively in Chinese cooking. Small amounts of chicken, pork, eggs, fish, and shellfish are usually stir-fried with vegetables. Milk, cheese, and beef are not common foods. Soy sauce is used extensively. Common seasonings include almonds, MSG, sesame seeds, and ginger. Sesame oil, peanut oil, and lard are often used in food preparation. Tea is the common beverage.

An important principle of Chinese eating patterns involves balancing "yin" (cold) and "yang" (hot) foods. "Hot" foods include fried, spicy, and rich foods. "Cold" foods are generally leafy green vegetables. Many Chinese believe that proper balance of hot and cold foods is necessary for good health and that an excess of either will cause poor health.[3]

Geographic Region

In addition to the sharing of cultural food patterns within the United States' melting pot, advances in food technology and transportation have vastly increased the variety and availability of food across the country. Although "regional" foods are available anywhere, certain areas of the country are noted for certain foods:

- New England: Boston baked beans, clam chowder, lobster, and clam cakes
- Pennsylvania Dutch: shoofly pie, scrapple, and German-style sausage
- The South: grits, fried chicken, hot biscuits, greens, sweet potatoes, and corn bread
- Louisiana: French and Creole-style cooking
- Texas: chili con carne
- The Southwest: Mexican foods such as tortillas, tamales, enchiladas, and refried beans
- The Far West: citrus fruit, fresh produce, salads, and Oriental cooking
- The Midwest: dairy products and beef

Religion

Religion may assign a particular meaning to food or restrict its use, and religious affiliation may have a greater impact on food habits than nationality or culture (*e.g.*, Orthodox Jews follow Kosher dietary laws regardless of their national origin).

- *Roman Catholics* do not eat meat on Ash Wednesday or Good Friday.
- *Muslims* cannot eat pork in any form. Alcohol is prohibited. Eating is a matter of worship.
- *Hindus* are vegetarians; beef is especially sacred.
- *Seventh Day Adventists* are lacto-ovovegetarians. Coffee, tea, and alcohol are prohibited. An interval of 5 to 6 hours between meals is recommended, with no snacking between meals.
- *Mormons (Church of Jesus Christ of the Latter-Day Saints)* do not use coffee, tea, alcohol, or tobacco.
- *Orthodox Jews* can eat only kosher meat and poultry that has been slaughtered according to ritual, soaked in water, salted, and washed. Shellfish and all pork products are prohibited. Milk and dairy products are used widely but cannot be consumed at the same meal as meat or poultry. Dairy products are not allowed within 6 hours after eating meat or poultry; meat and poultry cannot be eaten for 30 minutes after dairy products have been consumed. Separate utensils must be used for preparing and serving meat and dairy products.

    Food preparation is prohibited on the Sabbath. Religious holidays are celebrated with certain foods; for example, only unleavened bread is eaten during Passover; a 24-hour fast is observed on Yom Kippur.

    Because of the rigid dietary laws, Orthodox Jews rarely eat outside the home, with the exception of homes or restaurants with kosher kitchens.
- *Conservative Jews* may follow the Jewish dietary laws at home, but take a more liberal attitude on social occasions.
- *Reform Jews* may not follow any religious dietary laws.

FOOD QUALITY AND SAFETY CONSIDERATIONS

Planning an adequate diet relates not only to nutritional adequacy and an individual's psychosocial and cultural needs, but also to food quality and safety concerns. Proper storage and preparation are vital to ensure that the vitamin and mineral content of a food is retained. Food-borne illness represents a threat when food is improperly handled or stored, and naturally occurring toxicants may be a much greater threat to health than man-made pesticides.

Retaining the Nutrient Content of Food

Even when carefully planned, there are no guarantees that a diet will provide optimal amounts of all nutrients, especially if the food eaten has been improperly stored or overly processed. Generally, food begins to lose its nutrients the moment that harvesting or processing begins,[4] and the more that is done to a food before it is eaten, the greater the nutrient loss. Heat, light, air, soaking in water, mechanical injury, dry storage, and acidic or alkaline food processing ingredients can all hasten nutrient losses. Vitamins, minerals, and fiber are particularly vulnerable to the effects of food processing (see box, Retaining Nutrients in Food, for ways to minimize nutrient losses).

Food-Borne Illness

Pathogenic microorganisms are the leading cause of food-borne illness in the United States and may account for 24 million to as many as 80 million cases of diarrheal illness annually.[16] Most food-borne illness is caused by long-recognized bacterial species, namely *Salmonella*, *Staphylococcus aureus*, *Clostridium botulinum*, and *Clostridium perfringens*. However, it is estimated that in more than half the cases of food-related disease the pathogen is not known. "New" disease organisms have been identified within the last 15 years, and there has also been an increase in reporting of virus involvement and some new manifestations of long-recognized species of food-borne pathogens.[9] Food-borne illness outbreaks related to seafood consumption have also increased dramatically.

Worldwide, the majority of food-borne illness are caused by salmonellae, which are found in the intestinal tracts of humans and domestic and wild warm-blooded animals.[2] Salmonellae can easily pass from the intestinal tract to food during preparation without proper hand washing. In the United States, there have been large increases in *Salmonella enteritidis* infections caused by shell eggs: Salmonellae on the shells can contaminate the egg during preparation and service. Even uncracked eggs have been implicated in recent years for the sudden increase *S. enteritidis* infections. Salmonellae infects about half of poultry broiler carcasses, but only about 1% of beef and lamb carcasses.

Symptoms of *S. enteritidis* infection usually appear within 12 to 36 hours after infection and last from 2 to 5 days. Estimated annual total costs in the United States because of treatment, lost wages, and all related expenses is about $1.4 billion.

S. aureus, present on the skin and in boils, pimples, and throat infections, can produce a toxin at warm temperatures. It is easily spread to food when sanitary food handling practices are not followed. Meat, poultry, salads containing meat or poultry, cheese, egg products, starchy salads, custards, and cream-filled desserts are most often implicated. Symptoms of vomiting and diarrhea may last 1 to 2 days.

C. botulinum produces a toxin so potent that it is usually fatal. Home-canned, low-acid foods that have not been properly processed are a frequent cause of botulism. However, unexpected foods such as fried onions and chopped garlic have also caused outbreaks.[9] As

Retaining Nutrients in Food

Food Purchasing

Don't buy produce that is damaged or wilted, or that has been improperly stored.

Whenever possible, buy frozen foods instead of canned foods. Canning procedures (blanching, sterilizing, and soaking) destroy nutrients.

Whenever possible, buy produce that was picked when fully ripe. It is higher in nutrients than produce picked when green.

Food Storage

Avoid storing foods for a long time.

Avoid exposing food to light, especially milk. As little as 2 hours of light can decrease the riboflavin content of milk by 20% to 80%.

Keep milk cold and covered.

Refrigerate fruits and vegetables immediately to slow enzyme activity and retain nutrients; keep produce in the refrigerator crisper or in moisture-proof bags.

Avoid storing vegetables after they have been cut, since air can destroy nutrients (oxidation).

Store frozen foods at 0°F or below; even the nutrients in canned foods will be preserved better if stored below 65°F.

Food Preparation

Wash produce, but don't soak, to avoid leaching nutrients.

Use the dark outer leaves of salad plants whenever possible. They are higher in vitamins and iron than the light inner leaves.

Avoid peeling and paring vegetables before cooking because a valuable layer of nutrients is stored directly beneath the skin. If necessary, scrape or pare as thin a layer as possible.

Avoid cutting produce into small pieces: The larger the surface area, the greater the nutrient loss.

Prepare vegetables as close to serving time as possible to avoid excessive exposure to light and air.

Inactivate oxidative enzymes with an acidic solution (*e.g.,* lemon juice, salad dressings) because oxidation destroys vitamins and causes fruits (*e.g.,* bananas) and vegetables to brown.

(continued)

Retaining Nutrients in Food (*continued*)

Cooking

Eat some fruits and vegetables raw.

Cook produce in as little water as possible to avoid leaching vitamins. Stir-fry, steam, microwave, or pressure-cook vegetables.

Shorten cooking time as much as possible by

Cooking vegetables to the tender–crunchy, rather than to the mushy stage of doneness

Covering the pan to retain heat

Starting foods in a hot pan or hot water to speed heating time

Use aluminum, stainless steel, glass, or enamel cookware to retain vitamin C because cooking in copper pots can destroy vitamin C.

Cook vegetables in their skin whenever possible.

Don't thaw frozen vegetables before cooking.

If water is used in cooking, save and use as stock for soups, gravies, or sauces.

Cook only as much as needed at a time: Reheating vegetables causes considerable loss of vitamins.

Do not add baking soda to vegetables while cooking: Alkaline solutions destroy thiamine (vitamin B_1), riboflavin (vitamin B_2), and vitamin C.

Do not toast or brown dry rice before steaming so that the thiamine content can be retained.

Cook meat at simmering temperatures and just until tender because cooking meat by moist heat methods (braising, stewing) increases mineral losses.

Cook oven roasted meats only to the rare or medium stage of doneness.

a precaution, cans whose clear liquids have turned milky, cans that are swollen or dented, jars with cracks or loose-fitting lids, and any can or jar that has an off-odor when opened should all be discarded.

C. perfringens, a spore-forming bacterium, most often occurs when large amounts of food cool slowly, either in the refrigerator or in chafing dishes or steam tables that fail to keep food hot enough. Diarrhea usually lasts less than a day; however, consequences can be serious for the elderly and people with ulcers.

Escherichia coli was once considered an infrequent cause of food-borne illness. However, in 1982 a strain of *E. coli* was identified as a food-borne pathogen responsible for beef- and raw milk-linked cases of hemorrhagic colitis and hemolytic uremic syndrome.[5] In addition, food and water fecally contaminated with *E. coli* are blamed for travelers' diarrhea.

"Newer" pathogenic bacteria have been identified within the last 15 years as significant agents in food-borne illness. *Listeria monocytogenes*, recognized as an animal pathogen for more than 50 years, has only recently been identified as a serious food-borne pathogen. Infection can cause abortion in pregnant women and meningitis in infants and immunocompromised adults. Contaminated coleslaw, milk, and cheese are blamed for recent outbreaks of listeriosis that resulted in more than 100 deaths.[16] As a result of these fatalities, the FDA increased its surveillance and found *Listeria* in a variety of dairy products. Numerous recalls followed for chocolate milk, ice cream mix, ice cream novelties, and brie and other soft-ripened cheeses. Because *Listeria* is so widespread and appears to be able to survive short-term pasteurization temperatures used in processing, it poses a serious threat to public health.

Yersinia enterocolitica, an anaerobic organism that is able to grow in normal refrigeration, is most often found in pork, but outbreaks have been linked to contaminated milk, chocolate milk, and tofu. Symptoms of infection include diarrhea, fever, and severe lower abdominal pain that mimics acute appendicitis. Young children appear most vulnerable.

Campylobacter jejuni is the leading cause of acute gastroenteritis in humans.[16] *C. jejuni* is found primarily in the intestines of mammals and birds; fecal excrement can contaminate foods. Raw milk, cake icing, eggs, poultry, and beef all have been vehicles for transmission. Symptoms of infection—diarrhea, pain, fever, nausea, and vomiting—can range from mild to severe.

A strain of *Vibrio cholerae* is responsible for mild gastroenteritis, soft tissue infections, and septicemia. Outbreaks, related to eating undercooked, contaminated crabs and raw oysters or other shellfish, are generally limited in the United States to the coastal areas.

The major cause of food-borne infections is unsanitary food handling. To reduce the risk of contamination (see box, Safe Food Handling), proper personal hygiene and handwashing must be practiced by all food handlers. Steps must also be taken to prevent cross-contamination between raw and cooked foods and through food handlers. Thorough cooking of meat and fish is vital, as is pasteurization of all milk products, and adequate refrigeration. Infants, the elderly, and people with compromised immune systems are particularly vulnerable to the effects of food poisoning.

Naturally Occurring Toxicants in Foods

"Natural" ingredients in food include the energy nutrients (carbohydrates, protein, fat, and alcohol), essential nutrients (vitamins and minerals), dietary fiber, and naturally occurring compounds like caffeine and sterols.[14] However, certain toxins and antinutrients may also be natural ingredients in foods; as such, "natural" foods are not synonymous with "safe" foods.

Naturally occurring toxicants are present as normal ingredients in many plant foods (Table 8-6), since plants produce these toxins to protect themselves from predators. It is estimated that we consume 10,000 times more natural toxins by weight than man-made pesticides.[1] Still, the quantity of natural toxins consumed is generally so small that health is not endangered unless large amounts are eaten over a long period of time. A varied diet is the best assurance against untoward effects of both natural and "unnatural" toxins. Goitrogens can be classified as antinutrients because they induce goiter by their antithyroid action. Goitrogens are prevalent in members of the *Brassica* genus: cabbage,

Safe Food Handling

- Do not work with food if you have an infectious disease or infected cuts or other skin infections.
- Always work with clean hands, clean fingernails, and clean hair, and wear clean clothing.
- Wash hands thoroughly after handling raw meat, poultry, or eggs and before working with other food.
- Keep hands away from the mouth, nose, and hair.
- Avoid using the same spoon more than once for tasting food while preparing, cooking, or serving.
- Do not serve baby foods directly from the jar or can to avoid contaminating any remaining food.
- Never store cleaning supplies, pesticides, and drug with food or in food containers such as soda bottles and food jars.
- Refrigerate perishable foods at 40°F or below. Store perishable and frozen foods in the refrigerator and freezer as soon after shopping as possible.
- Keep hot foods hot—above 140°F—and cold foods cold—below 40°F. Foods that are held for more than 2 or 3 hours at a temperature between 60°F and 125°F may not be safe to eat.
- Keep food that contains milk or egg products and little vinegar or other acids refrigerated. This includes cream, custard, and meringue pies; foods that contain custard filings, such as cakes, cream puffs, and eclairs; and salads and sandwich fillings. If taken on summer outings, these foods should be kept in a cooler with ice or reusable cold packs.
- Cook commercially frozen stuffed poultry from the frozen state and keep it in the refrigerator until time to start cooking. If stuffing is made in advance at home, store it separately in the refrigerator. Stuff the bird just before putting it into the hot oven.
- Remove the stuffing from all leftover cooked meat, poultry, or fish before storing, and store it in the refrigerator in separate container.
- Refrigerate leftover meat, fish, poultry, broth, and gravy immediately after a meal. Freeze them if they are to be kept longer than a few days.
- Clean all dishes, utensils, and work surfaces thoroughly with soap and water after each use. It is especially important to clean equipment and work surfaces that have been used for raw food, such as raw poultry or meat, before they are used for cooked food or foods such as salads that are eaten without cooking. A solution prepared with 1 tbsp chlorine laundry bleach in 1 quart of cold water destroys bacteria. This solution can be used for rinsing utensils and work surfaces. Equipment such as cutting boards, meat grinder, blenders, and can openers particularly need to be sanitized in this way.

(continued)

Safe Food Handling (*continued*)

- Serve foods immediately after cooking or refrigerate promptly. Hot foods can be placed in the refrigerator as long as they do not raise the temperature of the refrigerator above 45°F. Large quantities of food can be cooled more quickly if refrigerated in shallow containers.
- Thaw frozen meat, fish, and poultry in the refrigerator. These meats may be cooked from the frozen state if cooked for at least 1½ times as long as required for the unfrozen product. Undercooked foods may be unsafe. Cook stuffing to a temperature of at least 165°F, even if you are cooking it separately. Use a meat thermometer.
- Heat leftovers thoroughly; boil broths and gravies for several minutes before reusing.
- Handle foods to be put in your home freezer as little as possible to keep bacteria at a minimum before freezing. Freezing does not kill bacteria but merely stops their growth; the bacteria then continue to multiply when the food is thawed.
- Avoid home canning of meat and poultry. It is too risky.
- Can low-acid vegetables in a pressure canner at the proper temperature and for the time specified in the directions. The boiling-water-bath method is safe only for fruits, high-acid red tomatoes, and jellies and jams.
- Simmer all home-canned vegetables, meat, and poultry for 10 to 20 minutes befor tasting.
- Heating makes the odor of spoilage more noticeable. If a food looks spoiled, foams, or has an off-odor, destroy it without tasting.
- Do not eat moldy foods. Discard the entire food, including those portions on which the mold is not apparent.
- Do not use fresh raw eggs in eggnog or soft custard, especially when serving the food to small children or persons in a weakened condition. Use pasteurized dried egg powder instead.
- Use cracked eggs only if thoroughly cooked, as in hard-cooked eggs or baked dishes.

(Eschelman MM: Introductory Nutrition and Diet Therapy, 2nd ed. Philadelphia: JB Lippincott, 1991)

turnip, mustard greens, and radish. Avidin, another antinutrient that destroys the vitamin biotin, is found in raw egg white.

ECONOMIC FEASIBILITY

Consumers are faced with the challenge of selecting an adequate diet, usually within a given food budget, from approximately 12,000 different items found in the average

Table 8-6
Naturally Occurring Plant Toxins

Toxin	Effect	Food Source
Protease inhibitors	Inhibit proteolytic enzyme activity of certain enzymes	Legumes, including a trypsin inhibitor in raw soybeans Also in wheat, oats, barley, rice, and potatoes
Hemagglutinins	Agglutinate RBC; cause inflammation of GI tract, local hemorrhages	Mainly found in seeds, with lesser amounts in leaves, bark, roots, and tubers Found in soybeans, kidney beans, black beans, and wax beans Largely destroyed in the GI tract; only small amounts are absorbed
Favism	Hemolytic anemia in sensitive individuals with inherited metabolic deficiency Most common among people from Mediterranean area or Asia	Fava or broad beans
Hepatotoxins (*Senecio* alkaloids)	Delayed liver damage Potent liver toxins at low to moderate exposure	Seeds of the *Senecio* genus, which grow interspersed with grains, contaminate grains or corn during mechanical harvest
Aflatoxin	Hepatoxic and carcinogenic	Fungal mold on peanuts and corn

supermarket. The following shopping suggestions are appropriate for anyone concerned with getting the most nutrition for their food dollar.

Supermarket Savvy[17]

Eat before you shop.

Shop without the children whenever possible.

Note special sales and stock up on nonperishables as much as storage space and budget will allow.

Do not go down an aisle more than once.

Read labels and compare prices.

Do not be an impulse buyer.

Ask for a raincheck if the store runs out of a sale item.

Make sure items on sale are properly priced to avoid paying the regular price.

Plan Ahead

Make a list and stick to it.

Organize items on your list according to the store's layout to save time and energy and reduce the risk of impulse buying while looking for needed items.

Coupons

Only clip and use coupons for items that you normally purchase. You don't save any money if you use a coupon to purchase something you don't use or need.

Use coupons for a competitor's brand of an item only if it saves you money and the quality is comparable. Getting a few cents off an overpriced item isn't much of a bargain.

If possible, shop at a store that doubles or triples coupons.

Generic Brands

Try various products to see if the quality is acceptable.

Use generic brands when acceptable. Nutritionally, generic foods are similar to name brands—the difference is in the size and uniformity of the pieces. Use generic products in recipes in which appearance and uniformity are not important, such as casseroles and soups.

Avoid Waste

Do not buy spoiled food, bulging cans, or produce that is wilted, decayed, bruised, or filled with soft spots.

Buy perishables, especially frozen foods, last and put them away first.

Avoid buying frozen food that has been partially thawed.

Check expiration dates (usually a "sell by" date).

Rotate food at home, using the oldest food first.

Comparison Shop

Check unit prices to compare values.

Be aware that the economy size is not always cheaper.

Buy the economy size if it is cheaper and you can use it or store it without wasting it.

Cans of sliced or diced fruits and vegetables are generally cheaper than whole or half styles.

Frozen vegetables sold with sauces, nuts, or other ingredients cost more per serving than plain vegetables. Add your own toppings.

Compare price per serving for meats, not price per pound.

In general, the larger cuts of meat and whole chickens are cheaper than smaller pieces. If freezer space allows, buy large cuts and cut them up yourself.

Shop in a store that regularly offers lower prices instead of choosing a store that has one or two items you need on sale.

Marked-Down Items

Buy day-old bread that has been marked down to use for stuffing, bread crumbs, bread pudding, or casseroles.

Buy marked-down undamaged produce only if you intend to use it immediately.

Bulk Foods

Compare prices: the savings on some bulk items may be up to 50%, whereas other items (such as flour) may cost more.

Buy only as much as you need.

For added safety, look for items dispensed by gravity or from containers with close-fitting covers.

Avoid bins that do not have scoops attached because unattached scoops could fall on the floor or get buried in the food.

Food Warehouses

(No-frills stores with minimal service)

Bring your own bags or boxes and be prepared to pack them yourself.

Although brand names are available, the variety is less than in a supermarket and usually is inconsistent.

Food Co-ops

(Nonprofit stores run by members)

Take advantage of this opportunity if you can.

Be prepared to volunteer several hours a month in order to join, but the savings are worth it, especially for perishables.

Change Your Eating Habits for Better Health and Bigger Savings

Consider using nonfat dry milk for cooking or drinking. It has all the nutrients of whole milk with none of the fat.

Eat less red meat and more poultry.

Serve an occasional meatless meal based on eggs, cheese, or dried beans and peas.

Avoid packaged items and convenience products that are often laden with salt and cost more than the homemade version.

Buy fruits and vegetables in season.

Avoid empty calorie extras such as soft drinks, candy, cakes, pies, doughnuts, sweet rolls, cookies, and traditional snack foods.

Beware of Supermarketing

The dairy case is usually located farthest from the front door so that people just wanting to buy milk have to walk through the entire store, giving them the opportunity to buy something else.

The prime selling area is at eye level (adult height for adult items and child height for child items). Bargains may be available at higher and lower levels.

End-of-aisle displays are not always sale items.

Checkout line goodies are obvious temptations to impulse buying: Resist the urge.

BIBLIOGRAPHY

1. Alfin-Slater RB (ed): Food-borne diseases. Nutrition and the M.D. 16(6):3, 1990
2. Baird-Parker AC: Foodborne salmonellosis. The Lancet 336:1231, 1990
3. Chau P, Lee H, Tseng R, et al: Dietary habits, health beliefs, and food practices of elderly Chinese Women. J Am Diet Assoc 90:579, 1990
4. Derelian D: The four food groups: An instructional tool for adults. Nutrition News 51(1):1, 1988
5. Doyle MP: Foodborne illness: Pathogenic *Escherichia coli, Yersinia enterocolitica,* and *Vibrio parahaemolyticus.* The Lancet 336:1111, 1990
6. Eschelman MM: Introductory Nutrition and Diet Therapy. 2nd ed. Philadelphia: JB Lippincott, 1991
7. Geiger CJ, Wyse BW, Parent CRM, et al: Review of nutrition labeling formats. J Am Diet Assoc 91:808, 1991
8. Hansen RG: An index of food quality. Nutr Rev 31:1, 1973
9. Liston J: Current issues in food safety-especially seafoods. J Am Diet Assoc 89:911, 1989
10. Mayer J (ed): The dietary guidelines become more user friendly. Tufts University Diet and Nutrition Letter 8(11):4, 1991
11. Monsen ER: What's in a food? J Am Diet Assoc 91:777, 1991
12. National Research Council: Recommended Dietary Allowances. 10th ed. Washington, DC: National Academy Press, 1989
13. Pennington JAT, Church HN: Food Values of Portions Commonly Used. 14th ed. Philadelphia: JB Lippincott, 1985
14. Pennington JAT, Wilkening VL, Vanderveen JE: Descriptive terms for food labeling. Journal of Nutrition Education 22(1):51, 1990
15. Public Health Service, United States Department of Health and Human Services: The Surgeon General's Report on Nutrition and Health: Summary and Recommendations. DHHS (PHS) Publication no. 88-50211. Washington DC: Government Printing Office, 1988
16. Ryser ET, Marth EH: "New" food-borne pathogens of public health significance. J Am Diet Assoc 89:948, 1989
17. Smith SM (ed): Supermarket savvy—how to save money. Environmental Nutrition Newsletter 8(3):S-1, 1985
18. United States Department of Agriculture, and United States Department of Health and Human Services: Nutrition and Your Health: Dietary Guidelines for Americans. 3rd ed. Home and Garden Bulletin no. 232, 1990
19. United States Department of Health and Human Services: A Consumer's Guide to Food Labels. DHHS Publication no. (FDA) 90-2083. Rockville, MD: Government Printing Office, 1990
20. Watt BK: Tables of food composition: Uses and limitations. Contemporary Nutrition 5(2), 1980

9 Assessing Nutritional Status

Nutritional status, or the state of balance between nutrient supply (intake) and demand (requirement), has a significant impact on both health and disease. For the "well" client, an optimum nutritional status helps maintain health, promotes normal growth and development, and protects against disease. During illness, an optimum nutritional status can reduce the risk of complications and hasten recovery. Conversely, a poor nutritional status (malnutrition) increases morbidity and mortality.

Malnutrition, a general term that literally means "bad" nutrition, may be caused by nutritional excesses (*e.g.*, obesity) or deficiencies (other variables and classifications of malnutrition are listed in Table 9-1). Severe deficiencies of specific nutrients (*e.g.*, vitamin C) can produce specific nutritional disorders (*e.g.*, scurvy); mild nutritional deficiencies in general can interfere with the ability to function, the quality of life, and the sense of well-being. Various nutritional assessment techniques can be used to identify deficiencies at certain stages of development, because the effects of nutrient deficiencies progress in a sequential and predictable manner (see box, Sequential Development of Malnutrition/Nutritional Assessment Methods).

Nutritional assessment is the process of collecting and interpreting data in order to evaluate an individual's nutritional status and identify nutritional needs. The focus of assessment in the hospital setting is to identify protein–calorie malnutrition. The process of assessment is followed by planning (determining what actions are necessary to achieve nutritional goals, when and how the actions are to be taken, and who should implement the actions), implementation (putting the plan into action), and evaluation (determining the effectiveness of the plan and revising the plan as needed) (see box, Nutritional Care Process).

Nutritional assessment is more than simply looking at diet to see if nutrient intake is adequate, although dietary evaluation is certainly a component of a nutritional assessment. Nutritional assessment criteria, frequently referred to as the ABCDs, include **a**nthropometric measurements, **b**iochemical data, **c**linical observations, and **d**ietary data; they may be used individually or collectively. Obviously, the more information obtained from a variety of sources (Table 9-2), the more accurate and reliable the assessment will be.

Table 9-1
Variable Classifications of Malnutrition

Variables	Classifications
Type	Overnutrition (*i.e.,* obesity) or undernutrition
Cause	Endogenous (*i.e.,* faulty metabolism) or exogenous (*i.e.,* inadequate intake)
Nutrients	Specific (*i.e.,* one nutrient) or multiple
Degree	Mild, moderate, or severe
Duration	Acute or chronic
Outcome	Reversible or irreversible

However, comprehensive nutritional assessments are not always appropriate or necessary, depending on the purpose of the assessment and the availability of equipment, time, personnel, and funds. Assessment levels range from minimal (screening) to in-depth (comprehensive) and can be "custom-made" for a particular population or setting.

In most health care facilities, the responsibility for nutritional assessment and support is shared by the physician, the dietitian, and the nurse. By using their communication and diagnostic skills, nurses are able to obtain screening data through routine nursing histories and physical examinations. Depending on the setting and availability of personnel, the nurse may assist and coordinate nutritional care activities or may be responsible for identifying high-risk clients. The nurse's ability to coordinate activities among health care team members, and close, continual interaction with the client and family place him or her in an ideal position to facilitate the nutritional care process, make appropriate referrals as needed, or initiate nutritional care.

LEVELS OF ASSESSMENT

Screening

Screening is a simple, easy, and cost-effective assessment tool that uses a minimum amount of data to assign relative risk; nutritional screening is used to identify clients with actual or potential nutritional problems who require nutritional intervention to either treat or prevent malnutrition. Screening can be custom-designed for a particular population (*e.g.,* pregnant women) or for a specific disorder (*e.g.,* cardiac disease).

To be both useful and efficient in the clinical setting, screening tools generally rely on data routinely available on admission to a hospital or health care facility. Much controversy exists about the accuracy and validity of screening data, especially anthropometric and biochemical data. Some studies have found that anthropometric measurements alone, such as weight loss greater than 10 pounds, are sufficient to predict mortality.[2] Other clinical studies have shown that both anthropometric and biochemical measures are necessary to evaluate the nutritional status of hospitalized clients.[2] Most experts agree that the most accurate method of identifying future nutritional risk is a combination of both selected anthropometric and biochemical data.

Sequential Development of Malnutrition/Nutritional Assessment Methods

Sequential Development of Malnutrition	Assessment Methods
Inadequate nutrient intake→ primary deficiency	Dietary data, medical–socioeconomic data
and/or	
Altered nutrient digestion, absorption, metabolism, excretion→ secondary deficiency	
↓	
Decreased nutrient content in cells and tissues	Biochemical data
↓	
Biochemical lesions and abnormal metabolism	Biochemical data
↓	
Anatomic lesions and signs of deficiency	Anthropometric measurement, clinical findings

Actual screening data obtained and evaluated vary among settings, the population group being screened, the availability of data, and the screening objectives. For instance, a hospital screening tool for medical–surgical patients is likely to focus on significant unintentional weight loss, serum albumin, total lymphocyte count, and possibly other biochemical data or clinical indicators, such as nausea, vomiting, diarrhea, and fever. A sample screening tool appears in Figure 9-1. A different setting, such as an obstetrics clinic, may concentrate on prepregnancy weight, pattern of weight gain, blood pressure, presence of edema, 24-hour food intake, alterations in gastrointestinal (GI) function, and hemoglobin and hematocrit.

Regardless of what data are gathered, the screening process is not complete until it is evaluated and a relative level of risk is assigned. Interpretation of risk usually is facility-defined, based on the number of abnormal measurements obtained. For instance, in the screening tool that appears in Figure 9-1, the degree of nutritional risk is defined as follows: 0–1 abnormal findings = no nutritional risk, 2 abnormal findings = mild risk, 3 = moderate risk, and 4 or more = severe risk.[2] Clients identified to be at no or mild risk may need only to be reassessed later during their admission to monitor for any deterioration in their nutritional status. An in-depth nutritional assessment is indicated for clients determined to be at moderate or severe risk in order to quantify the degree of malnutrition and to provide a baseline for subsequent nutrition intervention.[6]

Nutritional Care Process: Assessment→ Planning→ Implementation→ Evaluation

The nutritional care process, like the nursing process, is a systematic approach used to identify the client's needs, formulate plans to meet those needs, initiate a plan or assign others to implement it, and evaluate the effectiveness of the plan. As such, it is appropriate for all clients. The following format, which is used throughout the life cycle and clinical practice units of this book, serves as a guideline for determining optimum nutritional care.

Assessment

Assessment is a two-step process that involves both the collection and interpretation of data. In addition to the general assessment criteria listed in each clinical chapter, dietary and nutritional risk factors and signs and symptoms of health disorders should be evaluated for their impact on intake and nutritional status.

Nursing Diagnosis

Nursing diagnoses may relate to nutrition either directly (*i.e.,* altered nutrition is a problem) or indirectly (*i.e.,* change in diet is one of several interventions that will help eliminate a "non-nutritional" problem). "Altered Nutrition: Less than Body Requirements" applies most obviously to people who are underweight. However, less obvious is the impact health alterations and medical treatments have on nutrient intake, digestion, absorption, metabolism, and excretion. For instance, "Altered Nutrition: Less than Body Requirements" may also be appropriate for clients with malabsorption syndrome secondary to pancreatic disease who are unable to digest and absorb adequate calories and nutrients.

Likewise, because nutrition is important all along the wellness–illness continuum, nutrition intervention may be appropriate not only for restoring health in an "ill" client, but also for maintaining or improving health status in a "well" individual. For instance, a "healthy" man with a high cholesterol level who expresses interest in a low-fat, low-cholesterol diet may have the nursing diagnosis of "Health Seeking Behaviors, related to lack of knowledge of a heart-healthy diet and a desire to learn."

Throughout the clinical section of this book, only one nursing diagnosis is given as an example for each medical disorder discussed. Obviously, they represent only one way of looking at a problem; they may not be appropriate or specific for *individuals,* nor are they meant to exclude other diagnoses. In clinical practice, a nursing diagnosis is identified only after thorough analysis of the data.

(continued)

Nutritional Care Process: Assessment→ Planning→ Implementation→ Evaluation (*continued*)

Planning and Implementation

From a nutritional perspective, client goals are objectives that may be achieved through dietary intervention; they are determined on an individual basis after priorities are established. Although planning for high-risk clients may be the responsibility of the dietitian, the nurse may do the planning for healthy clients and those with minor problems.

General short-term client goals that may be appropriate for all clients are to maintain/restore optimal nutritional status and to allow as normal an intake as possible by individualizing the diet according to the client's food habits, preferences, and tolerances. A general long-term goal is to promote good nutritional practices to reduce the risk of chronic diet-related diseases such as obesity, diabetes, hypertension, atherosclerosis, and certain kinds of cancer. Additional goals that may be appropriate for hospitalized clients are to alleviate side effects of the disease or its treatment, if possible, and to prevent complications or recurrences of the disorder, if appropriate.

Inherent in planning individual client goals are the following general considerations:

- Diet orders are not always appropriate.
- Eating behaviors and food preferences may revert to childhood patterns during illness and stress.
- It is not only important that the proper food be served, but moreso that it be consumed. The manner in which food is presented and the attitudes of the health care team members regarding the diet may have a large influence on the client's acceptance.
- Restrictive diets should be progressed as soon as possible to ensure an adequate intake and increase the client's sense of well-being.
- Communication between other members of the health care team is vital.
- Assessment and evaluation are ongoing processes.
- The optimal diet in theory may not be practical for an individual in either the clinical or home setting, depending on the client's prognosis, support systems, level of intelligence and motivation, willingness to cooperate, emotional health, financial status, religious or ethnic background, and other medical conditions.

The *Nursing Interventions* sections of this book deal with diet management, client teaching, and monitoring. *Diet management* provides general guidelines for health maintenance or restoration through general dietary changes, such as increase/decrease, limit/reduce, avoid/encourage, modify/ maintain, promote, and monitor. Specific levels of nutrients or foods allowed

(continued)

Nutritional Care Process: Assessment→ Planning→ Implementation→ Evaluation (*continued*)

depend on the client's condition and the physician's discretion and should be revised as needed.

Client teaching is another important facet of nursing intervention; it may be the nurse's responsibility to provide or reinforce diet instructions to the client and family. Diet instructions are generally most effective when both verbal and written instructions are provided. Clients should always be advised to eliminate any foods not tolerated and to alert the physician if a conflict exists between the diet and religious beliefs, if adverse side effects to the diet develop, or if special foods required by the diet are difficult to locate or are too costly. Compliance should be encouraged, and support and assistance offered. Ideally, teaching should occur over time.

Monitoring is done on an ongoing basis to evaluate the client's tolerance and compliance to the diet and the effectiveness of the diet interventions. Other individual-, disease-, and symptom-related criteria may be indicated.

Evaluation

The effectiveness of the nutritional care plan is evaluated by examining the client's progress toward achieving the stated goals. Findings should be communicated to the other members of the health care team, and the nutritional plan of care should be revised as needed.

In-Depth or Comprehensive Nutritional Assessment

Screening data that indicate a client is at moderate or severe risk for nutritional problems should be followed by an in-depth nutritional assessment. Using the screening data as a foundation, additional anthropometric measurements, biochemical data, and a diet history

Table 9-2
Sources of Data Collection

Source	Data Collected
Client/family interview	Dietary data
	Medical–socioeconomic data
Physical examination	Medical–socioeconomic data
	Anthropometric and physiologic measurements
	Clinical observations
Laboratory studies	Biochemical data

```
┌─────────────────────────────────────────────────────────────┐
│              Nutrition Assessment Screening Sheet             │
│                                                               │
│  1. Height                              ☐  ☐   inches         │
│  2. Admission weight                 ☐  ☐  ☐   pounds         │
│  3. Usual weight                     ☐  ☐  ☐   pounds         │
│  4. Weight change in last 6–12 months?  ☐ yes  ☐ no          │
│  5. Change in appetite or food tolerance?  ☐ yes  ☐ no       │
│     If yes, specify _____   │
│                                                               │
│     _____  │
│                                                               │
│  6. Laboratory values:                                        │
│       Serum albumin value            ☐  ☐   g/dl             │
│       Hemoglobin level               ☐  ☐   g/dl             │
│       Total lymphocyte count    ☐  ☐  ☐   cu mm              │
│       Blood urea nitrogen            ☐  ☐   mg/dl            │
│  7. Is this patient at nutritional risk?  ☐ yes  ☐ no        │
│  Severity of risk:  ☐ mild  ☐ moderate  ☐ severe            │
│  Patient's name _____        │
│                                             MD initials       │
│  Recorder: _____        │
│  Date: _____        │
│  Physician's name: _____        │
└─────────────────────────────────────────────────────────────┘
```

Figure 9-1
A copy of the East Orange Nutritional Screening Form. *Reprinted from March, 1983 Quality Review Bulletin.*

can be added to provide a more complete client profile from which goals and interventions can be developed (see box, Nutritional Assessment of Adults). Unfortunately, in-depth nutritional assessments can be costly and time-consuming, and require extensive training to ensure accuracy.

In-depth nutritional assessment is used most effectively to assess and monitor moderate- to high-risk clients who have suspected or confirmed protein–calorie malnutrition, such as clients with hypermetabolic illness and injuries; cancer victims; people with altered liver, pancreatic, or GI function; obese clients; clients with kidney disease, diabetes, or other chronic diseases; the elderly; and people who have lost more than 20% of their usual body weight.[6]

NUTRITIONAL ASSESSMENT DATA AND METHODS

Because no single method currently available can assess nutritional status reliably and accurately, a combination of methods is recommended. The following descriptions of anthropometric measurements, biochemical data, clinical observations, and dietary data are intended to make the reader aware of the types of criteria that can be used to evaluate nutritional status; not all criteria are appropriate or useful for all situations. Exactly which

Nutritional Assessment of Adults: Suggested Data to Collect and Interpret

Anthropometric measurements

Screen:
    Height
    Weight
    Ideal body weight (IBW)
    Usual body weight (UBW)
    Recent weight history

In-depth: add
    Triceps skinfolds (TSF)
    Mid-arm circumference (MAC)
    Mid-arm muscle circumference (MAMC)

Biochemical data

Screen:
    Serum albumin
    Total lymphocyte count (TLC)

In-depth: add
    Serum transferrin
    Possibly thyroxin-binding prealbumin or retinol-binding protein
    24-hour urinary creatinine excretion, creatinine height index (CHI)
    Urinary urea nitrogen (UUN), state of nitrogen balance
    Antigen skin testing

Clinical observations

Screen and in-depth:
    Observe for signs and symptoms of malnutrition

Dietary data

Screen:
    24-hour food recall
    Food frequency record

In-depth: add
    Food diary
    Diet history, including medical–socioeconomic data and the effect of
        culture, religion, and psychological influences of food habit
        and choices

criteria are evaluated varies among facilities and is influenced by assessment objectives and other factors previously mentioned.

Anthropometric Measurements

Anthropometric measurements are measurements of body dimensions, such as size and weight, used to monitor growth and development in children and indirectly assess protein and calorie reserves in adults. Accurate equipment and standardized procedures must be used to ensure accurate and precise data collection. In addition, the data must be evaluated according to the appropriate reference standards for the client's age and sex.

Anthropometric measurements have the advantage of being objective, noninvasive, and relatively quick, easy, and inexpensive to obtain. In addition, when taken periodically, they can be used to monitor a client's progress. However, because changes in anthropometric measurements may be slow to occur, they are more reflective of chronic, not acute, changes in nutritional status.

Although weight is considered an important indicator of nutritional status, it does not provide qualitative information about the type of tissue lost (*i.e.*, whether weight loss is related to a decrease in muscle or fat tissue). Also, a client can be malnourished without showing significant weight loss; conversely, the extent of weight loss does not necessarily correlate with the degree of malnutrition.[6]

Unfortunately, inexperience on the part of the assessor, an uncooperative client, and inaccurate equipment are all frequent sources of error. However, self-reported height and weight often are inaccurate and should be used only when actual measurements cannot be obtained. Also, reference standards may not be appropriate for all populations—anthropologic differences may exist among races. Reference standards must also be adjusted for clients who have had amputations.

Height (Adults) and Length (Children)

Equipment

Adults: measuring tape or stick affixed to a vertical device or wall. A movable headpiece that slides easily should be attached at a right angle to the vertical surface.

Infants and children: should be measured lying down on a measuring board with a movable footboard and an immovable headboard.

Procedure

Adults

The client stands erect with feet flat on the floor and slightly apart, legs and back straight, and arms at sides. Shoulder blades, buttocks, and heels should touch the wall or surface of the measuring device.

The movable headboard is lowered until it firmly touches the crown of the head.

Record the measurement immediately.

Infants and children

The child's head should be held gently against the immovable headboard while the knees are pushed against the measuring board (to fully extend the legs).

Slide the movable footboard until it touches both heels. The child's feet are immediately removed and the footboard held securely so that the measurement can be
read and immediately recorded.

Weight

Equipment

Adults: beam-balance scale (or metabolic scale if client is bedridden), which is checked
frequently for accuracy. Bathroom scales are inaccurate and should not be used.
Infants and children who are too young to stand up or walk should be weighed lying down
on a pediatric scale with a pan.

Procedure

Weigh the client
- On the same scale each time.
- At the same time of day, preferably before breakfast.
- With the same amount of clothing on each time and without shoes.
  Record the weight immediately.

Interpretation

Children: based on the child's age and sex, plot measurements on the appropriate growth
chart: length/age, weight/age, weight/length. Data can be compared to either reference
standards (*i.e.*, percentile growth charts) or the child's previous measurements.

The following criteria reflect a potential problem and require further evaluation and
counseling:[8]

Weight/height at the 5th percentile or below may indicate underweight or wasting.
Height/age at the 5th percentile or below indicates a risk of growth retardation or stunting.
Weight/height at the 95th percentile or above indicates overweight or possibly obesity.
Deviations in the growth pattern or the child's normal percentile channels over time (*i.e.*,
falling from the 50th percentile for weight down to the 10th percentile).

Adults: weight may be compared to either of the following:
"Ideal" body weight (IBW), which is based on the client's height (see Chap. 4) or
"desirable" weight range based on height, sex, and frame size (see Appendix 10).
Actual weight that is 120% or more of "ideal" indicates obesity. Weight that is 90% or
less of "ideal" indicates undernutrition and warrants further evaluation.

$$\% \text{ IBW} = \frac{\text{actual weight}}{\text{ideal body weight}} \times 100$$

Usual body weight, or the client's normal weight. Recent weight changes can be evaluated
by comparing the client's actual present weight to his usual weight. Any recent
unintentional weight loss more than 10% of usual weight warrants further evaluation.

$$\% \text{ UBW} = \frac{\text{actual present weight}}{\text{usual weight}}$$

Head Circumference

(For infants up to the age of 2 years only): may indicate chronic undernutrition, or be used to screen for microcephaly or hydrocephalus.

Equipment

Nonstretchable tape, preferably insertion tapes for easy reading.

Procedure

Measure the circumference of the head around the middle of the forehead, making sure the ears are not under the tape and all headwear is removed.

Interpretation

Growth in head circumference usually parallels weight gain. Two standard deviations below the mean may indicate protein–calorie malnutrition; however, head circumference is not recommended as a screening device for malnutrition because it may vary for non-nutritional reasons (*i.e.*, microcephaly and macrocephaly).

Mid-Arm Circumference (MAC)

Measures skeletal muscle mass.

Equipment

Nonstretchable tape, preferably insertion tapes for easy reading (available from Ross Laboratories, Columbus, Ohio).

Procedure

Measure the midpoint of the nondominant arm between the top of the acromion process of the scapula and the olecranon process of the ulna with the forearm flexed at 90°. Mark the midpoint with a felt-tipped pen.

With the arm in the dependent position, gently and firmly draw the tape around the mid-upper arm; do not compress the soft tissue.

Record the reading to the nearest millimeter.

Interpretation

Compare measurements to previous MAC to identify any change.

Compare to reference standard (Table 9-3).

Measurements less than 90% of reference standard may indicate the need for nutritional support.

Triceps Skinfold (TSF)

Measures subcutaneous fat stores and is therefore an index of total body fat, because more than half the total body fat is subcutaneous.[6]

Equipment

Flexible, nonstretchable tape measure and a skinfold caliper.

Table 9-3
Standard Values and Deficiency Levels for Anthropometric Measurements for Adults

	Standard	*90% of Standard*	*80% of Standard*	*70% of Standard*	*60% of Standard*
MID-ARM CIRCUMFERENCE (cm)					
Male	29.3	26.3	23.4	20.5	17.6
Female	28.5	25.7	22.8	20.0	17.1
TRICEPS SKINFOLD (mm)					
Male	12.5	11.3	10.0	8.8	7.5
Female	16.5	14.9	13.2	11.6	9.0
MID-ARM MUSCLE CIRCUMFERENCE (cm)					
Male	25.3	22.8	20.2	17.7	15.2
Female	23.2	20.9	18.6	16.2	13.9

Procedure

Determine the midpoint of the nondominant arm while it is hanging freely.

Grasp a fold of skin and subcutaneous fat between the thumb and forefinger 1 cm above the midpoint mark. Gently pull the skin away from the underlying muscle, apply the caliper, wait 2 to 3 seconds and read the measure to the nearest one-fifth of an inch (0.5 cm).

Repeat the procedure two more times; calculate and record the average measurement.

Interpretation

Compare the measurement to previous TSF measurements to identify any change.
Compare to reference standard (Table 9-3).
TSF less than 90% of reference standard may indicate the need for nutritional support.

Mid-Arm Muscle Circumference (MAMC)

Measures skeletal muscle mass and fat stores.

Calculation

$$\text{MAMC (cm)} = \text{MAC (cm)} - [3.14 \times \text{TSF (cm)}]$$

Interpretation

Compare to previous MAMC to identify any change.
Compare to reference standards (Table 9-3).
MAMC less than 90% of reference standard may indicate the need for nutritional support.

Biochemical Data

Biochemical tests, which are used to measure blood and urine levels of nutrients or to evaluate certain biochemical functions that depend on an adequate supply of essential nutrients, can objectively detect nutritional problems in their early stage before anthropometric and clinical changes occur.[4] Most routine tests are aimed at assessing protein–calorie malnutrition; specialized tests to measure vitamin, mineral, and trace element status are also available.

Unfortunately, abnormal laboratory results are not always diet- or nutritionally related, and the tests do not indicate whether the cause is malnutrition, an outcome of disease, or the result of medical–surgical treatments. Laboratory results also can be affected by genetics, sex, age, physical activity, infection, stress, and even last night's dinner; therefore, reference standards may not be appropriate for all people at all times. What's more, "normal" values for blood and urine constituents vary depending on the laboratory performing the test and the method used.

Because the body can store some nutrients, a low serum level may not necessarily reflect a deficiency (e.g., the level of vitamin A may be low in the bloodstream but liver stores may be adequate). Also, there is not a definite value for a laboratory test that distinguishes between a deficient and nondeficient state (e.g., is less than 95% of normal considered deficient?).

Cost, availability, and the invasive nature of blood tests may be disadvantages.

Measures of Visceral Proteins

Because the primary objective of nutritional therapy is to preserve or restore body protein, assessment of this compartment is essential. Ideally, the serum proteins that are assessed should have a short half-life, should respond to a protein-deficient diet, and should decrease in the blood stream only in response to calorie and protein deficiency.[6] However, studies indicate that concentrations of serum proteins show significant decline only after protein deficiency is prolonged and severe. In addition, they are not specific indicators of protein deficiency because other factors, like zinc deficiency, energy deficiency, liver disease, renal disease, and infections may also contribute to their decline.

Serum albumin

Normal value: 3.5 to 5 g/dl (Table 9-4)

Albumin, the most abundant form of protein in the blood, helps maintain oncotic pressure and transport other nutrients, drugs, and hormones through the blood. Albumin synthesis depends on functioning liver cells and an adequate supply of amino acids.

Malnutrition and depletion of visceral protein stores is reflected in low serum albumin concentrations. However, because albumin is degraded slowly (it has a half life of 20 days) and the body has a large extravascular pool that can be mobilized to maintain serum

Table 9-4
Evaluation of Visceral Protein Depletion

Test	Mild Depletion	Moderate Depletion	Severe Depletion
Serum albumin (mg/dl)	3.5–3.2	3.2–2.8	< 2.8
Transferrin (mg/dl)	200–180	180–160	< 160

(*Keenan RA: Assessment of malnutrition using body composition analysis. Clinical Consultations in Nutritional Support 1:10, 1981*)

concentrations during periods of protein depletion, serum albumin concentrations are preserved until malnutrition is in a chronic stage.

Besides malnutrition, a low serum albumin may also be caused by liver disease, renal disease, congestive heart failure, and excessive protein losses (*e.g.*, burns, major surgery, infection, and cancer).

Transferrin

Normal levels: 200 to 400 mg/dl (Table 9-4)

Transferrin is a transport protein that binds and carries iron from the intestine through the serum. Because it has a shorter half-life than albumin (8 days), transferrin is likely to respond more quickly to protein depletion than albumin. Although serum transferrin levels fall in severe protein–calorie malnutrition, it is not known whether they are sensitive indicators of less severe or chronic malnutrition.

Besides malnutrition, a decrease in transferrin levels may be related to liver disease, nephrotic syndrome, anemia, or neoplastic disease. Furthermore, transferrin is inversely related to iron status: As iron storage increases, transferrin decreases because the body requires that less iron be absorbed. Conversely, iron deficiency causes an increase in serum transferrin.

Thyroxine-binding prealbumin

Normal levels: 15.7 to 29.6 mg/dl

Thyroxine-binding prealbumin transports thyroxine through the blood and is also a carrier for retinol-binding protein, the transport protein of vitamin A. Because its half-life is only 1.9 days and the body pool is small, it is a much more sensitive indicator of protein depletion than either albumin or transferrin. However, some studies show that it is a better measure of dietary intake than nutritional status,[6] and it is not often available from the standard hospital laboratory. Renal disease and iron can alter serum prealbumin levels.

Retinol-binding protein

Normal levels: 2.6 to 7.6 mg/dl

With a shorter half-life (12 hours) and smaller body pool than prealbumin, retinol-binding protein may be a better indicator for monitoring short-term acute changes in protein status. Serum concentration of retinol-binding protein quickly declines in response to both calorie and protein deficiency; however, it may also decline secondary to vitamin A deficiency, hyperthyroidism, chronic liver disorders, zinc deficiency, and cystic fibrosis.

Retinol-binding protein testing is not routinely available from most hospital laboratories.

Measures of Protein Metabolism: 24-Hour Urine Tests

Urinary creatinine and creatinine–height index (CHI)

CHI(%) = creatinine collected (mg/24 hr) divided by expected creatinine (mg/24 hr) × 100

Every day, about 2% of the creatine phosphate in muscle tissue undergoes an irreversible conversion to creatinine. Creatinine circulates in the blood and is excreted in the urine

Table 9-5
Ideal Urinary Creatinine Values

Height (cm)	Ideal Creatinine for Men (mg)*	Ideal Creatinine for Women (mg)†
147.3		830
149.9		851
152.4		875
154.9		900
157.5	1288	925
160.0	1325	949
162.6	1359	977
165.1	1386	1006
167.6	1426	1044
170.2	1467	1076
172.7	1513	1109
175.3	1555	1141
177.8	1596	1174
180.3	1642	1206
182.9	1691	1240
185.4	1739	
188.0	1785	
190.5	1831	
193.0	1891	

Creatinine coefficient for men = 23 mg/kg of ideal body weight.
†*Creatinine coefficient for women = 18 mg/kg of ideal body weight. (Keenan RA: Assessment of malnutrition using body composition analysis. Clinical Consultations in Nutritional Support 1:10, 1981)*

at a constant rate that depends on the amount of muscle mass; the more muscle mass, the greater the excretion of creatinine.

Creatinine–height index (CHI) combines an anthropometric measurement (height) and biochemical value (creatinine) to measure protein reserves. By collecting a 24-hour urine sample, the amount of creatinine can be measured and compared to normal ranges based on height and sex (Table 9-5). Values less than normal may indicate protein malnutrition and loss of lean body mass (muscle protein depletion) (Table 9-6). However, creatinine excretion tests may be invalid if renal function is altered because it requires a 24-hour urine collection. Although creatinine excretion decreases with increasing age, there are no age-adjusted reference standards for the elderly.

Urinary urea nitrogen

The state of nitrogen balance can be determined by comparing nitrogen intake (grams of protein divided by 6.25) to nitrogen output over a 24-hour period. A factor of 4 is added to urinary urea nitrogen (UUN) to account for nitrogen lost through the lungs, hair, skin, feces, and nonurea nitrogen in the urine. A positive nitrogen balance (anabolism) exists when intake exceeds nitrogen output; conversely, negative nitrogen balance (catabolism) is indicated when output exceeds nitrogen intake. For UUN to be valid, protein intake must be accurately recorded and kidney function must be normal.

$$\text{Nitrogen balance} = \frac{\text{g protein}}{6.25} - (\text{UUN} + 4)$$

Table 9-6
Evaluation of Protein Depletion Based on Creatinine Height Index (CHI)

	Protein Depletion		
	Mild	*Moderate*	*Severe*
CHI (%)	<90	<80	<70

Measures of Immune Function Status

Malnutrition has a serious effect on immunocompetence; in fact, it is recognized to be the most common cause of secondary immune deficiency.[6] The following tests may be used to test the body's immunocompetence.

Total lymphocyte count

$$TLC \ (cells/mm^3): TLC = WBC \times \% \ lymphocytes$$

Normal levels: 1500 mm to 1800 mm (Table 9-7)

Total lymphocyte count (TLC) is obtained from a complete blood count (CBC) and differential and is therefore usually available for most hospitalized clients. Malnutrition, especially inadequate intakes of calories and protein, decreases the total number of lymphocytes, which impairs the body's ability to fight infection. Total lymphocyte count is useful for both initial and ongoing assessment.

Antigen skin testing

Cellular immunity can be evaluated by placing small amounts of recall antigens, such as *Candida*, mumps, purified protein derivative of tuberculin (PPD), and streptokinase-streptodornase (SKSD), under the skin. Clients who are immunocompetent will exhibit a positive reaction within 24 to 48 hours, that is, a red area of 5 mm or more will appear around the test site. Because malnutrition delays antibody synthesis and antibody response to stimulation, clients with malnutrition may experience a delayed reaction, a reaction to only one of the antigens, or a negative (no) reaction.

Clinical Observations

Physical signs and symptoms of malnutrition may be visually apparent on inspection (Table 9-8). Abnormal findings should be closely scrutinized to determine whether they are (1) caused by a nutritional deficiency, (2) possibly related to a nutritional deficiency and require further study, or (3) unrelated to a nutritional deficiency.

Clinical observations are noninvasive and inexpensive to obtain. However, they involve a subjective evaluation of "normal" versus "abnormal" findings. Most signs cannot be considered diagnostic, but, rather, suggestive of malnutrition. Confirmation of malnutrition should be obtained with laboratory and dietary data.

Unfortunately, signs of malnutrition may be nonspecific. For instance, dull, dry hair may be related to kwashiorkor (severe protein depletion) or to overexposure to the sun.

Table 9-7
Evaluation of Protein Depletion Based on Total Lymphocyte Count

	Protein Depletion		
	Mild	*Moderate*	*Severe*
Total lymphocyte count (number/mm³)	1800–1500	1500–900	<900

Table 9-8
Clinical Observations for Nutritional Assessment

Body Area	*Signs of Good Nutritional Status*	*Signs of Poor Nutritional Status*
General appearance	Alert, responsive	Listless, apathetic, and cachexic
General vitality	Endurance, energetic, sleeps well, vigorous	Easily fatigued, no energy, falls asleep easily, looks tired, apathetic
Weight	Normal for height, age, body build	Overweight or underweight
Hair	Shiny, lustrous, firm, not easily plucked, healthy scalp	Dull and dry, brittle, loss of color, easily plucked, thin and sparse
Face	Uniform skin color; healthy appearance, not swollen	Dark skin over cheeks and under eyes, flaky skin, facial edema (moon face), pale skin color
Eyes	Bright, clear, moist, no sores at corners of eyelids, membranes moist and healthy pink color, no prominent blood vessels	Pale eye membranes, dry eyes (xerophthalmia); Bitot's spots, increased vascularity, cornea soft (keratomalacia), small yellowish lumps around eyes (xanthelasma), dull or scarred cornea
Lips	Good pink color, smooth, moist, not chapped or swollen	Swollen and puffy (cheilosis), angular lesion at corners of mouth or fissures or scars (stomatitis)
Tongue	Deep red, surface papillae present	Smooth appearance, beefy red or magenta colored, swollen, papillae, hypertrophy or atrophy
Teeth	Straight, no crowding, no cavities, no pain, bright, no discoloration, well-shaped jaw	Cavities, mottled appearance (fluorosis), malpositioned, missing teeth
Gums	Firm, good pink color, no swelling or bleeding	Spongy, bleed easily, marginal redness, recessed, swollen and inflamed
Glands	No enlargement of the thyroid, face not swollen	Enlargement of the thyroid (goiter), enlargement of the parotid (swollen cheeks)
Skin	Smooth, good color, slightly moist, no signs of rashes, swelling, or color irregularities	Rough, dry, flaky, swollen, pale, pigmented, lack of fat under the skin, fat deposits around the joints (xanthomas), bruises, petechiae
Nails	Firm, pink	Spoon shaped (koilonychia), brittle, pale, ridged
Skeleton	Good posture, no malformations	Poor posture, beading of the ribs, bowed legs or knock–knees,

(continued)

Table 9-8 (*continued*)

Body Area	Signs of Good Nutritional Status	Signs of Poor Nutritional Status
		prominent scapulas, chest deformity at diaphragm
Muscles	Well developed, firm, good tone, some fat under the skin	Flaccid, poor tone, wasted, underdeveloped, difficulty walking
Extremities	No tenderness	Weak and tender, presence of edema
Abdomen	Flat	Swollen
Nervous system	Normal reflexes, psychological stability	Decrease in or loss of ankle and knee reflexes, psychomotor changes, mental confusion, depression, sensory loss, motor weakness, loss of sense of position, loss of vibration, burning and tingling of the hands and feet (paresthesia)
Cardiovascular system	Normal heart rate and rhythm, no murmurs, normal blood pressure for age	Cardiac enlargement, tachycardia, elevated blood pressure
GI system	No palpable organs or masses (liver edge may be palpable in children)	Hepatosplenomegaly

(Adapted from Christakis G [ed]: Nutritional Assessment in Health Programs. Washington, DC: American Public Health Association, 1973; and Williams SR: Nutrition and Diet Therapy. 5th ed. St. Louis: Times Mirror/Mosby, 1985)

Also, the intensity of symptoms can vary among population groups because of genetic and environmental differences. Another disadvantage of using clinical observations is that they cannot detect subclinical malnutrition, which is more common than clinical (overt) malnutrition, because it does not produce any physical signs or symptoms.

Dietary Data

Dietary data can be collected through a variety of methods depending on the scope of the assessment. Data can be evaluated to determine the sources and amounts of nutrients consumed, which can help identify potential and actual nutritional problems and classify them as primary (caused by a poor intake) or secondary (caused by alterations in digestion, absorption, metabolism, or excretion of nutrients). As with any information obtained through an interview, the data are highly subjective and may not be reliable or precise. In addition, acute or chronic debilitating disease may make data collection difficult.

24-Hour Food Recall

A 24-hour food recall, obtained through questionnaire or by interview, asks the client to recall the quantity and quality of all foods eaten during the previous or any typical 24-hour period (see box, 24-Hour Food Recall). The data obtained usually are evaluated according to the Food Guide Pyramid to estimate overall adequacy (see Chap. 8); the data generally are considered incomplete or too imprecise to evaluate according to the RDAs. It is the

24-Hour Food Recall

Name: _____ Date: _____
Day of week of recall: _____

24-Hour Food Recall Record

Directions: In the space provided below, record all food and beverages consumed in the previous 24-hour period or in any typical 24-hour period. Include estimated amounts and the time and place when they were eaten.

Food and Beverage Consumed

Type	Amount	Method of Preparation*	Time	Place

Was this a typical day?   Yes _____   No _____
If not, why not?

Do you take a vitamin or
mineral supplement (pill)?   Yes _____   No _____

If yes, how often? _____
          what kind? (i.e., multivitamin, iron, potassium. Give brand name if
known.)

*Fried, baked, broiled, boiled, creamed, toasted.

easiest and quickest method of evaluating dietary intake, and is a good screening tool for assessing the average intake of a group of people.

Unfortunately, the 24-hour recall relies on memory and accurate interpretation of portion sizes; underreporting of food consumed may occur. The underlying assumption in using the 24-hour recall method is that a single day closely represents the usual pattern of intake over an extended period of time.[1] However, numerous studies have shown that it does not, and that a 24-hour recall is not an appropriate tool for assessing the usual diet of an individual.[1]

Food Frequency Record

Components of Diet History

Collect	Evaluate
Data Base	
Age, sex	Effect on nutritional requirements
Position in family; number in family; life style	Outside support systems; social aspects of eating
Occupation; frequency and intensity of physical exercise; usual number of hours of sleep/day	Effect on calorie requirements and meal timing
Religious affiliation, cultural and ethnic background	Effect on food choices and aversions
Educational background	Ability to comprehend diet instruction; appropriate teaching materials and methods
Use of alcohol and tobacco	Effect on food intake, food budget, and nutrient requirements
Dietary Data	
24-hour recall of typical food eaten, including	Adequacy according to
Usual portion sizes	Food Guide Pyramid
Usual meal and snack patterns	U.S. Dietary Guidelines
Usual meal timing	Recommended Dietary Allowances (RDA)
Place where most meals are eaten	
Food frequency record	
Present intake, if different from usual intake	Reason for change, for example: loss of appetitie, changes in smell, appetite or taste, difficulty chewing and swallowing, hospitalization, modified diet
Food likes, dislikes, intolerances, allergies	Impact on food choices
Information on who does the food shopping and preparation	Responsible person's nutrition knowledge, need for diet instruction
Information on food preparation and storage facilities	Impact on intake; need for social assistance
Present and past use of therapeutic diets	Client compliance and knowledge; effectiveness of the diet; need for diet revisions or follow-up teaching
Present and past use of food fads, such as fad dieting, health foods, self-prescribed vitamin/mineral supplements	Rationale; potential risks/benefits
Medical–Socioeconomic Data	
Past medical history: type of disorder, treatment (including diet and drug)	Effect on intake, digestion, absorption, metabolism, and excretion of nutrients;
Current illness or chief complaint	The need for diet modifications
Family medical history	
Past surgical history: type, date, length of hospitalization, development of complications	
Past and present drug history: name of prescription and nonprescription drugs used on a regular basis, purpose, dosage, duration of use	Potential or actual effects on nutritional status; need for diet modification

(continued)

Components of Diet History (*continued*)

History of drug dependence; drug abuse	
Ability to chew and swallow (Does the client have missing teeth? Full or partial dentures? Do the dentures fit?)	Impact on food intake
Appetite, bowel habits	Normal pattern, recent changes, impact on intake and nutritional status, need for diet modification
Source of income	Reliability and adequacy; eligibility for social assistance
Food budget	Adequacy

Food Frequency Record

A food frequency record is a checklist that indicates how often specific foods or general food groups are eaten; that is, times/day, times/week, times/month, or frequently, seldom, never (see box, Food Frequency Record). It provides information on the types of foods eaten, but not the quantities. A selective food frequency record may focus on specific foods or nutrients suspected of being deficient or excessive in the diet; a general one may be based on major food groups. Questionnaires may be completed relatively quickly and easily by the client or through an interview, and thus they are often used in large-scale epidemiologic studies.

Because portion sizes are not stressed, a food frequency record may be less intimidating than a 24-hour recall. When used together, a food frequency record and 24-hour recall complement each other and present a more complete dietary intake pattern than either method used alone. Unfortunately, this method also relies on memory.

Food Record

A food record is a detailed diary of all food and beverages consumed and measurements of portion sizes during a specified period of time, usually 3 to 7 days, depending on the regularity of food habits. In theory, an average daily intake can be calculated by totaling the nutrients consumed during the entire period and dividing by the total number of days. In practice, food records appear to be relatively valid for obtaining the mean intakes of nutrients consumed by groups of people, but individual food records tend to become unreliable after the first few days because accuracy of recording deteriorates.[1] Another disadvantage is that the client may modify usual intake during the recording period.

Diet History

A diet history is a time-consuming method of assessment requiring an extensive interview by a trained nutritionist or dietitian to determine a client's usual pattern of intake over time (see box, Components of Diet History). It is a complete and comprehensive assessment

Food for Thought	**Hair Analysis: Reliable or Ridiculous?**

Although hair analysis has limited applications as a screening tool for heavy metal exposure, many commercial laboratories are promoting hair analysis to health food stores, beauty shops, chiropractors, and "nutrition consultants" as a method of evaluating a person's mineral status and managing a wide variety of illnesses.

The results of a study that sent hair samples from two healthy teenagers to 13 commercial laboratories showed that there was little agreement between laboratories regarding the mineral levels present in identical samples of hair. Even more interesting is that two identical samples sent to the same lab yielded different results. The laboratories surveyed also disagreed as to what are the "normal" or "usual" levels of many minerals. Most reports were extensive computerized interpretations of absurd and potentially frightening findings. Six of the laboratories recommended food supplements, but the types and amounts varied from report to report and from laboratory to laboratory. Needless to say, commercial hair analysis is at best unscientific, a waste of money, and possibly even illegal.

tool that contains a data base (age, sex, activity, etc.) and food intake data (24-hour food recall, food frequency record). In addition, medical, social, and economic factors, as well as cultural and psychological influences, are evaluated for their impact on nutritional requirements and food habits, choices, and attitudes.

Dietary data collected through a diet history can be evaluated according to the Food Guide Pyramid (see Chap. 8), the Dietary Guidelines for Americans (see Chap. 8), the RDAs appropriate for the client's age and sex, or estimated requirements based on the client's condition. Diet histories appear to be a reliable method of assessment; however, it is not possible to know whether they are precise or accurate, because validation is so difficult and because food habits are not static.

BIBLIOGRAPHY

1. Block G: A review of validations of dietary assessment methods. Am J Epidemiol 115:492, 1982
2. Brown CSB, Stegman MR: Nutritional assessment of surgical patients. QRB 14:302, 1988
3. Cerrato PL: The most overlooked aspect of nursing. RN Aug 1988:69, 1988
4. Christakis G (ed): Nutritional Assessment in Health Programs. Washington, DC: American Public Health Association, 1979
5. DeHoog S: Nutritional screening and assessment in a university hospital. In Nutritional Screening and Assessment as Components of Hospital Admission: Report of the Eighth Ross Roundtable on Medical Issues. Columbus, OH: Ross Laboratories, 1988
6. Haider M, Haider SQ: Assessment of protein–calorie malnutrition. Clin Chem 30:1286, 1984
7. Page CP, Hardin TC: Nutritional Assessment and Support: A Primer. Baltimore: Williams & Wilkins, 1989
8. Simko MD, Cowell C, Gilbride JA: Nutrition Assessment: A Comprehensive Guide for Planning Intervention. Rockville, MD: Aspen, 1984

10 Pregnancy and Lactation

It has long been recognized that nutrition plays an important role in the progression and outcome of pregnancy. Women who enter pregnancy with adequate nutrient reserves and good eating habits are better prepared for pregnancy and lactation. Women who consume an adequate diet during pregnancy provide the fetus, placenta, and maternal tissues with the nutrients necessary for normal growth and development.

Indeed, the incidence of fetal and infant morbidity and mortality is significantly higher among women who are malnourished. Malnutrition occurring before the placental growth is complete (*i.e.*, during the first trimester) results in a small placenta, which remains undersized regardless of how well the mother eats later in the pregnancy. If the placenta is small, the fetus is usually small, possibly because a small placenta may not be able to nourish the fetus adequately.

Likewise, malnutrition occurring during the critical period of hyperplastic growth (increase in cell number) of any fetal organ may reduce the number of cells formed and may permanently impair the organ's growth and development. Malnutrition during hypertrophic (increase in cell size) growth results in a small cell size, which can be reversed with adequate nutrition.

Studies show that gestational weight gain, especially during the second and third trimesters, is an important determinant of fetal growth.[16] Low weight gain increases the chances of delivering a low-birth-weight (LBW) infant (a baby weighing less than 2500 g or 5.5 lbs). Low-birth-weight babies tend to be malnourished, especially if born full-term, and they have a high incidence of postnatal complications and mortality. In fact, birth weight may be the most important predictor not only of mortality, but also of subsequent development.

However, adequate weight gain during pregnancy cannot by itself ensure the delivery of a normal-birth-weight infant. A growing body of evidence shows that prepregnancy weight for height influences fetal growth beyond the effect of gestational weight gain; that is, women who are thinner before pregnancy tend to have smaller babies compared to their heavier counterparts with the *same* gestational weight gain.[16] Recent recommendations on weight gain during pregnancy stress the importance of individualizing weight gain goals based on an accurate assessment of prepregnancy weight.

NUTRITION AND PREGNANCY

Nutrient requirements increase during pregnancy to support optimal fetal growth and development (Table 10-1), and to maintain maternal homeostasis despite physiologic changes that involve all body systems. Alterations in metabolism, body composition, gastrointestinal function, and an expanded blood volume account for some of the maternal changes with nutritional implications (Table 10-2).

Table 10-1
Stages of Fetal Growth

Stage	Duration	Characteristics
Implantation Stage	Two-week period following conception	Fertilized egg undergoes cell division, differentiates into three distinct germinal layers, and implants itself into the uterine wall. During this critical period preceding growth, insults, including malnutrition, can cause birth defects or prevent implantation.
Organogenesis	Six-week period following implantation	Differentiation and development of various organs and tissues occurs. Adequate nutrient reserves established before conception can be used by the embryo for nourishment if maternal intake is impaired because of nausea and vomiting. Maternal intake is more important if preconceptual reserves are marginal.
Growth Stage	The remaining 7 months of pregnancy	The most intense period of anabolism in the life cycle, characterized by the extensive growth and development of tissues. During this period, the placenta nourishes the fetus by transferring nutrients and oxygen from maternal circulation. The placenta also removes fetal wastes.

Table 10-2

Maternal Physiologic Changes of Pregnancy With Nutritional Significance

Physiologic Change	Rationale
ALTERED METABOLISM	
Basal metabolic rate increases	Increased oxygen consumption related to the increase in maternal cardiac output and the oxygen needs of the placenta and fetus. The rate usually increases by the fourth month of gestation and rises to 15% to 20% above normal by term.
Fat becomes the major source of fuel	To conserve glucose for the fetus: Glucose is the only fuel the fetus can utilize to meet its energy requirements.[18]
Decrease in insulin efficiency develops during the latter part of pregnancy	May be a compensatory mechanism to provide the growing fetus with an adequate supply of glucose.
Total body water increases throughout pregnancy: It is estimated that 62% of weight gain at term is from the increase in water[16]	Minor edema may be considered normal if not accompanied by hypertension and proteinuria.
GASTROINTESTINAL CHANGES	
Nausea and vomiting are common in the first trimester; so are increases in appetite and thirst	Hypoglycemia, decreased gastric motility, relaxation of the cardiac sphincter, or anxiety may contribute to nausea and vomiting.
Decreased tone and motility of the smooth muscles of the GI tract may lead to esophageal reflux with heartburn and constipation	Increased progesterone production slows GI motility. Displaced stomach and intestines related to enlarging uterus.
Nutrient absorption increases	Increased progesterone production, which slows GI motility.
BLOOD VOLUME CHANGES	
Physiologic anemia of pregnancy	The increase in blood volume exceeds the increase in red blood cell production, resulting in hemodilution.

Recommended Dietary Allowances for Pregnancy

With the exception of vitamins A and K, the requirements of all nutrients with defined RDA increase during pregnancy over the RDA for nonpregnant women aged 25 to 50 (Table 10-3).[10] However, the degree and timing vary considerably among nutrients. For instance, the RDA for iron triples during pregnancy, yet only 10% more vitamin B_{12} is needed. Likewise, the RDA for calories is specified for each trimester; no other RDA distinguish between trimesters. The 10th edition of the *Recommended Dietary Allowances* lists absolute amounts of nutrients required during pregnancy, instead of additional amounts needed. For instance, the previous allowance for calcium during pregnancy was +400 g; in the 10th edition the RDA is a total of 1200 g. The change reflects the precision with which the additional costs of pregnancy are known.[10] However, calories are listed as an incremental increase.

Because calorie needs increase relatively little compared to the increased requirements for other nutrients, like calcium, iron, and folic acid, nutrient density is important. Table 10-4 outlines the sources and functions of calories and selected nutrients that are important during pregnancy.

Table 10-3

Recommended Dietary Allowances for Pregnancy and Lactation

	Nonpregnant Women			Lactation	
	Ages 19–24	Ages 25–50	Pregnancy	1st 6 months	2nd 6 months
Calories	2200	2200	1st tri:+0 2nd tri:+300 3rd tri:+300	+500	+500
Protein, g	46	50	60	65	62
Vit A, μg	800	800	800	1300	1200
Vit D, μg	10	5	10	10	10
Vit E, mg	8	8	10	12	11
Vit K, μg	60	65	65	65	65
Vit C, mg	60	60	70	95	90
Thiamine, mg	1.1	1.1	1.5	1.6	1.6
Riboflavin, mg	1.3	1.3	1.6	1.8	1.7
Niacin, mg	15	15	17	20	20
Vit B_6, mg	1.6	1.6	2.2	2.1	2.1
Folate, μg	180	180	400	280	260
Vit B_{12}, μg	2.0	2.0	2.2	2.6	2.6
Calcium, mg	1200	800	1200	1200	1200
Phosphorus, mg	1200	800	1200	1200	1200
Magnesium, mg	280	280	320	355	340
Iron, mg	15	15	30	15	15
Zinc, mg	12	12	15	19	16
Iodine, μg	150	150	175	200	200
Selenium, μg	55	55	65	75	75

Although the RDA for pregnancy may help health professionals assess, plan, and evaluate dietary data, especially for a high-risk client, the following limitations must be considered:

- The RDA represents allowances, not requirements. Actual requirements during pregnancy vary among individuals and are influenced by prior nutritional status, chronic illnesses, multiple pregnancies, and closely spaced pregnancies.
- The requirement for one nutrient may be altered by the intake of another (*i.e.*, protein requirements increase if calorie needs are not met).
- Nutrient needs are not constant throughout the course of pregnancy.
- The evaluation of a client's diet using the RDA is complex and time-consuming. Many daily food guides for pregnancy have been developed for simple, quick, routine assessments and client teaching.

The Food Guide Pyramid Approach for Pregnancy and General Dietary Suggestions

Numerous federal, state, and private agencies have published sound daily food guides for choosing a healthy diet that promotes adequate weight gain during pregnancy. Most food guides are based on the food group approach to eating, with additional information

Table 10-4

Functions of Calories and Selected Nutrients During Pregnancy

Nutrient and Sources	% Increase in RDA Above Nonpregnant Adult Female Aged 25–50	Rationale for Increase	Possible Outcome of Deficiency
Calories (It is recommended that CHO supply approximately 50% of total calories, mostly in the form of complex CHO)	1st trimester: no increase 2nd & 3rd trimesters: 14% increase	To spare protein for tissue synthesis; to meet increased BMR and increased energy expenditure related to increased body weight; to store calorie reserves for lactation	Inadequate weight gain increases the risk of low birth weight, fetal growth retardation, and fetal and neonatal death
Protein High biologic sources: eggs, milk, yogurt, cheese, meat, poultry, seafood Low biologic sources: nuts, seeds, grains, legumes	20%	Fetal growth and development; formation of the placenta and amniotic fluid; growth of breast and uterine tissue; expanded blood volume	Associated with toxemia, anemia, poor uterine muscle tone, abortion, decreased resistance to infection, and shorter, lighter infants with low Apgar scores
Folic acid Liver Beef Legumes Wheat germ Eggs Dark-green leafy vegetables	122%	Important for DNA and RNA synthesis, and therefore cell proliferation related to growth and development; plays a role in the maturation of RBC	Maternal megaloblastic anemia, nausea, third trimester bleeding; may be related to congenital malformations or impaired fetal growth
Vit D Sunlight Vitamin D fortified milk Margarine Breakfast cereals Liver Egg yolks	100%	Needed for fetal bone mineralization and normal calcium metabolism	Associated with neonatal hypocalcemia, tetany, and tooth enamel hypoplasia; may lead to maternal osteomalacia
Iron Liver Red meat Dried fruit Egg yolk Enriched and whole grain breads and cereals Leafy vegetables Nuts Legumes (The absorption of iron from plant sources is greatly enhanced when a rich source of vitamin C is eaten at the same meal.)	100%	Increased maternal blood volume and hemoglobin; fetal iron storage	Maternal iron deficiency anemia; infants born to anemic mothers have decreased iron reserves and are more prone to anemia in the first year of life. Effect of maternal iron deficiency on infant birth weight is controversial; maternal iron deficiency may increase the incidence of prematurity.

(continued)

Table 10-4 (*continued*)

Nutrient and Sources	*% Increase in RDA Above Nonpregnant Adult Female Aged 25–50*	*Rationale for Increase*	*Possible Outcome of Deficiency*

Calcium
  Milk
  Yogurt
  Cheese
  Ice cream
  Green leafy vegetables
  Legumes
	50%	Formation of fetal skeleton and teeth; maintenance of maternal serum and bone calcium	Decreased maternal bone density → osteomalacia; decreased infant bone density → congenital rickets; may be a major factor in the development of toxemia

provided regarding weight gain, meal frequency, water intake, and the use of vitamins, salt, alcohol, and caffeine.

There are relatively few differences between the Food Guide Pyramid recommendations for nonpregnant adults and the Daily Food Guide recommendations for pregnancy. (Table 10-5). One notable distinction is that the recommended number of servings from the milk group doubles during pregnancy; milk is an excellent source of protein, vitamin D, calcium, and other minerals. In fact, two additional glasses of 2% milk supplies 240 calories (an extra 300 calories/day is recommended during the 2nd and 3rd trimesters of pregnancy) and 16 g of protein (the RDA for protein increases by only 10 g during pregnancy). Obviously, little more is needed to fulfill the requirement for extra calories; however, milk does not supply adequate amounts of *all* essential nutrients. Consequently, wise food selections from the remaining food groups are needed to ensure nutritional adequacy.

Weight Gain

Since 1970, there has been a shift away from limiting weight gain during pregnancy and an increase in average gestation weight gain. Interestingly, there has also been a decrease in the infant mortality rate, an increase in average birth weights, and a lower incidence of LBW infants.[16] Although the increase in gestational weight gain cannot be solely credited for the positive changes, evidence suggests that it is an important determinant of fetal growth.

Conversely, very high gestational weight gain increases the incidence of high birth weight, which is associated with some increase in the risk of fetopelvic disproportion, operative delivery, birth trauma, and asphyxia and mortality.[16] The effect seems to be greatest in women less than 62 inches tall. Some studies also indicate that excessive weight gains during pregnancy contributes to maternal obesity.[11] Currently, the Weight Gain Subcommittee of the Institute of Medicine recommends desirable ranges of total weight gain based on prepregnancy weight status, which can be evaluated by body mass index (BMI) (Table 10-6). Body mass index is defined as weight/height squared × 100, and can be calculated using either English or metric units. For women of normal prepregnancy weight carrying a single fetus, a total gain of 25 to 35 lbs is recommended; optimal weight

Table 10-5
Daily Food Guide for Pregnancy and Lactation

Food Group	Serving Size of Representative Foods	No. of Servings Recommended for Adults (Food Guide Pyramid)	No. of Servings Recommended for Pregnancy	No. of Servings Recommended for Lactation
Bread, Cereal, Rice, and Pasta	1 slice bread ½ hamburger bun or English muffin 3–4 small or 2 large crackers ½ cup cooked cereal, pasta or rice 1 oz ready-to-eat cereal	6–11	6–11	6–11
Vegetable	½ cup cooked or chopped raw vegetables 1 cup leafy raw vegetables ¾ cup vegetable juice	3–5	3–5 (Include at least 2 servings of dark green leafy, yellow, or orange vegetables	3–5 (Include at least 2 servings of dark green leafy, yellow, or orange vegetables
Fruit (Include at least one citrus fruit or juice)	¾ cup juice 1 medium apple, banana, or other fruit ½ cup fresh, cooked, or canned fruit	2–4	2–4	2–4
Milk, Yogurt, and Cheese	1 cup milk 1 cup buttermilk 8 oz yogurt 1½ oz natural cheese 2 oz processed cheese	2–3	4	4
Meat, Poultry, Fish, Dry Beans, Eggs, and Nuts	Total of 5–7 oz cooked lean meat/poultry/fish/other protein sources daily 1 oz = 1 egg ½ cup cooked beans 2 tablespoons peanut butter	2–3 (5–7 oz)	2–3 (6–7 oz)	2–3 (5–7 oz)
Fats, Oils, and Sweets	Limit fats and sweets; avoid alcohol during pregnancy and lactation.			

Source: March of Dimes Birth Defects Foundation, International Food Information Council: Healthy Eating During Pregnancy, 1991 and USDA, prepared by Human Nutrition Information Service: USDA's Food Guide Pyramid Home and Garden Bulletin number 249. Hyattsville, MD, 1992.

gain for women underweight before conception may be 28 to 40 lbs, and obese women should gain at least 15 lbs.[16] Within each weight category, young adolescent and black mothers should be encouraged to strive for weight gains toward the upper range.[16] Women carrying twins should gain 35 to 45 lbs.

The pattern and source of weight gain may be more meaningful than the total amount. During the first trimester, a 2- to 4-lb weight gain is considered normal.[8] Thereafter, weight gain for normal-weight women is approximately 1 lb per week. Underweight women should gain slightly more than 1 lb per week, and overweight women should gain about

Table 10-6
**Recommended Weight Gain During Pregnancy Based
on Body Mass Index (BMI)**

Prepregnancy BMI	Classification	Recommended Total Weight Gain Range
<19.8	Underweight	28–40 pounds
19.8–26.0	Normal weight	25–35 pounds
>26.0–29.0	Overweight	15–25 pounds
>29.0	Obese	At least 15 pounds

*Source: Subcommittee of Nutritional Status and Weight Gain During Pregnancy,
Food and Nutrition Board, National Academy of Sciences: Nutrition During
Pregnancy. Washington, DC: National Academy Press, 1990.*

0.66 lb/week. The rate of weight gain for severely obese women should be determined on an individualized basis; however, weight reduction should never be undertaken during pregnancy. Although slightly higher or lower rates of weight gain can be considered normal, obvious or persistent deviations warrant further investigation.[16] For example, after the 20th week of gestation, a sudden weight gain of 2 lbs or more per week, accompanied by generalized edema and an elevated blood pressure, may signal preeclampsia.

Meal Frequency

Fasting, especially after midgestation, can result in hypoglycemia, hyperketonemia, acetonuria, and other signs of metabolic acidosis within 24 hours. It is not known if the fetus can use ketones for fuel as efficiently as glucose, and chronic ketosis can cause impaired mental and intellectual development.[18] Therefore, women are advised to avoid periods of hunger by eating three meals and two to three nutritious snacks. Small, frequent meals may also help alleviate nausea in the first trimester and heartburn during the second half of pregnancy.

Water Intake

Women are encouraged to drink six to eight glasses of fluid daily, either in the form of water, fruit juice, or milk. Empty calorie drinks like carbonated beverages and fruit-ades provide little more than calories.

Vitamin Supplements

The Subcommittee on Dietary Intake and Nutrient Supplements During Pregnancy considers food the ideal source of nutrients.[16] The committee states that the use of supplements "should be based on evidence of a benefit as well as a lack of harmful effects." They recommend that multivitamin and mineral supplements not be used routinely, nor should they replace food. However, supplements may be appropriate for certain nutrients and certain population groups. For instance, a low-dose multivitamin–mineral supplement is recommended for women in high-risk categories (*i.e.*, heavy smokers, drug abusers, and

Table 10-7

Recommendations for Nutrient Supplements During Pregnancy

Supplement	Indications
Iron	30–60 mg of ferrous iron is recommended for all pregnant women during the second and third trimesters. Absorption is enhanced on an empty stomach; however, it may be better tolerated with food. Vitamin C does not improve absorption of ferrous iron supplements.
Folic acid	300 µg/day may be used only when dietary intake appears inadequate.
Multivitamin and mineral supplements	Indicated beginning at the second trimester for women with inadequate intakes and for high-risk women: heavy cigarette smokers, alcohol and drug abusers, or women carrying more than one fetus. Supplements are better absorbed on an empty stomach.
Vit D	10 µg (400 IU) are recommended for complete vegans and others who do not consume adequate amounts of vitamin D fortified milk. Adequate dietary/supplement intake is especially important for women with minimal exposure to sunlight.
Calcium	600 mg/day is recommended for women under 25 years of age who consume less than 600 mg of calcium/day. Calcium supplements should be taken with meals to enhance absorption and reduce interaction with iron supplements.
Vitamin B_{12}	2.0 µg/day is recommended for complete vegans.
Zinc and copper	Because iron can interfere with their absorption and utilization, 15 mg of zinc and 2 mg of copper are recommended for women who take more than 30 mg of iron/day for the treatment of anemia.

Source: Subcommittee on Nutritional Status and Weight Gain During Pregnancy, Food and Nutrition Board, National Academy of Sciences: Nutrition During Pregnancy. Washington, DC: National Academy Press, 1990.

those carrying twins) and for those unlikely to consume an adequate diet despite dietary advice or counseling.[16] Other indications for supplements are outlined in Table 10-7.

Based on dietary intake studies, the Subcommittee determined that iron is the only nutrient for which requirements *cannot* be met by diet alone. A daily supplement of 30 mg of ferrous iron is recommended for all women during the second and third trimesters, preferably between meals or at bedtime on an empty stomach to maximize absorption.

Salt

Sodium needs increase during pregnancy to maintain normal sodium levels in the expanded blood volume and tissues. Restricting sodium intake may adversely affect both mother and fetus; therefore, a moderate intake of iodized salt is recommended.

Alcohol

Because alcohol is a potent teratogen and a "safe" level of consumption is not known, women are advised to avoid alcohol during pregnancy. Alcohol may do damage by dehydrating fetal cells, leaving them dead or functionless, or by causing secondary nutrient deficiencies related to poor intake, decreased absorption, altered metabolism, or increased excretion.

Chronic alcohol consumption can result in fetal alcohol syndrome (FAS), a condition characterized by varying degrees of physical and mental growth failure and birth defects.

Unlike other small-for-gestational-age infants, infants with FAS do not experience normal "catch-up" growth. Some degree of intellectual impairment is frequently reported in children with FAS.[16]

Not all alcoholic mothers deliver FAS infants, yet even alcoholics who abstain during pregnancy have a higher incidence of LBW infants than women who do not have a history of alcoholism. Although chronic alcohol abuse clearly increases the risk of growth failure and birth defects, and the effects of alcohol appear to be dose-related, when and how much alcohol is safe has not been established. Studies on the effects of low doses of alcohol on fetal growth have been limited and inconsistent. Although an occasional drink may not do damage, abstinence is recommended.

Caffeine

Although conclusive evidence that coffee or caffeine causes birth defects in humans is lacking, some studies suggest that moderate to heavy coffee and caffeine consumption may lower infant birth weight.[16] Moderate use of coffee and caffeine (the equivalent of four cups of coffee or less per day) during pregnancy is prudent, even though an official recommendation has not been made.

NURSING PROCESS

Initial assessment of anthropometric, biochemical, clinical, and dietary data, including medical–socioeconomic information, should be performed to identify clients at risk for poor nutritional status during pregnancy (see box, Risk Factors for Poor Nutritional Status During Pregnancy) and also to establish baseline data. Ongoing nutritional assessment and evaluation performed regularly throughout the course of pregnancy provides continuing surveillance and identifies clients in need of diet teaching or community assistance.

Assessment

In addition to the general pregnancy and lactation assessment criteria, assess for the following factors:

Weight, quantity and rate of weight gain. Figures 10-1, 10-2, and 10-3 are provisional weight gain graphs based on prepregnancy body mass.

Usual 24-hour intake according to the Daily Food Guide for Pregnancy, including foods from the "Fats, Oils, and Sweets" group and fluids consumed. A food frequency record or food record is obtained to provide more specific information. Pay particular attention to total quantity of food consumed (calories), as well as the number of servings consumed from each of the food groups. Determine what interventions are needed to improve intake.

Gastrointestinal (GI) side effects of pregnancy (nausea, vomiting, constipation, heartburn, increased appetite); assess onset, frequency, causative factors, severity, interventions attempted and the results.

Dietary changes made in response to pregnancy or diet-related complications of pregnancy (*i.e.*, foods avoided, foods preferred) (see box, Nutrition-Related Problems and Complications During Pregnancy). Determine foods best and least tolerated.

Risk Factors for Poor Nutritional Status During Pregnancy

Anthropometric Data

Prepartum weight <85% or >120% of ideal weight

Inadequate weight gain: <10 lb weight gain during the first 20 weeks of
    pregnancy; <2 lb weight gain/month after the first trimester

Excessive weight gain: >2 lb/week

Biochemical Data

Low or deficient hemoglobin and hematocrit

Dietary Data

Use of a therapeutic diet for a chronic disease

Substance abuse: tobacco, alcohol, drugs

Food faddism, unbalanced diet, pica (ingestion of nonfood items)

Medical–Socioeconomic Data

Age ≤15 years or ≥35 years

Poor obstetrical history

Repetitive pregnancies at short intervals

Economically deprived

Chronic systemic disease

The frequency of eating; assess for periods of fasting.

Cultural, familial, religious, and ethnic influences on eating habits. Determine what specific beliefs the client has regarding diet during pregnancy, including the practice of pica, and how they affect intake and the need for diet counseling (see box, Common Myths About Nutrition During Pregnancy).

The use of vitamin or mineral supplements—type, amount, and frequency. Evaluate their safety and effectiveness; determine if they are being used appropriately or whether they are being used as a substitute for a healthy diet.

History of food intolerances (especially lactose intolerance) or allergies; evaluate their impact on overall intake.

The client's nutritional knowledge and ability/willingness to implement dietary changes.

Plan to breastfeed; consider whether the client is carrying more than one fetus.

The client's use of alcohol, tobacco, caffeine, and drugs.

Financial status. Women determined to be at nutritional risk because of inadequate nutrition and inadequate income may be eligible for Women, Infants and Children (WIC), a supplemental food program for pregnant and postpartum women (up to 1 year if breastfeeding, up to 6 months if bottle-feeding), infants, and children up to age

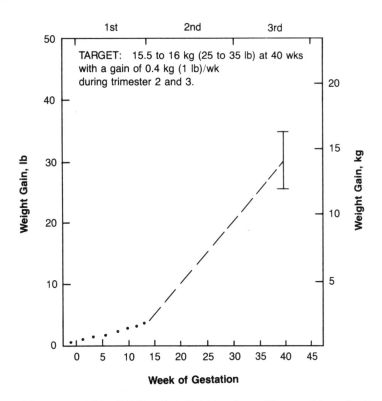

^a Assumes a 1.6-kg (3.5-lb) gain in first trimester and the remaining gain at a rate of 0.44 kg (0.97 lb) per week.
^b Assumes a 2.3-kg (5-lb) gain in first trimester and the remaining gain at a rate of 0.49 kg (1.07 lb) per week.
^c Assumes a 0.9-kg (2-lb) gain in first trimester and the remaining gain at a rate of 0.3 kg (0.67 lb) per week.

Figure 10-1
Provisional weight gain graph for normal weight women with BMI of 19.8 to 26.0 (metric).

5. WIC provides nutritional counseling and vouchers for specified foods of high nutritional quality.

Nursing Diagnosis

Health Seeking Behaviors, as evidenced by a lack of knowledge of diet for pregnancy and a desire to learn.

Planning and Implementation

For the optimal impact on maternal and infant health, nutritional counseling ideally should begin before conception. However, before counseling can begin, the client's attitudes, beliefs, and fears must be ascertained in order to determine the client's emotional as well as nutritional needs.

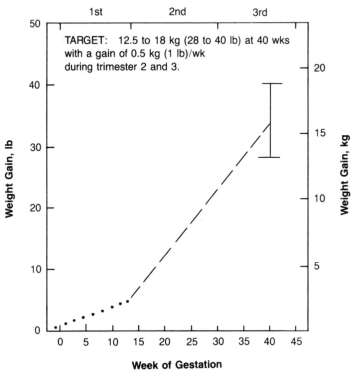

Figure 10-2
Provisional weight gain graph for underweight women with BMI less than 19.8 (metric).

The most effective approach to nutritional counseling begins with a 24-hour recall to determine usual intake, food preferences and aversions, and to identify potential nutritional problems. Individualized diet teaching, initiated during the first prenatal visit and continued throughout the course of pregnancy, should stress the continuance of good dietary habits and should recommend realistic ways to improve intake. A variety of teaching materials are available; select those appropriate for the client's level of understanding.

Because the risk of low gestational weight gain is higher among unmarried women, adolescents, black and Hispanic women, cigarette smokers, and women with low levels of education, these women should receive additional nutritional counseling to ensure an adequate weight gain during pregnancy.[16]

Client Goals

The client will:

Explain the importance of diet to her health and to fetal growth and development.

Plan _____ days' menus that are nutritionally adequate, using the Daily Food Guide for Pregnancy.

Consume an adequate, varied, and balanced diet based on the Daily Food Guide for Pregnancy.

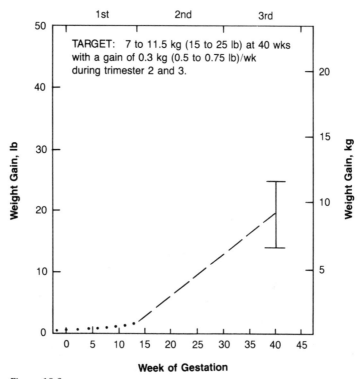

Figure 10-3
Provisional weight gain graph for overweight women with BMI of more than 26.0 to 29.0 (metric).

Avoid periods of fasting by consuming three meals per day plus two to three nutritious snacks.

Gain weight within the recommended range and rate, as determined by her assessment data.

Have an absence of nutrition-related problems or complications of pregnancy (see box, Nutrition-Related Problems and Complications During Pregnancy).

Nursing Interventions

Diet management

Set a mutually agreeable weight gain goal (range), based on the client's prepregnancy weight for height.

Promote the intake of a varied, nutrient-dense diet based on the Daily Food Guide for Pregnancy (see Table 10-5). Although the actual nutrient content of the diet will vary with the foods chosen, using the guide will help ensure an average adequate intake.

Modify the diet, as needed, to avoid or alleviate nutrition-related problems or complications of pregnancy.

(*Text continued on page 251*)

Nutrition-Related Problems and Complications During Pregnancy

Common Gastrointestinal Discomforts

NAUSEA AND VOMITING

Nausea and vomiting, common during the first trimester, may be related to hypoglycemia, decreased gastric motility, relaxation of the cardiac sphincter, or anxiety.

Nursing Interventions
Encourage the client
- To eat small frequent meals every 2 to 3 hours
- To increase CHO intake; in addition to leaving the stomach quickly, CHO also raise blood glucose levels
- To eat CHO before rising, like dry crackers, melba toast, dry cereal, hard candy
- To avoid drinking liquids with meals
- To avoid coffee, tea, and spicy foods
- To avoid high-fat foods because they delay gastric emptying time
- To eliminate individual intolerances

CONSTIPATION

Constipation during pregnancy may be caused by relaxation of GI muscle tone and motility related to elevated progesterone levels, or may result from pressure of the fetus on the intestines. Other contributing factors may include a decrease in physical activity and an inadequate intake of fluid and fiber. Constipation is also a common side effect of iron supplements.

Nursing Interventions
Encourage the client
- To increase fiber intake, especially whole-grain breads and cereals high in bran (see Chap. 15)
- To drink at least six to eight glasses of water daily
- To try hot water with lemon or prune juice on waking to help stimulate peristalsis

Recommend regular exercise. Reduce the dosage or frequency, if possible, if iron supplement is contributing to constipation.

HEARTBURN

A decrease in gastric motility, relaxation of the cardic sphincter, and pressure of the uterus on the stomach are contributing factors to heartburn.

Nursing Interventions

Encourage the client
- To eat small frequent meals and eliminate liquids immediately before and after meals to avoid gastric distention

(continued)

Nutrition-Related Problems
and Complications During Pregnancy (*continued*)

- To avoid coffee, high-fat foods, and spices
- To eliminate individual intolerances

Advise the client not to lie down or bend over after eating.

Nutritional Complications

IRON DEFICIENCY ANEMIA

Although iron absorption increases during pregnancy and losses through menstruation cease, maternal stores and diet are not likely to be sufficient to meet the increased demands for iron related to expanded blood volume and fetal requirements.

Nursing Interventions

Advise the client that

- Liver and red meats are the best sources of iron.
- Iron absorption from plant sources can be maximized by eating them with a rich source of vitamin C or with red meat.
- Iron aborption from plant sources is impaired when consumed with coffee and tea.

Encourage the client to take iron supplements as prescribed. See *Drug Alert* for possible adverse side effects and nursing actions related to iron supplements.

INADEQUATE WEIGHT GAIN

Inadequate weight gain may occur secondary to a poor appetite related to nausea, vomiting, heartburn, or smoking, or from an inadequate intake related to lack of knowledge, fear of gaining weight, or in inadequate food budget. Women who mistakenly believe that the fetus is a perfect parasite and will be adequately nourished regardless of maternal intake may also experience inadequate weight gain.

Although a short-term goal is to promote weight gain, the timing and the source of the weight gain are more important than the total amount. On a long-term basis, an improvement in overall eating habits will benefit both the health of the family and any subsequent pregnancies.

Nursing Interventions

Encourage the client to continue good eating practices and recommend specific ways to improve other habits.

Set mutually agreeable weight gain goals.

Depending on the cause, make appropriate diet modifications to improve appetite. Advise the client to quit smoking, not only to improve appetite, but because smoking is detrimental to both maternal and infant health.

(continued)

Nutrition-Related Problems
and Complications During Pregnancy (*continued*)

Counsel the client on the recommended rate and quantity of weight gain associated with optimal maternal and infant health and the ability to successfully breastfeed. Explain how the weight gain is distributed between the fetus, placenta, and maternal tissues. Encourage the client to ask questions and verbalize feelings. Advise the client that extra weight gained during pregnancy is quickly lost during lactation or through dieting *after* pregnancy.

Advise the client that

- If her diet is inadequate in calories, it also probably is inadequate in other nutrients.
- All nutrient requirements increase during pregnancy to support the growth of the fetus, placenta, and maternal tissues.
- Although the fetus can utilize maternal nutrient stores if her diet is inadequate, many nutrients are not stored by the body and a daily dietary intake is necessary.
- An inadequate intake can adversely affect maternal health (*i.e.*, poor iron intake→ anemia, poor calcium intake→ increased chance of bone loss later in life) and infant health (low birth weight, anemia, other postnatal complications)
  Refer the client to social services; determine if the client is eligible for WIC.

EXCESSIVE WEIGHT GAIN

After the 20th week of gestation, rapid weight gain may be a sign of fluid retention and preeclampsia.

Women who overeat may do so because they lack knowledge concerning recommended weight gain, or may believe that a pregnant woman must "eat for two." Stress may add to overeating; a decrease in physical activity can contribute to weight gain.

Although it is prudent to limit excessive weight gain, weight reduction diets should *never* be undertaken because of the risk of ketonemia and its potential damage to the fetus. Also, counting calories may take priority over the nutritional value of foods and result in a nutrient-poor diet. Again, a long-term objective of diet counseling is to improve eating habits for family health and any subsequent pregnancies.

Nursing Interventions

Notify the physician if signs of preeclampsia are observed: hypertension, fluid retention, albuminuria, complaints of headaches, blurred vision or visual disturbances.

Counsel the client on the recommended rate and quantity of weight gain

(continued)

Nutrition-Related Problems
and Complications During Pregnancy (*continued*)

associated with optimal maternal and infant health and the ability to successfully breastfeed. Explain how the weight gain is distributed between the fetus,
placenta, and maternal tissues. Set mutually agreeable weight gain goals. Recommend specific ways to limit the rate of weight gain without compromising
nutrient intake.

Substitute skim or low-fat milk for whole milk.

Bake, broil, or steam foods instead of frying.

Eliminate empty calories: carbonated beverages, candy, rich desserts, traditional
snack foods.

Limit portion sizes to those recommended by the Daily Food Guide for
pregnancy.

Use fats and oils sparingly.

**INADEQUATE INTAKE OF VITAMIN B_{12}, CALCIUM, VITAMIN D, RIBOFLAVIN,
AND POSSIBLY CALORIES RELATED TO PURE VEGETARIANISM/VEGANISM
(ELIMINATION OF ALL ANIMAL PRODUCTS)**

Vegan diets are lacking in vitamin B_{12} because it is found only in animal products (and fortified soybean milk). Also, diets lacking in milk and dairy products
are likely to be deficient in calcium, vitamin D, and riboflavin, particualrly during pregnancy. In addition, vegetarian diets tend to be lower in calories than
normal mixed diets.

Nursing Interventions

Explain the importance of obtaining adequate amounts of vitamin B_{12}, calcium,
vitamin D, riboflavin, and calories during pregnancy, and the difficulty in
obtaining these nutrients through a vegan diet.

　　Encourage the client

• To include milk, dairy products, and eggs in her diet during pregnancy and
lactation

• To eat a variety of foods and choose the proper combinations of *vegetable
proteins to complement one another (see Chap. 2)*

• To take vitamin B_{12}, calcium, and vitamin D supplements if milk and dairy
product intake is deficient

• To replace sea salt with iodized salt, if appropriate

**INADEQUATE INTAKE OF CALCIUM, VITAMIN D, RIBOFLAVIN, AND POSSIBLY PROTEIN
RELATED TO LACTOSE OR MILK INTOLERANCE**

Clients with lactose or milk intolerance avoid milk because they experience
gas, distention, cramping, and diarrhea to some degree after ingesting lactose
(milk sugar). Diets lacking in milk and dairy products are likely to be deficient
in calcium, vitamin D, and riboflavin.

(continued)

Nutrition-Related Problems
and Complications During Pregnancy (*continued*)

Nursing Interventions

Obtain a history to determine the extent of milk or lactose intolerance.

Many people with milk intolerance (milder form of lactose intolerance) can tolerate milk if consumed slowly and with food. Encourage the maximum intake of milk tolerated.

Advise the client of the importance of an adequate calcium intake during pregnancy (and lactation) and suggest other dairy products that may be tolerated: LactAid milk (commercially treated to reduce the lactose content), yogurt, buttermilk. (Other sources of calcium are listed in Appendix 13; see Chap. 15 for more information on lactose intolerance.)

Provide a calcium supplement, if appropriate.

PICA

Pica is a psychobehavioral disorder characterized by the ingestion of nonfoodstuffs—dirt, clay, starch, and ice are the most common items ingested. Eating these items may displace the intake of nutritious foods or interfere with nutrient absorption. Other potential complications vary with the items ingested and include lead poisoning, fecal impaction, parasitic infections, prematurity, and toxemia.

Iron deficiency may be a risk factor for pica; however, studies suggest it is more likely a consequence. Pica can be a strongly rooted social tradition and is more prevalent among blacks and rural residents. Other suggested risk factors include low socioeconomic status, inadequate nutritional status, and a childhood or family history of pica. Pica is surrounded by misconceptions about pregnancy and childbirth.

Some women who practice pica claim that it "helps" babies, cures swollen legs, relieves nausea and vomiting, ensures beautiful children, helps infants "slide out" more easily, and prevents birth marks. Pica may also be used to relieve tension or hunger, and some women claim they are merely satisfying cravings for clay or starch.

Some studies indicate anemia, iron deficiency, and toxemia are the most common outcomes in mothers with pica; dysfunctional labor related to fecal impaction, maternal death, premature birth, perinatal mortality, low birth weight, and anemia in the infant have also been reported.

Nursing Interventions

Determine what is being ingested and why. Refer the client to social services or WIC if appropriate.

Remain nonjudgmental but stress the importance of an adequate diet during pregnancy and the potential dangers of pica.

(continued)

Nutrition-Related Problems
and Complications During Pregnancy (*continued*)

Offer economical ways to obtain an adequate diet.

Provide an iron supplement if appropriate.

Encourage a high-fiber, high-fluid diet if the client experiences constipation.

Observe for diarrhea and vomiting, which may indicate a parasitic infection or lead poisoning.

Medical Complications

MATERNAL PHENYLKETONURIA

Phenylketonuria (PKU) is an inborn error of phenylalanine (an essential amino acid) metabolism that results in retardation and physical handicaps in newborns if not treated with a low-phenylalanine diet shortly after birth. Women who have PKU and who consume a normal diet during pregnancy have a high risk of delivering an infant with microcephaly, mental retardation, and LBW, even though the infant does not have PKU. The incidence of spontaneous abortion also increases.

Animal studies indicate that the fetus is more vulnerable to phenylalanine than the PKU mother and that a safe maternal intake may be harmful to the fetus.[7] Also, low-phenylalanine diets initiated after conception may be of little value; in order to prevent mental and physical handicaps, rigid diets may be necessary before conception.

Nursing Interventions

Obtain a complete history to determine if the client has PKU. Many adults may not be aware of their history of PKU if the diet was discontinued early in childhood. Maternal PKU may present a bigger problem for adolescents with unexpected pregnancies who may hide the pregnancy until late in gestation.

Advise the client

- That complete understanding and strict adherence to the diet are vital.
- That protein foods are high in phenylalanine and must be eliminated: meat, fish, poultry, eggs, dairy products, and nuts.
- That the special PKU formula is expensive and often offensive to adult palates, but must be consumed in adequate amounts both to support fetal growth and to prevent maternal tissue breakdown, which would have results similar to those from cheating on the diet.
- That an adequate calorie intake is necessary for normal protein metabolism.
- On the importance of close monitoring and periodic evaluations.

DIABETES MELLITUS

Diabetes mellitus, which is characterized by abnormal glucose tolerance, requires dietary management, whether it was present before conception

(continued)

Nutrition-Related Problems
and Complications During Pregnancy (*continued*)

(established diabetes) or develops during gestation (gestational diabetes) as a result of the metabolic changes of pregnancy. Diabetes increases the risk of infection, especially urinary tract infection, preeclampsia, and eclampsia. Diabetics tend to have large infants, which may complicate delivery and increase the risk of postpartum hemorrhage. The incidence of spontaneous abortion, hydraminios, extrauterine and neonatal deaths, and congenital abnormalities is higher among established diabetic patients than gestational diabetic patients.

Diabetic management during pregnancy includes diet therapy and, possibly, multiple daily doses of insulin.

Nursing Interventions

Monitor the progress and course of pregnancy of established diabetics. Screen all women for gestational diabetes at about the sixth month of pregnancy; check for ketonuria regularly.

Advise the client

- That pregnant diabetics require the same nutrients, and probably the same weight gain, as nonpregnant women.
- That weight loss and fasting should never be undertaken during pregnancy.
- That a 2000-calorie diet containing approximately 100 g of protein, 200 to 250 g of CHO, and 60 g of fat is recommended for normal-weight women who are hospitalized; women who are active need additional calories.
- That a liberal CHO intake (not less than 200 g/day) is necessary to prevent ketonemia and that it is better to eat too many calories than not enough.
- To distribute the CHO and calories as follows: 2/7 for breakfast, 2/7 for lunch, 2/7 for dinner, and 1/7 at bedtime. Smaller, more frequent feedings may be needed to better control and to alleviate other discomforts of pregnancy; periods of hunger should be avoided.
- That close monitoring and periodic evaluations are necessary throughout the course of pregnancy to meet nutritional needs and to control blood glucose levels.

PREGNANCY-INDUCED HYPERTENSION

Pregnancy-induced hypertension (PIH or toxemia) is a hypertensive syndrome occurring in approximately 6% to 7% of all pregnancies. Severe cases are associated with an increased risk of maternal, fetal, and neonatal deaths.

Preeclampsia is characterized by hypertension accompanied by proteinuria, edema, or both. A sudden weight gain (>2 lb/week after the 20th week of gestation) may indicate preeclampsia.

Eclampsia develops with the occurrence of one or more convulsions resulting from preeclampsia.

(continued)

Nutrition-Related Problems
and Complications During Pregnancy (*continued*)

> Although the exact cause is unknown, the development of PIH is strongly correlated to poverty and malnutrition, especially inadequate intakes of calories, protein, sodium, and possibly calcium. Good nutrition can prevent toxemia, and prevention is far more effective than treatment. Women at risk include those who are poorly nourished, primigravida, economically deprived, very young or very old, obese and gain too much weight, or underweight and fail to gain enough weight.
>
> *Nursing Interventions*
> Screen women at risk for toxemia and monitor for signs and symptoms: hypertension, facial edema, proteinuria (especially albumin), headaches, blurred vision or visual disturbances.
>
> Obtain a 24-hour recall and evaluate the diet according to the Daily Food Guide for Pregnancy, paying particular attention to calorie, protein, calcium, and sodium intakes.
>
> Advise clients at risk for preeclampsia to consume a liberal intake of calories, protein, and calcium, and to salt their food to taste. Sodium-restricted diets and diuretics are not advised.
>
> Recommend ways to improve the diet that are acceptable to the client.
>
> Identify and refer women who are eligible for social service programs or WIC.

Client teaching

Instruct the client and family

On the importance of adequate nutrition and weight gain for maternal and infant health. Describe the optimal rate of weight gain. Explain that weight gain during pregnancy is not synonymous with "getting fat," and that weight reduction should never be undertaken during pregnancy, even by overweight women. Overweight women who require less weight gain than normal should be instructed on how to choose a nutrient-dense diet for a controlled amount of high-quality weight gain.

On how to achieve nutritional adequacy by using the Daily Food Guide for Pregnancy. Stress the principles of variety, balance, and moderation; items from the "Fats, Oils, and Sweets" group should be used sparingly. Counsel the client on meal frequency, fluid requirements, and the use of salt, alcohol, and caffeine.

To take supplements only as prescribed by the physician. Discourage the use of supplements not prescribed by the physician and stress the importance of taking only the prescribed dosage because megadoses of some vitamins and minerals may cause fetal malformations. Advise against the use of dolomite and bone meal as calcium supplements; they may contain high levels of lead, and other heavy metals, which pose a hazard to both mother and fetus.

Common Myths About Nutrition During Pregnancy

You can eat anything you want because you're eating for two.

You can eat double portions because you're eating for two.

You should eat whatever you're craving; your body must need it.

If you take prenatal vitamins, you don't have to worry about what you eat.

You must take vitamins to have a healthy baby.

The baby gets what he or she needs first, the rest goes to the mother.

If you breast feed, you can lose all the weight you gain in pregnancy.

Obese women don't need to gain weight during pregnancy.

It doesn't matter what you eat because the baby will take what it needs from your body.

As long as you take vitamins, it's all right to skip meals.

When you are pregnant, you will crave pickles and ice cream.

Gaining lots of weight makes a healthy baby.

You lose a tooth with every baby if you don't drink milk.

Beets build red blood.

Food cravings during pregnancy will determine your child's like and dislikes later in life.

Give in to your cravings or you will mark the baby.

Do not eat fish and milk at the same meal.

Do not eat egg yolks because they will rot the uterus.

If you crave sweets, the baby will be a girl; if you crave pickles, the baby will be a boy.

(Carruth BR, Skinner JD: Practitioners beware: Regional differences in beliefs about nutrition during pregnancy. J Am Diet Assoc 91:435, 1991)

To avoid alcohol, tobacco, and drugs during pregnancy because of the actual or potential adverse health effects on both mother and baby.

That although coffee and caffeine are not necessarily contraindicated during pregnancy, they should be used sparingly.

That cravings during pregnancy do not appear to have a physiologic basis; rather, they are likely to be influenced by culture, geography, social traditions, the availability of foods, and previous experience. Satisfying cravings for foods is relatively harmless, as long as the overall impact on nutrient intake is not negative (*e.g.*, an occasional dill pickle is okay; eating an entire jar of them is not). Cravings for nonfood items should be investigated (see box, Nutrition-Related Problems and Complications During Pregnancy, for discussion of pica). Dispel myths about diet during pregnancy (see box, Common Myths About Nutrition During Pregnancy).

On how to modify her diet to alleviate or avoid nutrition-related problems and complica-

Assessment Criteria	**General Pregnancy and Lactation Assessment Criteria**
	Prepregnancy weight, preferably from a previously recorded measure
	Height
	Present weight
	BMI
	Blood pressure
	Hemoglobin, hematocrit to detect preexisting anemia. (Many laboratory values change during pregnancy due to normal adjustments in maternal physiology, and therefore laboratory tests during pregnancy cannot be validly compared to nonpregnancy standards. Biochemical norms have not been established for lactating women; hence laboratory tests are not indicated for routine assessments.)
	Severe dependent edema
	Other clinical signs that may occur during pregnancy (*i.e.*, bleeding gums) may be related to normal physiologic changes, not to nutritional deficiencies. However, a general examination of the skin, mucous membranes, gums, teeth, tongue, eyes, and hair that reveals abnormal findings may indicate potential nutritional problems and warrants further investigation.
	History of chronic illness, use of medications

tions of pregnancy (see box, Nutrition-Related Problems and Complications During Pregnancy), as appropriate.

To avoid all medications unless approved by the physician.

That once labor begins, no food or liquids should be consumed in order to prevent aspiration if anesthesia is used.

Monitor

Monitor for the following signs or symptoms:

Monthly weight gain. Monthly weight gains less than 1 pound per month by obese women or less than 2 pounds for all other women warrant further investigation.[17]

Food intolerances, especially lactose intolerance, and the overall impact on diet adequacy.

Ongoing compliance and tolerance of diet; evaluate adequacy and the need for further diet counseling or WIC participation.

Evaluation

Evaluation is ongoing. Assuming the plan of care has not changed, the client will achieve the goals as stated above.

DRUG ALERT: IRON SUPPLEMENTS

Use

Prevention and treatment of iron deficiency anemia

Possible Adverse Side Effects

May cause diarrhea, constipation, dark-colored stools, and GI upset. Although better absorbed when taken in between meals, iron supplements are less irritating to the GI tract when taken with food.

Actions

Observe for diarrhea and constipation. If constipation is not alleviated with a high-fiber diet, consider reducing the dosage or frequency.

If supplements are irritating to the GI tract when taken between meals, advise the client to take them with food.

Advise the client that a change in stool color is to be expected.

ADOLESCENT PREGNANCY

According to the American Dietetic Association, any pregnant adolescent is at nutritional risk because her own growth and development are compromised by the extra demands of fetal growth and development.[1] The incidence of low birth weight and infant mortality is high among pregnant adolescents, especially those under age 15. However, biologic age appears to be a more valid predictor of pregnancy outcome than chronologic age. Adolescents who conceive less than 4 years after the onset of menses have a higher risk of delivering a LBW infant than teenagers who become pregnant after the completion of the adolescent growth spurt.[1] Health risks to both mother and infant are lower in teenagers who seek early prenatal care and who are well nourished before conception. Compared to adult women, however, adolescents differ in the following ways:

- Are more likely to be physically, emotionally, financially, and socially immature. Low-income pregnant teens are especially likely to be at dietary risk.
- Have higher requirements for some nutrients. In addition, maternal–fetal competition for nutrients can develop if pregnancy occurs before completion of the adolescent growth spurt.
- Are more likely to be underweight at the time of conception and gain less than 16 pounds during pregnancy. Schneck reported that 40% of the pregnant teens in her study gained less than adequate weight.[13]
- Are more likely to have inadequate nutrient reserves.
- May not know how to choose a nutritious diet and tend to have poor eating habits. In one study,[13] pregnant teens frequently reported drinking three to four cans of soda a day and substituting chips, candy, and soda for a meal. More than 40% of the teens studied indicated that they did not make any dietary changes while pregnant, although other studies indicate much higher percentages.[13]
- Are more reluctant to take supplements, making adequate dietary intake essential.
- Seek prenatal care later and have fewer total visits.

Nutritional Requirements

The RDA for pregnancy are not categorized according to maternal age. For instance, the RDA for calcium for nonpregnant women aged 11 to 24 is 1200 mg, the same amount recommended during pregnancy. Obviously, teenagers require more than their normal RDA during pregnancy; however, actual nutrient needs depend more on biologic age than chronologic age and should be determined on an individual basis.

Nutrient requirements during pregnancy also are influenced by preconception nutritional status. Nutrients most often lacking in adolescent diets are iron, calcium, and vitamin A. Pregnant adolescents from low socioeconomic groups also may have inadequate intakes of protein, calories, and folic acid. Like pregnant adults, adolescents need supplements of iron in addition to a nutritious diet.

Diet Counseling

Diet management and client teaching outlined above are also appropriate for adolescent pregnancies. However, to maximize the effectiveness of nutritional counseling of adolescents, it is particularly important to establish a rapport in a relaxed, nonthreatening, nonjudgmental environment. In addition to assessing the client's nutritional needs, her attitudes, interests, beliefs, fears, and lifestyle must also be evaluated. Many teens have limited reading skills, therefore, teaching materials must be appropriate for their level of understanding. The Daily Food Guide for Pregnancy is useful both for assessing dietary strengths and weakness, as well as serving as a framework for implementing dietary changes at a level the teenager can understand.[13]

Set mutually agreeable realistic goals for weight gain and food intake. Diet recommendations must be concrete and reasonable,[13] and achievable given the client's financial status and lifestyle. Because teens living with one or more parents may have little control over what food is available to them, parents and significant others should be encouraged to attend counseling sessions.

Ideally, the client should be monitored at frequent periodic intervals to evaluate the effectiveness of the nutritional care plan and redefine needs as the pregnancy progresses.

LACTATION

Data on the incidence and duration of breastfeeding are limited; however, women who breastfeed are more likely to be well educated, older, and white.[15] Despite efforts by the Surgeon General and leading health agencies to promote breastfeeding, the incidence of breastfeeding has declined since the early 1980s.

Breast milk is recognized as the optimal food for infants (see box, Composition of Breast Milk). Because it imparts benefits to both mother and infant, breastfeeding is recommended for all normal full-term infants for the first 4 to 6 months of life (see box, Advantages and Disadvantages of Breastfeeding).

Although almost all women have the potential to breastfeed successfully, lactation may fail because of inadequate knowledge, lack of adequate support, or conflict with lifestyle and career. Counseling on the importance of breastfeeding and how best to initiate and

Composition of Breast Milk

Protein

Provides 6% to 7% of total calories.

Content is adequate to support growth and development without contributing to an excessive renal solute load.

The amino acid patterns are ideal for infants. Breast milk contains small amounts of amino acids that may be harmful in large amounts (*i.e.*, phenylalanine) and high levels of amino acids that infants cannot synthesize well (*i.e.*, taurine).

Fat

Provides about 50% of total calories.

Content is high in linoleic acid, the essential fatty acid.

Is easily digested because of fat-digesting enzymes contained in the milk.

Contains high levels of cholesterol, which may help infants develop enzyme systems to handle cholesterol later in life.

CHO

Provides about 42% of total calories.

Lactose is the most abundant CHO, which stimulates the growth of friendly GI bacteria and promotes calcium absorption.

Antibodies

Although more abundant in colostrum, antibodies and anti-infective factors are present in mature breast milk.

Minerals

Content is adequate for growth and development but not excessive to the point of burdening immature kidneys with a high renal solute load.

The calcium-to-phosphorus ratio is 2:1, ideal for calcium absorption.

Iron absorption is about 49%, compared to an absorption rate of about 4% for iron-fortified formulas.

Zinc absorption is better from breast milk.

Low in sodium.

Vitamins

All vitamins needed for growth and health are contained in adequate amounts in breast milk if the mother's diet is adequate. Vitamin C, riboflavin, and thiamine are the vitamins most affected by maternal diet.

(continued)

Composition of Breast Milk (*continued*)

Renal Solute Load

Suited to the immature kidneys' inability to concentrate urine.

Other Compounds

Bifidus factor promotes the growth of friendly GI bacteria (*Lactobacillus*), which protect the infant against harmful GI bacteria.
Several enzymes.
Several hormones.

continue lactation should begin early in pregnancy to promote the greatest chance of success.

Composition of Breast Milk

The composition of breast milk is ideally formulated to promote normal infant growth and development. Human milk, which differs from milk of other mammals, is unique in the type and concentrations of macronutrients (CHO, protein, fat), micronutrients (vitamins and minerals), enzymes, hormones, growth factors, host resistance factors, inducers/modulators of the immune system, and anti-inflammatory agents.[15]

The composition of breast milk may vary not only among individuals but also with the time of day, maternal age, and parity. Other significant variables include the stage of lactation, maternal diet, and the duration of the feeding.

Stage of Lactation

Breast milk varies considerably with the stage of lactation. Preterm milk, secreted in small amounts before delivery, is higher in nitrogen (protein) than milk produced after a term delivery.

Colostrum, which is secreted during the first few postpartum days, is a yellowish fluid that is higher in protein and lower in CHO, fat, and calories than mature milk. Colostrum is also rich in antibodies and anti-infective factors that protect the infant against certain viral and bacterial diseases.

Colostrum begins to change to transitional milk 3 to 6 days postpartum as the protein content decreases and the CHO and fat content increases. Major changes in the milk take place by the 10th day and mature milk is stable by the end of the first month.

Maternal Diet

Almost all women are capable of producing enough high-quality breast milk to promote infant growth and development. In well nourished women, neither the volume nor caloric density of breast milk is affected by excessive or inadequate calorie intakes. Likewise, the

Advantages and Disadvantages of Breastfeeding

Advantages

For the infant:

- "Breast is best"—breast milk contains all essential nutrients in optimum amounts and in forms the infant can easily tolerate and digest. Breast milk is recommended as the sole source of nutrition for the first 4 to 6 months of life.
- Breast milk is a "natural" food that contains no artificial colorings, flavorings, preservatives, or additives.
- Colostrum and breast milk contain antibodies and anti-infective factors that protect the infant against certain viral and bacterial diseases. Studies suggest that breastfed infants are less prone to both wheezing and stomach and intestinal illnesses.
- Breast milk is sterile, is at the proper temperature, and is readily available.
- Breastfeeding promotes better tooth and jaw development than bottle feeding because the infant has to suck harder.
- Breastfeeding avoids nursing-bottle caries.
- Breastfeeding is protective against allergies.
- Overfeeding is not likely with breastfeeding.
- Breastfeeding promotes optimal maternal–infant bonding.

For the mother:

- Breastfeeding can mobilize fat stores to help women lose weight.
- Early breastfeeding stimulates uterine contractions to help control blood loss and regain prepregnant size.
- Breast milk is readily available and requires no mixing or dilution.
- Breastfeeding may be less expensive than purchasing bottles, nipples, sterilizing equipment, and formula.
- Breastfeeding may decrease the risk of thromboembolism, especially after operative deliveries.
- Childbirth and breastfeeding may be protective against breast cancer.
- Although not reliable, breastfeeding affords some contraceptive protection.

Disadvantages

Others cannot share in feeding the infant unless breast milk is manually expressed.

Breastfeeding may be uncomfortable, particularly in women with inverted nipples.

Drugs and environmental contaminants can be transmitted through breast milk.

Vegan mothers may produce milk that is deficient in vitamin B_{12} and vitamin D.

(continued)

Advantages and Disadvantages of Breastfeeding (*continued*)

Breast feeding is contraindicated when
- The infant has an inborn error of metabolism (*i.e.*, galactosemia, phenylketonuria).
- The mother has a chronic illness or must use medications that can harm the infant.
- The mother has a serious psychiatric disorder.
- The mother has cancer and is being treated with chemotherapeutic drugs or radiotherapeutics.
- The mother's milk is contaminated with environmental pollutants.
- The mother becomes pregnant, because the combined demands of pregnancy and lactation on maternal tissues are great.

concentration of CHO, protein, major minerals (calcium, phosphorus, magnesium), and most trace elements in breast milk is stable regardless of whether the maternal diet is inadequate or excessive in those nutrients. However, some studies indicate that poor maternal nutrition decreases the concentrations of certain host resistance factors.[15]

The concentrations of some nutrients in breast milk are maintained at the expense of maternal reserves when intake is inadequate. However, the concentrations of fatty acids, vitamins, iodine, and selenium in breast milk do vary with maternal intake.

Fatty acids

The fat and calorie content of the mother's diet influences the fatty acid patterns of breast milk; that is, a diet high in polyunsaturated fats results in a high polyunsaturated fat content in the milk. The fatty acid composition of milk produced by women on low-calorie diets (*i.e.*, women mobilizing their fat stores for energy) is similar to the fatty acid composition of stored fat. Women who consume low-calorie diets and have inadequate fat reserves may produce milk significantly reduced in fat content.

Vitamins

The vitamin content of breast milk depends on maternal intake and reserves, although the magnitude of the dependency varies among vitamins.[15] Chronic poor vitamin intake, especially poor intakes of vitamin C, riboflavin, and thiamine, results in vitamin-poor milk.

Unusually high intakes of most vitamins, either through food or supplements, do not increase their concentration in breast milk; the exceptions are vitamins B_6 and D.

Iodine and selenium

Studies have shown that the concentrations of iodine and selenium in breast milk increase in response to a high maternal intake. It is not known whether high levels pose a risk to the infant.

Duration of the Feeding

Fore-milk, the milk secreted as each feeding begins, is lower in fat than hind-milk, the milk secreted at the end of each feeding. The increase in fat content may be a physiologic mechanism designed to provide satiety and signal the infant to stop nursing.

Recommended Dietary Allowances for Lactation

The RDA for lactation are based on the nutritional content of breast milk and the nutritional "cost" of producing milk. Compared to the RDA for nonpregnant, nonlactating women, breastfeeding significantly increases the requirements of all nutrients with established RDA (see Table 10-3), with the exception of iron. In fact, the RDA for lactation are equal to or higher than those for pregnancy for all nutrients except vitamin B_6, folic acid, and iron.

New to the 10th edition of the *Recommended Dietary Allowances* are two separate categories for lactation: the first 6 months and the second 6 months of breastfeeding. The differences in recommendations between the two groupings reflect the variation in the average amount of milk produced (750 ml and 600 ml, respectively).

Calorie requirements while breastfeeding are proportional to the amount of milk produced.[10] The average calorie content of breast milk produced by well-nourished mothers is 70 cal/100 ml, and approximately 85 calories are needed for every 100 ml produced. The average woman uses approximately 640 calories/day for the first 6 months and 510 calories/day during the second 6 months to produce a normal amount of milk; women who only partially breastfeed use fewer calories.

The RDA recommends that women who gained the appropriate amount of weight during pregnancy increase their calorie intake by 500 per day for both the first and second 6 months of lactation. This allows women to mobilize fat accumulated during pregnancy and may help achieve prepregnancy fat stores and weight. Women who failed to gain enough weight during pregnancy or who have inadequate fat reserves should consume a total of 650 additional calories per day during the first 6 months of breastfeeding. Theoretically, women who breastfeed can consume more calories and still lose weight easier than women who do not breastfeed. In fact, women eating self-selected diets tend to lose approximately 1 to 2 lbs/month during the first 4 to 6 months of breastfeeding. However, studies indicate about 20% of lactating women maintain or gain weight.

Assuming lactating women follow an eating pattern similar to nonlactating women but with additional calories to meet their energy requirements, the nutrients most likely to be consumed in inadequate amounts are calcium, magnesium, zinc, folic acid, and vitamin B_6.[15] Women who voluntarily restrict their calorie intake to promote weight loss may obtain less than optimal amounts of other nutrients.

The Food Group Approach for Lactation and General Dietary Suggestions

Although actual nutrient content of the diet will vary with the foods chosen, using the Daily Food Guide for Lactation will help ensure an average adequate intake (see Table 10-5). As in the guidelines for pregnancy, there are few changes during lactation. Again, the most notable difference is that four or more servings of milk are suggested in order to meet calcium requirements. The extra servings of milk also provide the extra protein to meet the increased requirements. Liberal amounts of fruits and vegetables, whole-grain breads and cereals, and protein-rich foods are encouraged to meet additional requirements imposed by lactation.

Another nutritional consideration during lactation is fluid intake. It is suggested that women drink 2 to 3 quarts of fluid daily, preferably in the form of water, milk, and fruit juices instead of carbonated beverages, sweetened fruit drinks, and caffeine-containing beverages. Thirst is a good indicator of need; fluids consumed in excess of thirst do not increase milk volume.[15]

NURSING PROCESS

The reliability and validity of using anthropometric and biochemical methods for assessing the nutritional status of lactating women have not been proven. Therefore, the only criteria recommended for routine screening for nutritional problems are maternal weight and dietary intake.

Assessment

In addition to the general pregnancy and lactation assessment criteria, assess for the following factors:

Weight. Studies on American women indicate that weight is the only anthropometric measurement useful for monitoring ongoing nutritional status during lactation.[15]

Usual 24-hour intake; a food frequency record or food record is also collected for additional information.

Usual intake of milk and other calcium-rich dairy products compared to the Daily Food Guide for Lactation. Also of particular importance are the use of vitamin D fortified foods and the intake of vitamin-rich fruits and vegetables.

Strict vegetarianism, or the elimination of whole food groups from the diet (*e.g.*, milk because of lactose intolerance).

Cultural, familial, religious, and ethnic influences on eating habits.

Voluntary restriction of calorie intake to lose weight or the use of a modified diet to treat a disease.

Adequacy of sunlight exposure.

The client's use of alcohol, tobacco, caffeine, and drugs.

Nursing Diagnosis

Health Seeking Behaviors, as evidenced by a lack of knowledge of diet during lactation and a desire to learn.

Planning and Implementation

Lactating women should be encouraged to consume at least 1800 calories per day to obtain adequate amounts essential nutrients. Because the vitamin content of the mother's diet influences the concentration of vitamins in breast milk, women should be encouraged to choose a varied diet and eat fresh fruits and vegetables with a minimal amount of preparation.

Multivitamin and mineral supplements are not recommended for routine use. However, specific supplements may be indicated when maternal intake is inadequate. For instance, a balanced multivitamin and mineral supplement may be necessary for women who consume fewer than 1800 calories. Women who are lactose-intolerant or who do not consume enough milk and other calcium-rich foods may require a calcium supplement. Supplemental vitamin D may be indicated for women who avoid vitamin D-fortified foods (*e.g.*, milk and cereals) and have limited exposure to the sun. Strict vegans need supplemental vitamin B_{12} if they do not regularly consume vitamin B_{12}-fortified plant products.

Ideally, preparation for breastfeeding should begin prenatally with counseling, guidance, and support throughout the gestational period. Postpartum teaching has been shown to have a significant impact on both the ability to breastfeed successfully and the duration of lactation. Individual or small group counseling sessions should first assess the couple's attitudes, fears, expectations, and knowledge, before providing information on how milk is produced and secreted, factors that impair lactation (see box, Factors That Impair Lactation), breast care, feeding positions, how to express milk manually, and how to stimulate the infant.

Some studies show that the most vulnerable period for lactation is the immediate postpartum period.[4] To establish lactation and promote the best chance of success, the infant should be offered the breast as soon as possible after birth and at frequent intervals. Hospital procedures should allow for immediate maternal–infant contact after delivery and true demand feedings.

Allergy to breast milk is uncommon, and some researchers believe it may not even exist.[18] However, the infant may develop an allergic reaction to breast milk if the mother ingests a protein that enters the breast milk intact; if this occurs, the protein can be identified and eliminated from the mother's diet.

Few foods are contraindicated during lactation. It is generally not necessary to eliminate any particular foods while breastfeeding unless the infant shows an intolerance, except for freshwater fish from water contaminated with dioxin, PCB, or other chemicals. Women should contact their State Health Department for recommendations regarding fish consumption during lactation. It may also be prudent to avoid saccharin while breastfeeding.

Garlic and onion oils may flavor the taste of breast milk. However, they need not be eliminated from the mother's diet unless the taste of the milk is objectionable to the infant.

Breastfeeding is contraindicated when the mother is being treated with antimetabolites or radiotherapeutics, or uses illicit drugs.[15] Medications that have the potential to enter breast milk and harm the infant should be avoided, if possible, and replaced with a safer acceptable one.[15] Although tobacco, caffeine, and alcohol are not absolutely contraindicated, they should be used as little as possible. Women who have been exposed to high levels of environmental toxins should have their milk analyzed for contaminants.

Client goals

The client will:

Explain the importance of diet to her health and to infant growth and development.

Plan _____ days' menus that are nutritionally adequate, using the Daily Food Guide for Lactation.

Factors that Impair Lactation

Failure to Establish Lactation Related to

Delayed or infrequent feedings
Weak infant sucking because of anesthesia during labor and delivery
Nipple discomfort or engorgement

Decreased Demand Related to

Supplemental bottles of formula or water
Introduction of solid food
The infant's lack of interest

Impaired Let-Down Related to

Tension
Fatigue
Negative attitude, lack of desire, lack of family support
Excessive intake of caffeine or alcohol
Smoking
Drugs

Consume an adequate, varied, and balanced diet based on the Daily Food Guide for
     Lactation.
Attain/maintain normal weight.

Nursing Interventions

Diet management

Promote the intake of a varied, nutrient-dense diet based on the Daily Food Guide for
     Lactation (see Table 10-5). Although the actual nutrient content of the diet will vary
     with the foods chosen, using the guide will help ensure an average adequate intake.
Individualize the diet as much as possible to correspond with the client's likes, dislikes, and
     eating pattern. Special attention should be given to calcium intake among women who
     are lactose-intolerant.

Client teaching

Principles of breastfeeding

Instruct the client
On the benefits of breastfeeding to both mother and infant.
That even a short period of breastfeeding is better than not nursing at all.

On normal physiology of lactation, the role of hormones, and factors that may inhibit lactation (see box, Factors That Impair Lactation).

That all women have the ability to breastfeed if given proper instruction and encouragement.

That the infant should be allowed to nurse for 5 minutes on each side on the first day in order to achieve let-down and milk ejection. By the end of the first week, the infant should be up to 15 minutes per side.

That the supply of milk is equal to the demand; the more the infant sucks, the more milk produced. Six- and 12-week-old infants who suck more are probably experiencing a growth spurt and hence need more milk.

That once the milk supply is established and let-down is functioning, the infant will be able virtually to empty the breast within 5 to 10 minutes. However, the infant needs to nurse beyond that point to satisfy his need to suck and for emotional and physical comfort.

That feeding the infant more frequently and manually expressing milk will help increase the milk supply.

That a warm bath, gentle massages, and a relaxed atmosphere may help achieve let-down.

That because breast milk is easier to digest than formula, breastfed babies usually need to nurse at shorter intervals than bottle-fed babies.

That early substitution of formula or introduction of solid foods may decrease the chance of maintaining lactation.

That breast pumps are available for manual expression of milk. Milk expressed into a sanitary bottle should be refrigerated or frozen immediately. Milk should be used within 24 hours if refrigerated, within 3 months if stored in the freezer compartment of the refrigerator, and within 2 years if maintained at 0°.

Role of nutrition in lactation

Instruct the client

On the importance of eating a diet adequate in calories, fluid, calcium, and vitamins, and how to use the Daily Food Guide for Lactation in meal planning.

That even if a mother has adequate fat stores, calorie intake should increase because fat is mobilized slowly.

That lactating women may experience a 1- to 2-lb weight loss per month, although some women may lose up to 4 lbs per month.[15] Normal weight loss does not adversely effect milk production. Excessive maternal weight gain during pregnancy increases the likelihood of postpartum weight retention despite breastfeeding.

That appetite and thirst are generally good indicators of need; consuming excesses of either will not produce "better" or more milk.

To avoid freshwater fish and saccharin. Other foods may be eliminated if the infant appears to develop an intolerance.

That although moderate amounts of alcohol may help let-down, large amounts can enter breast milk and should be avoided.

To avoid large amounts of caffeine because it also enters breast milk, although at very low levels. However, infants are unable to metabolize caffeine as well as adults, and over time caffeine can accumulate in the infant's bloodstream.

General information related to lactation

Instruct the client

Not to take drugs or medications unless approved by the physician.

Can Vitamins Prevent Spina Bifida?

Spina bifida, the second most common birth defect in the United States, is characterized by the incomplete closing of the bony casing surrounding the spinal cord. Two thirds of infants born with neural tube defects (NTD) survive into childhood; many of its victims lack bowel and bladder control or suffer paralysis from the waist down. In some cases, mental retardation results from the excess accumulation of fluid in the brain.

A hot topic of recent research is whether multivitamin supplements, especially those containing folic acid, can prevent NTD when taken before conception and/or during the first 6 weeks of pregnancy when the spinal cord (neural tube) is closing. Earlier studies showed that women who had babies with NTD consumed folic acid-deficient diets and had low-serum folic acid levels. A British study found that folic acid supplements decreased the risk of spina bifida in subsequent babies born to women who had already given birth to a baby with a NTD. A newer study at the Boston University School of Medicine found that 100 μg of folic acid taken during the first 6 weeks of pregnancy reduced the risk of NTD by 50% to 70%.

However, other studies have found no correlation between supplements and NTD. As of yet, it is not clear whether folic acid alone, or taken together with other vitamins, offers protection against NTD.

Unfortunately, controlled studies on supplement use before conception and during the first 6 weeks of pregnancy are difficult to conduct, largely because many women may not even realize they are pregnant.

At the very least, women planning to become pregnant should make improvements in their diets if folic acid intake appears to be inadequate: liver, eggs, broccoli, kale, dried peas and beans, whole-grain breads, fruits, vegetables, and orange juice are the best sources of folic acid. Even though conclusive evidence is lacking, it may be prudent for all women planning to become pregnant to take a multivitamin supplement that provides 100% of the USRDA of folic acid; vitamin supplements taken in larger doses have the potential to cause harm. Even if future research disproves the role of vitamins in the prevention of NTD, taking a multivitamin of this potency is harmless.

On breast care, positioning of the infant, ways to stimulate the infant, how to end a feeding, and advice on weaning.

That the La Lèche League is an international organization founded for the purpose of helping nursing mothers. The League prints a bimonthly newsletter, holds conventions and monthly group meetings, and is available as a source of information and advice 24 hours a day.

That numerous instructional materials and books are available on breastfeeding from community organizations and bookstores.

Monitor

Monitor for the following signs or symptoms:

Weight changes

Food intolerances, especially lactose intolerance, and the overall impact on diet adequacy

Ongoing compliance to diet; evaluate adequacy and the need for further diet counseling

Evaluation

Evaluation is ongoing. Assuming the plan of care has not changed, the client will achieve the goals as stated above.

BIBLIOGRAPHY

1. American Dietetic Association: Position of the American Dietetic Association: Nutrition management of adolescent pregnancy. J Am Diet Assoc 89:104, 1989

2. American Dietetic Association: Nutrition management of adolescent pregnancy: Technical support paper. J Am Diet Assoc 89:105, 1989

3. Carruth BR, Skinner JD: Practitioners beware: Regional differences in beliefs about nutrition during pregnancy. J Am Diet Assoc 91:435, 1991

4. Ferris AM, McCabe LT, Allen LH, et al: Biological and sociocultural determinants of successful lactation among women in eastern Connecticut. J Am Diet Assoc 87:316, 1987

5. Haase TB: Study aims to reduce mental retardation in children of PKU mothers. J Am Diet Assoc 85:307, 1985

6. Horner RD, Lackey CJ, Kolsa K, et al: Pica practices of pregnant women. J Am Diet Assoc 91:34, 1991

7. Liebman B: Can vitamins prevent birth defects? Nutrition Action Health Letter 18:8, 1990

8. March of Dimes Birth Defects Foundation, International Food Information Council: Healthy Eating During Pregnancy. White Plains, NY, 1991.

9. Mayer J (ed): Strictly supplemental. Tufts University Diet and Nutrition Letter 7(12):1, 1990

10. National Research Council: Recommended Dietary Allowances. 10th ed. Washington, DC: National Academy Press, 1989

11. Parham ES, Astrom MF, King SH: The association of pregnancy weight gain with the mother's postpartum weight. J Am Diet Assoc 90:550, 1990

12. Public Health Service, United States Department of Health and Human Services: The Surgeon General's Report on Nutrition and Health: Summary and Recommendations. DHHS (PHS) Publication no. 88-50211. Washington, DC: Government Printing Office, 1988

13. Schneck ME, Sideras KS, Fox RA, et al: Low-income pregnant adolescents and their infants: Dietary findings and health outcomes. J Am Diet Assoc 90:555, 1990

14. Skinner JD, Carruth BR: Dietary quality of pregnant and nonpregnant adolescents. J Am Diet Assoc 91:718, 1991

15. Subcommittee on Nutrition During Lactation, Food and Nutrition Board, National Academy of Sciences: Nutrition During Lactation. Washington, DC: National Academy Press, 1991

16. Subcommittee on Nutritional Status and Weight Gain During Pregnancy, Food and Nutrition Board, National Academy of Sciences: Nutrition During Pregnancy. Washington, DC: National Academy Press, 1990

17. Suitor CW: Perspectives on nutrition during pregnancy: Part I: Weight gain; Part II: Nutrient supplements. J Am Diet Assoc 91:96, 1991

18. Worthington-Roberts BS, Verseersch J, Williams SR: Nutrition in Pregnancy and Lactation. 4th ed. St. Louis: CV Mosby, 1989

11 Growth and Development: Infancy Through Adolescence

RELATIONSHIP BETWEEN GROWTH, DEVELOPMENT, AND NUTRITION

Growth is defined as an increase in the number and size of cells. Development is the increase in function and complexity that occurs through growth, maturation, and learning. Mental, emotional, social, and physical growth and development occur throughout the life cycle. The timing and rate of growth and development are influenced by genetic, hormonal, behavioral, and environmental factors, including diet.

An optimum diet provides adequate, but not excessive, amounts of all the nutrients essential for growth and development. Early in life, nutrition is important for enabling a child to reach his genetic potential for physical and mental growth and development. Average increases in height (length) and weight can be predicted according to the child's age (Table 11-1). Actual assessment of an individual's physical growth and growth pattern should be done periodically by measuring and plotting height (length), weight, and weight for height (length) on the National Center for Health Statistic (NCHS) growth grids (Figs. 11-1 to 11-8). Normally, an individual's percentile status for height (length) and weight remains fairly constant throughout childhood. A deviation of more than 2 percentile channels warrants a more in-depth assessment of growth and nutritional status. An increase in weight percentile may suggest the development of obesity; a decrease may indicate undernutrition, an undiagnosed chronic disease, or emotional problems.

(*Text continued on page 277*)

Table 11-1
Average Increases in Weight and Height (Length) Based on Age

Age	Average Weight Gain	Average Height Gain (inches)
Birth–6 months	140–200 g/week (5–7 oz) Birthweight doubles between 4–6 months.	2.5 cm (1 in)/month
6–12 months	85–140 g/week (3–5 oz) Birthweight triples by the end of the first year.	1.25 cm (½ in)/month Birth length increases by about 50% by the end of the first year.
1–3	2–3 kg (4.4–6.6 lb)/year Birthweight quadruples by age 2½.	12 cm (4.8 in) during second year; 6–8 cm (2.4–3.2 in) during third year. Height at 2 years is about 50% of eventual adult height.
3–6	2–3 kg (4.4–6.6 lb/year)	6–8 cm (2.4–3.2 in)/year
6–pubertal growth spurt	2–3 kg (4.4–6.6 lb)/year	5 cm (2 in)/year after age 7
Pubertal growth spurt Females between 10–14 years old	7–25 kg (15–55 lb) Mean = 17.5 kg (38.1 lb)	5–25 cm (2–10 in) Mean = 20.5 cm (8.2 in) Approximately 90% of mature height is attained by onset of menarche or skeletal age of 13 years.
Males between 11–16 years old	7–30 kg (15–65 lb) Mean = 23.7 kg (52.1 lb)	10–30 cm (4–12 in) Mean = 20.5 cm (8.2 in) Approximately 95% of mature height is attained by skeletal age of 15 years.

(Adapted with permission from Whaley LF, Wong DL: Nursing Care of Infants and Children, 4th ed., St. Louis: Mosby–Year Book, 1991)

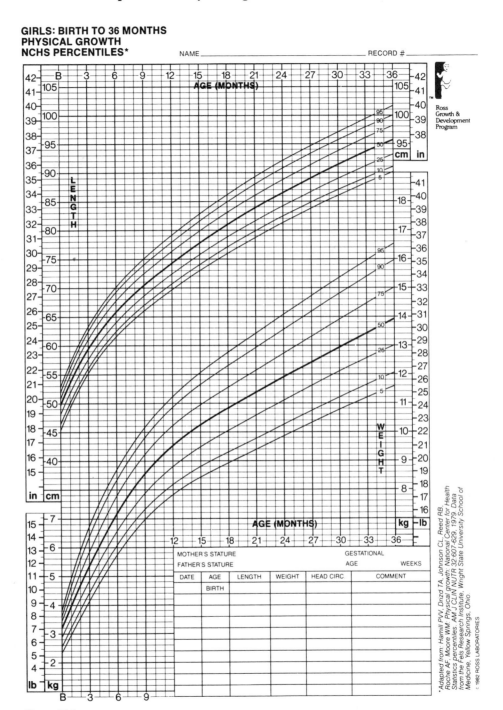

Figure 11-1

NCHS percentiles for physical growth of girls aged from birth to 36 months. (Adapted from Hamill PVV, Drizd TA, Johnson CL et al: Physical growth: National Center for Health Statistics percentiles. Am J Clin Nutr 32:607, 1979. Data from the Fels Research Institute, Wright State University School of Medicine, Yellow Springs, Ohio.)

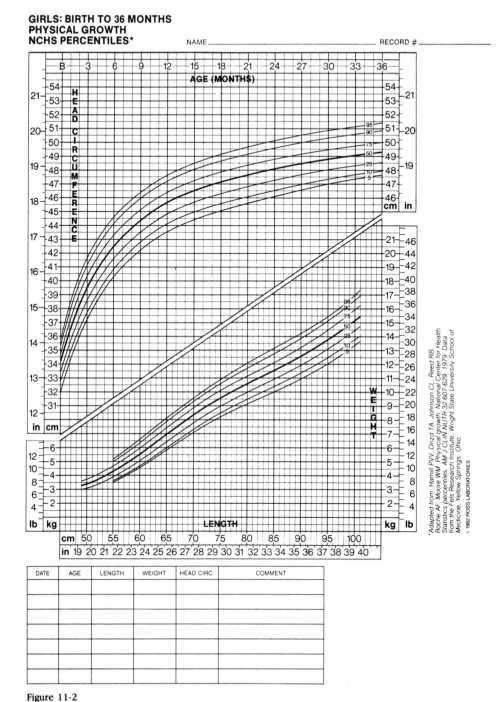

Figure 11-2

NCHS percentiles for physical growth of girls aged from birth to 36 months. (Adapted from Hamill PVV, Drizde TA, Johnson CL et al: Physical growth: National Center for Health Statistics percentiles. Am J Clin Nutr 32:607, 1979. Data from the Fels Research Institute, Wright State University School of Medicine, Yellow Springs, Ohio.)

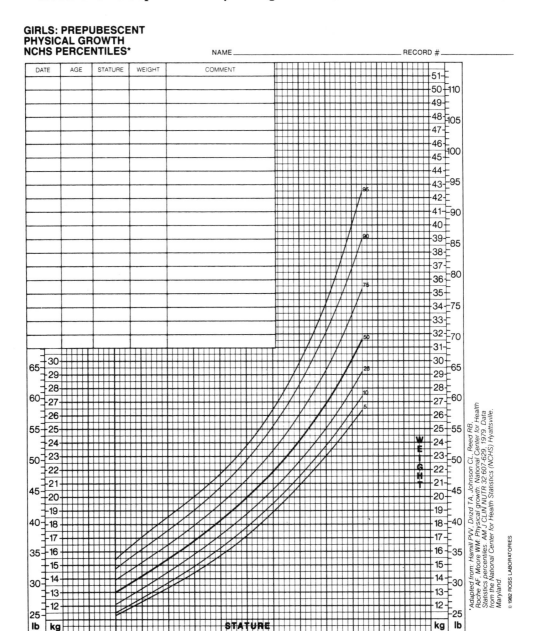

Figure 11-3

NCHS percentiles for physical growth of prepubescent girls. (Adapted from Hamill PVV, Drizd TA, Johnson CL et al: Physical growth: National Center for Health Statistics percentiles. Am J Clin Nutr 32:607, 1979. Data from the National Center for Health Statistics, Hyattsville, Maryland.)

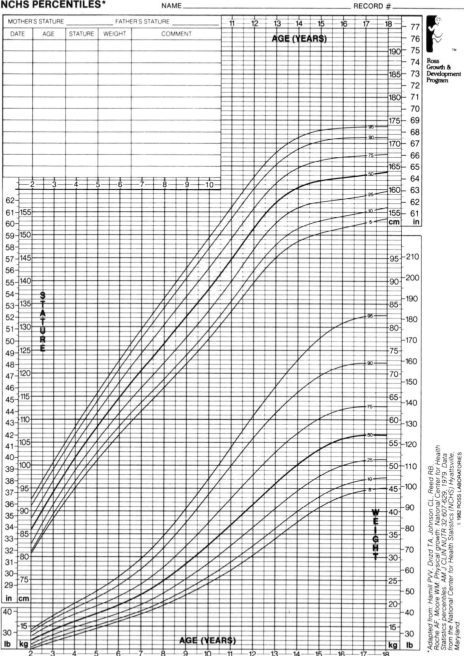

Figure 11-4

NCHS percentiles for physical growth of girls aged from 2 to 18 years. (Adapted from Hamill PVV, Drizd TA, Johnson CL et al: Physical growth: National Center for Health Statistics percentiles. Am J Clin Nutr 32:607, 1979. Data from the National Center for Health Statistics, Hyattsville, Maryland.)

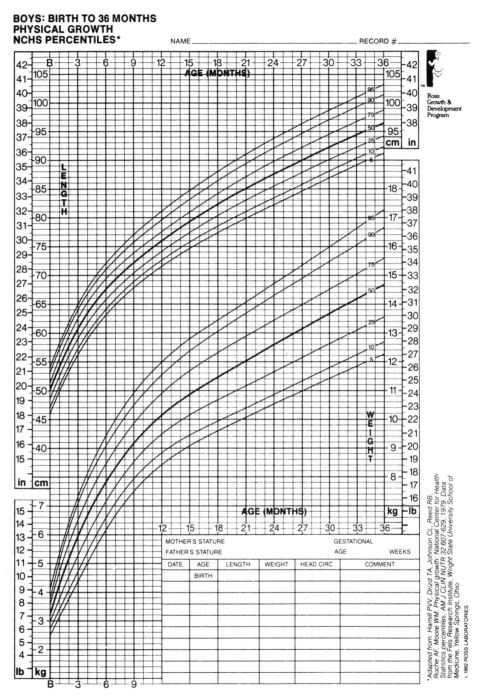

Figure 11-5

NCHS percentiles for physical growth of boys aged from birth to 36 months. (Adapted from Hamill PVV, Drizd TA, Johnson CL et al: Physical growth: National Center for Health Statistics percentiles. Am J Clin Nutr 32:607, 1979. Data from the Fels Research Institute, Wright State University School of Medicine, Yellow Springs, Ohio.)

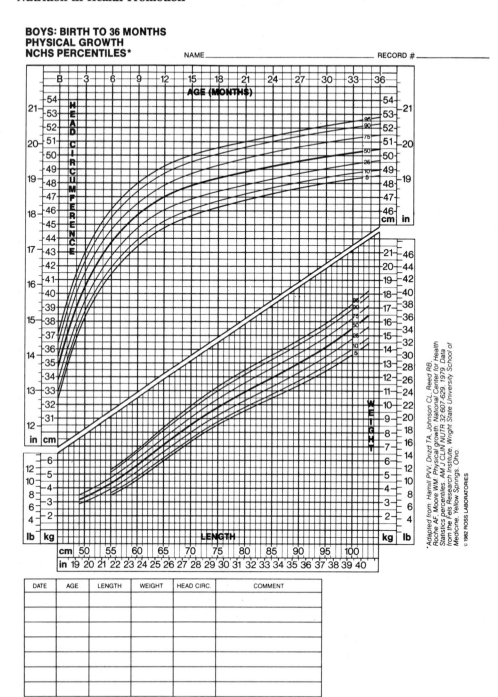

Figure 11-6

NCHS percentiles for physical growth of boys aged from birth to 36 months. (Adapted from Hamill PVV, Drizd TA, Johnson CL et al: Physical growth: National Center for Health Statistics percentiles. Am J Clin Nutr 32:607, 1979. Data from the Fels Research Institute, Wright State University School of Medicine, Yellow Springs, Ohio.)

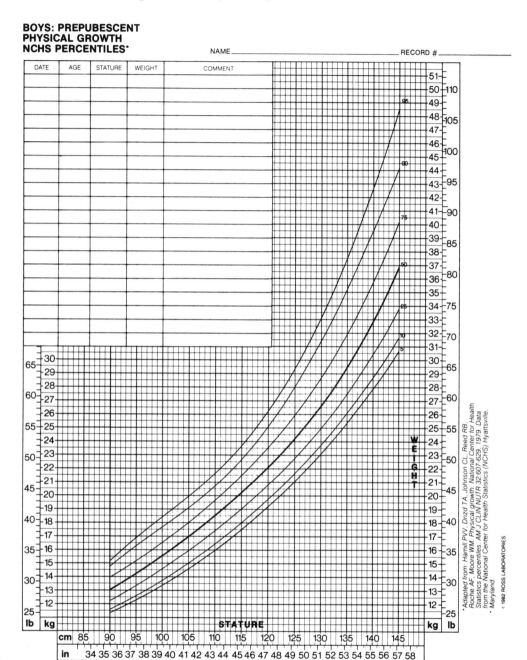

Figure 11-7
NCHS percentiles for physical growth of prepubescent boys. (Adapted from Hamill PVV, Drizd TA, Johnson CL et al: Physical growth: National Center for Health Statistics percentiles. Am J Clin Nutr 32:607, 1979. Data from the National Center for Health Statistics, Hyattsville, Maryland.)

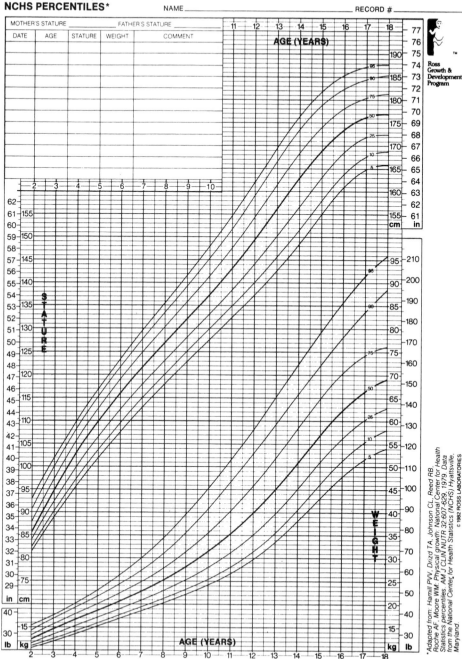

Figure 11-8

NCHS percentiles for physical growth of boys aged 2 to 18 years. (Adapted from Hamill PVV, Drizd TA, Johnson CL et al: Physical growth: National Center for Health Statistics percentiles. Am J Clin Nutr 32:607, 1979. Data from the National Center for Health Statistics, Hyattsville, Maryland.)

Table 11-2
RDAs of Selected Nutrients for Infants, Children, and Adolescents

Age (Years)	Protein (g)	Iron (mg)	Calcium (mg)	Vitamin C (mg)	Vitamin D (μg)*
Birth–0.5	13	6	400	30	7.5
0.5–1.0	14	10	600	35	10
1–3	16	10	800	40	10
4–6	24	10	800	45	10
7–10	28	10	800	45	10
Males					
11–14	45	12	1200	50	10
15–18	59	12	1200	60	10
Females					
11–14	46	15	1200	50	10
15–18	44	15	1200	60	10

As cholecalciferol. 10 μg cholecalciferol = 400 IU vitamin D. (Food and Nutritional Board, National Academy of Sciences–National Research Council: Recommended Daily Dietary Allowances. Revised 1989)

Other benefits to be gained from a well-balanced diet in childhood include health and vigor, a foundation of healthy eating habits, and the prevention of nutrition-related problems common among the healthy pediatric population (see box, Nutrition-Related Problems Among the Healthy Pediatric Population).

Nutrient requirements and eating behaviors vary according to health status, activity patterns, and growth rate; the greater the rate of growth, the more intense the nutritional needs. Although a child's growth is individualized, predictions can be made based on age about the sequence, patterns, and rate of growth and development, and therefore nutritional needs. The RDA are based on age from birth through age 10; thereafter, they are grouped according to age and sex (Table 11-2). At best, the RDA are rough estimates of actual needs; recommended nutrient allowances are less precise for children than adults because of individual variations in growth rate and activity patterns. A more appropriate nutrition teaching tool is the Daily Food Guide, which recommends the number of servings from food groups children at various ages should eat daily (Table 11-3).

Table 11-3
Daily Food Guide for Children and Adolescents

Group	Number of Servings (based on age)			
	1–5	6–11	Teen	Adult
Bread, Cereal, Rice, and Pasta	6–11 (¼ to ½ adult size)	6–11*	6–11*	6–11
Vegetable	3–5†	3–5*	3–5*	3–5
Fruit	2–4†	2–4*	2–4*	2–4
Milk, Yogurt, and Cheese	2 cups	2 cups	4 cups	2–3 servings
Meat, Poultry, Fish, Dry Beans, Eggs, and Nuts‡	2–3 oz	2–3 oz	4–5 oz	5–7 oz

Serving sizes for 6–11 year olds and teens are about the same as those of an adult.
† Serving sizes for ages 1–5 years are about 1 level tablespoon per year of age; e.g., 1 serving is 3 tablespoons for a 3-year old, 5 tablespoons for a 5-year old.
‡ Nuts are not recommended for children under 4 because they are a choking hazard.
Source: Dray J: Mealtime Family Time, Manhattan, Kansas: Cooperative Extension, 1992.

Nutrition-Related Problems Among the Healthy Pediatric Population

Iron Deficiency Anemia

Iron stores of formula-fed infants become depleted between 3 and 6 months after birth if not supplemented.

Six-month to 2½-year-old may develop "milk" anemia related to excessive milk intake (*i.e.*, >32 oz/day), displacing other iron-rich foods.

In childhood, iron deficiency anemia is commonly related to finicky eating habits; there are relatively few rich sources of iron that are acceptable to children.

Adolescent boys can develop iron deficiency quickly after the onset of puberty because of the increased need for iron related to expanding blood volume and muscle mass.

Adolescent girls tend to develop iron deficiency slowly after puberty related to poor eating habits, chronic fad dieting, and menstrual losses.

NURSING IMPLICATIONS AND CONSIDERATIONS

To prevent iron deficiency among infants, encourage mothers

- To give iron-fortified formula to breastfed infants who are weaned before 1 year of age; iron-fortified formula should be used until the infant is 1 year old.
- To use iron-fortified infant cereals until the infant is 12 to 18 months old because its iron is absorbed more readily than the iron in other cereals.
- To limit milk consumption to amounts recommended in the infant feeding schedule or daily food guide (for toddlers) because milk can displace iron-rich food from the diet.

To prevent iron deficiency in children and adolescents, encourage

- A liberal intake of high-iron foods: liver, organ meats, dried fruit, iron-fortified cereals, whole grains.
- A rich source of vitamin C at every meal to enhance iron absorption from plant sources.

NURSING CONSIDERATIONS

Studies suggest that hemoglobin alone may not be sensitive enough to identify iron deficiency; iron supplements given to babies whose hemoglobin was normal but whose total iron-binding capacity was elevated resulted in improved attention spans and performances on mental development tests. Because iron deficiency is so prevalent and may affect learning ability, iron status should be carefully monitored.

Cow's milk should not be given to infants younger than 1 year of age because it is a poor source of iron, and may promote occult blood loss.

Infants born to iron-deficient mothers may have inadequate iron stores.

(continued)

Nutrition-Related Problems Among the Healthy Pediatric Population (*continued*)

Once anemia develops, diet alone cannot cure anemia, and supplements are
needed (see Chap. 16).

Obesity

Obesity is loosely defined as weight above the 95th percentile for age, or body
weight >20% above ideal weight for height. It develops when calorie intake
exceeds energy expenditure. Inactivity appears to be an effect rather than a
cause of childhood obesity.

The causes of obesity may be multifactorial and difficult to determine;
genetic, physiologic, environmental, psychological, behavioral, or a combination of factors may be implicated. Children from low socioeconomic backgrounds tend to become overweight before adolescence, whereas children
from higher socioeconomic backgrounds tend to become overweight during
or after the onset of adolescence.

NURSING IMPLICATIONS AND CONSIDERATIONS

Before a child is labeled as obese or overweight, assess
- The age of onset. Obesity in infants less than 1 year old is not predictive of
  obesity later in life; however, childhood fatness does predict adolescent
  fatness. The later the age of onset, the less likely a spontaneous remission
  will occur. Eighty percent of obese adolescents remain obese as adults.
  Because obesity may be easier to prevent than treat, overweight children
  (who are likely to become obese adolescents and adults) should be identified and treated.
- The degree and duration of the obesity. Fat stores that increase before puberty
  in preparation for the adolescent growth spurt may cause transient excess
  body weight and resolve itself as the child grows taller while maintaining
  body weight.
- Family history for genetic or endocrine problems that may be the cause of
  obesity.
- Health status for medical complications. In children, obesity is the major cause
  of hypertension, and increases the risk of cardiovascular disease, diabetes
  mellitus, joint diseases, and other chronic illnesses.
- Family dynamics and attitudes toward body weight. Unresolved crisis and
  conflicts within the family may contribute to eating problems and complicate weight control. Tolerance toward body weight varies considerably
  among families; weight status acceptable to one family may not be tolerated by another. Children with two normal-weight parents have a 10%
  chance of becoming obese, one obese parent increases the chance of

(*continued*)

Nutrition-Related Problems Among
the Healthy Pediatric Population (*continued*)

obesity to 40%, and if both parents are obese, children have an 80% chance of becoming obese.

The social and psychological impact of obesity is greater on children than on adults. Overweight or obese children

- Tend to have poorer academic performance than normal-weight children of the same intellectual ability.
- May be teased and psychologically abused by peers and adults, which leads to social isolation, depression, and low self-esteem.
- May actually consume fewer calories than their thin counterparts, but because they are social outcasts, a perpetuating cycle of weight gain→ inactivity→ weight gain makes weight control difficult.
- May be discriminated against in school, and later in college and at work. Studies have found that most preschoolers believe a fat child is ugly, stupid, mean, sloppy, lazy, dishonest, forgetful, naughty, sad, lonely, and poor at sports. Both children and adults ranked a chubby child lower on a scale of preference than a child with crutches and a brace, a child in a wheelchair, a child missing the left hand, or a child with a facial disfigurement.

To prevent obesity

- Parents should recognize that infants cry for reasons other than hunger and should not be fed every time they cry. Overfeeding is one of the biggest hazards of formula feeding.
- Infant formula should be properly diluted; concentrated formulas are a source of concentrated calories.
- Infants should not be forced to finish their bottle.
- Solid foods should not be introduced before the infant is developmentally ready (4 to 6 months old).
- Children should be allowed to eat in a relaxed atmosphere at their own pace.
- Children should be allowed to stop eating when they are full and should not be made to eat until their "plate is clean."
- Healthy "thin" eating habits should be learned by parental example, because young children tend to imitate their parents.
- Avoid empty-calorie foods.
- Children should not be given food rewards for good behavior, denied food as punishment, bribed with food, or given food for comfort.

To treat obesity

- Assess the child's normal daily intake, eating behaviors and attitudes, and activity patterns.
- Individualize the plan of care for the child and his family.

(continued)

Nutrition-Related Problems Among the Healthy Pediatric Population (*continued*)

- If possible, it is best to allow children to "outgrow" obesity by maintaining their weight as they grow taller, rather than actually losing weight.
- Children should not be put under pressure to lose weight; resentment and rebellion may cause extreme behavior resulting in anorexia nervosa, bulimia, or compulsive eating. Subtle changes such as limiting portion sizes, eating baked instead of fried foods, substituting fresh fruits and nutritious desserts for pies, cakes, and cookies, and eliminating traditional empty-calorie snack foods is more effective than measuring food and counting calories.
- Encourage exercise that an obese child will feel comfortable doing, for example, exercise that does not require a lot of skill or a change of clothes, such as walking and bowling.
- Group support is most effective at achieving and maintaining weight loss in overweight adolescents.

Dental Caries

Sugar (sucrose, lactose, fructose) plus bacteria found in plaque produce acids that destroy tooth enamel, leading to tooth decay (dental caries). A high intake of sugars, especially between meals, increases the risk of caries. Although on an ounce-for-ounce basis sticky foods are more likely to cause caries than liquids, the frequency and quantity of soft drinks consumed may make them equally as damaging. "Nursing bottle caries" occur when infants or children are put to bed with a bottle of milk, juice, or any other sweetened liquid.

NURSING IMPLICATIONS AND CONSIDERATIONS

Protein, calcium, vitamins A, C, D, and fluoride are important for dental health. Fluoride has been shown to prevent tooth decay by incorporating itself into the structure of the teeth as they form during infancy and childhood. Sources of fluoride include fluoridated water; concentrated liquid or powdered formula mixed with fluoridated water, and fluoride supplements. Breast milk and ready-to-use formulas may be inadequate sources of fluoride. The American Academy of Pediatrics recommends fluoride supplements be given to formula-fed infants living in areas with unfluoridated water and breastfed infants.[3]

Advise parents
- That only bedtime bottle feedings of plain water should be given to infants after the teeth erupt.
- Not to give their infants more than the prescribed dose of fluoride, because it may cause spots to form on the teeth.

(continued)

Nutrition-Related Problems Among the Healthy Pediatric Population (*continued*)

- That because young children tend to swallow toothpaste, avoid giving fluoridated toothpaste to children under age 3.
- That if sweets are consumed, they are less damaging when eaten with other foods and liquids than when eaten alone.
- That so-called "healthy" snacks may be high in sugar: granola, dried fruit, anything made with molasses or honey.
- That a good diet must also be accompanied by good dental hygiene to be most effective against dental caries.

INFANT NUTRITION (BIRTH TO 1 YEAR)

Growth Characteristics and Nutritional Implications

Physical and Physiologic Growth	*Nutritional Implications*
Excluding fetal growth, growth in the first year of life is more rapid than at any other time in the life cycle (see Table 11-1).	Although the total amount recommended for most nutrients during infancy is less than adult requirements, the amount needed per unit of body weight is greater than at any other age.

EXAMPLE	174 lb Adult Male (79 kg)	13 lb Infant (6 kg)
Calories		
Per kg:	37 cal/kg	108 cal/kg
Total:	2900 cal	650
Protein		
Per kg:	0.8 g	2.2 g
Total:	63 g/day	13 g/day

Birthweight doubles in 4 to 6 months and triples by age 1.	Nutritional deficits can impair growth and development.
Length increases 50% during the first year.	
The percentage of both lean body mass and body fat increase.	
Muscular control of the head, neck, jaw, and tongue develops, as well as hand-eye coordination, and the ability to sit, grasp, chew, drink, and self-feed.	Because of inborn reflexes, the most appropriate feeding for an infant is milk (breast milk or commercial formulas).
	Between 4 to 6 months, reflexes disappear, head control develops and the infant is able to sit, mak-

(*continued*)

Physical and Physiologic Growth	*Nutritional Implications*
	ing spoon-feeding possible. (see Table 11-8 for developmental landmarks and the introduction of solids.)
At birth, the kidneys are immature and unable to concentrate urine; by 4 to 6 weeks of age, urine concentrating ability approximates adult levels.	Excess protein and mineral intake (*i.e.,* cow's milk) can tax kidney function and lead to dehydration.
	Infants need more water per unit of body weight (150 ml/kg) than adults related to their immature renal function and the high percentage of body weight from water.
Stomach capacity is limited to about 90 ml at birth. Emptying time is short (about 2½ to 3 hours), and peristalsis is rapid.	Initially, small frequent feedings are necessary; the amount of food/feeding increases with age and increased stomach capacity.
The GI tract is sterile at birth	Lack of gut bacteria that synthesizes Vit K necessitates an IM injection of Vit K shortly after birth to prevent hemorragic disease
Decreased quality and quantity of pancreatic amylase (starch-digesting enzyme), pancreatic lipase (fat-digesting enzyme) and bile (fat digestion) limits digestion and absorption of nutrients.	Infants are unable to digest starch (cereal) until about 3 months of age; bile composition reaches maturity around 6 months of age.
Susceptibility to food allergies decreases between 4 to 6 months as the immune system matures.	Introducing solid foods (beikost) before 4 to 6 months increases the risk of food allergies.
Teeth erupt.	The texture of food progresses from strained to mashed to chopped fine to regular as the ability to chew improves.

Infant Feeding

Breastfeeding

Because of the advantages to both mother and infant, the American Academy of Pediatrics recommends that infants should be breastfed for the full first year of life (see Chap. 10). Even low-birth-weight (LBW) infants weighing less than 1250 g have been shown to tolerate breast milk better than formula.[22] However, formula feeding is an acceptable alternative if lactation is contraindicated or the mother is unwilling/unable to breastfeed.

Formula Feeding

Infant formulas are designed to resemble breast milk and provide comparable nutritional benefits (Table 11-4). Standards for levels of nutrients in formulas have been established by the Infant Formula Act and are mostly based on recommendations of the Committee on Nutrition of the American Academy of Pediatrics. With the exception of fluoride, supplements are not necessary for infants given iron-fortified formula. Milk-based and whey-adjusted formulas are available for full-term infants. Infants intolerant of the protein or lactose in cow's milk may be given formulas made with soy isolates, casein hydrolysates, or meat (Table 11-5).

A variety of formulas have been developed for infants with special needs, such as LBW infants. Numerous physiologic and developmental problems may make feeding the premature infant difficult (see box, Feeding the Premature Infant). Studies indicate that the nutrient needs of premature infants differ with regard to rate of growth, body composition,

Table 11-4

Comparison Between Breast Milk and Cow's Milk, and How Cow's Milk Is Modified in the Production of Milk-Based Formula

Nutrient	Mature Breast Milk	Whole Cow's Milk	How Cow's Milk Is Modified to Resemble Breast Milk
% Protein whey: casein	7 70:30	20 18:82	Total protein control is reduced to 7% to 16%.
			Milk is homogenized and treated with heat to reduce curd tension and increase digestibility. Some formulas combine demineralized whey with nonfat milk to approximate the whey/casein ratio of breast milk. Taurine (an amino acid that infants cannot efficiently synthesize) is being added to many milk-based and soy formulas to approximate the levels found in breast milk.
% Fat P : S ratio % Lineolic acid	50 0.32 4	50 0.06 1	Butterfat is removed (difficult to digest) and replaced with vegetable oils to increase polyunsaturated fat, which is more easily digested by infants.
% Lactose	42	30	Lactose is added.

Minerals (mg/liter)
  Sodium
  Calcium
  Phosphorus
  Ca : P ratio
  Iron
	
	150
	340
	140
	2.4
	0.3
		
		506
		1200
		955
		1.3
		0.5
			Total mineral content is reduced.
			  Calcium : phosphorus ratio is adjusted to be no less than 1.1 and no greater than 2.0.
			
			Formulas may be fortified with additional iron.

Cal/liter	690	660	Standard formulas contain the same amount of calories as cow's milk.

and physiologic maturity; thus, the nutritional requirements of LBW infants are not precisely defined. Compared to routine formulas for full-term infants, LBW formulas generally contain more calories (24 cal/oz instead of 20 cal/oz), more whey protein, more vitamins and minerals (except iron, which can interfere with vitamin E absorption and result in hemolytic anemia), less lactose, and contain medium-chain triglyceride (MCT) oil as part of the fat source.

Incomplete formulas are also available for infants with inborn errors of metabolism, such as phenylketonuria (PKU) and maple syrup urine disease. These specialized formulas are intentionally lacking or deficient in one or more nutrients and therefore do not supply adequate nutrition for normal infants; they must be supplemented with small amounts of regular formula.

Formula feeding offers the advantage of allowing others to share in infant feeding, which gives the mother more freedom. In addition, the supply of formula is unlimited.

Although designed to resemble breast milk, formulas lack the unique nutrient content, ease of digestibility, enzymes, hormones, and anti-infective properties of breast milk. There is also a greater chance of overfeeding, and it must be properly prepared; too dilute → failure to thrive, too concentrated → excess weight gain, obesity. Depending on the form of formula used, it may be expensive or require refrigeration (Table 11-6).

Table 11-5
Comparison Between Various Types of Formulas

Type of Formula	Source of Protein	Source of Fat	Source of CHO
REGULAR			
Milk-based (Manufacturer: cal/oz)	Nonfat cow's milk	Vegetable oils	Lactose (Milumil is the only low lactose milk-based formula available; contains lactose, starch, and corn syrup solids)
Similac 20 (Ross) 20			
Similac 13 (Ross) 13			
Similac 24 (Ross) 24			
Similac 27 (Ross) 27			
Similac LBW (Ross) 24			
Enfamil 13 (Mead) 13			
Enfamil 24 (Mead) 24			
SMA 13 (Wyeth) 13			
SMA 24 (Wyeth) 24			
SMA 27 (Wyeth) 27			
Milumil (Milupa) 20			
Uses: Routine			
Whey-adjusted (Manufacturer: cal/oz)	Nonfat cow's milk plus demineralized whey	Vegetable and oleo oils	Lactose
Similac with whey (Ross) 20			
Similac PM 60/40 (Ross) 20 (low mineral)			
Enfamil 20 (Mead) 20			
SMA (Wyeth) 20			
Uses: Routine			
Soy isolate (Manufacturer: cal/oz)	Soy protein isolate	Vegetable oils	Corn syrup solids and/or sucrose
ProSobee (Mead) 20			
Nursoy (Wyeth) 20			
Isomil (Ross) 20			
Isomil SF (Ross) 20 (sucrose free)			
Soyalac (Loma Linda) 20			
I-Soyalac (Loma Linda) 20 (low sucrose)			
Uses: Lactase deficiency related to diarrhea, congenital lactose intolerance, or galactosemia; infants born to vegetarian families			
Casein hydrolysate (Manufacturer: cal/oz)	Casein hydrolysate or sodium caseinate	Corn oil or corn oil and medium-chain triglycerides	Corn syrup solids and modified corn starch or sucrose
Nutramigen (Mead) 20			
Pregestimil (Mead) 20			
Portagen (Mead) 20			
Uses: Cow's milk allergy, protein sensitivity, galactosemia, persistent diarrhea, malabsorption			
FORMULAS FOR PREMATURE INFANTS*			
(Manufacturer: cal/oz)	Whey and nonfat milk	Vegetable oils with MCT oil	Lactose with corn syrup solids or glucose polymers
Similac Special Care 20 (Ross) 20			
Similac Special Care 24 (Ross) 24			
Enfamil Premature Formula 20 (Mead) 20			
Enfamil Premature Formula 24 (Mead) 24			
Use: Preterm infants under 2 kg			

(*continued*)

Table 11-5 (*continued*)

Type of Formula	Source of Protein	Source of Fat	Source of CHO
INCOMPLETE FORMULAS (must be supplemented with regular formula)			
Lofenalac (Mead) (20 cal/oz)	Hydrolyzed casein with most of the phenylalanine removed	Corn oil	Corn syrup solids and modified tapioca starch
Use: Phenylketonuria (PKU)			
MSUD Diet Powder (Mead) (20 cal/oz)	Amino acids without any branched-chain amino acids	Corn oil	Corn syrup solids and modified tapioca starch
Use: Maple syrup urine disease (disorder of branch-chain amino acid metabolism)			

* Except for iron (which may interfere with vitamin E absorption), the levels of many vitamins and minerals are increased to support the rapid growth rate. Initial feedings are diluted. (American Dietetic Association: Manual of Clinical Dietetics, 1988)

Formula preparation

A single bottle or whole day's supply of formula can be prepared by either the clean technique or by sterilization. Recently, experts have questioned the necessity of sterilization. Surveys indicate that although sterilization techniques often are not properly followed or are totally disregarded, infant gastrointestinal (GI) disorders are attributed infrequently to formula contamination, possibly because almost all formulas are already treated with heat, refrigeration is widely available, and water supplies supposedly are free of bacteria.

If done properly, the "clean" technique of formula preparation may be as safe as sterilization (see box, Formula Preparation).

(*Text continued on page 290*)

Table 11-6
Formula Varieties

	Advantages	Disadvantages
Powder	Unprepared powder does not require refrigeration; can be stored in a cool, dry place Least expensive form of formula	Requires proper dilution with water
Liquid concentrate	Less expensive than ready-to-use formula	Must be refrigerated after opening Requires proper dilution with water
Ready-to-use	Convenient: no preparation, no dilution with water Easy: poured directly into clean bottles	Most expensive form of formula Must be refrigerated after opening

Feeding the Premature Infant

Potential Problem/Rationale

Failure to achieve adequate "catch-up" growth related to high nutrient requirements combined with limited tolerance to feedings. Premature infants are usually expected to "catch up" to normal weight by 24 months of age and to height by 36 months.

Normally, weight gain between 26 to 36 weeks of gestation is greater than at any other time in the life cycle; the earlier the infant is born before term, the greater the impact on nutritional status and requirements. Calorie requirements are higher than normal because of the following:

Most of the fat stores are laid down during the last 6 weeks of pregnancy. In a premature infant, fat may comprise less than 1% of total body weight, compared to 16% of total body weight in a term infant. A lack of fat stores leaves the infant dependent on exogenous sources of calories.

Glycogen stores are usually deposited during the last 4 weeks of a term pregnancy. Without adequate glycogen reserves, the infant does not have a readily available source of stored energy and is at risk of hypoglycemia.

Even labored breathing related to an immature respiratory function can increase calorie requirements.

NURSING INTERVENTIONS AND CONSIDERATIONS

Individualize the diet according to the infant's physiologic and developmental status. Most preterm infants are unable to tolerate enteral feedings in the early neonatal period and are therefore given intravenous fluid, glucose, and electrolytes to maintain fluid balance and promote metabolic homeostasis.[17] Partial or total parenteral nutrition may be necessary until GI tolerance is established, especially in preterm infants with limited metabolic reserves. Usually enteral feedings can begin after the initial acute treatment of respiratory distress, perinatal sepsis, or other stressful events.[13]

Although breast milk has numerous benefits (low renal solute load, anti-infective properties, easily digested fat, a high nitrogen content, unique amino acid composition, and a high whey/casein ratio), some researchers believe that, even if consumed in high-volume amounts, preterm breast milk lacks sufficient amounts of calcium, phosphorus, and, possibly, some essential vitamins. Further compounding the problem is the inability of many preterm infants to consume enough milk to meet their nutritional needs.[21]

To boost its nutritional value, calcium, phosphorus, and vitamins can be added to breast milk through nasogastric or bottle feedings; however, GI intolerance often results because of the increase in osmolarity. Another option, alternating breast milk feedings with premature formula, falls short of providing

(continued)

Feeding the Premature Infant (*continued*)

adequate amounts of calcium and phosphorus; although preterm milk formula provides adequate amounts of calcium and phosphorus when used as the sole source of nutrition, it cannot compensate for their low content in breast milk when used as a supplemental feeding. Relatively new to the market are human milk fortifiers (Enfamil Human Milk fortifier powder and liquid Similac Natural Care Low Iron Human Milk Fortifier), designed to supplement breast milk given to preterm infants whose tolerance for enteral feedings has been established.[21] Along with calcium and phosphorus, the human milk fortifiers also provide protein, carbohydrates, fat, vitamins, and minerals. Because they may lack sufficient quantities of some nutrients (*i.e.*, vitamin D) and have the potential to contribute excessive amounts of other nutrients when consumed in large quantities (*i.e.*, potassium), their use should be closely monitored. Human milk fortifiers are not necessary for every preterm infant and are not used once the infant weights 2 kg.

Although exact nutritional requirements are unknown, a premature infant may need

Three grams of protein/kg of body weight. Even if premature infants need more protein than this, they should not receive more than 4 to 5 g of protein/kg because their immature kidneys are unable to handle large amounts of nitrogenous waste generated from protein metabolism.

A whey-to-casein ratio of 60:40, which is typical of breast milk and LBW formulas. This ratio is easily digested and provides adequate amounts of the nonessential amino acids cystine and methionine, which premature infants may have difficulty synthesizing. In addition, the nonessential amino acids taurine and tyrosine may be essential for premature infants.

Ninety to 120 cal/kg of body weight to promote growth. After the first week of life, the calorie requirements of premature infants are greater than those of term infants. Standard LBW formulas supplying 24 cal/oz should be used until the infant weighs 2 kg.

Thirty-five percent to 55% of total calories in the form of CHO. Because lactase activity may be inadequate, glucose polymers are the major form of CHO in premature formulas.

Adequate amounts of essential fatty acids in a form of fat that the infant can easily absorb. Because of premature infants' impaired fat digestion, premature formulas contain a combination of MCT oil and vegetable oil; excessive intake of PUFA should be avoided because they increase the risk of vitamin E deficiency and hemolytic anemia.

Vitamin and mineral supplements. Compared to term infants, preterm infants have notably higher mineral requirements, especially for calcium, phosphorus, zinc, copper, and initially, sodium.[13] Vitamins A, D, and C (ADC) usu-

(*continued*)

Feeding the Premature Infant (*continued*)

ally are given to all premature infants. Iron supplements may be initiated as early as 2 weeks after birth, but not later than 2 months of age.

Monitor nutritional status for several years after birth, basing the assessment on the infant's corrected age (chronologic age minus the number of weeks the infant was born prematurely). Neonates' postnatal growth should parallel in utero growth at term, that is, a weight gain of approximately 14 to 36 g/day.

Potential Problem/Rationale

Maldigestion or malabsorption related to an insufficient amount or potency of digestive enzymes. Inadequate lactase, amylase, and lipase may cause maldigestion of lactose, starch, and lipids and the fat-soluble vitamins, respectively.

NURSING INTERVENTIONS AND CONSIDERATIONS

Observe for signs of maldigestion/malabsorption, such as diarrhea and steatorrhea.

Potential Problem/Rationale

Aspiration, which may be related to delayed or incomplete gastric emptying, leading to gastric residuals and abdominal distention. Immature sucking or swallowing reflexes (if less than 32 to 34 weeks of gestation) also increase the risk of aspiration.

NURSING INTERVENTIONS AND CONSIDERATIONS

If possible, premature infants are given small, frequent feedings by mouth. Gavage feedings by continuous infusion or bolus may be needed for very small premature infants. Check for gastric residuals before administering a feeding to avoid distention and possible aspiration.

Parenteral nutrition is required if enteral feedings are contraindicated or if growth falls below established minimum standards.

Potential Problem/Rationale

Vitamin E deficiency leading to hemolytic anemia. Vitamin E deficiency may occur secondary to fat malabsorption (vitamin E is a fat-soluble vitamin) and/or to excessive iron supplementation, which interferes with vitamin E absorption.

NURSING INTERVENTIONS AND CONSIDERATIONS

Vitamin E deficiency can be prevented by giving water-soluble supplements of vitamin E orally and by avoiding excess iron supplementation.

Monitor the infant for signs of vitamin E deficiency (hemolytic anemia is the first sign), especially at 6 to 10 weeks of age.

(*continued*)

Feeding the Premature Infant (*continued*)

Potential Problem/Rationale

Dehydration related to immature renal function and a low renal solute toler-ance. In particular, the high osmolalities of concentrated LBW formulas (24 cal/oz) increase the risk of dehydration.

NURSING INTERVENTIONS AND CONSIDERATIONS

Fluid requirements vary with the infant's condition and treatment. Initially, 100 ml/kg/day may be given and adjusted as needed.

Monitor the infant's intake and output and serum BUN levels. Observe for signs and symptoms of hypernatremia and dehydration.

Potential Problem/Rationale

Hypoglycemia, which may be related to (1) immature hepatic function→ inadequate enzymes for glycogenolysis and gluconeogenesis→ tendency toward hypoglycemia; (2) inadequate glycogen reserves; (3) respiratory distress syndrome; or (4) hypothermia, which occurs due to inadequate brown fat reserves.

NURSING INTERVENTIONS AND CONSIDERATIONS

Monitor the infant's serum glucose levels.

To prevent hypoglycemia, frequent and adequate feedings containing a readily utilized source of carbohydrate are needed.

NURSING PROCESS

Assessment

In addition to the general growth and development assessment criteria, assess for the following factors:

Length of gestation. Determine whether there were complications during pregnancy, labor, or delivery.

Growth rate, weight status, and weight fluctuations.

Sleeping habits; determine whether the infant is given a bottle at bedtime, and if so, what it contains.

Type of feeding (formula, breast milk, beikost).

The use of vitamin/mineral supplements; type, amount, and frequency. Determine if the local water is fluoridated.

For breastfed infants, assess the mother's prepregnancy nutritional status, weight gain pattern, food allergies, and adequacy of present intake. Assess maternal use of alcohol, tobacco, caffeine, and drugs.

Formula Preparation

"Clean" Technique

Wash hands thoroughly.

Wash top of formula can with soap and water and rinse thoroughly.

Open can with a clean opener.

Pour ready-to-use formula directly into clean bottle.

Pour liquid concentrate formula directly into clean bottle and add equal amounts of water.

Pour proper amount of water into clean bottle or container and add correct amount of powdered concentrate. Allow the formula to settle for a few minutes before shaking to mix.

Sterilization

Pour the required amount of water into each of the bottles.

Place nipples on the bottles and put the caps on loosely.

A jar with extra nipples may be placed in the center of the sterilizer. Put the jar lid inside the sterilizer but not on the jar.

Pour 2 to 3 inches of water into the sterilizer.

Put the lid on the sterilizer and place on the stove. Boil for 10 minutes after the water begins to boil.

After the sterilizer has cooled, remove the bottles, tighten the caps, and store in the refrigerator.

At feeding time, add the required amount of liquid concentrate or powder.

Put the nipple and cap on and shake to mix.

For formula-fed infants, assess the type of formula used, the frequency, and the method of preparation. Determine if the formula used is iron-fortified.

For infants receiving solid foods, determine what is given, at what age each item was introduced in the diet, the frequency of use, and whether it is age-appropriate. Determine if any untoward side effects occurred, such as diarrhea, fussiness, skin rash, etc.

Familial attitudes about food, eating, and body weight.

Whether the infant has received immunizations.

Nursing Diagnosis

Health Seeking Behaviors, as evidenced by the lack of knowledge of infant nutritional requirements and feeding practices and the desire to learn.

Planning and Implementation

The objective of diet intervention for infants is to promote normal growth and development. Breastfeeding should be encouraged as the main source of nutrition for the first 6 months of life. If breastfeeding is contraindicated or has failed because of maternal anxiety or misconceptions, the mother should be assured that infant formula will supply adequate nutrition (see Chap. 10).

The amount of formula per feeding and the frequency of feeding depends on the infant's age and individual needs. Feeding guidelines are listed in Table 11-7. Evaporated milk is not recommended as a substitute for breast milk because it does not meet the minimum standards set by the Infant Formula Act. Even when correctly diluted and mixed with CHO, additional vitamins and some minerals are required. Also, the only source of fat is butterfat, which is poorly tolerated by infants, and the concentration of some minerals is too great.

Infants generally are not developmentally ready for solid foods until 4 to 6 months of age (see Table 11-8); feeding solids before the infant is ready may contribute to overfeeding, may increase the chance of food allergies, and may frustrate both the mother and the infant. There is no evidence to support the belief that solids help the infant sleep through the night. The early introduction of cow's milk and solid foods should be discouraged. Conversely, the introduction of solids should not be delayed beyond 7 to 9 months of age in order to provide a nutritionally adequate intake and promote normal development.

Breast milk/formula intake should decrease after 6 months of age to avoid displacing the intake of other iron- and nutrient-rich foods. Iron-fortified infant rice cereal is recommended as the first solid because it is not likely to cause an allergic reaction (hypoallergenic). The cereal may be mixed with breast milk, formula, or water. New foods, in plain and simple forms, should be introduced one at a time for a period of 5 to 7 days to observe for possible allergic reactions, which may be exhibited as a rash, fussiness, vomiting, diarrhea, and constipation. The amount of solids taken at a feeding may vary from 1 to 2 teaspoons initially, to one-quarter to one-half cup as the infant gets older.

Because cow's milk is a poor source of iron, may cause occult blood loss (possibly from an allergic response to the protein), and provides an unsuitably high potential renal solute load related to its protein, phosphorus, and electrolyte composition, it is an undesirable feeding for infants.[23] Many experts recommend delaying the introduction of

Table 11-7
Guidelines for Formula Feeding*

Age	Feedings/ 24 Hours	Amount/Feeding	Amount/Day
1 week–1 month	6–8	4–5 oz	21–24 oz
1–3 months	5–6	5–7 oz	24–32 oz
3–6 months	4–5	6–7 oz	24–32 oz
6–12 months (feedings from the cup and bottle if the infant is not completely weaned)	3–4	6–8 oz	16–24 oz

*Actual number of feedings and amount/feeding depends on the infant's rate of growth and size. Never force infants to finish a bottle.

Table 11-8
Introduction of Solids Based on Development

Age (Months)	Feeding Skills	Approriate Foods to Introduce
0–3	Sucking reflex Rooting reflex Swallowing reflex	Breast milk; formula
4–6	Sucking, rooting, and biting (clamps down on spoon) reflexes disappear between 3 to 5 months. Head and neck control develop. Can transfer food to the back of the mouth for swallowing Can sit with support	Introduce iron-fortified infant cereals between 4 to 6 months for formula-fed infants: after 6 months for exclusively breast-fed infants.

5–8	Brings hand to mouth
	Grasps and reaches for objects in sight; can feed self finger foods
	At 7 months, grasps spoon, nipple, cup rim
	Drinks from cup when held to lips
	Interested in biting and chewing: begins chewing movements
		5–7 months
		  Strained vegetables, fruits, and fruit juices (noncitrus)
		  Sips of water, juice, milk, formula, from cup
		6–8 months
		  Ready for finger foods between 24 to 28 weeks of age: arrowroot biscuits, crackers, dry toast
		  Begin protein foods: strained meats, egg yolk, cheese, yogurt
		  Rice, noodles, potatoes
		  Citrus juices
		  Plain desserts: pudding, custards, ice cream, plain cookies
		  May give whole milk if taking more than 1.5 jars strained baby food

9–12	Increased ability to chew Increased pincer grasp	Gradually increase texture by replacing strained foods with finely chopped, mashed, or soft vegetables, fruit, and meat. Prefer finger foods: can give smaller-sized finger foods Can drink from cup alone
12	Chewing more refined, especially after molars erupt Increasingly independent Drinks from cup without sucking; blows bubbles in cup	Limit milk to 16–24 oz/day, all by cup. Because the risk of allergy is diminished, egg white may be added. Using molars, can eat regular solid foods and teething crackers Continue iron-fortified infant cereal until 18 months old, if possible.

cow's milk until after the age of 1; quantities should be limited to 1 quart or less daily. Skim milk lacks fat, the essential fatty acid, and sufficient calories for the amount of protein it supplies and therefore is rarely indicated before the age of 2.

Adequacy of growth is the best indicator of whether an infant is receiving sufficient nutrition. However, it should be noted that breastfed infants usually have a slower growth rate than formula-fed infants. Also, infants who have suffered impaired growth related to undernutrition or illness experience "catch-up" growth, which usually is completed by age 2. Generally, weight gain increases rapidly until the child reaches his normal weight percentile; thereafter, weight and height increase together at a slower rate. However, depending on the timing, severity, nature, and duration of the malnutrition, growth may or may not be permanently affected.[18]

Iron is the nutrient most commonly deficient during infancy. The American Academy of Pediatrics recommends that iron-fortified formula be used for formula-fed infants. Long-standing beliefs that iron added to formula increased the incidence of GI problems (colic, constipation, cramping, diarrhea, gas, regurgitation) or that it interferes with the absorption of other minerals have not been proven in case studies.

Although approximately one third to one half of infants over 6 months old receive nutrient supplements, their use is controversial.[5] From birth to 6 months of age, breastfed infants may be given fluoride and vitamin D; iron may be given after 4 months of age.[3] Formula-fed infants may be given iron, if the formula is not iron-fortified, and fluoride, if the local water supply is not fluoridated. The American Academy of Pediatrics has stated that vitamin and mineral supplements are "usually not required" by normal, healthy infants during the second 6 months of life; however, it is important that vitamin D-fortified milk be used, that the diet provide adequate vitamin C, and that iron is supplied from iron-fortified formula or infant cereals. High-risk infants may be given a multivitamin/multi-mineral supplement.

Vegan diets (no animal products) are not recommended for infants and young children because certain vitamins and minerals are likely to be deficient if not properly supplemented, namely riboflavin, vitamin D, calcium, iron, zinc, and vitamin B_{12}. In addition, the intake of protein, fat, and calories may be inadequate, and the high-fiber content may increase satiety (further reducing calorie intake) or interfere with the absorption of some vitamins and minerals.

Client Goals

The caretaker will:

Describe the principles and rationale of infant feeding, and practice age-appropriate feeding.

Delay the introduction of solids until the infant is 4 to 6 months old.

The infant will:

Experience normal growth and development.

Avoid nursing bottle caries, if formula-fed.

Consume an age-appropriate intake.

Nursing Interventions

Diet management

The RDA for protein, calories (see Table 11-2), and most nutrients for infancy can be obtained either through breast milk or formula; breastfeeding is recommended as the main source of nutrition for the first 6 months of life.

Delay the introduction of solids until the infant is developmentally ready, usually between

4 to 6 months of age. Introduce one new food at a time and observe for an allergic response.

Advance the diet according to the infant's feeding skills (see Table 11-8).

Client teaching

Instruct the family

On formula feeding

Infants should not be given supplements unless prescribed by the physician.

Formula may be given at room temperature, slightly warmed, or directly from the refrigerator; however, it should always be given at approximately the same temperature.

Each feeding should last 20 to 30 minutes.

Hold the infant closely and securely. Position the infant so that his head is higher than the rest of his body.

Avoid jiggling the bottle and extra movements that could distract the infant from feeding.

Never prop the bottle or put the infant to bed with a bottle. Giving the infant a bottle of anything but plain water at bedtime can cause tooth decay (nursing bottle caries) once the teeth erupt.

Check the flow of formula by holding the bottle upside down. A steady drip from the nipple should be observed. If the flow is too rapid because of too large a nipple opening, the infant may overfeed and develop indigestion. If the flow rate is too slow because of too small a nipple opening, the infant may tire and fall asleep without taking enough formula. Discard any nipples with holes that are too large; enlarge holes that are too small with a sterilized needle.

There is no danger of "spoiling" an infant by feeding him when he cries for a feeding.

Burp the infant half-way through the feeding, at the end of the feeding, and more often if necessary, to help get rid of air swallowed during the feeding. Infants can be burped by gently rubbing or patting the infant's back as he is held on the shoulder, laying over the lap, or sitting in an upright position.

One of the greatest hazards of formula feeding is overfeeding. Never force the infant to finish a bottle or take more than he wants. Signs that an infant is finished include biting the nipple, facial puckering, and turning away.

Discourage the misconception that a "fat baby = a healthy baby = good parents."

During hot weather the baby may want supplemental bottles of water.

Spitting up a small amount of formula during and after a feeding is normal. Feeding the infant more slowly and burping more frequently may help alleviate spitting up.

On proper handling and storage of formulas

Before beginning, wash hands thoroughly with soap and hot water.

Prepare formula by either the clean technique or sterilization.

Use standard measuring devices to ensure accuracy.

Fill bottles with just the amount of formula the infant will need at one feeding; discard formula left over after a feeding.

Formula should be immediately used or stored in the refrigerator after preparation; formula in a bottle or can left at room temperature for more than an hour should be discarded (bacteria thrive on warm formula).

Maintain the refrigerator temperature between 32°F and 40°F.

Discard refrigerated cans of opened formula if not used within 2 days.

On adding solids to the infant's diet

Always feed the infant in an upright position; do not feed the infant solids from a bottle.

Infant rice cereal is recommended as the first solid feeding; follow with other iron-fortified infant cereals.

Before giving cereal the first few times, give the infant a small amount of formula or breast milk to take the edge off hunger and increase the likelihood of acceptance. After the infant is accustomed to solids, introduce new foods at the beginning of the feeding (when the infant is most hungry) and with a familiar favorite.

Infants vary in the amount of food they want or need at each feeding; let the baby determine how much food he needs.

Respect the infant's likes and dislikes; rejected foods may be reintroduced at a later time.

If there is a positive family history for food allergies, delay introducing milk, eggs, wheat, and citrus fruits, which tend to cause allergic reactions in susceptible infants.

Infants can be given the same plain, pure fruit juices as the rest of the family instead of expensive infant juices. Avoid sweetened fruit drinks.

Except for mixed dinners (little meat content) and desserts (highly sweetened), commercially prepared baby food is nutritious and safe for infant use (sodium was removed in 1976). Read the label to determine if sugar or fillers have been added.

Homemade baby food can be prepared by blending, mashing, or grinding food to the proper consistency for the infant's stage of development. However:

- Do not salt the food or use spicy or high-fat foods.
- Do not use canned vegetables because of the high sodium content, possibility of lead contamination, and generally lower water-soluble vitamin content than fresh and frozen vegetables.
- Do not make baby-food carrots, beets, or spinach because they may have a high nitrite content.
- Do not give honey to infants under 1 year old because of the risk of infant botulism.

Between 6 to 8 months of age, the infant may be ready for three meals with three planned snacks.

When the infant is ready for finger foods, try ripe banana, cheerios, toast strips, graham or soda crackers, cubes of cheese, noodles, and chunks of peeled apple, pears, or peaches.

To decrease the risk of choking:

- Avoid foods that are most often the cause of choking: hot dogs, candy, nuts, and grapes. Other offenders include raw carrots, tough meat, watermelon with seeds, celery, biscuits, cookies, popcorn, and even peanut butter.
- Always supervise meals and snacks.
- Do not allow the infant to eat or drink from a cup while lying down, playing, or strapped in a car seat.
- Cook foods well and serve in small pieces.
- Do not give a child food he cannot chew, or food you are unsure of.
- Topical teething anesthetics that numb the gums can interfere with the ability to swallow foods that require chewing.

Avoid foods that may be difficult to digest: bacon, sausage, fatty or fried foods, gravy, spicy foods, and whole-kernel corn.

How to avoid common nutrition-related problems of iron deficiency, obesity, and dental caries (see box, Nutrition-Related Problems Among the Healthy Pediatric Population).

Monitor

Monitor for the following signs and symptoms:
Growth and development, and weight status
Diet progressions
The development of food allergies
The need for follow-up family diet counseling

Evaluation

Evaluation is ongoing. Assuming the plan of care has not changed, the client will achieve the goals as stated above.

NUTRITION FOR TODDLERS (AGED 1 TO 3 YEARS) AND PRESCHOOLERS (AGED 3 TO 6 YEARS)

Growth Characteristics and Nutritional Implications

Physical and Physiologic Growth	*Nutritional Implications*
Growth rate decreases dramatically (see Table 11-1).	Appetite decreases dramatically; becomes erratic. Interest in food declines → "physiologic anorexia"
Maturation of biting, chewing, and swallowing abilities continues.	Can eat a variety of textures, table food
Develops greater mobility, coordination, and autonomy	Self-feeding skills improve, can completely self-feed by the end of the second year. Can seek food independently May use food to express autonomy and manipulate parents; finicky food habits and food jags may begin around 15 months
Muscle mass and bone density increase.	Need adequate amounts of protein, calcium, and phosphorus to support normal bone growth.
Language skills increase.	Between the age of 1 to 3, associate food with taste and name; between the age of 4 to 6 begin verbalizing food dislikes and preferences
Between the age of 3 to 5, develop attitudes about food and eating	Inappropriate use of food (*i.e.,* to reward, punish, convey love, bribe) may lead to inappropriate food attitudes.

(Text continued on page 304)

Nursing Interventions and Considerations for Disorders of Infancy and Childhood

Failure to Thrive

Failure to thrive is generally defined as an inadequate gain in weight and/or height compared to growth and development standards. It may be caused by clinical diseases, such as CNS disorders, endocrine disorders, congenital defects, or intestinal obstructions, or occur secondary to an inability to suck, chew, or swallow related to neuromuscular problems. An inadequate calorie intake related to inappropriate formula selection, improper formula dilution, or alterations in digestion or absorption (*i.e.*, lactose intolerance) can lead to failure to thrive. Family problems, such as inadequate nurturing and infant stimulation, may also be implicated.

NURSING INTERVENTIONS AND CONSIDERATIONS

To develop a plan of care, the cause(s) of failure to thrive must first be identified.

Diet interventions depend on the infant's age and stage of development. Generally, a high-calorie, high-protein diet is indicated.

Physical, emotional, and intellectual growth may be permanently affected if failure to thrive becomes a chronic problem.

Colic

Colic is characterized by intermittent periods of profuse crying. It most often affects the first-born child, is more common in formula-fed infants than breast-fed infants, and usually resolves itself by the time the infant is 3 months old. The exact cause of colic is unknown, but it may be related to overfeeding, underfeeding, feeding too quickly, swallowed air, or maternal or infant anxiety.

NURSING INTERVENTIONS AND CONSIDERATIONS

Assess feeding practices: frequency of burping, type of feeding used, volume, concentration, frequency of feedings, and size of nipple opening (formula-fed infants). If no feeding problems are identified, assure the parents that colic is transient and not indicative of health problems or parental ineptness.

Cleft Palate

Numerous combinations of developmental defects involving the lip and palate may occur, resulting in an opening in the roof of the mouth or incompletely formed lips. The cause may be hereditary or unknown.

NURSING INTERVENTIONS AND CONSIDERATIONS

Depending on the type of defect, infants with a cleft palate may be unable to suck. Soft nipples or nipples with enlarged holes may help the infant to feed.

(continued)

Nursing Interventions and Considerations
for Disorders of Infancy and Childhood (*continued*)

Maintaining good nutritional status is especially important for infants who require multiple surgeries over an extended period of time.

Advise parents to

- Feed the infant in an upright position and direct the formula to the side of the mouth to prevent formula from entering the nasal passage.
- Feed the infant slowly and burp the infant frequently. Feeding may be a long and tiring process for both the infant and parents.
- Follow the normal diet progression and introduction of solids based on the child's development and nutritional needs. Assure the parents that children with a cleft palate can handle solids better than liquids.

Pyloric Stenosis

Pyloric stenosis is characterized by an obstructive narrowing of the pyloric opening, resulting in projectile vomiting within 30 minutes after feeding, weight loss, dehydration, and poor nutritional status. It is caused by excessive thickening of the pyloric muscle or hypertrophy and hyperplasia of mucosa and submucosa.

NURSING INTERVENTIONS AND CONSIDERATIONS

The major goal of nutritional therapy is to achieve fluid and electrolyte balance so that the infant can undergo surgery.

After surgery, the infant is given glucose water and is advanced to full-strength formula as tolerated, after which the infant can be breastfed, if desired.

Vomiting

Vomiting, characterized by the ejection of stomach contents through the mouth, may occur secondary to viral infections, formula contamination, food poisoning, or intestinal obstructions.

NURSING INTERVENTIONS AND CONSIDERATIONS

Food intake is unimportant. The major nutritional concern for prolonged vomiting is fluid and electrolyte replacement.

Advise parents

- To withhold solid food and offer the child small amounts of clear liquids.
- To progress the diet as tolerated after the vomiting subsidies.

Mild Diarrhea (1 to 4 Days' Duration)

Mild diarrhea may be related to numerous causes, such as viral infections, formula contamination, food poisoning, overfeeding, excessive fat intake, exces-

(continued)

Nursing Interventions and Considerations for Disorders of Infancy and Childhood (*continued*)

sive fiber intake, and food allergies. Sorbitol (sugar alcohol used as a sweetener) may cause osmotic diarrhea if consumed in large amounts. In infants, a frequent cause of mild diarrhea is the introduction of solid food (cereal) before enzyme levels are adequate, leading to CHO fermentation within the GI tract.

NURSING INTERVENTIONS AND CONSIDERATIONS

Diarrhea may cause intestinal inflammation, resulting in the loss of the enzyme lactase. Decreased lactase → lactose intolerance → increased bowel aggravation and permeability of the GI wall → possibility of protein leakage through the bowel into the bloodstream, setting up an allergic reaction. An allergy to protein and impaired ability to digest lactose (milk) may persist for a few days after diarrhea subsides.

Obtain a diet history to rule out diet-related causes.

Prolonged or severe diarrhea can be serious in infants and young children; hospitalization may be required to correct fluid and electrolyte imbalances parenterally.

Advise parents
- To withhold all food for 12 to 24 hours, then offer small amounts of clear liquids (avoid iced liquids). However, clear liquids lack the proper balance of electrolytes; therefore, a commercial electrolyte solution (Pedialyte, Resol, Lytren) may be indicated for electrolyte replacement. It is recommended that a total of 1 cup of commercial oral rehydration mixture be given between each loose bowel movement, perhaps 1 teaspoon at a time if necessary, until diarrhea subsides, to prevent dehydration.[11]
- That it may be necessary to withhold milk and lactose-containing formulas for at least a week if diarrhea is severe. Soy or casein formulas are used until the infant is able to tolerate lactose.
- That when milk-based formula is reintroduced, it should be diluted and gradually progressed to full strength (*i.e.,* 1 part formula to 3 parts water for one day, followed by 1:2 → 1:1 → full strength)
- That older children should be given foods high in pectin to help firm the stools: firm **B**ananas; plain **R**ice; firm, scraped, skinless **A**pples; **T**oast (BRAT diet).

Constipation

Formula that is too concentrated or inadequae in CHO may contribute to constipation in formula-fed infants; constipation is rare in breastfed infants. In older children, constipation may be caused by an excessive milk intake, inadequate fluid and fiber intake, irregular bowel habits, or may be labeled psychogenic constipation related to toilet-training trauma.

(continued)

Nursing Interventions and Considerations for Disorders of Infancy and Childhood (*continued*)

NURSING INTERVENTIONS AND CONSIDERATIONS

Daily bowel movements are not necessary as long as the stools are easily passed.

Obtain a diet history to determine the cause of constipation.

Advise parents how to modify the diet to prevent constipation, such as

- Properly diluting the formula. Some physicians recommend adding corn syrup to formula to increase the CHO content. Honey should never be added because of the risk of infant botulism.
- Limiting milk intake to the recommended amount for the child's age.
- Adding fiber to the diet: whole grain breads and cereals, fresh fruits and vegetables, and dried peas and beans (see Chap. 15 for more on high-fiber diet).

Phenylketonuria

Phenylketonuria (PKU) is an inborn error of metabolism (autosomal-recessive hereditary trait) characterized by a defect in phenylalanine (an essential to amino acid) metabolism that prevents the conversion of phenylalanine to tyrosine (a nonessential amino acid), which is normally converted to thyroxine, melanin, and catecholamines. Tyrosine becomes an essential amino acid. Phenylketonuria causes the accumulation of toxic phenylalanine in the tissues, bloodstream, and CNS, resulting in mental retardation and urinary excretion of phenylketones.

NURSING INTERVENTIONS AND CONSIDERATIONS

Because early diagnosis and initiation of the diet can prevent mental retardation, all infants should be tested for PKU immediately after birth. Diet cannot reverse brain damage after it occurs.

The diet for PKU is low in phenylalanine, not phenylalanine-free. Because phenylalanine is an essential amino acid, it must be supplied in the diet for tissue growth and repair to occur. If the phenylalanine content of the diet is inadequate, the body will catabolize its own body protein to supply the missing amino acid; the effect is the same as cheating on the diet, namely an increase in blood and urine phenylalanine levels. Therefore, the phenylalanine content of the diet, as well as the child's blood and urine phenylalanine levels and physical and mental growth and development, must be closely monitored and evaluated. The diet is continuously modified to provide enough phenylalanine to support growth and development without causing a build-up of phenylketones.

(continued)

Nursing Interventions and Considerations
for Disorders of Infancy and Childhood (*continued*)

The diet must be adequate in protein-sparing calories to prevent the use of protein for energy, which would also result in body protein catabolism.

The age at which the diet can be discontinued is controversial. From a practical standpoint, some physicians recommend discontinuing the diet when the child enters school (4 to 6 years of age) because brain growth is at least 90% completed. However, a study of school-aged children who followed the diet from the first few weeks of life until age 6 showed that although discontinuing the diet did not affect baseline IQ, the children performed less well in school, which could be as damaging to the child's overall development as a decrease in IQ. Some researchers are recommending that the diet be followed to adolescence or even later.

Women with PKU have a high incidence of aborted pregnancies and infants born with mental handicaps, unless they follow a low-phenylalanine diet during pregnancy or possibly before conception (see Chap. 10).

Lofenelac (Mead), the formula specially prepared for infants with PKU, has 95% of the phenylalanine removed. It may need to be supplemented with small, controlled amounts of formula or milk to supply the proper amount of phenylalanine. Unfortunately, it is expensive and older children and adults find the taste objectionable, although it is usually well accepted by infants.

Once solid foods are added to the infant's diet (at 4 to 6 months of age), parents may be given meal patterns and exchange lists of foods grouped according to their phenylalanine content to aid in diet planning.

Comprehensive and frequent diet counseling is necessary to assess the child's intake, monitor progress, and allay the parents' fears.

Advise parents

- That following the diet is essential to prevent mental retardation and other problems of PKU.
- That although other infant formulas or milk may *supplement* Lofenalac, they cannot *replace* Lofenalac in the infant's diet.
- That the diet is low in phenylalanine, not phenylalanine-free, and must provide adequate calories.
- That phenylalanine is an amino acid and, therefore, is found in greatest concentrations in high-protein foods such as meat, fish, poultry, milk, dairy products, and eggs. These products are eliminated or restricted.
- That vegetables, fruits, some cereals, breads, and other starches are low in phenylalanine and are used in measured amounts.
- That label reading is essential; for example, aspartame (NutraSweet) is not appropriate for phenylketonurics because it contains phenylalanine.

(continued)

Nursing Interventions and Considerations for Disorders of Infancy and Childhood (*continued*)

Cystic Fibrosis

Cystic fibrosis (CF), inherited as a recessive trait, is a metabolic disease characterized by excessive exocrine secretions (especially mucous) that form plugs. The sites most commonly affected by mucous plugs are the bronchi, leading to chronic pulmonary infections and fibrosis of the lung tissue, the intestines, creating problems with nutrient absorption, and the pancreatic and bile ducts, which impairs pancreatic enzyme secretion and results in protein and fat malabsorption (steatorrhea), secondary nutrient deficiencies, malnutrition with possible growth retardation, and glucose intolerance related to impaired insulin secretion. In addition, sweat gland secretions contain excessive amounts of sodium and chloride.

NURSING INTERVENTIONS AND CONSIDERATIONS

Monitor fluid and electrolyte balance, and growth and development.

Fat malabsorption, leading to steatorrhea, malabsorption syndrome, and malnutrition, is the greatest nutritional problem of CF. Fat tolerance varies considerably among individuals.

Clients with CF need to take pancreatic enzyme supplements with all meals and snacks to enhance fat digestion and absorption.

Because protein requirements are greatest during the first year of life, infants are particularly susceptible to protein deficiency and malnutrition.

Clients with CF excrete high concentrations of sodium in their sweat. However, except for hot climates, sodium supplements are usually not necessary because the average American diet provides up to ten times more sodium than needed.

Although diet therapy is an important component of treatment, there is no evidence that good nutrition has a significant impact on the course of CF.

Advise parents

- That a high-protein, high-calorie diet is necessary to replace losses. The Daily Food Guide can be used to plan a varied, balanced diet.
- That although fats are a concentrated source of calories and are needed for the essential fatty acid, fat may not be well tolerated and may need to be restricted; medium-chain triglycerides (MCT) are readily absorbed and may be given for additional calories (see Chap. 3).
- That simple sugars are better tolerated than starches.
- To give the child water-soluble supplements of the fat-soluble vitamins and a multivitamin, as prescribed.
- To give the child pancreatic enzyme supplements with all meals and snacks.
- That children with CF need more fluid and sodium; encourage a liberal intake of both.

NURSING PROCESS

Assessment

In addition to the general growth and development assessment criteria, assess for the following factors:

Growth rate, weight status, and weight fluctuations

Pattern of meals and snacks

Adequacy of intake based on the Daily Food Guide (see Table 11-3), paying particular attention to iron intake: meat, shellfish, enriched and fortified breads and cereals, dried peas and beans, and dried fruit

Feeding skills and "feeding problems"

Pica. If the child/family practices pica, determine what items are consumed, how frequently, and the rationale

Dental health

The frequency and intensity of physical activity

Nursing Diagnosis

Health Seeking Behaviors, as evidenced by a lack of knowledge of age-appropriate eating behaviors and nutritional requirements, and the desire to learn.

Planning and Implementation

Parents are the primary gatekeepers and role models of their young children's food intake and habits. Encourage parents to set a good example.

The usual meal pattern is three small meals with three planned snacks. Milk intake decreases to about 16 oz/day by age 2, which is adequate. Excessive milk intake can contribute to iron deficiency anemia by displacing iron-rich foods in the diet (see box, Nutrition-Related Problems Among the Healthy Pediatric Population). Liquids should be withheld until half-way through the meal or until the end of the meal to avoid replacing the intake of nutrient-rich foods.

Appetite fluctuates widely because of erratic growth patterns. Children eat to satisfy hunger and should not be forced to overeat. Although there are individual differences, usually a larger child eats more than a smaller one, an active child eats more than a quiet one, and a happy, content child eats more than an anxious one.

The most common concerns of parents are of limited intakes of milk, rejection of meat and vegetables, and excessive intake of sweets. However, feeding problems tend to be a product of culture, economic status, and parental nutrition knowledge, and often occur because parents overestimate the amount of food children need and force them to overeat. Assure parents that if the child's growth chart shows a consistent and reasonable rate of growth, nutritional intake is probably adequate.

Nutrients most likely to be consumed in inadequate amounts are iron and vitamin B_6.[18] However, supplements are generally not needed unless the child has a chronic illness or is a particularly poor eater.

Client Goals

The child will:

Experience normal growth and development, and maintain optimal nutritional status.

Avoid common nutrition-related problems: iron deficiency anemia, obesity, and dental caries (see box, Nutrition-Related Problems Among the Healthy Pediatric Population).

Avoid milk anemia.

Begin to establish lifelong healthy eating patterns.

Engage in regular physical activity.

Nursing Interventions

Diet management

Provide a varied, nutrient-dense diet, based on the Daily Food Guide for Childhood (see Table 11-3).

Provide three meals daily plus two to three planned snacks.

Modify the diet, as needed, to avoid common nutrition-related problems (see box, Nutrition-Related Problems Among the Healthy Pediatric Population). Limit milk intake to 16 oz/day.

After age 2, limit fat intake to 30% of calories (see Food for Thought: Preventative Nutrition for Children).

Allow children to choose their own food likes and dislikes, and vary their intake according to appetite.

Client teaching

Instruct the family

On eating behaviors characteristic of this age

Food "jags" are a normal expression of autonomy as the child develops a sense of independence. As long as the diet is adequate but not excessive in water, calories, and all essential nutrients, food jags should not be a cause of concern.

Foods most commonly rejected are as follows:

- Meats (with the exception of chicken, hamburger, and hot dogs). The iron status of children who refuse animal sources of iron may require monitoring.
- Cooked vegetables. Serve vegetables raw if possible, or serve more fruit.
- Casseroles or mixed dishes. Serve plain, simple foods.

Avoid encouraging the inborn preference for sweets. Sweets can displace other nutrient-rich foods and contribute to nutrient deficiencies, dental caries, and obesity.

Children may refuse to eat for the following reasons:

- Too excited or distracted. Allow the child time to calm down before eating and try to minimize mealtime commotion.
- Too tired. A brief rest or quiet time before mealtime may help.
- Not hungry. Remove the child's plate without comment. If the child wants a snack later, make it nutritious. Try spacing meals further apart and limit snacking so the child will be hungry at mealtime.
- Seeking attention. Provide attention other than at mealtimes. Do not tolerate manipulative behavior.

Food for Thought

Preventive Nutrition for Children

Numerous studies indicate that atherosclerosis and heart disease begin in childhood. For instance, more than half the soldiers who died in Korea, at an average age of 22, had some degree of atherosclerosis at the time of autopsy. In another study conducted in Louisiana, autopsies performed on 88 children who had died of illness or in an accident showed that almost 40% had fibrous plaques or fatty streaks in the walls of blood vessels; these children also had high serum cholesterol levels.[12] It is estimated that 30% to 40% of all children have high serum cholesterol levels, and 80% of them will continue with high serum cholesterol as adults.[12]

A strong relationship exists between diet and serum cholesterol levels, even in childhood. Studies show that, generally, children with high total serum cholesterol levels have higher intakes of cholesterol and fat, especially saturated fat, and eat less carbohydrates than children with the lowest cholesterol levels.

Because atherosclerosis can begin in childhood, and because diet can reduce the risk of atherosclerosis by reducing serum cholesterol, many experts believe children should adopt a heart-healthy diet, namely, limiting total fat intake and avoiding obesity. In April of 1991, a panel of the National Cholesterol Education Program (NCEP) published the following diet recommendations for all children over the age of 2:

- Eat a variety of foods for a nutritionally adequate diet.
- Eat adequate calories to support normal growth and development, and to attain or maintain desirable body weight.
- Limit total fat intake to 30% of total calories or less, saturated fat intake to 10% of total calories, and cholesterol to less than 300 mg/day.

To limit fat without compromising calories and essential nutrients, researchers suggest that children switch to low-fat dairy products, trim visible fat from meat, limit their intake of highly processed meats such as luncheon meats and hot dogs, and substitute low-fat snacks for those high in fat. No dietary modifications are recommended for children under the age of 2 because of the potential negative impact on growth and development related to an inadequate intake of calories and nutrients.

- Expressing independence. Accept it as a normal phase of development and do not make it an issue.

Appetite is often least at dinner.

Ritualistic eating may become apparent.

On how to foster good eating habits

Offer the proper food.

Using the Daily Food Guide, offer a variety of nutritious foods. It is not important if a child refuses to eat a particular food (*e.g.*, spinach), as long as he has a reasonable intake from each of the major food groups.

Encourage the child to taste new foods but respect individual likes and dislikes.

Introduce a small amount of a new food with a familiar favorite.

Children usually prefer mild-flavored foods.

Make dessert a nutritious part of the meal (such as pudding, fruit, nutrient-rich cookies) instead of a bribe, reward, or routine bedtime snack.

Serve nutritious planned snacks (see box, Nutritious Snacks).

Offer child-sized servings. Generally, a serving size equals 1 tablespoon of food/year of age (*e.g.*, the serving size for a 3-year-old is 3 tablespoons). It is better to serve seconds than to overwhelm the child with too much food. Parents should decide *what* the child should eat, the child should decide *how much*. Instead of "clean your plate," the rule should be "try a little bit of everything."

Offer foods the child can easily chew and digest.

Use child-sized utensils and small, unbreakable cups and plates.

Serve colorful foods (red tomatoes, orange slices, green peas) of various textures (smooth mashed potatoes, crunchy raw vegetables, tender meats) attractively (shaped sandwiches made with cookie cutters, carrot curls).

Children prefer finger foods. Allow children to explore foods by touching. Children learning to use utensils often place the food on the utensil by hand.

Provide an enjoyable atmosphere.

Never force a child to eat; if a healthy child is hungry, he will eat.

Do not use food to reward, punish, bribe, or convey love.

Mealtime should be relaxed, pleasant, and unhurried. Allow 20 to 30 minutes per meal.

Eat with the child.

Provide comfortable, child-sized tables and chairs. If the child refuses to sit while eating, remove him from the table.

Minimize confusion and excess noise at mealtime. Keep mealtime conversation pleasant, do not use it as a time for discipline.

Expect occasional table accidents as a part of growing up.

Encourage children to participate in food preparation and clean-up.

Praise good eating behaviors and do not scold children for not eating.

On how to avoid common nutrition-related problems of
healthy children (see box, Nutrition-Related Problems Among the Healthy Pediatric Population)

Monitor

Monitor for the following signs or symptoms:
Growth and development, and weight status
Overall intake according to the Daily Food Guide
Iron status
Dental health
The development of food allergies
The need for follow-up family diet counseling

Evaluation

Evaluation is ongoing. Assuming the plan of care has not changed, the client will achieve the goals as stated above.

NUTRITION FOR SCHOOL-AGED CHILDREN (AGED 6 TO 12 YEARS)

Growth Characteristics and Nutritional Implications

Physical and Physiologic Growth	Nutritional Implications
Latent period of growth, characterized by erratic, uneven growth pattern	Nutrient needs per unit of body weight continue to decline; dietary intake is regular and appetite gradually increases in preparation for the adolescent growth spurt
Wide variations in growth rates among individuals	
Digestive system matures; can handle larger meals and eat less frequently.	Meal pattern: 3 meals with 2 snacks
Permanent teeth erupt.	Nutrients important for dental health include fluoride, vitamin A, vitamin D, calcium, and phosphorus.
Increased socialization, growing sense of independence	Parents role as gatekeepers declines; advertising has an impact on food choices; variety of food increases.
Reserves are laid down for upcoming adolescent growth spurt.	Toward the end of the school-age period, nutrient needs increase in preparation for the adolescent growth spurt.

NURSING PROCESS

Assessment

In addition to the general growth and development assessment criteria, assess for the following factors:

Growth rate, weight status, and weight fluctuations

Pattern of meals and snacks

Adequacy of intake based on the Daily Food Guide for the child's age, paying particular attention to the sources of calories, iron, and protein

The use of vitamin/mineral supplements; type, amount, and frequency

Frequency and intensity of physical activity

Nursing Diagnosis

Health Seeking Behaviors, as evidenced by a lack of knowledge of normal nutritional requirements of children and a desire to learn.

Nutritious Snacks

Snacks

Are an excellent way to provide additional protein, calories, and essential nutrients to children who cannot eat a lot at mealtime.

Should be offered at least 1.5 hours before mealtime to avoid interfering with appetite.

Should be based on the child's appetite, preferences, and ability to chew and digest.

Suggestions

Unsweetened cereal, with or without milk

Meat or cheese on whole-grain bread or crackers

Graham crackers, fig bars

Whole-grain cookies or muffins made with oatmeal, dried fruit, or iron-fortified cereal

Quick breads like banana, date, pumpkin

Raw vegetables, vegetable juices

Fresh fruit or canned fruit without sugar

Pure fruit juice as a drink or frozen on a stick

Plain low-fat yogurt, with or without fresh fruit added

Chunks of cheese, cottage cheese

Popcorn, nuts, sunflower or pumpkin seeds (not before age 3)

Hard-cooked or deviled eggs

Peanut butter on bread, crackers, celery, apple slices

Milk shakes made with fruit and ice cream or frozen yogurt

Low-fat ice cream, frozen yogurt, ice milk, sherbet

Planning and Implementation

School-aged children maintain a relatively constant intake in relation to their age group, that is, children who are considered big eaters in second grade are also big eaters in sixth grade.

A child's genetic potential for growth is reached only if nutrient needs are met. A calorie deficit of as little as 10 cal/kg can result in malnutrition.

Generally, eating is still a ritual for 6- and 7-year-olds, 8-year-olds tend to have large appetites, and 9-year-olds have firmly established likes and dislikes and may be very resistant to change; vegetables are the least favorite foods.

Breakfast skipping is a concern of parents of school-aged children. Studies show that breakfast-skipping impairs attitudes, work output, problem-solving performance, and grades. Traditionally, breakfast supplies 100% of the RDA for vitamin C (orange juice) and one third of the day's requirement for protein, calories, and other nutrients.

Another consideration is the effect of advertising on children's food choices. Nine out of 10 Saturday-morning food commercials on the major networks advertise high-sugar, high-fat, and high-sodium items. Breakfast cereals are the first or second most frequently advertised products on Saturday-morning children's television.[10]

Food additives are a concern of parents with hyperactive children. Although difficult to define objectively, common characteristics of hyperactivity (or attention deficit disorder—ADD—with or without concurrent hyperactivity) include specific learning deficits, impulsivity, hyperkinesis, short attention span, motor and coordination deficits, and aggression. In 1973, the late Dr. Ben Feingold proposed that food additives and salicylates may be responsible for about 25% of the cases of hyperactivity with learning disability among school-aged children. Numerous studies indicate that the Feingold diet (a diet devoid of artificial colors, flavors, BHT, BHA, and salicylate-containing fruits, vegetables, and spices) rarely helps control hyperactivity. However, the Feingold diet is probably not nutritionally harmful (as long as fruits and vegetables containing vitamin C are allowed) and may have a placebo effect on behavior.

Food allergies, which are most commonly caused by protein substances in food (*i.e.*, the protein component of milk, wheat, eggs, corn), are influenced by a variety of environmental, emotional, genetic, and physical factors. Introducing solids into the diet before the immune system matures increases the likelihood of food allergies. Fortunately, most children tend to outgrow food allergies as they get older. Because allergies may be difficult to diagnose, foods should be introduced in the diet one at a time for 5 to 7 days so that if a reaction occurs, the offending item can be identified easily (see box, Allergic Reactions). Older children suspected of having food allergies may benefit from eliminating common allergens from the diet (Table 11-9). If the food allergy persists, it may be necessary to use skin testing or elimination diets to diagnose the offending item. Initially, children on elimination diets receive foods that are relatively hypoallergenic (rice, tapioca), after which other foods are introduced singly and the child is observed for a reaction.

Client Goals

The child will:
Experience normal growth and development, and maintain optimal nutritional status.

Allergic Reactions

- May be immediate (within 1 hour) or delayed (within 24 to 48 hours)
- May be cyclical (not always occurring after the offending item is eaten) or fixed (always occurring after the offending item is eaten)
- May produce skin, GI, respiratory, or CNS symptoms

Table 11-9
Common Food Allergens

Bacon	Peanut butter
Chocolate	Pineapple
Citrus fruit	Pork
Cocoa	Seafood
Eggs	Strawberries
Milk and milk products	Tomatoes
Nuts	Wheat

Avoid common nutrition-related problems: iron deficiency anemia, obesity, and dental caries.

Continue to establish lifelong healthy eating patterns.

Engage in regular physical activity.

Nursing Interventions

Diet management

Provide a varied, nutrient-dense diet, based on the Daily Food Guide for Childhood (see Table 11-3).

Modify the diet, as needed, to avoid common nutrition-related problems (see box, Nutrition-Related Problems Among the Healthy Pediatric Population).

Limit fat intake to 30% of calories (see Food for Thought: Preventative Nutrition for Children).

Allow children to choose their own food likes and dislikes, and vary their intake according to appetite.

Client teaching

Instruct the child/family

On the importance of nutrition in normal growth and development, and overall health and well-being.

On the principles and rationale of the Daily Food Guide, and how to choose an adequate diet.

How to modify the diet, as needed, to avoid common nutrition-related problems (see box, Nutrition-Related Problems Among the Healthy Pediatric Population).

On the relationship between nutrition, physical activity, and health status. Encourage regular physical activity.

Monitor

Monitor for the following signs or symptoms:

Growth and development, and weight status

Overall intake according to the Daily Food Guide for childhood

Iron status

Dental health

The need for follow-up family diet counseling

Evaluation

Evaluation is ongoing. Assuming the plan of care has not changed, the client will achieve the goals as stated above.

ADOLESCENT NUTRITION (AGED 12 TO 18 YEARS)

Growth Characteristics and Nutritional Implications

Physical and Physiologic Growth	*Nutritional Implications*
Rapid period of physical, emotional, social, and sexual maturation	To support adequate growth and development, nutritional needs increase, especially for calories, protein, calcium, and iron
Growth begins at different times in different individuals; therefore, physiologic age is a more valid indicator of need than chronological age.	Because the RDAs are based on chronological, not physiologic age, they may be invalid for some or many adolescents, depending on when the growth spurt begins (the increase in nutritional requirements is dependent on the timing and duration of the growth spurt)
Generally, the growth spurt begins in females around age 10 to 11, peaks at age 12, and is completed by age 15.	Nutritional needs increase earlier for girls than boys.
Menstruation begins.	To replace monthly losses, the requirement for iron increases and remains high until menopause
Girls experience fat deposition, especially in the abdomen and pelvic girdle; the pelvis widens in preparation for childbearing. Girls experience less growth of lean body tissue and bones than boys.	Fat requires fewer calories to be maintained than does lean body tissue; therefore, girls have lower calorie requirements than boys and may have difficulty meeting nutrient needs without exceeding calorie needs. Girls tend to become weight and figure conscious and often voluntarily restrict the amount and types of food eaten.
Generally, the growth spurt begins in males around age 12 to 13, peaks at age 14, and is completed by age 19.	Nutritional needs increase later for boys than girls.
Boys experience an increase in muscle mass, lean body tissue, and bones.	Lean body tissue requires more calories to be maintained than fat tissue; therefore, boys have higher calorie needs than girls. During the growth spurt, adolescent males need the same amount of iron as menstruating females because of the increase in muscle mass and blood volume; iron need decreases to below female requirement after the growth spurt is complete.
Period of intense psychosocial growth, family conflict, social and peer pressures.	Nutritional needs may be difficult to meet because Fewer meals are eaten at home. Of strong peer influence Of busy schedules Adolescents may express their independence through the diet.

NURSING PROCESS

Assessment

In addition to the general growth and development assessment criteria, assess for the following factors:

Growth rate, weight status, and weight fluctuations

Pattern of meals and snacks

Adequacy of intake based on the Daily Food Guide for Adolescents, paying particular attention to iron and protein intake

The use of vitamin/mineral supplements; type, amount, and frequency

The use of alcohol, tobacco, and drugs

Familial attitude toward weight, thinness, and the client's weight[4]

The use of any fad diets; assess the age at which dieting began and associated events, the methods/patterns of dieting, and the client's feelings/beliefs about food and dieting.[4]

The frequency and intensity of physical activity

Nursing Diagnosis

Health Seeking Behaviors, as evidenced by a lack of knowledge of normal nutritional requirements for adolescents and the desire to learn.

General Growth and Development Assessment Criteria

Age

Height (length in infants)

Weight

Weight for height and head circumference (for infants)

Hemoglobin

Hematocrit

Clinical observations: skin color, pallor, turgor; gross deformities; subcutaneous fat; dental caries

Chronic illness, family history of chronic illness

Use of medication for chronic illness

Allergies, nature of allergic reactions

Socioeconomic status

Developmental status

Planning and Implementation

Because of varying growth rates, a wide range of weights is considered normal during adolescence.

Childhood nutritional problems tend to intensify during adolescence. Mild nutrient deficiencies may be common; for example, laboratory values may indicate a deficiency but overt clinical symptoms are not apparent. Nutrients most likely to be consumed in inadequate amounts are iron (particularly in girls), calcium, and energy.[7]

Peer and social pressures and enjoyment often have a greater impact on adolescent food choices than the nutritional quality of the food and health implications of diet.

Effective adolescent nutrition education programs are those that allow adolescents to express their attitudes, beliefs, concerns, and feelings regarding food, food choices, eating, and diet, and are tailored to meet the needs and interests of the individual or group. They also encourage self-direction and responsibility for food choices based on an adequate knowledge base, and allow the educator to be a facilitator of learning, not a "teacher." Nutrition education programs should also encourage physical activity for overall health.

Nutritional concerns among this age group include the following:

- *Meal skipping:* Some studies report up to 50% of the adolescents surveyed skipped breakfast because of the lack of time or desire to lose weight.
- *Snacking:* Snacks may contribute 30% or more of adolescents' total calorie intake each day. Unfortunately, snacks are often high in fat, sugar, or sodium, and may increase the risk of obesity and dental caries. Adolescents should be encouraged to take responsibility for choosing healthy snacks.
- *Dieting:* Many adolescents are preoccupied with dieting because of concerns about their appearance. Also, many girls do not understand that increases in fat tissue during puberty are necessary for normal growth and development; boys may have the mistaken belief that dieting will improve athletic performance. Regardless of the motivating factor, adolescents should be counseled on realistic views of desirable weight, and the importance of regular physical activity. For extreme eating disorders, see section on anorexia and bulimia.
- *Adolescent pregnancy:* Adolescent pregnancy is associated with increased medical, nutritional, social, and economic risks depending on biologic maturity, ethnic background, economic status, prenatal care, and life style (see Chap. 10).
- *Acne:* There is no scientific evidence to support the belief that chocolate, soft drinks, or peanut butter cause acne. Although vitamin A is important for normal skin integrity, vitamin A supplements are not effective in treating acne and are toxic in large amounts. A compound related to vitamin A (13-*cis*-retinoic acid or Accutane) has been approved for treatment of severe cystic acne but is available only through prescription and must be used with caution.
- *The use of alcohol, tobacco, marijuana, oral contraceptives:* Alcohol, especially in growing adolescents, can produce nutritional deficiencies related to decreased food intake, decreased absorption, increased excretion, decreased storage, or altered metabolism of nutrients. Likewise, tobacco and marijuana can alter food intake. Oral contraceptives alter serum levels of some nutrients and may increase the requirement for folic acid and vitamin B_6, although clinical observations of deficiencies are rare and vitamin supplements are unnecessary.

- *Nutrition for the growing athlete:* Diet guidelines for growing athletes suggest a balanced, varied diet with adequate fluid and calories to meet increased needs. During training, the diet should be composed of about 15% protein, 55% CHO, and 30% fat. Young athletes may develop a transient low hemoglobin related to a greater increase in plasma volume than in red blood cell mass, or from true iron deficiency anemia. Amenorrhea is also common among adolescent female athletes and may be related to the stress of physical training and competition or to a reduction in body fat. Regular menstrual activity returns after intense training is reduced and body fat level increases. Misconceptions regarding the role of nutrition and diet in athletic competition should be dispelled (see box, Misconceptions About Sports Nutrition).

Client Goals

The client will:

Consume adequate calories, protein, and nutrients to support the adolescent growth spurt.

Prevent or correct nutritional deficiencies.

Avoid common nutrition-related problems: iron deficiency anemia, obesity, and dental caries.

Engage in regular physical activity.

Continue to establish lifelong healthy eating patterns.

Nursing Interventions

Diet management

Provide a varied, nutrient-dense diet based on the Daily Food Guide for Adolescents.

Modify the diet, as needed, to avoid common nutrition-related problems.

Limit fat intake to 30% of total calories.

Client teaching

Instruct the client

On the principles and rationale of the Daily Food Guide, and how to choose an adequate diet.

On the relationship between diet, health, weight control, and physical fitness. Explain that an increase in fat tissue before the adolescent growth spurt is a normal physiologic occurrence. Encourage regular physical activity.

On how to modify the diet, as needed, to avoid common nutrition-related problems.

On the importance of not skipping meals, especially breakfast.

To choose nutritious snacks.

That limiting fat intake may help prevent heart disease later in life.

Monitor

Monitor for the following signs or symptoms:

Growth and development, and weight status

Overall intake according to the Daily Food Guide for Adolescents

Iron status

Dental health

The need for follow-up family diet counseling

Misconceptions About Sports Nutrition

Fallacy: Extra protein builds muscles.

Fact: Muscle mass increases only through repeated exercise, providing that a sufficient supply of calories is available. According to the American Dietetic Association, the RDA for protein may be inadequate for adult endurance athletes, who may actually need 1.0 g of protein/kg, instead of the RDA of 0.8 mg/kg. However, because most American diets provide more protein than is needed, young athletes are probably consuming enough. Protein taken in excess of need is not magically converted to muscle, rather, it is converted to and stored as fat, just like an excess intake of CHO or fat.

Fallacy: Carbohydrate foods are fattening and should be avoided by athletes.

Fact: The primary muscle fuel during exercise is carbohydrates, in the form of blood glucose or stored glycogen. When low-CHO diets are consumed during training, the body's storage of fuel may not be adequate to sustain an athlete through prolonged competition, resulting in weakness, the inability to perform, or "hitting the wall." Carbohydrates also provide the same amount of calories as an equivalent amount of protein and less than half the calories in an equal measure of fat.

Fallacy: CHO loading can be used routinely to increase athletic performance.

Fact: CHO loading is based on the idea that glycogen stores can be maximized, and, therefore, endurance improved, in a step-by-step process involving training and diet. Traditionally, CHO loading involved depleting glycogen stores followed by loading, in which the athlete exercised to a minimum and ate a high-CHO intake to supersaturate the muscles with glycogen.

Unfortunately, carbohydrate loading is beneficial only to athletes participating in long-duration endurance or multiple-event competitions.[2] Also, it is now recommended that athletes follow a high-CHO diet throughout training and begin a tapered rest approximately 7 days before the competition, with complete rest the day before the event.[2] CHO loading is not recommended for growing athletes.

Fallacy: The less body fat, the better the athlete.

Fact: Different sports require different amounts of body fat for optimum performance; for example, the ideal percentage of body weight as fat for male distance runners is 4% to 8%, and for male tennis players, 14% to 16%. While it is true that too much body fat means excess body weight and interferes with the body's ability to dissipate heat, too little fat should also be avoided. Adjusting body weight is a gradual process; rapid weight loss results in a greater loss of lean body tissue than fat tissue, can impair performance, may endanger health, and could adversely effect growth. Likewise, rapid weight gain usually means fat gain, not an increase in lean body tissues.

(continued)

Misconceptions About Sports Nutrition *(continued)*

Fallacy: Salt tablets are needed to replace sodium lost through perspiration.

Fact: Salt tablets are not recommended; sodium chloride taken without adequate amounts of water can further aggravate intracellular dehydration caused by sweating. Dehydration can impair physical performance, and thirst is not always a reliable indicator of need. Plain water is probably the most important substance for replacing fluid loss. Prepubescent athletes are particularly susceptible to heat stroke or heat-induced collapse because of their inability to produce sweat effectively and, thus, cool the body through evaporation.

Fallacy: Supplements of vitamin B_6 and other vitamins will improve performance.

Fact: An increase in calorie intake does warrant a higher intake of vitamins used to metabolize calories, namely thiamine, riboflavin, and niacin. However, sufficient amounts of these vitamins can easily be obtained by the increase in calorie (food) intake. These and other water-soluble vitamins taken in excess of need do not enhance energy metabolism but are excreted in the urine. Megadoses of the fat-soluble vitamins and some water-soluble vitamins can cause toxic or adverse effects and should not be used.

Fallacy: The precompetition meal should be high in protein.

Fact: High-protein meals can lead to mild dehydration because the kidneys must excrete the nitrogenous wastes resulting from protein metabolism. In addition, high-protein meals may also be high in fat, which delays gastric emptying. A meal high in complex CHO should be eaten 3.5 to 4 hours before competition to ensure gastric emptying and to avoid discomfort and cramping. Although the meal may contain between 300 to 1000 calories, generally, the lighter the better.[2]

Evaluation

Evaluation is ongoing. Assuming the plan of care has not changed, the client will achieve the goals as stated above.

EATING DISORDERS: ANOREXIA, BULIMIA, AND BULIMIA NERVOSA

Anorexia nervosa and bulimia are two distinct eating disorders with common characteristics. Anorexia nervosa is a condition of self-imposed fasting or severe self-imposed dieting characterized by dramatic weight loss. Thinness is pursued compulsively, and self-perception of body weight is distorted. Bulimia is a binging–purging syndrome characterized by self-induced vomiting and/or laxative, emetic, diuretic, or diet pill abuse. Unlike anorexics, bulimics experience weight fluctuations and may appear to have normal weight. Both eating disorders are related to a preoccupation with food and an irrational fear of being fat and may coincide; anorexics may develop bulimia, bulimics may develop anorexia.

Bulimia nervosa, considered a variant of anorexia nervosa, was first described as a distinct psychiatric illness in 1979.[15] It is characterized by recurrent binge eating episodes, at which time the client feels a lack of control over the eating behavior. Self-induced vomiting, laxative abuse, strict dieting, fasting or vigorous exercise are used to prevent weight gain. Like anorexics, clients with bulimia nervosa are preoccupied with body shape and weight. Bulimia nervosa is now the most common eating disorder.[8]

Although extensively studied, the basic causes of anorexia nervosa remain unknown.[21] However, studies strongly indicate a relationship between depression and eating disorders; many anorexics suffer from low mood, loss of interest, shortened attention span, disrupted sleep patterns, and suicidal tendencies.[23] Studies suggest that alcohol and drug abuse may be four to five times higher in women with eating disorders than in the general population. Indeed, psychological and social factors, especially problems with family dynamics, are generally considered to be central to the problem. Major stressors, such as the onset of puberty, parents' divorce, death of a family member, broken relationships, and ridicule of being or becoming fat are frequent precipitating factors. Eating disorders are most likely to occur immediately before or after the onset of puberty, and are often preceded by prolonged "dieting."[19] Athletes, like dancers and gymnasts, may develop eating disorders to improve their performance.

Some experts believe anorexia and bulimia are reaching epidemic proportions; anorexia may affect 1 of every 100 teenage girls and young women; bulimia 1 of every 5 women in college. Approximately 90% of the cases of anorexia and bulimia are female, with a peak age of onset between 12 to 13 and 19 to 20 years. Anorexics typically are from white, middle- to upper-middle-class families that place heavy emphasis on high achievement, perfection, and physical appearance. Anorexics are often described as "model" children, although they tend to be immature, need parental approval, and lack independence. Bulimics tend to be extroverted, have a history of being overweight before their illness, and have voracious appetites.

Numerous physical and mental signs and symptoms may be observed in people with eating disorders (see box, Physical, Mental, and Behavioral Signs and Symptoms of Anorexia). Severe or chronic eating disorders may lead to permanent brain damage, permanent sterility, chronic invalidism; damage to vital organs, including gastric and esophageal rupture; heart failure, and rupture or erosion of the esophagus, fluid and electrolyte imbalances, and destruction of tooth enamel secondary to vomiting. As many as one out of five to seven clients with chronic anorexia may die from complications.

Treatment seeks to restore normal nutritional status through an oral diet, enteral feedings, or hyperalimentation if necessary. Step-by-step goals of diet therapy designed to meet the client's physiologic and psychological needs are as follows:

1. Prevent further weight loss. Because of low body weight and decreased metabolic rate, initially, small quantities of food are sufficient to prevent weight loss and are more acceptable to the client than above-average quantities.
2. Improve nutritional status while low weight is maintained.
3. Gradually increase weight by reestablishing normal eating behaviors. Initially, clients may respond to nutritional therapy better if they are allowed to exclude high-risk binge foods from their diet. However, the binge foods should be reintroduced later so that the "feared food" idea is not promoted.[15]

Physical, Mental, and Behaviorial Signs and Symptoms of Anorexia

Physical Symptoms

- Extreme weight loss and muscle wasting (anorexics may lose 25% of their body weight over a period of months); bulimics experience weight fluctuations, but may appear normal weight
- Arrested sexual development, amenorrhea
- Dry, yellow skin related to the release of carotenes as fat stores are burned for energy
- Loss of hair or change in hair texture
- Pain on touch
- Hypotension, bradycardia
- Anemia
- Constipation
- Severe sleep disturbances, insomnia
- Dental caries and periodontal disease

Mental and Behavioral Symptoms

- Bizarre eating habits, refusal to eat
- Feelings of failure, low self-esteem, social isolation
- Perfectionist, overachiever
- Preoccupation with food, dieting, and death
- Intense fear of becoming fat that does not lessen with weight loss
- Distorted body image and denial of eating disorder
- Frantic pursuit of exercise
- Frequent weighing
- Use of laxatives, diuretics, emetics, and diet pills
- Manipulative behavior

4. Maintain a set weight goal that has been agreed on by the health care team and the client. Sometimes a lower-than-ideal weight is selected as the initial weight goal (*i.e.*, enough weight to regain normal physiologic function and menstruation). When achieved, the goals may be reevaluated. Many recovered clients have chronic problems with eating and weight.

The underlying problem of the eating disorder may be treated with a multidimensional approach, including behavior modification, individual psychotherapy, family counseling, and group therapy. Antidepressant drugs effectively reduce but do not eliminate the frequency of problematic eating behaviors.[15] Depending on the severity of the eating disorder, clients may be treated on either an outpatient or an inpatient basis. All aspects of treatment (dietary, behavioral modification, psychotherapy) must be highly individualized; treatment is often time-consuming and frustrating. Because the eating and behavior patterns of bulimics are usually altered for a longer time, bulimia may be more difficult to treat than anorexia.

NURSING PROCESS

Assessment

Assess for the following factors:
Signs and symptoms of eating disorder: onset, causative factors, severity
Food fears and eating behaviors: determine what foods are "feared"
The use of laxatives or diuretics; determine if self-induced vomiting is practiced
Weight status and adequacy of growth, if appropriate
Fluid and electrolyte balance

Nursing Diagnosis

Altered Nutrition: Less than Body Requirements, related to anorexia nervosa.

Planning and Implementation

Initially, the diet should be low in calories and progressed slowly to promote compliance and gain the client's trust. Because gastrointestinal intolerance may exist, gassy and high-fat foods should be limited in the early stages of treatment.

Serve small, attractive meals based on individual food preferences. Never force the client to eat, and minimize the emphasis on food.

As the treatment progresses, calorie intake is gradually increased. A high-fiber or low-sodium diet may be helpful to control symptoms of constipation and fluid retention, respectively. A multivitamin and mineral supplement may be prescribed.

Tube feedings or parenteral nutrition should be used only if necessary to stabilize the client medically.

Prevention may be far more effective than the treatment of eating disorders. Encourage parents, teachers, and significant others

- To help children and adolescents establish a strong positive self-image and sense of worth regardless of their weight.
- Not to expect perfection and to avoid putting pressure on children to excel beyond their capabilities.
- To give adolescents an appropriate amount of independence, responsibility, and accountability for their own actions.
- To recognize stresses in the child's life and provide support and encouragement.
- To teach the basis of good nutrition and normal exercise.
- To avoid putting pressure on young people to lose weight. If weight control is really indicated, a medically supervised plan of weight loss and weight maintenance should be followed.
- To recognize the signs and symptoms of eating disorders.
- To seek professional help if eating disorders are suspected.

Client Goals

The client will:

Gain 1 to 2 lbs/week until reasonable weight goal is achieved; achieve normal growth and development, if appropriate.

Be free of signs and symptoms of eating disorders.

Adopt and maintain normal eating behaviors.

Nursing Interventions

Diet management

Provide basal calorie requirements plus 300 to 400 calories initially; gradually increase to a high-calorie diet to promote weight gain.

Provide small frequent feedings to maximize intake.

Limit fat intake initially if GI intolerance exists.

Limit sodium intake if fluid retention is a problem.

Avoid caffeine, which acts as both a stimulant and diuretic.

Client teaching

The diet counselor should promote self-esteem in clients with eating disorders by using a positive approach, providing support and encouragement, fostering self-decision-making, and offering the client choices.[17] Avoid preaching rules and reinforcing the client's preoccupation with food.

Instruct the client and family

On the principles of "good" nutrition, "healthy" weight, and weight maintenance.

On the principles and rationale of the Daily Food Guide, and how to choose an adequate diet.

To eat regular balanced meals. Structured meal-planning techniques are one of the most effective ways to encourage bulimics to eat balanced meals.[15]

On how to recognize signs of hunger.

That the following volunteer organizations have information on treatment centers, hospitals, clinics, groups, and doctors specializing in anorexia nervosa:

American Anorexia Nervosa Association, Inc
133 Cedar Lane
Teaneck, NJ 07666
National Anorexic Aid Society, Inc (NAAS)
PO Box 29461
Columbus, OH 43229
Anorexia Nervosa and Associated Disorders (ANAD)
Suite 2020
550 Frontage Rd
Northfield, IL 60093

Monitor

Monitor for the following signs or symptoms:

Tolerance to fat (*i.e.*, absence of GI upset, bloating) and sodium (absence of fluid retention) in the diet

Compliance to diet, and the need for follow-up diet counseling
Weight, weight gain
Eating behaviors
The effectiveness of the diet, and the need for further diet modifications
The client's attitude about food, dieting, and weight

Evaluation

Evaluation is ongoing. Assuming the plan of care has not changed, the client will achieve the goals as stated above.

BIBLIOGRAPHY

1. American Dietetic Association: Position of The American Dietetic Association: Nutrition intervention in the treatment of anorexia nervosa and bulimia nervosa. J Am Diet Assoc 88:68, 1988
2. American Dietetic Association: Position of the American Dietetic Association: Nutrition for physical fitness and athletic performance for adults. J Am Diet Assoc 87:33, 1987
3. The Chicago Dietetic Association and The South Suburban Dietetic Association, American Dietetic Association: Manual of Clinical Dietetics. Chicago: The American Dietetic Association, 1988.
4. Carruth BR: Nutritional assessment: A guide for nutrition educators. Journal of Nutrition Education 20:280, 1988
5. Curtis DM: Infant nutrient supplementation. J Pediatr 117:S110, 1990
6. Escott-Stump S: Nutrition and Diagnosis-Related Care. 2nd ed. Philadelphia: Lea and Febiger, 1988
7. Gong FJ, Spear BA: Adolescent growth and development: Implications for nutritional needs. Journal of Nutrition Education 20:273, 1988
8. Krey SH, Palmer K, Porcelli KA: Eating disorders: The clinical dietitian's changing role. J Am Diet Assoc 89:41, 1989
9. Lucas AR: Update and review of anorexia nervosa. Contemporary Nutrition 14(9), 1989
10. Mayer J (ed): T.V. feeds kids steady diet of sugary-food ads. Tufts University Diet and Nutrition Letter 9(9):7, 1991
11. Mayer J (ed): The best way to treat your child's diarrhea. Tufts University Diet and Nutrition Letter 8(2):7, 1990
12. Mayer J (ed): When deciding between feeding by breast or by bottle. Tufts University Diet and Nutrition Letter 8(10):3, 1990
13. Mayer J (ed): Making sure your children's hearts stay healthy. Tufts University Diet and Nutrition Letter 7(2):3, 1989
14. Merritt RJ: Nutritional management of low-birth weight infants. Nutrition and the MD 15(10):1, 1989
15. Mitchell JE: Bulimia nervosa. Contemporary Nutrition 14(10):XX 1989
16. Nicklas TA, Arbeit ML, Srinivasan SR, et al: Cardiovascular risk factors in children and prevention of adult atherosclerosis. Contemporary Nutrition 16(3):XX 1991
17. Omizo SA, Oda A: Anorexia nervosa: Psychological considerations for nutrition counseling. J Am Diet Assoc 88:49, 1988
18. Pipes PL: Nutrition in Infancy and Childhood. 4th ed. St. Louis: CV Mosby, 1989

19. Sedlet KL, Ireton-Jones CS: Energy expenditure and the abnormal eating pattern of a bulimic: A case report. J Am Diet Assoc 89:74, 1989
20. Splett PL, Story M: Child nutrition: Objectives for the decade. J Am Diet Assoc 91:665, 1991
21. Tolstoi LG: The role of pharmacotherapy in anorexia nervosa and bulimia. J Am Diet Assoc 89:1640, 1989
22. Wink DM: Better breast milk for preemies? Am J Nurs 89:48, 1989
23. Ziegler EE: Milks and formulas for older infants. J Pediatr 117:S76, 1990

12 Aging and the Aged

The elderly, especially those over 85 years old, represent the fastest-growing segment of the American population. Today, approximately 12% of Americans are over age 65; by 2030, the percentage is expected to increase to almost 22%.[20] Currently, life expectancy is 72 years for men and 77 years for women, compared to 45 years in 1900. The increase can be attributed to improvements in health care, immunizations, hygiene, and nutrition.

Aging is a gradual, inevitable, complex process of progressive physiologic, cellular, cultural, and psychosocial changes that begin at conception and end in death. As cells age, they undergo degenerative changes in structure and function, which eventually impair organ, tissue, and body functioning. Exactly how and why aging occurs is unknown, although most theories are based on either genetic or environmental causes (Table 12-1).

Despite the misconceptions and stereotypes people have of the elderly, they are a heterogeneous group that vary in age, marital status, social background, financial status, living arrangements, and health. Only 5% of the elderly are institutionalized. Although 86% of all elderly have at least one chronic disease,[16] only 21% consider their health poor, possibly because they define wellness/illness differently and accept changes in health as normal aspects of aging.

Genetic and environmental "life advantages," such as genetic potential for longevity, intelligence, motivation, curiosity, good socialization, religious affiliation, marriage and family, physical activity, avoidance of substance abuse, availability of health care, adequate sleep, rest, and relaxation, and good eating habits have a positive effect on both the length and quality of life.

Throughout the life cycle, nutrition has a significant impact on health and the quality of life. Studies suggest that good eating habits established early in life influence health maintenance in old age.[18] Clearly, the development and progression of certain degenerative disorders associated with aging, such as diabetes mellitus, atherosclerosis, hypertension, and obesity, are influenced by lifelong eating habits. Although diet modifications

Table 12-1
Theories of Aging

Proposed Cause of Aging	Theory
Genetic	Genes fail to function normally, possibly due to radiation or faulty selection of amino acids for protein synthesis, which leads to defective replication, transcription, or translation of DNA.
Immunologic	As immune function decreases with age, the incidence of autoimmune reactions increases; that is, the body makes antibodies against its own tissue. It is speculated that the process of aging can be delayed by manipulating the immune system through diet modification, temperature regulation, or avoidance of illness.[4]
Free radical	Due to a force on the polyunsaturated fats in the cell, unstable free radicals are released and peroxidized, resulting in destruction of cell structure. Vitamin E, vitamin C, and selenium (antioxidants) may all inhibit the production of free radicals and thus delay aging.
Cross linkage	Aging molecules link together to form complexes that cannot function normally. This theory has been observed in collagen in aging organisms.
Biologic clock	Each cell is believed to be programmed, through DNA, to self-destruct, that is, certain cells are known to multiply and divide a fixed number of times and then self-destruct.
Aging pacemakers	Pacemakers in the brain initiate a neurohormonal response, possibly through serotonin, dopamine, norepinephrine, or tryptophan, that results in aging.

initiated late in life may not prevent or delay the development of disease, they may influence disease progression and improve the quality of life.

NUTRITIONAL IMPLICATIONS OF AGING

Predictable changes in physiology and function, income, health, and psychosocial well-being are associated with aging, although the rate and timing at which they occur vary among individuals. Changes with a potential impact on diet and nutritional status include the following.

Changes in Physiology and Function	Nutritional Implications
BODY COMPOSITION AND ENERGY EXPENDITURE	
Energy expenditure decreases related to the following:	Calorie requirements decrease in response to the decrease in REE, decrease in physical activity, and change in body composition. Studies show that people tend to eat less as they get older.
Decrease in BMR of about 20% from age 20 to 90	
Decrease in physical activity related to retirement or physical impairments (cardiovascular or pulmonary disorders, arthritis, bone fracture, poor vision)	
Changes in body composition:	
Loss of lean body mass. Muscle mass is replaced by fat and connective tissue.	Loss of muscle mass → loss of muscle strength → loss of range of motion and mobility → impaired ability to purchase, prepare, and eat food
Increase in adipose tissue, which requires fewer calories to be maintained than muscle tissue	

(continued)

Changes in Physiology and Function	*Nutritional Implications*
ORAL AND GI CHANGES	
Difficulty chewing related to loss of teeth and periodontal disease. 50% of Americans have lost all their teeth by age 65. Jaw bone deterioration may be related to osteoporosis.	If intake is limited to soft, easy-to-chew foods, some essential nutrients may be deficient. Meat is the food most commonly eliminated by people who have difficulty chewing.
Constipation is 5 to 6 times more frequent in the elderly than in younger adults, and may be related to the following:	40% to 50% of the elderly reportedly use laxatives. A high-fiber diet with an adequate fluid intake can help relieve constipation.
Decreased peristalsis related to loss of abdominal muscle tone	
Inadequate fluid and fiber intake	
Secondary to drug therapy: antihypertensives, diuretics, sedatives, laxative dependence	
Decrease in physical activity	
Digestive disorders may develop related to the following:	Diet modification may be necessary if food intolerances or impaired nutrient absorption develop.
Decreased secretion of hydrochloric acid (stomach) and digestive enzymes (pancreatic and intestinal)	
Altered esophageal motility	
Nutrient absorption may decrease due to decreased mucosal mass and decreased blood flow to and from the mucosal villi.	
METABOLIC CHANGES	
Altered glucose tolerance. The underlying reason is unclear; may be due to a decrease in insulin secretion or a decrease in tissue sensitivity to insulin.	Nutritional implications are not clear.
CNS CHANGES	
Tremors, slowed reaction time, short-term memory deficits, personality changes and depression may be related to a decrease in the number of brain cells or the decrease in blood flow to the brain and nervous system. Between 1% and 6% of people over 65 have severe dementia, another 2% to 15% have mild dementia.	Food purchasing, preparation, and eating may all be impaired.
RENAL CHANGES	
Decreased ability to excrete nitrogen and other metabolic wastes related to:	If renal failure develops, protein, sodium, and other nutrients may need to be restricted in the diet.
Decreased capillary blood flow	
Decreased glomerular filtration rate (GFR)	
Inability to regenerate nephrons	
Urinary incontinence may develop related to impaired bladder sphincter function.	The elderly may voluntarily restrict fluid intake to cope with incontinence.
SENSORY LOSSES	
Gradual progressive sensory losses may be related to impaired nerve cell function.	
Hearing loss begins around age 30.	Socialized eating may be difficult or intimidating: Lack of socialization can significantly impair appetite and intake in the elderly.[1]
Loss of visual acuity, visual accommodation, ability to see in low light, ability to distinguish color in-	Food purchasing and preparation may be impaired.

(continued)

Changes in Physiology and Function	*Nutritional Implications*
tensities, and decrease in depth perception begins at age 50.	
Loss of taste begins between 55 to 59 years of age and becomes increasingly severe after age 70. Contributing factors include:	Studies show that average detection threshold for elderly people was 2.72 times higher for sweeteners, more than 11 times higher for sodium salts, and 4 times higher for acids.
Sensory losses can cause a decrease in salivation, gastric secretion, pancreatic enzyme secretion, and pancreatic hormone secretion, which could alter nutrient utilization.	
A decrease in the number of taste buds and papilla. Sweet and salty tastes are lost first, followed by bitter and sour.	
Oral infections, poor hygiene, decreased flow of saliva	
Decreased ability to smell is significant at age 60 and becomes increasingly severe after age 70.	
Decreased sensation of thirst, which may be due to changes in the thirst center in the hypothalamus.	The elderly are prone to dehydration.

Change in Income Related to Retirement	
More than 50% of the elderly population are estimated to be economically deprived; 25% have annual incomes under $10,000.	The first items sacrificed when food budget is limited are milk and meats, which are rich sources of calcium, protein, zinc, iron, and B vitamins.[11]
	The lower the income, the less likely an adequate and varied diet will be consumed.

Changes in Health	
Degenerative diseases like diabetes, atherosclerosis, hypertension, and cancer are more common among the elderly, as are disabling disorders like bone fractures, arthritis, and strokes.	May affect nutrient requirements, intake, digestion, absorption, metabolism, and excretion
	Disabling disorders may impair food purchasing, preparation, or eating.
Reliance on drugs. The elderly, who comprise 11% of the population, account for approximately 25% of all drugs used. Compared to younger adults, the elderly are more likely to use drugs, to use a combination of drugs, and to take drugs over a longer period of time.[13]	Drugs may affect nutritional status by altering appetite, the ability to taste and smell, or the digestion, absorption, metabolism, and excretion of nutrients (Appendix 5). Likewise, food intake can increase or decrease the effectiveness of some drugs by altering the rate of absorption. If a large percentage of a fixed income is spent on medication, less money is available for food.
Alcohol abuse. Some segments of the elderly population may rely on alcohol to relieve boredom, loneliness, depression, or pain.	Alcohol abuse may cause nutrient deficiencies, particularly of folic acid and thiamine, by altering
	Food intake through a decrease in appetite, food budget, or alertness
	Nutrient digestion, absorption, metabolism, and excretion

Psychosocial Changes	
Social isolation related to	The elderly frequently complain that they do not
Death of spouse; death of friends	like to cook for one person or eat alone, either at
Living alone	home or in a restaurant. Studies indicate that
Impaired mobility	elderly living alone do not make poorer food

(*continued*)

Psychosocial Changes

	choices than those living with a spouse, but they do eat fewer calories.
Poor self-esteem related	Poor self-esteem may lead to lack of interest in eating.
To change in body image	
To lack of productivity	
To feelings of aimlessness	
Institutionalized	Generally, elderly who are institutionalized are more likely to have an inadequate diet than those living independently, especially in terms of calories, thiamine, niacin, and vitamins C and D.[9]

NUTRITION FOR THE ELDERLY

Although the nutritional needs of the elderly have been studied with more frequency within the last 20 years, there are limited data available on the nutritional requirements of relatively healthy people over 70 years of age. Most large-scale national surveys on food consumption have had few participants over the age of 74, and most studies conducted on the nutritional status of the elderly focus on people confined to nursing homes or hospitals.

Recommended Dietary Allowances

The current RDA divide the mature adult population into two age groups: those who are 25 to 50 and those aged 51 and above. However, one would expect the nutritional requirements of 51-year-olds to be different from those of 60-, 70-, 80-, and 90-year-olds.[3] Unfortunately, there are insufficient data available to break down recommendations and requirements further into more precise age groupings.

Compared to younger adults aged 25 to 50, the only RDA that differ for older adults are for calories, certain B vitamins, and iron (for women only) (Table 12-2). The RDA of all other essential nutrients remain constant from age 23 throughout adulthood.

However, for any elderly individual, the RDA may be inappropriate because they are not based on studies of nutrition in the elderly but are, instead, extrapolated from studies of younger adults; the elderly differ from younger adults in the way they absorb some nutrients, their gastric acidity, and in their overall nutrient utilization. Also, the RDA are

Table 12-2
Adult RDA for Calories, Certain B Vitamins, and Iron

	Men		Women	
	Age 25–50	*Age 51+*	*Age 25–50*	*Age 51+*
Total calories	2900	2300	2200	1900
Thiamine (mg)	1.5	1.2	1.1	1.0
Riboflavin (mg)	1.7	1.4	1.3	1.2
Niacin (mg N.E.)	19	15	15	13
Iron (mg)	10	10	15	10

intended to meet the needs of healthy people and do not take into account the effects chronic diseases or medications may have on nutritional needs.

Calories

Beginning in early adulthood, lean body mass (muscle and bone) declines whereas the proportion of fat increases, resulting in a decrease in resting energy expenditure (REE). Physical activity also declines with aging, although this is neither desirable nor inevitable.[4] Together, the decline in REE and physical activity causes a decrease in energy requirements. However, because rates of decline vary significantly among individuals, chronologic age is not always a good predictor of energy requirements.

The RDA for calories for men and women of "reference size" over age 50 are 2300 and 1900, respectively, or 30 cal/kg of body weight (see Table 12-2). The NAS-NRC Subcommittee notes that the calorie requirements of people over 75 are likely to be less because of the decrease in lean body mass, REE, and physical activity. However, no specific recommendations were made. As calorie requirements decline, it becomes increasingly difficult to consume adequate amounts of all essential nutrients.

Thiamine, Riboflavin, and Niacin

Because these B vitamins are involved in energy metabolism, lesser amounts are needed when calorie intake is reduced. Only minor reductions are suggested in the RDA for people over age 51 (see Table 12-2).

Iron (for Women)

Physiologic data (cessation of growth and menstruation) and measurements of body iron stores in the elderly indicate that iron requirements are lowest in old age. The RDA for iron in women decreases from 15 mg (23- to 50-year-olds) to 10 mg (51 + -year-olds) (see Table 12-2).

However, some segments of the elderly population may be at risk for developing iron deficiency and iron deficiency anemia because of a decrease in iron availability or absorption. Compared with younger adults, the elderly often eat less red meat, which is the best source of heme iron in the diet. Difficulty in chewing and economic factors are often to blame. Iron absorption may be impaired by the decrease in gastric HCl secretion (achlorhydria), which occurs with aging, or secondary to a partial or complete gastrectomy, malabsorption syndrome, or chronic use of antacids. Reliance on "tea and toast" may also be a factor—tea is a potent inhibitor of iron absorption. Finally, chronic blood loss due to hemorrhoids, ulcers, renal disease, neoplasms, or medications such as aspirin, anticoagulants, and drugs for arthritis may result in iron deficiency anemia.

The RDA for the elderly are especially controversial with regard to protein and calcium.

Protein

Despite the fact that protein metabolism changes with aging, there is little agreement on protein requirements in the elderly. Whereas some studies have shown that the elderly require more protein based on nitrogen balance studies, others studies indicate protein requirements decrease because of the reduction in muscle mass and the decrease in renal function. The most recent studies suggest the elderly may need more protein than the current recommendation of 0.8 g/kg, and that people over age 65 may need 2 g of protein/kg body weight. Although the NAS-NRC Subcommittee states that aging may alter protein requirements, the RDA for people aged 51 and older are not different than those for younger adults.

Calcium

The elderly are at risk of calcium deficiency because both calcium intake and efficiency of calcium absorption decrease with age. Studies suggest a strong relationship between calcium deficiency and the development of osteoporosis, a metabolic bone disease of the elderly characterized by a negative calcium balance and loss of bone mass.

Some researchers believe the current RDA for calcium (800 mg) may be too low to maintain normal calcium balance, especially for postmenopausal women and men over age 60 who may need 1000 to 1500 mg/day. However, because prevention is far more effective than treatment, good eating habits and weight-bearing exercise should be encouraged early in life to attain maximum bone density (see Chap. 19 for more information on osteoporosis).

Dietary Guidelines

The *Dietary Guidelines for Americans*, prepared by the United States Department of Agriculture and United States Department of Health and Human Services, offer suggestions on how to modify the typical American diet to improve overall health and reduce the risk of certain chronic diseases such as obesity, heart disease, certain types of cancer, and diabetes.[21] To "eat a variety of foods," "choose a diet with plenty of vegetables, fruits, and grain products," and "if you drink alcoholic beverages, do so in moderation" is clearly good advice for people of all ages. The applicability of other guidelines to the elderly population is less obvious.

Because the focus of diet modification for the elderly is on improving the quality of life and maintaining the person's ability to function, preventative nutrition may no longer be appropriate. At best, there may be little value in adopting the guidelines late in life, and some studies indicate some of the guidelines may even adversely affect the health of the elderly.

For instance, "choose a diet low in fat, saturated fat, and cholesterol" may not be appropriate for the elderly as a group. Some epidemiologic evidence indicates that the importance of serum cholesterol levels as a risk factor for chronic heart disease decreases beginning at age 44 and virtually disappears after age 64.[1] Some animal, epidemiologic, and clinical studies suggest that a modified fat diet should not be used by the elderly because the potential benefit from reducing serum cholesterol decreases progressively with age; that is, the diet may decrease serum cholesterol levels in the elderly but may not reduce the incidence of cardiovascular mortality. Also, overly restrictive diets should be avoided because of the potential negative impact on calorie and protein intake.

Another guideline advises Americans to "maintain healthy weight." However, healthy body weight and ideal percentage of body fat have not yet been determined for the elderly.

The assumption that excess weight reduces longevity may be true for younger adults but not necessarily true for the elderly. Some studies suggest that elderly who are underweight (75% to 95% of ideal weight) actually have a higher morbidity and mortality than those who are moderately overweight (up to 130% of ideal weight). Therefore, except for clients with debilitating arthritis aggravated by obesity, weight reduction may not be prudent in elderly who are moderately overweight. Elderly who are underweight should be encouraged to gain weight.

To "use sugars only in moderation" may be difficult for some elderly. True, sugar intake, just like fat intake, should be limited because it provides calories with few other nutrients; sugar should not supply more than 5% to 10% of the total calorie intake. However, as the taste sensitivity for sweetness declines with age, the elderly may use more sugar. Most older people like sweet desserts and candy; denying the elderly these foods, especially those who are underweight or have a poor appetite, is not justified.

Another controversial guideline for the elderly is to "use salt and sodium only in moderation." Younger adults are advised to reduce their intake of sodium because excessive sodium may increase the risk of hypertension in some people. Sodium restriction, however, may not be appropriate for the elderly because studies indicate the risk of stroke from hypertension is less in the elderly than other age groups. Also, a diet low enough in sodium to lower blood pressure effectively (2 to 3 g sodium) would limit food choices and may make the diet less palatable, and would complicate meal planning for someone underweight or anorexic. In addition, because taste sensitivity for salt decreases with age, compliance is difficult.

The Food Guide Pyramid and Daily Food Guide

Because few RDA change with aging except calories, it is important for the elderly to choose a nutrient-dense diet composed of a variety of foods from the major food groups. Although the Food Guide Pyramid is still appropriate, the elderly may need to limit the number of servings from each major food group to the least amount recommended, so as not to exceed calorie requirements (Table 12-3). Elderly who require more calories should eat more from the major food groups and not fill up on "Fats, Oils, and Sweets."

Table 12-3
Daily Food Guide for the Elderly

Food Group	Number of Servings Recommended in the Food Guide Pyramid	Number of Servings Appropriate for the Elderly (about 1600 calories)
Bread, Cereal, Rice, and Pasta Group	6–11	6
Vegetable Group	3–5	3
Fruit Group	2–4	2
Milk, Yogurt, and Cheese Group	2–3	2–3
Meat, Poultry, Fish, Dry Beans, Eggs, and Nuts Group	2–3 (5–7 ounces)	2 (5 ounces)
Fats, Oils, and Sweets	Use sparingly	Use sparingly

NURSING PROCESS

A large portion of elderly Americans are at greater risk for nutritional problems than the general population, and many have poor nutritional status requiring nutrition intervention.[12] Studies suggest that specific nutritional deficiencies exist in as many as 50% of the independent-living elderly in the United States,[10] and that as many as 30% of the elderly skip meals almost daily.[12] Two criteria highly predictive of mortality and morbidity in the elderly are low body weight and rapid unintentional weight loss[7] (see box, Risk Factors in Poor Nutritional Status Among the Elderly).

For the "well" elderly, nutrition screening may be used quickly and cost-effectively to identify clients at risk before they become malnourished. A sample tool appears in Figure 12-1. Additional assessment data may be needed for clients identified to be at risk for actual or potential nutritional problems.

Major indicators of poor nutritional status in older Americans appear in the following box. However, because of age-related changes, assessment data of the elderly may be unreliable or invalid. For instance, accurate anthropometric measurements and dietary information may be difficult to obtain because of illness or cognitive changes. Also, normal standards for laboratory tests used for younger adults may not be appropriate for the elderly. Standards of nutritional assessment specifically for the elderly need to be defined. Specific problems in assessing the nutritional status of the elderly are listed in the box, Problems With Nutritional Assessment of the Elderly.

Assessment

In addition to the general geriatric assessment criteria, assess for the following factors:

Significant, undesirable change in body weight within the last 6 months. Intervention should be initiated when weight loss exceeds 5% of usual body weight in 1 month or 10 pounds over a 5- to 6-month period.

Dentition and ability to swallow.

Usual 24-hour intake, including the frequency and pattern of eating, as well as the method of preparation. A food record or food frequency questionnaire may provide additional intake data. If malnutrition is suggested, intake and output may be carefully monitored to calculate actual nutritional intake.

Adequacy of the client's usual intake based on the Food Guide Pyramid/Daily Food Guide for the Elderly (see Table 12-3); pay particular attention to nutrient density and the intake of foods from the "Fats, Oils, and Sweets" group that supply little more than calories.

Appetite. Determine if there have been any recent significant changes in eating patterns and, if so, why.

The use of a modified diet and, if so, the rationale, duration, level of understanding, and compliance.

Cultural, familial, religious, and ethnic influences on eating habits.

The use of vitamin or mineral supplements. Evaluate their safety and appropriateness.

The use of medications and over-the-counter drugs. Find out if any food–drug interactions are affecting nutritional status or drug effectiveness.

The client's use of alcohol, tobacco, caffeine, and drugs.

Risk Factors in Poor Nutritional Status Among the Elderly

Anthropometric Data

Weight loss of 10% or more within 6 months

Weight 95% less than or 120% greater than ideal

Dietary Data

Numerous food intolerances

Inability to self-feed

Missing or ill-fitting dentures

Loss of appetite, refusal to eat

Unbalanced diet

Consumption of megadoses of vitamins, health foods, or food supplements

NPO longer than 2 days

Medical–Socioeconomic Data

Institutionalized

Living alone

Recently widowed

Mental or physical handicap that interferes with food purchasing, preparation, or eating

Inadequate food budget

Inadequate facilities for food storage and preparation

Acute diseases that affect nutritional status by altering appetite (*i.e.*, influenza) or increasing nutritional requirements (*i.e.*, fever)

Chronic diseases with nutritional implications: Diabetes, renal disease, hypertension, heart disease, GI disorders, or cancer

Chronic use of prescriptions or over-the-counter drugs that affect nutritional status

Alcohol abuse

Biochemical Data

Hemoglobin less than 10 mg/100 ml in women or 12 mg/100 ml in men

Nutrition screening is a quick and easy way to find out if you are at risk because of poor nutrition. If you are well nourished, your body is better able to resist illnesses. By completing this nutrition screening form, you can help your doctor tell if you are in good nutritional health.

Below are 10 questions. Fill in the date and your name. Then circle either Yes or No for each question.

Date _____ Name _____

		(Circle)	
1. Do you often skip meals?		Yes	No
2. Is your appetite poor?		Yes	No
3. Do you have problems chewing or swallowing?		Yes	No
4. Have you been told to cut down on salt, sugar, fat, or protein in your diet?		Yes	No
5. Have you lost more than 10 pounds in the last 6 months without trying?		Yes	No
6. Have you been told you have diabetes, kidney disease, liver disease, gastrointestinal disease, or cancer?		Yes	No
7. Have you recently had surgery in the last month or an illness lasting more than 3 weeks?		Yes	No
8. Do you take any prescription or nonprescription medicines or vitamins?		Yes	No
9. Do you currently have problems with nausea or vomiting?		Yes	No
10. Do you experience diarrhea or constipation?		Yes	No

When you have answered all the questions, please give this form to your nurse or doctor.

Nutrition Screening Form: Part B

This part of the form will be filled out by your nurse or doctor.

Patient's current weight is _____ lb.
Has patient's weight decreased since last visit?
_____ No _____ Yes, by _____ lb.
                               (number)

If two or more of the answers on Part A (Table 20) are "yes," or if the patient has had involuntary weight loss:
_____ The patient is a candidate for further nutritional assessment.
_____ Other: _____
_____

Figure 12-1
Nutritional screening form.

Major Indicators of Poor Nutritional Status in Older Americans

Significant weight loss over time
- 5.0% or more of prior body weight in 1 month
- 7.5% or more of body weight in 3 months
- 10.0% or more of body weight in 6 months or involuntary weight loss

Significantly low or high weight for height
- 20% below or above desirable weight for height at a given age (considering loss of height due to vertebral collapse, kyphosis, and deformity)

Significant reduction in serum albumin
- Serum albumin of less than 3.5 g/dL

Significant change in functional status
- Change from "independent" to "dependent" in two of the ADLs or one of the nutrition-related IADLs

Significant and sustained inappropriate food intake
- Failure to consume the recommended minimum from one or more of the food groups suggested in the Dietary Guidelines for Americans (groups such as milk and milk products, cereals and grains, fruits, vegetables, meat/poultry/fish/eggs/legumes) or sufficient variety of foods for a period of 3 months or more
- Excessive consumption of fat, saturated fat, and/or alcohol (alcohol: >1 oz/day, women; 2 oz/day, men)

Significant reduction in mid-arm circumference
- To less than 10th percentile (NHANES standards)

Significant increase or decrease in triceps skinfolds
- To less than 10th percentile or more than 95th percentile (NHANES standards)

Significant obesity
- More than 120% of desirable weight or body mass index over 27 or triceps skinfolds above 95th percentile (NHANES standards)

Other nutrition-related disorders
- Presence of osteoporosis, osteomalacia, folate deficiency, or vitamin B-12 deficiency.

(Reprinted with permission: Nutrition Screening Initiative, Ham RJ. Indicators of poor nutritional status in Older Americans. Washington, DC; 1991. NHANES = National Health and Nutrition Evaluation Survey)

Problems With Nutritional Assessment of the Elderly

Anthropometric Measurement

Accurate weights may be difficult to obtain if the client
- Is bed-ridden.
- Has edema.

Accurate heights may be difficult to obtain if the client
- Is bed-ridden.
- Has curvature of the spine (kyphosis).

Accurate skinfold thickness may be difficult to obtain because of changes in compressibility of subcutaneous fat with aging.

Biochemical Data

Not all normal laboratory values for the elderly have been defined; therefore, interpretation of results is difficult.

Clinical Observations

Nonspecific signs of malnutrition (*i.e.*, anorexia, fatigue) may be attributed to other causes, for example, aging, chronic diseases, secondary to drug therapy.

Age-related changes in physiology and function may mimic signs of a nutritional deficiency (*i.e.*, loss of visual acuity in dim light occurs with aging and may not indicate a deficiency of vitamin A)

Most malnutrition in the United States is subclinical; that is, a deficiency may exist but physical signs are not apparent.

Dietary Assessment

A 24-hour recall or food-frequency record may be unreliable if the client has short-term memory deficits, confusion, or is hard of hearing.

EXAMPLE

Evaluating weight status:

$$\text{Percentage of usual body weight} = \frac{\text{current weight}}{\text{usual weight}} \times 100$$

$$\text{Percent weight change} = \frac{(\text{usual weight} - \text{actual weight})}{\text{usual weight}} \times 100$$

General Geriatric Assessment Criteria

Weight, weight status (see box, Evaluating Weight Status). For the non-ambulatory client, a bed or wheelchair scale is needed to accurately assess weight.

Hemoglobin, hematocrit

Serum albumin, lipids, glucose

Urinalysis for glucose, ketones, protein, occult blood

Skin turgor and appearance

Bowel and bladder function

Past and present medical history

Use of medications, laxative abuse

Physical disabilities

Living arrangements, social life, source of income, and how income is allocated

Activity pattern and frequency

Mental health status

Nursing Diagnosis

Altered Nutrition: Less than Body Requirements, related to inadequate intake secondary to poor dentition as evidenced by weight loss.

Planning and Implementation

Rather than a textbook approach, which may be appropriate for younger adults, nutritional care of the elderly should be client-centered and based on the individual's physiologic, pathologic, and psychosocial condition. With any diet intervention for the elderly, overall goals are to maintain or restore maximum independent functioning, and maintain the client's sense of dignity and quality of life by imposing as few dietary restrictions as necessary. Except for diet-related diseases such as severe hypertension, renal disease, ascites, brittle diabetes, and obesity in clients with debilitating arthritis, modified diets may be of little value. In fact, special diets are a major cause of malnutrition in the elderly.[15] Therefore, diet changes should only be undertaken when a significant improvement in health can be expected.[16] Any necessary dietary changes should be incorporated into the client's existing food pattern rather than by planning a completely new approach to eating.[13]

Like all age groups, the elderly need a balanced diet from all major food groups; however, some elderly may consume less than optimal intakes from one or more food groups. Studies indicate that the nutrients most often deficient in the diets of the elderly (when compared to the RDA) include calories, calcium, vitamin D, zinc, vitamin A, thiamine, and folic acid. Inadequate intakes from the meat group often occur secondary to a limited food budget or difficulty chewing. Many adults avoid milk, which is another source of high-quality protein, because of its association with childhood. The intake of fruits and vegetables may be limited because they are expensive or difficult to chew. Clearly, food choices of the elderly often are based on considerations other than food preferences, such as income, the client's physical ability to shop, prepare, chew, and swallow food, and food intolerances related to chronic disease or side effects of medications. The elderly at greatest risk for inadequate diets are female, poor and black, and the institutionalized.

Generally, food preferences in the elderly are a result of a lifetime of food habits influenced by cultural, social, and personal factors. To have the greatest impact on food habits and nutritional status of the elderly, nutrition education should be initiated at a young age and continued through life.[18]

The elderly should be encouraged to be as physically active as possible to improve calcium balance, to help promote gastrointestinal function, and to improve their sense of well-being. Exercise also increases energy expenditure, making a greater calorie (and therefore nutrient) intake possible.

The client's need for homemaker services, shopping assistance, transportation, food stamps, congregate meals, or Meals-on-Wheels should be evaluated and the appropriate referral made. Congregate meals and Meals-on-Wheels are federally funded nutrition programs specifically for the elderly, designed to provide low-cost, nutritious hot meals, food and nutrition education, the opportunity for socialization and recreation, and information on other health and social assistance programs. The congregate meal program provides a balanced, hot midday meal and the opportunity to socialize in senior citizen centers and other public or private facilities. Those choosing to pay may do so; otherwise the meal is free. Meals-on-Wheels is a home-delivered meal program for the elderly who are unable to get to congregate meal centers because they live in an isolated area or have a chronic illness or disability. Usually a hot meal is served at midday, with a bagged lunch for the evening meal. Modified diets, like diabetic diets and low-sodium diets, are provided as needed.

Client Goals

The client will:
Attain/maintain "healthy" weight.
Consume, on average, the recommended number of servings from each of the major food
   groups.
Modify food texture, as needed, to facilitate chewing and swallowing.

Nursing Interventions

Diet Management

Provide a varied, nutrient-dense diet based on the Daily Food Guide for the Elderly (see Table 12-3). Although the actual nutrient content of the diet will vary with the foods chosen, using the guide will help ensure an average adequate intake. A variety of foods should be selected from each food group; limiting food choices or eliminating a food group increases the risk of both nutrient deficiencies and excesses. If additional calories or protein are needed, encourage additional servings from the milk group; although two servings are recommended, five cups of milk or the equivalent may be needed to maintain calcium balance, especially in postmenopausal and osteoporotic women (see Appendix 13 for foods high in calcium).

Limit foods that are calorically dense but provide few other essential nutrients, such as foods high in sugar, fats, and oils. As calorie requirements decline with age, nutrient density (the nutritional value of a food compared to the amount of calories it provides) becomes increasingly important in order to meet nutritional needs without exceeding calorie requirements.

Discourage large or frequent use of alcohol. Small amounts of alcohol, however, such as an occasional glass of wine or beer, may help stimulate the appetite and enhance sleep. In an institutional setting, alcohol may improve socialization and food intake. However, alcohol contributes little nutritional value to the diet except calories and may cause multiple nutritional problems if used excessively. Even moderate use can displace the intake of nutrient-dense foods, especially in the diets of the elderly who have limited budgets, food intakes, and calorie requirements.

Increase fiber intake to prevent or alleviate constipation and laxative dependence. Substituting whole-grain breads and cereals for refined products is a subtle way to increase the fiber content of the diet that is realistic for elderly who have difficulty chewing or who are on a fixed income. If income and dental health allow, increasing the intake of fresh fruits and vegetables also will add fiber to the diet.

Avoid excessive salt intake. Opinions vary as to the optimal sodium content of the diet for the elderly. Recommendations on sodium intake should be made on an individual basis according to the client's cardiac and renal status, appetite, and drug therapy.

Drink six to eight glasses of water daily to maintain hydration and normal urine and fecal output. Thirst is not a reliable indicator of need in the elderly.

Take supplements only as prescribed by the physician. According to the National Institute on Aging (NIA), a balanced diet based on the Daily Food Guide is nutritionally adequate for most healthy elderly men and women. However, vitamin and mineral supplements are popular among the elderly. Estimates from survey populations indicate that 40% to 60% of the elderly use some form of vitamin and/or mineral supplement,[20] 56% of whom do so on the recommendation of family, friends, or the media. The elderly are particularly vulnerable to false nutritional claims that promise to restore youth, cure disease, and improve sense of well-being. The purchase of unnecessary and ill-advised supplements can displace the purchase of food if funds are limited; lead to toxic or adverse reactions from excessive intakes of certain vitamins and minerals; and prevent an individual from seeking sound medical advice if the supplements are used to "cure" illness.

Modify the texture of the diet as needed, if chewing or swallowing are compromised. Meats and vegetables may be served soft-cooked, chopped, ground, or puréed. Eggs and dairy products are good substitutes for meats and are easy to consume and relatively economical. Take care to avoid overprocessing foods because they may lose nutrients and appeal. Liquids thickened to the consistency of honey are easier to swallow than thin liquids. Other diet modifications to help relieve eating problems related to aging are listed in Table 12-4.

Client Teaching

Instruct the client and family

That a balanced diet based on the major food groups can help maximize the quality of life.

Stress the importance of consuming adequate protein, calcium, fiber, and fluid.

Table 12-4
Dietary Interventions for Eating Problems of the Elderly

Problem	Rationale	Dietary Interventions
Difficulty chewing	Missing or decayed teeth Peridontal disease Missing or ill-fitting dentures	Provide liquid, semisolid, mashed or chopped foods as tolerated. Progress liquid diet as soon as possible.
Difficulty swallowing	Paralysis related to stroke Parkinson's disease	Thickened and gelled liquids are usually better tolerated than thin liquids. Baby food can be used as a nutritious thickener. Avoid overuse of puréed foods because of the negative connotations associated with it.
Lack of appetite	Depression Acute or chronic disease Loss of sense of smell and taste Side effect of medication Loneliness Early satiety	Offer small frequent meals. Solicit food preferences. Allow plenty of time to eat. Because appetite is usually greatest in the morning, emphasize a nutritious breakfast. Encourage group eating.
Impaired ability to feed self	Poor vision Arthritis of the hands; stroke	Describe the meal and how it is arranged on the plate. Assist the client by opening packages of bread and crackers, buttering bread and vegetables, cutting meat, and opening milk cartons. Assess the client's ability to grasp utensils and guide food to the mouth. Refer the client to an occupational therapist to evaluate the need for assistive devices or retraining.
Loss of taste and smell	Normal aging Endocrine disorders secondary to drug therapy Certain nutrient deficiencies (zinc, vit B_{12}, niacin)	Add commercial flavors to foods to intensify smell. Add texture, when possible (*i.e.,* crunchiness, chewiness).

On how to modify the diet, as needed, to alleviate eating problems common in the elderly (see Table 12-4).

That unless prescribed by a physician, taking vitamin and mineral supplements may be unnecessary and potentially dangerous.

That eating alone does not have to be boring if you set a pretty table and use the good dishes. Meals that vary in color, texture, temperature, and flavor also add interest. Experiment with herbs and spices, or try a new recipe. Eat by a window, on the porch, or out in the yard. For company, listen to the radio or music, watch television, read, or eat with friends.

That making meals is less of a chore if you choose easy-to-prepare foods or make extra portions for homemade TV dinners that can be frozen and used later.

To stretch the food budget by buying only as much as needed, unless freezer and storage space is adequate. Although single-serving cans of vegetables cost more per unit of measure, they are less expensive than allowing unused portions of regular-size cans to spoil in the refrigerator. Large bags of frozen vegetables are economical because they allow you to cook only as much as you need. Ask the butcher to wrap individual portions of meat; freeze in freezer bags until needed.

Monitor

Monitor for the following signs or symptoms:
Compliance to the diet and the need for follow-up diet counseling
Effectiveness of the diet, and evaluate the need for additional diet changes
Weight, weight changes
Laboratory values, as available
Medical–social status, and periodically evaluate the need for Meals-on-Wheels or other assistance programs

Evaluation

Evaluation is ongoing. Assuming the plan of care has not changed, the client will achieve the goals as stated above.

NUTRITIONAL CONSIDERATIONS FOR THE INSTITUTIONALIZED ELDERLY

The typical long-term care resident has numerous psychosocial, functional, and medical problems that often are complicated by poor nutritional status. The incidence of protein–calorie malnutrition has been reported to range from 50% to 85% among nursing home residents,[7] and 40% or more residents are unable to feed themselves independently.[9]

Institutionalization often means a loss of independence and is viewed both as a punishment and going to a place to die. Nursing home residents generally tend to eat less food and have a greater risk of nutritional deficiencies than independently living elderly, possibly because of limited food choices and unfamiliarity with the foods offered. Loss of favorite or familiar foods, altered meal schedules, and a change in serving style can also contribute to poor intakes. Depression, anxiety, and feelings of hopelessness contribute to anorexia.

Nutrition intervention aimed at preventing overt malnutrition is economically, medically, and functionally desirable; a high-protein, high-calorie diet of small, frequent feedings is commonly used to prevent or treat weight loss and decubitus ulcers. In contrast, rigid or unnecessary dietary restrictions can compound the client's feelings of hopelessness and depression. Therapeutic diets should be used only when a significant improvement in health can be expected, as in cases of severe hypertension, ascites, congestive heart failure, constipation, brittle diabetes, and obesity if excess weight aggravates arthritis (see appropriate chapters in the section on Nutrition in Clinical Practice for possible diet modifications). The validity of other diet modifications to prevent or delay disease in the

Liberal Geriatric Diet

The Liberal Geriatric Diet is designed to meet the nutritional requirements of institutionalized elderly by offering a diet as close to the individual's usual diet as possible. It provides 1500 to 2000 cal/day using a variety of regular foods. Simple sugars are kept to a minimum and low-fat milk is used routinely. A moderate sodium intake of 3 to 4 g/day is achieved by eliminating salty foods and by using herbs and spices as alternatives to salt in many foods. An adequate fluid intake is encouraged. The fiber content of the diet is increased by emphasizing whole-grain breads and cereals, adding coarse raw bran, if needed, and offering fresh fruits and vegetables. Individual preferences should be honored whenever possible.

The Liberal Geriatric Diet can be modified as needed. For instance, texture can be altered for residents who have difficulty chewing or swallowing. Reducing portion sizes, eliminating sugar, and restricting sweets may be appropriate for clients with diabetes or obesity. For residents who require a sodium restriction, salt-containing condiments can be eliminated and salt-free breads and cereals used as needed. Residents with early satiety should receive small, frequent meals. More comprehensive modifications may be needed for residents with diet-related diseases or nutrient deficiencies.

Sample Liberal Geriatric Diet

Breakfast

Orange juice
Oatmeal
1 soft-cooked egg
1 slice buttered whole-wheat toast
Low-fat milk
Coffee/tea
Salt*/pepper/sugar*

Lunch

Grilled cheese sandwich made with two slices whole-wheat bread
Cream of broccoli soup
Sliced strawberries
½ cup low-fat milk
Coffee/tea
Salt*/pepper/sugar*

(continued)

Liberal Geriatric Diet (*continued*)

Dinner

Baked chicken
Steamed rice
Baked acorn squash
Fresh fruit salad
Ice milk
Coffee/tea
Salt*/pepper/sugar*

Snack

½ cup low-fat milk
Bran muffin

*Packages of salt and sugar may be omitted if a restriction of either is appropriate.

elderly is questionable, especially if diet restrictions are viewed as a "punishment" and discourage the client from eating.[16]

In place of standard therapeutic diets, many clinicians recommend a more progressive approach to feeding the elderly. Clients who receive a liberal geriatric diet (see box, Liberal Geriatric Diet) similar to what they were eating at home tend to eat better, have fewer bowel problems, enjoy their meals more, are more alert, and are generally happier than clients receiving therapeutic diets.[16]

Commercial supplements are often given between meals to increase the calorie and protein content of a client's diet. Although they may be temporarily useful, they are generally not well accepted, tolerated, or effective on a long-term basis. Taste fatigue and lack of hunger for the meal that follows often occur. Compliance may be better if relatively tasteless supplements are added to foods that the client normally eats, thereby increasing the nutrient density of the diet without increasing the volume of food consumed.

To promote optimal intakes in an institutionalized setting, the nurse should make mealtime as enjoyable an experience as possible, encourage independence in eating, or if necessary, provide assistance with eating. Food preferences should be honored whenever possible, and food from home should also be encouraged. Provide liberal intake of fluid and protein in clients who have, or are at risk of, decubitus ulcers. Vitamin C and zinc are also necessary for healing.

Ongoing monitoring may include intake observations or intake and output records when a problem is suspected. Because weight loss is one of the most important and sensitive indicators of malnutrition, obtaining accurate monthly weights is vital.[7] More frequent weights may be necessary if a nutritional problem is indicated. Communicate

Food for Thought

Nutrition Intervention for Alzheimer's Disease

Alzheimer's disease is the most common cause of dementia in the United States today and the fourth leading cause of death. Although the cause of Alzheimer's disease is unknown, there appears to be a genetic predisposition. Aluminum toxicity has been proposed as an etiologic factor. However, most researchers believe that the aluminum accumulation seen in Alzheimer's disease is not the cause of the disease but, rather, a consequence of it.

The course of Alzheimer's disease is progressive and nonreversible. Initially, the disease manifests itself with loss of memory, forgetfulness, and a decrease in social and vocational abilities.[11] The victim may become lost in familiar surroundings, and personality changes may develop. As the disease progresses, the victim can no longer cope without assistance, and he becomes disoriented to time and place. Delusions, depression, agitation, and language difficulties are noted. Finally, severe intellectual impairment and complete disorientation are seen. Verbal skills are lost, motor skills deteriorate, and self-care activities may be impossible. Urinary and fecal incontinence are common, and clients may become bedridden. Death usually results from infection.[11]

At present, there is no clear evidence that Alzheimer's disease alters nutritional requirements. However, it can have a devastating impact on nutritional status. Early in the disease, impairments in memory and judgment may make shopping, storing, and cooking food difficult. The client may forget to eat or may forget that he already ate and, consequently, eat again. Changes in the sense of smell and food preferences may also develop. A preference for sweets and salty foods is noted,[11] and unusual food choices may occur. Agitation increases energy expenditure, and calorie requirements may increase by as much as 1600/day.[11] Weight loss is common. Choking may occur if the client forgets to chew food sufficiently before swallowing, or if he hoards food in the mouth. Eating of nonfood items may occur, and eventually self-feeding ability is lost.

Nutrition interventions that may be appropriate for clients with Alzheimer's disease include the following recommendations:

- Closely supervise mealtime; check food temperatures to prevent accidental mouth burns.
- Serve meals in the same place at the same time each day, and keep distractions to a minimum.[2]
- Minimize confusion by offering a nonselect menu.
- Provide in-between meal snacks that are easy to consume such as sandwiches, beverages, and finger foods.
- Modify food consistency as needed, cutting food into small pieces and reminding the client to chew to avoid choking. Physical assistance (*i.e.*, light pressure applied to the underside of the chin to push up on the tongue) may be needed to promote swallowing.

(continued)

Nutrition Intervention for Alzheimer's Disease (*continued*)

Food for Thought (*continued*)

- Monitor weight closely.
- Clients in the latter stage of Alzheimer's disease are not only unable to feed themselves, but also no longer know what to do when food is placed in their mouth. When this occurs, a decision regarding the use of other means of nutritional support (*i.e.,* NG or PEG tube feedings) must be made.

feeding/eating problems, food intolerances, and significant weight changes to the dietitian for further assessment and intervention.

DRUG ALERT The elderly, who make up 12% of the population, use 20% to 25% of all prescription and over-the-counter drugs. Most elderly people take at least one prescription drug daily, and 45% take multiple prescription drugs that can interfere with appetite and nutrition absorption.[12] Because the elderly take more drugs than any other age group, they are particularly prone to nutritional problems related to drug use. Drugs may affect nutrition by inhibiting appetite, altering the sense of taste or smell, altering saliva secretion, irritating the stomach, or causing nausea.[15] Some drugs contribute directly to dietary deficiencies by altering nutrient absorption, utilization, or excretion.

Beside nutrient–drug interactions, the elderly also have a higher incidence of drug reactions than younger adults, possibly related to the chronicity and multiplicity of their diseases; drug misuse because of sensory impairment, confusion, personal choice, financial reasons, or lack of knowledge/instruction; delayed drug metabolism and excretion; popularity of over-the-counter drugs; sharing medications with others; consuming alcohol with medication; or food–drug incompatibilities.[16]

To avoid potential problems, the elderly should be informed about the side effects of medications they are using, that is, how their medications interact with food, alcohol, and other medicines and also about the proper dosage and timing of medications. They should be advised to consult their physician or pharmacist if problems arise.

BIBLIOGRAPHY

1. Allred JB, Gallagher-Allred CR, Bowers DF: Elevated blood cholesterol: A risk factor for heart disease that decreases with advanced age. J Am Diet Assoc 90:574, 1990
2. Betz A: Nutritional care for residents with Alzheimer's disease. The Consultant Dietitian 14(4):1, 1989
3. Butler RN: Geriatric nutrition: Advice from an expert panel. Geriatrics 45(10):17, 1990
4. Craig L: Nutrition and Aging. Columbus, OH: Ross Laboratories, 1991
5. Davis MA, Murphy SP, Neuhaus JM, et al: Living arrangements and dietary quality of older US adults. J Am Diet Assoc 90:1667, 1990

6. Delahanty LM: Geriatric team dynamics: The dietitian's role. J Am Diet Assoc 84:1353, 1984
7. Fischer J, Johnson MA: Low body weight and weight loss in the aged. J Am Diet Assoc 90:1697, 1990
8. Fournier CJ: Nutritional management of patients with Alzheimer's disease. Caring Magazine October:76, 1990
9. Gallagher-Allred CR, Bockus S: Specialized nutritional support in long-term care. The Consultant Dietitian 15(4):1, 1990
10. Goodwin J, Garry P: Association between nutritional status and cognitive functioning in a healthy elderly population. JAMA 249:2717, 1983
11. Gray GE: Nutrition and dementia. J Am Diet Assoc 89:1795, 1989
12. Hess MA: ADA as an advocate for older Americans. J Am Diet Assoc 91:847, 1991
13. Holmes S: Nutrition and the elderly. Nursing 3(37):18, 1989
14. Iverson-Carpenter M, Haskin MS, Maas M, et al: Fulfilling nutritional requirements. Journal of Gerontological Nursing 14(4):16, 1988
15. Lowenthal DT: Nutrition and the elderly. In The Mount Sinai School of Medicine Complete Book of Nutrition, Herbert V, Subak-Sharpe GJ (eds), Hammock DA, (assoc. ed). New York: St. Martin's Press, 1990
16. Luros E: A rational approach to geriatric nutrition. Dietetic Currents 8:25, 1981
17. National Research Council: Recommended Dietary Allowances. 10th ed. Washington, DC: National Academy of Sciences, 1989
18. Schiffman SS: Taste and smell losses with age. Contemporary Nutrition 16(2):1, 1991
19. Schneider EL, Vining EM, Hadley EC, et al: Recommended dietary allowances and the health of the elderly. N Engl J Med 314:157, 1986
20. United States Bureau of the Census: Statistical Abstract of the United States: 1990. 110th ed. Washington, DC: Government Printing Office, 1990
21. United States Department of Agriculture, and United States Department of Health and Human Services: Nutrition and Your Health: Dietary Guidelines for Americans. 3rd ed. Home and Garden Bulletin No. 232, 1990
22. White JV, Ham RJ, Lipschitz DA, et al: Consensus of the Nutrition Screening Initiative: Risk factors and indicators of poor nutritional status in older Americans. J Am Diet Assoc 91:783, 1991

III
Nutrition in Clinical Practice

13 Oral, Enteral, and Parenteral Nutrition

ORAL DIETS

ENTERAL NUTRITION

Oral Supplements
Modular Products
Tube Feedings

NURSING PROCESS

Assessment
Nursing Diagnosis
Planning and Implementation
Evaluation

PARENTERAL NUTRITION

Peripheral Nutrition
Central Vein Total Parenteral Nutrition

NURSING PROCESS

Assessment
Nursing Diagnosis
Planning and Implementation
Evaluation

Illness can have a significant impact on nutritional status by altering nutrient requirements, intake, absorption, metabolism, or excretion. Diagnostic procedures, medical treatments, and drug therapy (see Appendix 5) imposed on the emotional stress of hospitalization can create or compound nutritional problems. "Hospital food," which may be a vital component of treatment, may be rejected for social, religious, or personal reasons. Frequently, appetite decreases as nutritional requirements increase (see box, Risk Factors for Poor Nutritional Status).

Nutritional support must not only provide adequate amounts of required nutrients—it must also deliver those nutrients in a form that the client will accept, use, and tolerate. Nutrients can be delivered orally, enterally, parenterally, or by a combination of those methods. Figure 13-1 illustrates the step-by-step decision-making process involved in selecting the appropriate type and method of feeding.

ORAL DIETS

Obviously, oral diets are the easiest, least expensive, least risky, and most preferred method of delivering nutrients, not only from a physiologic standpoint, but also psychologically (see box, Normal and Modified Diets). Normal diets are intended to maintain health by meeting the recommended dietary allowances (RDA) for the client's age and sex. No foods are excluded and portion sizes are not restricted on a normal diet.

Risk Factors for Poor Nutritional Status

Anthropometric Risk Factors

Weight 20% greater than ideal or 10% less than ideal

Recent unintentional weight loss greater than 10% of weight

Arm muscle circumference or triceps skinfold <85% of standard

Inconsistent growth rates in children or abnormal weight for height

Dietary Risk Factors

Inadequate food intake, fad dieting, numerous food intolerances or allergies

Use of inadequate modified diet (*i.e.*, clear liquid) for more than 3 days without adequate supplementation

NPO with simple IV therapy for longer than 3 days

Inadequate tube feedings

Difficulty chewing or swallowing

Changes in taste, smell, or appetite

Medical–Socioeconomic Risk Factors

Medical conditions that alter intake or nutrient requirements: cancer, malabsorption, diarrhea, hyperthyroidism, severe infection, recent surgery, hemorrhage, physical or mental disabilities, multiple wounds or fractures, extensive burns

Persistent fever above 37°C for more than 2 days

Chronic use of drugs that affect nutritional status

Alcohol abuse

Inadequate food budget

Biochemical Risk Factors

Low hematocrit and hemoglobin

Decrease in lymphocyte count

Elevated or decreased serum cholesterol level

Serum albumin less than 3.5 g/dl

Modified diets are used for clients who are unable to tolerate a normal diet or who have altered nutritional requirements. Modified diets can differ from normal diets in their consistency (*i.e.*, liquid or pureed consistency), total calorie content (*i.e.*, high-calorie, low-calorie), the concentration of macronutrients (*i.e.*, high-protein, low-fat), or concentration of one or more micronutrients (*i.e.*, low-sodium, low-potassium). Combinations of diet modifications may be necessary to meet a client's needs. All diets should be individualized as much as possible to ensure optimal tolerance and compliance.

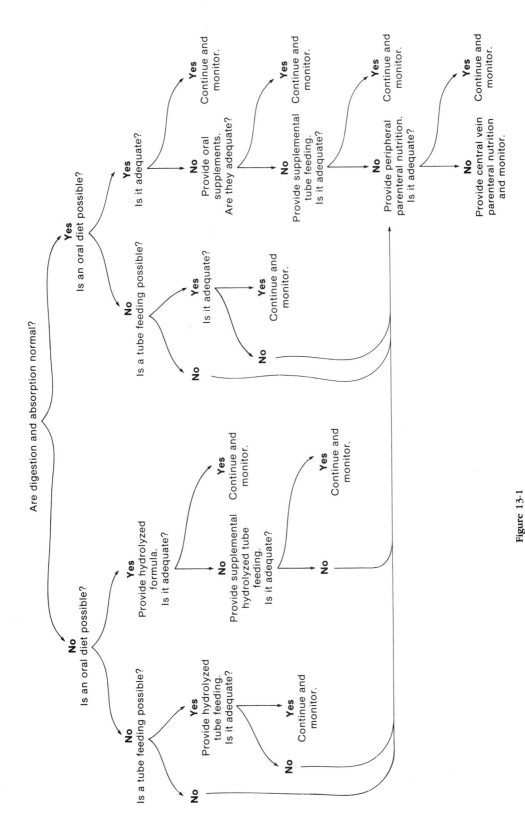

Are digestion and absorption normal?

Yes · Is an oral diet possible?

Yes · Is it adequate?
- **Yes** · Continue and monitor.
- **No** · Provide oral supplements. Are they adequate?
  - **Yes** · Continue and monitor.
  - **No** · Provide supplemental tube feeding. Is it adequate?
    - **Yes** · Continue and monitor.
    - **No** · Provide peripheral parenteral nutrition. Is it adequate?
      - **Yes** · Continue and monitor.
      - **No** · Provide central vein parenteral nutrition and monitor.
        - **Yes** · Continue and monitor.

No · Is a tube feeding possible?
- **Yes** · Is it adequate?
  - **Yes** · Continue and monitor.
  - **No**
- **No**

No · Is an oral diet possible?

Yes · Provide hydrolyzed formula. Is it adequate?
- **Yes** · Continue and monitor.
- **No** · Provide supplemental hydrolyzed tube feeding. Is it adequate?
  - **Yes** · Continue and monitor.
  - **No**

No · Is a tube feeding possible?

Yes · Provide hydrolyzed tube feeding. Is it adequate?
- **Yes** · Continue and monitor.
- **No**

No

Figure 13-1
Selecting the appropriate type and method of feeding.

351

Normal and Modified Diets

"Normal" ("Regular" or "House") Diets for

Adults
Infants, children, and adolescents
Pregnancy and lactation
Vegetarians

Diets Modified in Consistency and Texture

Clear liquid diet
Full liquid diet
Soft diet
Mechanical soft diet
Puréed diet
Tube feedings
Low-residue diet
High-fiber diet
Bland diet

Calorie Modified Diets

High-calorie diet
Low-calorie diet
Calorie-controlled diet (*i.e.*, diabetic diets)

Modified Nutrient Diets

High-CHO diet
Restricted CHO diet (*i.e.,* "anti-dumping" diets)
High-protein diet
Low-protein diet
Low-fat diet
Modified fat diet
Low-cholesterol diet
Low-potassium diet
Low-sodium diet
Fluid-restricted diet
Force fluids

(continued)

Normal and Modified Diets (*continued*)

Modified Diets Restricting or Eliminating Certain Foods

Gluten-free diet
Low-lactose or lactose-free diet
Purine-restricted diet
Elimination diets for allergies
Tyramine-restricted diet
Phenylalanine-restricted diet

When oral intake is resumed after acute illness, surgery, tube feedings, or total parenteral nutrition, clear liquids may be ordered and progressed to full liquids → soft diet → normal or modified diet (Table 13-1). Depending on the client's tolerance and condition, this routine progression may be accelerated by eliminating one or more of the transitional diets.

Various diagnostic tests performed in the hospital setting require specific diets be followed before the procedure. Although diet specifications vary among laboratories, examples of common "test" diets are outlined in Appendix 6.

Clients who are unable or unwilling to eat enough food to meet at least two thirds of their protein and calorie requirements may be given nourishment orally or through a tube to supplement their intake.

ENTERAL NUTRITION

Enteral nutrition is defined as the delivery of a liquid diet by mouth or tube into the gastrointestinal (GI) tract.[3] It may be used as a supplement to an oral diet or may provide total nutrition to clients who are unable to consume food orally. A wide variety of products are available commercially (see Appendix 7). Because enteral nutrition is easier, safer, better tolerated, and less expensive than parenteral nutrition, it should be used whenever the GI tract is functional (see box, Common Indications for Tube Feedings). If the client's nutritional requirements exceed those provided orally and/or enterally, parenteral nutrition may also be needed.

Oral Supplements

Plain or fortified milk, milk shakes, instant breakfasts, and eggnogs are high-protein, high-calorie "homemade" oral supplements that are palatable, relatively inexpensive, and suitable for boosting the protein and calorie intake in clients who are unable to meet their

(*Text continued on page 356*)

Table 13-1

Characteristics, Indications, and Contraindications for Liquid and Soft Diets

Diet Characteristics	Foods Allowed	Indications	Contra-indications
CLEAR LIQUID			
A short-term, highly restrictive diet composed only of clear fluids or foods that are fluid at body temperature. It requires minimal digestion and leaves a minimum of residue. Although it provides some electrolyte and carbohydrates, clear liquid diets are inadequate in calories and all nutrients except vitamin C. Be sure to include bouillon in the diet if electrolyte replacement is needed; eliminate bouillon if the client requires a sodium restriction (one bouillon cube provides 424 mg of sodium)	Bouillon Fat-free broth Carbonated beverages Coffee, regular and decaf Fruit juices, strained and clear (apple, cranberry, grape) Gelatin Popsicles Tea Sugar, honey, hard candy	Initial feeding after surgery or parenteral nutrition; in preparation for surgery and various diagnostic tests of the bowel	Long-term use
FULL LIQUID DIET			
Composed of foods that are liquid or liquefy at body temperature. Full liquid diets can be carefully planned or supplemented to approximate the nutritional value of a regular or high-calorie–high-protein diet, making it suitable for long-term use. Full liquid diets may be inadequate in folic acid, iron, vitamin B_6 and fiber. If the diet is used longer than 2 to 3 days, the following modifications may be needed to increase calories and protein: Add sugar and syrups whenever possible. Use whole-fat milk unless the client has hypercholesterolemia. Melt butter or margarine on soup and cereal. Add glucose supplements to fruit juices, milk, and milk drinks. Add skim milk powder to milk, milk drinks, soup, custard, puddings, cereal.	All the above plus: All milk and milk drinks, puddings, custards, desserts All vegetable juices All fruit juices Refined or strained cereals Eggs in custard Butter, margarine, cream	Used as a transitional diet between a clear liquid diet and a soft diet, and by clients who have difficulty chewing or swallowing	Severe lactose intolerance (diet relies heavily on milk and dairy products for protein and calories) Unless modified to decrease the cholesterol content, a liquid diet is not suitable for long-term use by clients with hypercholesterolemia

(continued)

Table 13-1 (*continued*)

Diet Characteristics	Foods Allowed	Indications	Contra-indications
Add instant breakfast or commercial supplements (Appendix 7). Lactose-reduced milk is available for clients with lactose intolerance. May be adapted for clients with diabetes mellitus, renal disease, and other disorders. Low-sodium soups, eggnogs, and custard should be used by clients who require a sodium restriction. To avoid salmonella infection, raw eggs should not be used.			

SOFT DIET

Diet Characteristics	Foods Allowed	Indications	Contra-indications
An adequate diet low in fiber, connective tissue, and fat. Restrictions vary considerably among institutions: Individual tolerances should determine the content of the diet.	All the above plus: Cooked vegetables as tolerated Lettuce in small amounts Cooked or canned fruit Avocado Banana Grapefruit and orange sections without membranes Whole grain or enriched breads and cereals Potatoes Enriched rice, barley, pasta All lean, tender meats, fish, poultry Eggs, mild cheese, smooth peanut butter Butter, margarine, mild salad dressings	Used for clients who have difficulty chewing or swallowing. A mechanical soft diet is used primarily by clients who have difficulty chewing because they are endentulous or have ill-fitting dentures. A regular soft diet is used as a transition between liquids and a regular diet.	None

Common Indications for Tube Feedings

Neurologic/Psychiatric

Post cerebrovascular accident

Neoplasms

Trauma

Inflammation

Demyelinating diseases

Severe depression, psychosis, other mental disorders

Anorexia nervosa

Gastrointestinal

Severe dysphagia

Pancreatitis

Inflammatory bowel disease

Short bowel syndrome

Malabsorption

Low-output enterocutaneous fistula

Other

Thermal injury

Chemotherapy

Radiotherapy

Sepsis

Head and neck surgery, trauma, and cancer

Postoperative nutritional support

Ventilator-dependent clients

Protein–calorie malnutrition with inadequate oral intake

nutritional requirements through food alone. For example, oral supplements are commonly used in conjunction with full liquid diets, and to meet increased requirements related to surgery or simple stress. However, these milk-based formulas are not appropriate for clients who (1) are lactose-intolerant (unable to tolerate milk sugar); (2) are unable to digest or absorb a normal diet; (3) need *complete* nutritional support in a liquid form; or (4) have metabolic disturbances that alter nutritional requirements. In addition, they may not be suitable for long-term use because of taste fatigue. Numerous commercial products, which vary in composition, characteristics, and cost, are available as alternatives (see Appendix 7).

Modular Products

Modular products are incomplete formulas that supply a single nutrient, either carbohydrate (*e.g.*, hydrolyzed cornstarch), protein (*e.g.*, whey protein), or fat (*e.g.*, MCT oil). They are not intended to be used as a sole source of nutrition but, rather, are used individually or in combination to alter the nutritional value of a food or enteral formula. For instance, a protein module may be added to a tube feeding to increase protein density without significantly effecting volume. Likewise, clients with chronic renal failure may receive CHO-fortified mashed potatoes and juices to increase calorie intake without increasing protein content.

Tube Feedings

Tube feedings may be "homemade" blenderized diets or commercial formulas used as a total or supplemental feeding, and are often used as a transition between parenteral nutrition and an oral diet (see Appendix 7). Compared to parenteral nutrition, enteral nutrition is safer, significantly less costly, and has the advantage of stimulating the GI tract. Because it helps maintain normal enzyme activity and gut mucosal integrity, nutrients are used better. Also, enteral nutrition helps maintain normal immune function by increasing IgA; IgA prevents absorption of enteric antigens. Parenteral nutrition does not increase IgA.

Although tube feedings are useful for a variety of clinical conditions (see box, Common Indications for Tube Feedings), they are contraindicated when the GI tract is nonfunctional, as in the case of gastric or intestinal obstruction, paralytic ileus, intractable vomiting, and severe diarrhea.

Types of Formulas

Complete tube feeding formulas provide adequate amounts of all required nutrients, and, although intended as a total feeding, they may also be given in smaller amounts to supplement an oral diet. The two major categories of commercial formulas are intact formulas and hydrolyzed formulas.

Intact protein (or intact nutrient) formulas contain whole complete proteins (*e.g.*, milk, meat, and eggs), or protein isolates (semipurified, high-biologic-value proteins that have been extracted from milk, soybean, or eggs). Standard formulas (milk-based and lactose-free) and blenderized formulas are categorized as intact formulas. Most intact formulas provide approximately 1 cal/ml, although high-density formulas that supply 2.0 cal/ml also are available.

Recently, there has been a proliferation of intact formulas enriched with dietary fiber. Although high-fiber formulas have been promoted as preventing/controlling both constipation and diarrhea in tube-fed clients, definitive studies on fiber's efficacy are lacking. However, because of its role in maintaining gut mucosal integrity, fiber may be a desirable component of a standard tube-feeding regimen.[13]

Because all intact formulas are made from complex molecules of protein, CHO, and fat, they require normal digestion before they can be absorbed. They are more palatable, less costly, and lower in osmolality (see box, Osmolality) than hydrolyzed formulas.

Osmolality

> *Osmolality* equals the number of particles (osmoles) per kg of water in solution.
>
> The concentration of CHO, amino acids, and electrolytes determines osmolality of nutritional formulas.
>
> A solution that is *isotonic* has approximately the same osmolality as blood, about 300 mOsm.
>
> The osmolality of a *hypertonic* or *hyperosmolar* solution is greater than that of blood (greater than 300 mOsm). If administered too rapidly or before the client has adapted to the high concentration of particles, hypertonic solutions can cause water to rush into the intestines to dilute particle concentrations, leading to cramping, nausea, and diarrhea ("dumping syndrome").

Hydrolyzed formulas are made from partially or totally "predigested" protein, carbohydrate, and fat, and require little or no digestion in order to be absorbed from the proximal small bowel. The osmolality of these products ranges from 300 to 810 mOsm/kg water. These formulas are often used as a transition diet between parenteral nutrition and a standard feeding. However, because most are hypertonic and relatively expensive, hydrolyzed formulas are contraindicated in clients who have a normally functioning GI tract.

Defined formula diets, sometimes referred to as *elemental* formulas, are the simplest type of hydrolyzed protein formulas, made from free amino acids, simple sugar, and very little fat. Some elemental formulas are designed to be used for "stress"; they are high in branched-chain amino acids, which are metabolized primarily in the peripheral muscle tissue and may be used preferentially for energy during stress. *Specially defined formula diets* are designed for clients with specific metabolic disorders such as renal failure or hepatic failure.

Feeding Tubes

Large-bore feeding tubes made of rubber or polyvinyl chloride were widely used in the past, even though they were extremely irritating to the nose and esophagus, needed to be replaced frequently because digestive juices caused them to stiffen, and interfered with normal cardiac sphincter function, which increased risk of gastric reflux and aspiration (see box, Ideal Tube Feeding Characteristics).

These problems, especially severe irritation, have been greatly reduced by the introduction of soft, pliable, small-bore feeding tubes. Newer tubes are also available with mercury-weighted tips to facilitate their passage into the intestines and help anchor them in position. The diameter of the tube used should be the smallest size possible that allows the formula to flow freely. Generally, the lower the residue content of a formula, the smaller the tube size needed (Table 13-2). Small-bore tubes used for supplemental tube feedings allow the client to consume food orally while the tubes are left in place. Regardless of the

"Ideal" Tube Feeding Characteristics

Provides nutrients in a form the client can digest and absorb; is free from
nutrients not tolerated by the client (*e.g.*, lactose)

Nutritionally balanced and calorically adequate

Provides 100% of the Recommended Dietary Allowances for vitamins and
minerals in an acceptable volume of formula

Well tolerated: The client does not experience diarrhea, nausea, constipation,
vomiting.

Low in osmolality and easy to digest

Easy to prepare and bacteriologically safe

Convenient and easy to administer

Of the proper viscosity to prevent clogging the tube

Affordable and readily available

type of tube used or its placement, proper care must be given to ensure that the tube does
not clog, break, fall out, or fall "in."

Feeding Tube Placement

The placement of the feeding tube depends on the client's medical status and the
anticipated length of time the tube feeding will be used. Generally, transnasal tubes, of
which nasogastric is the most common, are used for tube feedings of relatively short
duration. Ostomies, or stomas, are surgically created openings made to deliver feedings
directly into the stomach or intestines. They are the preferred method for permanent or
long-term feedings because they eliminate irritation to the mucous membranes. Percutaneous endoscopic gastrostomy tube feedings are placed nonsurgically with the aid of a
endoscope. The placement of any feeding tube should be determined by abdominal x-ray
before the first feeding is initiated.

Table 13-2
Feeding Tubes: Appropriate Sizes for Various Formulas

Formula	Residue Content	Appropriate Tube Size (French)*
Intact nutrient formulas (excluding protein isolates)	High	8 F–12 F
Protein isolate formulas	Medium	7 F–10 F
Hydrolyzed formulas	Minimal	5 F–6 F

* The smaller tube sizes can be used if the formula is delivered by pump.

Transnasal Tubes

Transnasal tubes are inserted nonsurgically through the nose and extended into either the stomach, duodenum, or jejunum. The client can participate actively in the procedure by swallowing small sips of water as the tube is passed, which will minimize discomfort and speed its passage. All transnasal tubes have the potential to irritate the nose and esophagus if used for prolonged periods or if the tube is too large. Uncooperative clients also are able to withdraw transnasal tubes.

Nasogastric (NG) tubes extend from the nose into the stomach. Formulas delivered through a NG tube generally are well tolerated because the stomach acts as a reservoir to hold and release the formula at a controlled rate, which prevents the "dumping syndrome." However, the risk of aspiration is high and NG feedings are contraindicated if the client has uncontrolled vomiting, inadequate gag reflexes, gastroesophageal reflux, inadequate gastric emptying, upper GI bleeding, or a complete intestinal obstruction.

Nasoduodenal (ND) tubes span from the nose through the pylorus into the duodenum. Nasoduodenal feedings are not likely to be aspirated because both the cardiac and pyloric sphincters work to inhibit gastric reflux; ND feedings can be adequately digested and absorbed if the correct formula is administered properly. Unfortunately, "dumping syndrome" may occur because the stomach is bypassed.

Nasojejunal (NJ) tubes extend from the nose through the pylorus into the jejunum; they are usually placed radioscopically. They are least likely to be aspirated because both the cardiac and pyloric sphincters work to inhibit gastric reflux. However, "dumping syndrome" may occur if the formula given is hyperosmolar or administered too rapidly.

Tube Enterostomy

Ostomy tubes are inserted through a surgical opening in the stomach, esophagus, or jejunum, usually under general anesthesia. Compared to transnasal feedings, ostomy feedings may be more successful in long-term use and more acceptable to the client because they are hidden under clothing.

Esophagostomy, a surgical opening made in the esophagus through which a feeding tube is passed into the stomach, is commonly used for clients with head and neck cancer. Esophagostomy feedings are generally well tolerated because the stomach is used to hold and release food at a controlled rate, which prevents the "dumping syndrome." However, the risk of aspiration is high, and the danger of hemorrhagic injury to the thoracic duct exists.

A surgical *gastrostomy* is performed by inserting a tube directly into the stomach. Gastrostomy feedings are well tolerated because they take advantage of the stomach's role in digestion to hold and release food at a controlled rate to avoid the "dumping syndrome." A disadvantage is the high risk of aspiration. Also, if the gastric contents leak, the skin surrounding the exit site may become irritated and infected; the danger of peritonitis exists.

A *jejunostomy* can be accomplished by way of a needle catheter placement, direct tube placement, or creation of a jejunal stoma that can be intermittently catheterized. Percutaneous endoscopic jejunostomy (PEJ), an extension of the percutaneous endoscopic gastrostomy procedure, is also performed. Jejunostomy feedings pose little risk of aspiration and have the advantage of using the GI tract for absorption even if digestion is impaired. Formula selection depends on where in the jejunum the tube is placed; intact formulas may be used if infused into the proximal jejunum, whereas hydrolyzed formulas are indicated for infusions into the mid- or distal jejunum and for needle catheter jejunostomies, because thicker formulas clog the small-bore tube. Jejunostomy feedings also require careful administration, that is, a slow, controlled, continuous drip by pump to avoid diarrhea.

Percutaneous Endoscopic Gastrostomy (PEG)

Percutaneous endoscopic gastrostomy (PEG) is a relatively new nonsurgical technique used to place a feeding tube directly into the stomach. Although there are several different techniques, all methods use an endoscope with a light to determine placement. A flexible guidewire is inserted percutaneously into the stomach, and a tube is then inserted over the wire and secured by rubber "bumpers" or an inflated balloon catheter.[1]

This procedure avoids laparotomy and usually can be performed under local anesthesia and intravenous sedation. As such, it is less costly and less risky than surgical gastrostomies, and feedings can be started sooner, usually within 24 hours after the procedure. Percutaneous endoscopic gastrostomy can also be used as a route of placement for a transpyloric feeding tube in clients with a contraindication for intragastric feedings. Percutaneous endoscopic gastrostomy feedings are contraindicated when an endoscopy cannot be performed, and in cases of active peptic ulcer disease or gastric outlet obstruction. Relative contraindications include previous gastric surgery, gastric or esophageal varices, ascites, severe gastroesophageal reflux, and gastroenteric fistulas.[18] Because it makes the procedure more difficult, obesity may also be considered a contraindication. The most common complications of a PEG are accidental tube removal, wound cellulitis, aspiration pneumonia, and clogged tubes.[19]

Method of Delivery

The three methods of delivering tube-feeding formulas are bolus administration, intermittent infusions, and continuous drip. The rates may be regulated by either a pump or by gravity drip. The type of delivery method used depends on the type and location of the feeding tube, the type of formula being administered, and the client's tolerance.

Bolus feedings can be used only when the tube is placed in the stomach. The feeding, poured into the barrel of a large syringe attached to a feeding tube, flows by gravity into the stomach. Generally, a 4- to 6-hour volume of formula is given four to six times a day. Intact formulas, either prepared commercially or "homemade," can be used. This method of feeding is most appropriate for clients who want to feed themselves and for disoriented clients who require observation throughout the feeding to ensure that the feeding actually is delivered.[16] Unfortunately, rapid, uncontrolled bolus feedings of 300 to 400 ml of formula given four to six times per day are poorly tolerated, often causing the dumping syndrome: nausea, diarrhea, glucosuria, distention, cramps, vomiting, and increased risk of aspiration.

Intermittent tube feedings, administered in equal portions four to six times a day, have the advantage of resembling a more normal pattern of intake and allow the client more freedom of movement between feedings. Tolerance of intermittent feedings is optimized by infusing the formula by slow gravity drip or by pump over a 30- to 60-minute period. Generally, no more than 300 ml of formula should be given in a single feeding, unless delivered very slowly. To decrease the risk of aspiration, gastric residuals should be checked before each feeding until tolerance is clearly established.

The continuous drip method of feeding is given over a 16- to 24-hour period to maximize tolerance and nutrient absorption; as such, it is the recommended method for feeding critically ill clients and for feedings delivered into the jejunum. It also is commonly used to begin a feeding into the stomach (*i.e.*, NG, gastrostomy, PEG), but may be replaced with intermittent feedings after 3 or 4 days without complications to resemble more closely a normal intake. Because consistent flow rates are difficult to achieve by gravity drip, infusion pumps are recommended. Pumps have significantly reduced the incidence of diarrhea, and should always be used to prevent "dumping syndrome" when feedings are infused into the distal duodenum or jejunum. Feedings should be interrupted every 6 hours to infuse water into the line to clear the tubing and hydrate the client.[16]

Administration

Before initiating a tube feeding, tube placement must be verified, preferably by x-ray, and bowel sounds must be present. Isotonic feedings (approximately 300 mOsm) should be given full-strength at 25 to 50 ml/hr and advanced by 25 ml/hr every 12 to 24 hours until the desired rate is achieved. Initially, hypertonic feedings should be diluted to approximate isotonicity (*i.e.*, one-quarter to one-half strength). After tolerance is established, the rate is advanced by 25 ml/hr every 8 to 12 hours until the desired rate is achieved. The concentration is increased every 8 to 12 hours only after the desired rate is achieved, in gradations of one-half to three-quarters strength, as tolerated. Rate and concentration should never be advanced at the same time, and neither should be progressed until 8 to 12 hours after tolerance is established. When a fluid restriction is required, tube feedings can be started at 30 ml/hr.

Although feedings infused by continuous drip can be given chilled, intermittent and bolus feedings are better tolerated at room temperature. To reduce the risk of bacterial contamination, closed feeding systems are recommended. Other precautions include changing the extension tubing and bag daily, refrigerating prepared formulas until they are needed, never adding a new supply of formula to old formula, and hanging feeding solutions for less than 6 hours.

To prevent aspiration, the head of the bed should be elevated at least 45° during the feeding and for 30 to 45 minutes afterward. Feedings should be held if gastric residuals are greater than 100 ml; aspirate should be replaced to reduce the loss of electrolytes and gastric juices. Some facilities color the feedings with food dye so that pulmonary secretions can be monitored for aspirated tube feedings. Although this practice may facilitate detection of aspirate, it does not protect against aspiration. In addition, blue food coloring will cause a false-positive result in a Hematest for occult blood, and red or orange food coloring added to the formula will make stool look bloody.[12] A better approach for testing pulmonary secretions for aspiration is to use a glucose dipstick—unless they are bloody, pulmonary secretions normally do not contain glucose, whereas enteral formulas do.

To help ensure tube patency, intermittent and bolus feedings should be followed by an infusion of 40 to 50 ml of warm water and continuous feeding tubes should be irrigated every shift with 40 to 50 ml of warm water. Likewise, every time the feeding is interrupted, the tube should be flushed with water.

Medications can become therapeutically ineffective if added directly to the enteral formula. A better approach is to administer the drug in a single bolus through the enteral tube, making sure the tube is flushed with water before and after the drug is administered.

If more than one drug is given, the tube should be flushed between doses. Drugs that are absorbed from the stomach should never be given through a nasoduodenal tube.[12]

Transition to Oral Diet

The goal of diet intervention during the transition period between enteral nutrition and an oral diet is to ensure an adequate nutritional intake while promoting an oral diet. To begin the transition process, the tube feeding should be stopped for 1 hour before each meal. Gradually increase meal frequency until six small oral feedings are accepted. Actual intake should be recorded and evaluated daily. When oral calorie intake is consistently 500 to 750 calories/day, tube feedings may be given only during the night. When the client consistently consumes two thirds of protein and calorie needs orally for 3 to 5 days, the tube feeding may be totally discontinued.

NURSING PROCESS

Assessment

Initial and ongoing assessments are vital to evaluate the success of a tube feeding. Because the majority of clients with tube feedings have had feeding difficulties or medical problems that place the client at increased risk, initial and periodic nutritional assessments should be performed. Although an in-depth nutritional assessment may be the dietitian's responsibility, the following screening data may be useful for the nurse.

Assess for the following factors:

Feeding route and the client's ability to digest and absorb nutrients (Table 13-3); compare these to the form and source of nutrients provided in the formula. Be aware that clients with altered renal, liver, or cardiac function may require specialized metabolic formulas. Other considerations include the goals of therapy, the availability and cost of

Table 13-3
Formula Selection Based on Tube Placement

Route	Recommended Type of Formula
Into the stomach (NG, esophagostromy, gastrostomy, PEG)	Intact formula. If a high-residue formula is indicated, consider a blenderized formula or fiber-enriched formula.
	If a low residue formula is indicated, choose a lactose-free protein isolate formula.
Into the duodenum to proximal jejunum with unimpaired digestion and absorption	Lactose-free protein isolate formula as near isotonic as possible
Into the mid to distal jejunum with normal or altered digestion	Hydrolyzed formulas

the formula, especially for home enteral nutrition, and "taste." Even though the client cannot truly taste a tube feeding, appearance and aroma may influence palatability and acceptance (see box, Ideal Tube Feeding Characteristics).

Weight status and any recent weight change.

Serum albumin and transferrin, if available, and evaluate any other abnormal laboratory values for their nutritional significance.

Outward signs of malnutrition.

Hydration status.

Adequacy of intake before the initiation of tube feeding. Assess cultural, familial, religious, and ethnic influences on eating habits and how they may affect formula selection. Ask the client if there is a history of food intolerances or allergies (*e.g.*, lactose, gluten).

Past medical history and current problems, and evaluate the impact on intake and nutritional status. Assess GI and major organ function (renal, hepatic, cardiac).

For clients who are candidates for home enteral nutrition, assess the client's motivational level, social support system, and financial status. Evaluate the home environment to assess the availability of running water, electricity, refrigeration, and storage space.[15]

Nursing Diagnosis

Altered Nutrition: Potential for More than or Less than Body Requirements, related to tube feeding.

Planning and Implementation

Fluid, calorie, and protein requirements are individualized according to the client's nutritional assessment data.

The normal fluid requirement for adults is about 1 ml/cal. Clients experiencing a fever, draining fistulas or surgical tubes, diarrhea, hemorrhaging, extensive tissue breakdown, increased perspiration, or an inability to concentrate the urine (*i.e.*, characteristic of some renal diseases and the elderly) will require more fluid. Clients with renal failure, liver failure, and heart disease may require less fluid. Generally, formulas providing 1 cal/ml contain approximately 850 ml of water per liter of formula. Additional water given between feedings and the water used to clean the feeding tube also contributes to fluid intake.

Estimate calorie and protein requirements based on weight status, serum protein values, medical history, and current illness. (For more precise information on calorie and protein requirements based on stress level, see Chap. 14.)

Be aware of the potential complications associated with tube feedings and nursing interventions to alleviate those problems (see box, Tube Feedings: Potential Problems, Rationale, and Nursing Interventions). In addition, clients who are receiving formula at a decreased volume or concentration may not be meeting their nutritional requirements and may need supplements.

Even though clients cannot taste tube feedings, the formula's appearance and aroma may influence the client's acceptance. For variety, add commercially available flavoring packets. If the formula's appearance is offensive, cover the feeding reservoir or remove it from the client's field of vision, if possible.

Estimated Enteral Calorie and Protein Requirements for Adults

Total calories/day for men and women:
25–30 cal/kg for weight loss
30–35 cal/kg for weight maintenance
35–40 cal/kg for weight gain

Grams of protein/day for men and women:
0.8–2.0 g/kg

Before a client is discharged on home tube feedings, a thorough evaluation of the client's tolerance of the formula, ability and motivation to learn, manual dexterity, attitude toward the tube feeding, willingness to comply, and family support is necessary to determine the best formula and delivery system for the client. In addition, the formula's cost and availability and the need for storage, electricity, running water, and refrigerator space must also be considered. Home health and community services can be used to provide additional support.[15]

Client Goals

The client will:
Attain/maintain "healthy" body weight.
Receive _____ calories in _____ ml/day of _____ (product used), as ordered.
Be free of any signs and symptoms of tube-feeding intolerance (see box, Tube Feedings: Potential Problems, Rationale, and Nursing Interventions).
Prepare, administer, and monitor tube feeding as ordered for use at home, when home enteral nutrition is indicated.
Resume oral intake when and if possible.

Nursing Interventions

Diet Management

Select an appropriate formula based on calorie and protein requirements, tube placement, medical status, and diet therapy objectives.
Initially, dilute the formula to approximate isotonicity and administer slowly to give the client time to adapt to the tube feeding. The small intestine can tolerate changes in volume better than changes in concentration; therefore, the volume should be in-

(Text continued on page 373)

Tube Feedings: Potential Problems, Rationale, and Nursing Interventions

Potential Problem

Diarrhea

Although properly administered tube feedings do not cause diarrhea, diarrhea frequently develops in tube-fed clients. Clients fed low-residue formulas cannot be expected to have firm stools; rather, their stools are likely to be pasty or gruel-like.[2] However, if it is established that the client is truly having diarrhea, the probable cause is investigated. If antidiarrheal medications are ordered by the physician, observe for constipation and signs of fecal impaction.

RATIONALE/NURSING INTERVENTION AND CONSIDERATIONS

1. Formula too cold

   Give canned formulas at room temperature; warm refrigerated formulas to room temperature in a basin of hot water.

2. Bacterially contaminated formula

   Hand washing and strict sanitation are required for formula preparation; equipment and utensils used in preparation should be washed in an automatic dishwasher or cleaned with hot, soapy water and rinsed thoroughly in boiling water; dry upside down.

   Administer formula promptly after opening; do not add newly opened formula to formula already in the feeding bag.

   Store unused formula in a tightly covered, dated container in the refrigerator; use within 24 hours or as recommended by the manufacturer.

   Rinse the equipment before each feeding with 30 ml to 50 ml of water.

   Replace the feeding bag and tubing every 24 hours.

   Be sure continuous drip feeding formulas do not hang at room temperature longer than 6 hours; do not hang "homemade" blenderized formulas longer than 4 hours.

3. Lactose intolerance

   Switch to a lactose-free formula.

4. Feeding rate too rapid

   Start initial feedings at 50 ml/hr and increase by 25 ml/hr every 12 hours depending on the client's tolerance.

   For existing feedings, decrease the rate of feeding to the level tolerated; increase by half the original increment.

5. Volume of formula too great

   Decrease the volume to a level tolerated by the client; gradually increase as tolerated.

   Feed smaller volumes of formula at more frequent intervals or switch to a continuous drip method of feeding.

(continued)

Tube Feedings: Potential Problems, Rationale, and Nursing Interventions (*continued*)

6. Hypertonic formula (concentrated solution of sugars, amino acids and electrolytes) delivered before adaptation has occurred

   Give initial feedings at one-quarter to one-half strength for a minimum of 8 hours and gradually increase to allow the client time to adjust to a hypertonic solution (do not increase the rate and strength at the same time).

   Deliver by continuous drip method.

   Switch to an isotonic solution, if possible.

7. Nasogastric feeding misplaced into the duodenum→ "dumping syndrome"

   Check the position of the tube before administering the formula.

8. Low serum albumin→ decreased oncotic pressure→ increased water within the bowel→ diarrhea. A low serum albumin, which may indicate malnutrition, may also be accompanied by (1) a decrease in intestinal border enzymes (protein molecules), and/or (2) a decrease or flattening of the microvilli lining the intestinal tract, both of which lead to diarrhea.

   Dilute the formula and increase the concentration gradually, or switch to an isotonic formula and infuse at slow rates.

   Consider parenteral administration of albumin.

9. Secondary to antibiotics or other drugs. The overgrowth of certain strains of intestinal flora that are not affected by antibiotics is believed to cause diarrhea. These flora digest formula, producing excess gas and acid and resulting in diarrhea. Antibiotic-associated diarrhea may also be related to a superinfection with *Clostridiam difficile* or *Staphylococcus aureus.* The use of undiluted, hypertonic oral electrolyte solutions and drugs, as well as sorbitol, has been implicated as a cause of diarrhea.

   Determine if the client is receiving antibiotics or other medications that may produce diarrhea: antiarrhythmic drugs (quinidine propranolol), aminophylline, digitalis, potassium supplements, phosphorus supplements, cimetidine. Investigate possible alternatives; administer antidiarrheals as ordered.

Potential Problem

Regurgitation of stomach contents→ aspiration penumonia

RATIONALE/NURSING INTERVENTION AND CONSIDERATIONS

1. Slowed gastric emptying time; that is, the gastric residual is greater than 100 ml

   Check gastric residual before each intermittent feeding and every 4 hours if continuous feeding is used. The physician should be notified and

(continued)

Tube Feedings: Potential Problems, Rationale, and Nursing Interventions (*continued*)

the feeding regimen should be evaluated if gastric emptying is consistently delayed.
   Switch to a continuous drip method of delivery.

2. Inhibited cough reflex related to debilitation, unconsciousness, or pulmonary complications
   Consider a nasoduodenal, nasojejunal, gastrostomy, or jejunostomy feeding.

3. Improper feeding position
   Elevate the head of the bed at least 30° during the feeding and for approximately 1 hour afterward.

4. Relaxed gastroesophageal sphincter related to a large-diameter feeding tube
   Switch to a pliable, small-diameter feeding tube.

5. High-fat content of formula (fat delays gastric emptying time)
   Switch to a low-fat formula.

Potential Problem

Nausea

Discontinue the feeding.

Administer antiemetics if ordered by the physician.

RATIONALE/NURSING INTERVENTION AND CONSIDERATIONS

1. Malplacement of the tube
   Check the position of the tube.

2. Feeding rate too rapid
   Slow the rate of feeding; switch to a continuous drip method of delivery.

3. Volume of formula too great→ delayed gastric emptying
   Check gastric residual and notify the physician if >100 ml.
   Reduce the volume and increase gradually.
   If distention is contributing to nausea, encourage ambulation.

4. Feeding too soon after intubation
   Allow approximately 1 hour between intubation and the first feeding.

5. Anxiety
   Explain the procedures to the client and encourage questions.
   Allow the client to verbalize his or her feelings; provide emotional support.

6. Intolerance to a specific formula, especially high-fat formulas
   Switch to a different formula.

(continued)

Tube Feedings: Potential Problems, Rationale, and Nursing Interventions (*continued*)

Potential Problems

Distention and bloating

RATIONALE/NURSING INTERVENTION AND CONSIDERATIONS

1. High-fat content of the formula
   Switch to a low-fat formula.
2. Decrease in GI function, especially among critically ill clients
   Check for active bowel sounds; switch to a hydrolyzed formula if the bowel sounds are hypoactive.

Potential Problem

Dehydration

Monitor fluid intake and output. Provide fluid to balance urine output plus insensible water losses (approximately 500 ml/day in uncomplicated cases)

Monitor serum BUN and sodium levels; elevated BUN and sodium level indicate that the kidneys are unable to adequately excrete the nitrogenous wastes resulting from a high-protein intake combined with an inadequate intake of fluid.

Monitor hematocrit and urine specific gravity, both of which increase as a result of dehydration.

RATIONALE/NURSING INTERVENTION AND CONSIDERATIONS

1. Diarrhea
   See above.
2. Excessive protein intake→ increase in urea formation (end products of protein metabolism)→ compensatory increase in urine output
   Switch to a formula with less protein.
   Increase water intake, if possible.
3. Inadequate fluid intake
   Increase fluid intake.
4. Glycosuria
   Test for glucose in the urine; notify the physician of glucosuria of 3+ or 4+.
   Administer insulin if ordered by the physician.
   Switch to a continuous drip method to avoid giving a high CHO load each feeding.

Potential Problem

Fluid overload

(continued)

Tube Feedings: Potential Problems, Rationale, and Nursing Interventions (*continued*)

Monitor serum sodium, BUN, and hematocrit—all will decrease as a result of overhydration.

Monitor intake and output.

RATIONALE/NURSING INTERVENTION AND CONSIDERATIONS

1. Excessive use of water to clean the tube after feedings
   Use only 30 ml to 50 ml of water to rinse the tube after each feeding.
2. Formula too dilute
   Check formula preparation for the proper dilution.

Potential Problem

Constipation

RATIONALE/NURSING INTERVENTION AND CONSIDERATIONS

1. Low-residue content of the formula
   Increase residue content if appropriate (*i.e.*, change to a formula with added fiber or increase fruits and vegetables in a blenderized diet).
2. Decreased activity related to feeding apparatus
   Encourage ambulation as much as possible.
3. Dehydration
   Monitor I & O. Add free water if intake is not greater than output by 500 to 1000 cc.
4. Obstruction
   Stop feeding and notify the physician.

Potential Problem

Nose irritation

RATIONALE/NURSING INTERVENTION AND CONSIDERATIONS

1. Presence of an NG tube
   Remove dry mucous secretions with warm water or a water-soluble lubricant.
   Lubricate the tube regularly with water or a water-soluble lubricant.
   For persistent discomfort, withdraw the tube, clean, and reinsert.
   Notify the physician if irritation or bleeding is observed.
2. Too large an NG tube
   Switch to a smaller-diameter tube.

Potential Problem

Skin irritation around the insertion site of a gastrostomy or jejunostomy tube

(continued)

Tube Feedings: Potential Problems, Rationale, and Nursing Interventions (*continued*)

RATIONALE/NURSING INTERVENTION AND CONSIDERATIONS

1. Leakage of gastric or intestinal contents through the ostomy opening or tension from the tube

    Clean the skin around the catheter daily with warm water and mild soap to prevent skin irritation.

    Observe for drainage and signs of infection: edema, tenderness, or redness. If drainage is present, remove immediately, apply gauze around the tube, and notify the physician.

Potential Problem

Gastric rupture

RATIONALE/NURSING INTERVENTION AND CONSIDERATIONS

1. Dangerous retention of feeding in the stomach related to gastric atony or obstruction

    Check for residual before beginning each feeding.

    Observe for signs of impending gastric rupture: distention, epigastric and upper quadrant pain, nausea, a large residual. If observed, discontinue feeding immediately and notify the physician.

Potential Problem

Dry mouth

RATIONALE/NURSING INTERVENTION AND CONSIDERATIONS

1. NPO→ irritation of the mucous membranes

    Apply petroleum jelly to the lips to prevent cracking.

    Allow ice chips, sugarless gum, and hard candies, if possible, to stimulate salivation.

    Encourage good oral hygiene to alleviate soreness and dryness: mouthwash, warm saline rinses, and regular brushing.
2. Breathing through the mouth

    Encourage the client to breathe through the nose as much as possible

Potential Problem

Clogged tube

RATIONALE/NURSING INTERVENTION AND CONSIDERATIONS

1. Feeding warmed formulas

    Do not heat formulas. Not only is the risk of clogging the tube

(continued)

Tube Feedings: Potential Problems, Rationale, and Nursing Interventions (*continued*)

increased, but water-soluble vitamins may be destroyed and the likelihood of bacterial contamination is increased.

2. Improper cleaning of the tube

Replace the feeding tube and bag every 12 to 24 hours.

Flush the tube before and after each infusion (regardless of the method) with 30 ml to 50 ml of water. If flushing fails to remove clog, the tube must be removed and replaced.

3. Formula too thick

High-viscosity formulas (*i.e.,* blenderized tube feedings or commercial formulas that provide 1.5 cal/ml to 2 cal/ml) should be infused by pump and possibly through a large-bore feeding tube to prevent clogging.

If possible, consider switching to a less calorically dense formula.

Because it is desirable to use the smallest size tube, viscous formulas may be delivered by a pump to help prevent clogging.

Potential Problem

Anxiety

RATIONALE/NURSING INTERVENTION AND CONSIDERATIONS

1. Deprivation of food → lack of sensory, social, and cultural satisfaction from eating

Allow oral intake of food that the client requests, if possible. If oral intake is contraindicated, allow the client to chew his or her favorite food without swallowing.

If possible, liquefy and add the client's favorite food to the tube feeding.

Encourage the client to leave the room when others are eating and find other enjoyable activities.

Encourage the client and family to view the tube feeding as another way of eating, rather than a form of treatment.[15]

2. Altered body image

Encourage the client to verbalize his or her feelings.

Stress the positive aspects of the tube feeding.

3. Loss of control and fear

Encourage the client to become involved in the preparation and administration of the formula, if possible.

Inform the client of potential problems that may occur and how to prevent or cope with them.

Encourage socialization with other well adapted tube-fed clients.

(continued)

Tube Feedings: Potential Problems, Rationale, and Nursing Interventions (continued)

> 4. Limited mobility
>   Encourage normal activity.
>   Control GI symptoms, such as diarrhea, nausea, vomiting, and constipation, that interfere with normal activity.
> 5. Discomfort related to the tube or formula
>   Observe for intolerances; alleviate with appropriate interventions.
>   Be sure to inspect and properly care for the tube exit site to avoid potential complications.

creased gradually to the optimal level before the concentration is increased. Isotonic formulas are given full strength.

Initiate continuous drip feeding at a rate of 25 ml/hour to 50 ml/hour for at least 8 hours. Increase the rate by 25 ml/hour every 8 to 12 hours as tolerated. If the client develops an intolerance (diarrhea, nausea, glucosuria), reduce the rate and then progress more slowly.

After the optimal volume is achieved, increase the concentration gradually, until full strength is achieved.

Flush tubing with water after every bolus or intermittent feeding, and every 3 to 6 hours with continuous feedings.

Encourage oral intake, if appropriate.

Client Teaching

Instruct the client

On the importance of tube feedings when oral intake is inadequate or impossible.

On the signs and symptoms of tube-feeding intolerance, and to alert the nurse if any problems arise.

To remain in an upright position or with the head elevated during and after the feeding to reduce the risk of aspiration.

Not to manipulate the flow rate unless otherwise instructed.

When home enteral nutrition is indicated, discharge teaching should encompass formula preparation, administration, and monitoring, as well as the rationale and interventions for tube feeding complications (see box, Client Teaching for Home Enteral Nutrition).

Monitor

Ongoing assessment is necessary to evaluate the client's tolerance and response to the tube-feeding formula.

Time	Procedure*
Before initiating a new or intermittent feeding	Check placement of an NG tube.
	Instill a small amount of water to make sure the tube is patent and to prevent the formula from sticking to it.
	Determine the amount of residual; if >150 ml, investigate reasons for delayed emptying.
Every ½ hour	Check gravity drip rates if applicable.
Every hour	Check pump drip rate if applicable.
Every 2 to 4 hours of continuous feeding	Check residual.
	After the first few days, residual should be checked at least once every 8 hours.
Every 4 hours	Check vital signs: blood pressure, temperature, pulse, and respiration.
	Check glucose and acetone in the urine.
	Discontinue nondiabetic monitoring if the client tests consistently negative for 48 hours. Monitor diabetic clients throughout the duration of the tube feeding.
	Refill feeding container.
Every 8 hours	Check intake and output and specific gravity of urine.
	Chart client's acceptance of and tolerance to the tube feeding.
Daily	Record the client's weight.
	Change feeding bag and tubing.
	Check serum electrolytes, BUN, and glucose until stabilized.
Every 3–4 days	Change irrigation set.
Every 7–10 days	Check all laboratory data.
	Reassess nutritional status.
PRN	Observe for intolerances: diarrhea, nausea, cramping, abdominal distention, vomiting, and glycosuria.
	Check NG tube placement, if appropriate.
	Check nitrogen balance and laboratory data.
	Perform delayed hypersensitivity skin testing.
	Clean feeding equipment.
	Chart significant information.

*From Cataldo CB, Smith L: Tube Feedings: Clinical Applications. Reprinted with permission of Ross Laboratories, Columbus, OH. © Ross Laboratories.

Evaluation

Evaluation is ongoing. Assuming the plan of care has not changed, the client will achieve the goals as stated above.

PARENTERAL NUTRITION

Parenteral nutrition, such as simple intravenous (IV) solutions, peripheral parenteral nutrition (PPN), and total parenteral nutrition (TPN), delivers nutrients directly into the bloodstream, thereby bypassing the GI tract. Parenteral nutrition is used when a client

Client Teaching for Home Enteral Nutrition

Provide verbal and written instructions to the client and family for the following:

Formula preparation, including handwashing techniques, how to clean equipment, proper measuring and mixing, and formula storage.

Enteral administration, including the proper procedure for intubation (if applicable), how to check for proper tube position and residuals, proper feeding technique, correct body position during feeding, flushing the tube, how to connect the feeding tube, capping/clamping the tube, and the feeding schedule (time/volume/rate).

Tube care, including the name of the tube and proper method of irrigation.

Equipment care, including how to clean the pump and tube.

Pump operation, including proper set up and alarms/batteries.

Problem solving, including how to manage cramps, bloating, diarrhea, constipation, nausea, tube malposition, tube breakage, a clogged tube, and mechanical problems with the pump.

Where to call for guidance, and when to call the physician. Unusual abdominal pain or distention, rapid weight gain or loss, GI bleeding, or vomiting require immediate professional attention.[15]

Exit site care, that is, nose care, care of ostomy site, oral hygiene.

How to collect data for follow-up care by consistently and regularly checking gastric residuals, sugar and acetone in the urine, and weight.

physically or psychologically cannot consume enough nutrients orally or enterally, or when altered GI functions precludes oral and enteral feedings.

The usual fluid volume given to adults over a 24-hour period is 3 liters. The composition of parenteral solutions is individualized according to the client's nutritional requirements and medical condition. However, because there are standard concentrations of protein, carbohydrate, and fat in standard volumes, individualization is somewhat limited.[14]

Sterile water, dextrose (available in 5%, 10%, 20%, 30%, 50%, and 70% solutions), amino acids (available in 3.0%, 3.5%, 5.0%, 7.0%, 8.5%, and 10% solutions), lipid emulsions(10% or 20% solutions), electrolytes, multivitamins, minerals, and trace elements may all be given intravenously. The actual composition of the parenteral solution depends on the site of infusion and the client's fluid and nutrient requirements.

Peripheral Nutrition

Solutions infused into peripheral veins must be isotonic (*i.e.*, must have low concentrations of dextrose and amino acids) to prevent irritation and eventual collapse of the small-diameter veins. Although lipid emulsions are isotonic and may be given for additional calories, the need to maintain isotonic concentrations of dextrose and amino acids while avoiding fluid overload limits the caloric value of peripheral solutions.

Simple IV Solutions

The primary objective of simple IV solutions is to maintain or restore fluid and electrolyte balance on a short-term basis. They are used most commonly before and after surgery, after trauma, and during childbirth. Simple IV solutions contain water with dextrose (usually 5%, sometimes 10%), electrolytes, or both.

A liter of 5% dextrose in water (D_5W) provides 50 g of dextrose. One gram of dextrose provides 3.4 calories, when administered parenterally, and therefore 1 liter D_5W = 170 calories; 2.5 to 3 liters/day = 425 cal/day to 510 cal/day. Because simple IV solutions have little nutritional and caloric value, they should not be used longer than 1 to 2 days or if nutritional requirements are high.

Protein-Sparing Therapy

Protein-sparing therapy solutions contain amino acids and water; vitamins and electrolytes may be added. A 3.5% crystalline amino acid solution provides 35 g amino acids/liter, or 5.9 g nitrogen/liter (g nitrogen = g protein divided by 6.25).

The purpose of protein-sparing therapy is to prevent or minimize the loss of lean body mass by allowing adaptation to short-term starvation to occur. Without a supply of dextrose, serum insulin levels drop, which allows body fat to be used for energy. The resultant ketosis indicates adaptation has occurred and body protein is being conserved. Also, some of the infused amino acids may be converted to glucose and used for energy, adding to the protein-sparing effect.

Studies show that amino acids are better at sparing protein than dextrose; however, it is not clear whether amino acids are more effective when given alone or when combined with dextrose. Therefore, protein-therapy solutions may also contain 5% to 10% dextrose or lipids.

Protein-sparing is controversial because amino acids are an expensive source of energy. Also, ketones inhibit normal appetite, which may delay the return to eating, and the long-term effects of ketosis are not known. Protein-sparing is not appropriate for debilitated clients who have inadequate fat stores, and more aggressive nutritional support is indicated if the client is unable to eat for more than 5 days.

However, protein-sparing therapy may be used for a few days after surgery by clients who have adequate fat stores or during the acute hypercatabolic phase after stress or illness.

Peripheral Parenteral Nutrition

Peripheral parenteral nutrition infuses a hypotonic or isotonic solution of dextrose (5% to 10%), amino acids (3% to 8.5%), vitamins, electrolytes, and trace elements into a peripheral vein. Up to 2 liters of 10% lipid emulsion may be given daily. Peripheral parenteral nutrition contains lesser concentrations of the same ingredients found in central vein TPN.

Peripheral parenteral nutrition provides temporary nutritional support to promote nitrogen balance and weight gain when oral intake is inadequate or is contraindicated. It may be used to supplement an oral diet or tube feeding, or as a transition from TPN to an enteral intake. Peripheral parenteral nutrition is used most effectively in clients who need short-term nutritional support (7 to 10 days) but do not require more than 2000 to 2500 cal/day. It may also be used in clients with a postsurgical ileus or an anastomotic leak, or in clients who require nutritional support but who are unable to use TPN because of limited accessibility to a central vein. Clients receiving peripheral parenteral nutrition should have normal kidney function and lipid metabolism. Peripheral parenteral nutrition is not adequate for clients who have increased nutritional requirements or who need more than 2000 to 2500 cal/day, and is contraindicated in clients with abnormal lipid metabolism (*i.e.*, elevated serum triglycerides) or poor peripheral veins.

Central Vein Total Parenteral Nutrition

Central vein total parenteral nutrition (TPN) is an infusion of a hypertonic solution through an indwelling catheter placed into a central vein, usually the internal jugular or subclavian, and passed into the superior vena cava. Large-diameter veins with a high blood-flow rate are needed to dilute the solution quickly to isotonic.

The actual TPN composition depends on the client's condition and nutritional requirements. Solutions may contain 5% to 25% dextrose, 2% to 10% amino acids, vitamins, minerals, electrolytes, and trace elements. A 10% to 20% lipid emulsion may be given twice weekly for additional calories and to prevent essential fatty acid deficiency (see box, Parenteral Lipid Emulsions). However, because lipid emulsions mixed with dextrose–amino acid mixtures are not stable, lipid solutions are infused from a separate container and tubing that joins the dextrose–amino acid mixture by way of a "Y" connector just before it enters the vein.

Total parenteral nutrition provides complete nutritional support for clients who cannot or will not consume an adequate oral or enteral intake. Indications include the following conditions:
* Severe malnutrition; weight loss of 10% or more
* GI abnormalities: obstruction, peritonitis, impaired digestion and absorption, enterocutaneous fistulas, chronic vomiting, chronic diarrhea, prolonged paralytic ileus
* Anorexia nervosa, coma
* Severely malnourished preoperative clients
* Supplementation of an inadequate oral intake in clients who are aggressively treated for cancer
* After surgery or trauma, especially extensive burns, multiple fractures, sepsis
* Acute liver and renal failure when amino acid requirements are altered

Because TPN is expensive, requires constant monitoring, and has potential infectious, metabolic, and mechanical complications (see box, Potential Complications of Total Parenteral Nutrition), it should be used *only* when an enteral intake is inadequate or contraindicated and when prolonged nutritional support is needed. Likewise, TPN should be discontinued as soon as possible. Gradual weaning to enteral nutrition or oral feedings is required to prevent metabolic complications and nutritional inadequacies. Total parenteral nutrition is never an emergency procedure and is always accompanied by potential risks.[11]

Administration

Catheter insertion, usually into the subclavian vein, is a surgical procedure performed under sterile conditions. The client is given a local anesthetic and should be instructed to expect some pain. The placement must be confirmed by x-ray before the solution can be

Parenteral Lipid Emulsions

Isotonic fat emulsions composed of 10% or 20% safflower or soybean oil, egg yolk phospholipids, and glycerin. Can be infused through either peripheral or central veins.

Indications

Can safely provide up to 60% of the total calorie intake
Used to correct or prevent essential fatty acid deficiency

Contraindications

Intravenous lipid emulsions should not be given to clients who have these conditions:
- Abnormal lipid metabolism, such as hyperlipidemia
- Severe liver disease
- Acute pancreatitis

Products Available With 10% Fat Emulsions

Product	Manufacturer	Cal/ml	Osmolarity (mOsm/L)
Liposyn 10%	Abbott	1.1	300
Travamulasion 10%	Travenol	1.1	270
Intralipid 10%	Cutter	1.1	280

Products Available With 20% Fat Emulsions

Liposyn 20%	Abbott	2.0	340
Intralipid 20%	Cutter	2.0	330

Nursing Assessment

Observe for the following adverse reactions:
Immediate reactions (occur with 2.5 hours after infusion)
- Fever
- Flushing, sweating
- Insomnia, dizziness
- Nausea, vomiting, headache
- Chest and back pains
- Dyspnea, cyanosis

Delayed reactions (occur within 10 days)
- Hepatomegaly
- Splenomegaly
- Thrombocytopenia

(continued)

Parenteral Lipid Emulsions (*continued*)

- Hyperlipidemia
- Seizures
- Shock
- Jaundice
- Leukopenia

Nursing Considerations

Intralipid must be refrigerated; let it stand at room temperature 30 minutes before using. Liposyn may be stored at room temperature.

Administer a test dose of 1 ml/min for 15 to 30 minutes and observe the client's tolerance. Notify the physician if adverse reactions develop. If no adverse reactions occur, the infusion rate can be increased.

Do not shake bottles of fat emulsions or combine with other solutions because the emulsion will "break" and separate. (Do not use solutions that appear separated.) A Y-connector is used to join the fat emulsion tubing at the TPN tubing just before the vein so that the solutions do not mix for very long.

administered, and the catheter should be checked periodically for proper position, leaks, and obstructions. Although the site of insertion should be routinely cleaned, dressed, and checked for signs of infection, dressings or adhesives should not be removed for 48 hours after the catheter is inserted.

To prevent contamination, the central line should not be used to administer drugs (except insulin), measure central venous pressure, or withdraw blood. Equipment and solution containers should always be checked for leaks and cracks before use.

Initially, the infusion is started slowly (*i.e.*, 25 to 50 ml/hr) to give the body time to adapt to the high concentration of glucose and the hyperosmolality of the solution. Continuous drip by pump infusion is needed to maintain a slow constant flow rate. After the first 24 hours, the rate of delivery is gradually increased over 4 to 5 days, until the optimal volume is achieved. If the rate falls behind or speeds up, the infusion rate may be adjusted up or down by 10% of the original rate to compensate for the deviation (if ordered by the physician). Because of the dangers of hyperosmolar diuresis from an excessive glucose infusion, attempts should not be made to "catch up" more quickly.

Cyclical TPN (10- to 16-hour infusion of amino acids and glucose followed by parenteral or enteral amino acids, amino acids and fat, or nothing for the remaining 24-hour period) may be used if the client is on home TPN, or if the client needs TPN only to support an inadequate oral intake. Cyclical TPN allows serum glucose and insulin levels to drop during the periods when TPN is not infused, thereby promoting fat and glycogen mobilization.

Clients must be weaned off TPN gradually to prevent rebound hypoglycemia. Enteral intake (either an oral diet or tube feeding) should increase as TPN decreases; enteral intake should be adequate before TPN is discontinued.

Potential Complications of Total Parenteral Nutrition

Infection and Sepsis Related to

Catheter contamination during insertion

Long-term indwelling catheter

Catheter seeding from blood-borne or distant infection

Contaminated solution

Metabolic Complications

Dehydration

Hyperglycemia

Rebound hypoglycemia

Hyperosmolar, hyperglycemic nonketotic coma

Azotemia

Electrolyte disturbances
  Hypocalcemia
  Hypophosphatemia, hyperphosphatemia
  Hypokalemia
  Hypomagnesemia

High serum ammonia levels

Deficiencies of
  Essential fatty acid
  Trace elements

Altered acid–base balance

Elevated liver enzymes

Mechanical Complications Related to Catheterization

Catheter misplacement

Hemothorax (blood in the chest)

Pneumothorax (air or gas in the chest)

Hydrothorax (fluid in the chest)

Hemomediastinum (blood in the mediastinal spaces)

Subcutaneous emphysema

Hematoma

Arterial puncture

Myocardial perforation

Catheter embolism

Air embolism

Endocarditis

Nerve damage at the insertion site

Laceration of lymphatic duct

Chylothorax

Lymphatic fistula

Thrombosis

NURSING PROCESS

Assessment

Ongoing assessment of the client's needs and tolerance to parenteral nutrition is necessary to ensure maximum benefit and prevent complications. Although an in-depth nutritional assessment may be the dietitian's responsibility, the following screening data may be useful for the nurse.

Assess for the following factors:

Weight status, any recent weight change.

Past medical history and current problems, and evaluate the impact on intake and nutritional status.

GI and major organ function (renal, hepatic, cardiac).

Serum albumin and transferrin, if available, and evaluate any other abnormal laboratory values for their nutritional significance.

Outward signs of malnutrition; assess hydration status.

For clients who are candidates for home parenteral nutrition, assess the client's motivational level, social support system, financial status, and home environment.

Nursing Diagnosis

Altered Nutrition: Potential for More than or Less than Body Requirements, related to total parenteral nutrition.

Planning and Implementation

Calculate parenteral calorie and protein requirements based on the client's assessment data and medical status (Table 13-4). Approximately 30 to 50 ml of fluid/kg should be provided.

Minimal fat requirements are 2% to 4% of calories as essential fatty acids; 1 to 2.5 g/kg is recommended as the maximum.

Because the exact requirements for vitamins, minerals, and trace elements given parenterally are not known, close monitoring of nutritional status is necessary to prevent the development of nutrient deficiencies or toxicities.

Change the infusion equipment as needed to help prevent contamination. The infusion bottle should be changed every 12 hours, even if it still contains some solution. Change the infusion tubing from the bottle to the catheter hub once every 24 hours.

Monitor the flow rate to avoid complications and ensure adequate intake. Solutions infused too rapidly can cause hyperosmolar diuresis, leading to seizures, coma, and even death; solutions administered too slowly prevent an optimal nutritional intake.

Some clients may feel hungry while receiving TPN and should be allowed to eat if possible. If an oral intake is contraindicated, give ice chips or allow the client to chew his favorite food without swallowing.

Begin weaning the client from TPN as soon as possible; enteral nutrition may be indicated until oral intake is adequate.

Table 13-4
Parenteral Calorie and Protein Requirements
Based on Weight and Stress Level

	Calories/kg/day	Grams Protein/kg/day
Resting state (i.e., medical clients)	20–30	0.8–1.0
Uncomplicated postoperative clients	25–35	1.0–1.3
Depleted clients	30–40	1.3–1.7
Hypermetabolic clients	35–45	1.5–2.0

Food for Thought	## Hospital Malnutrition

Nutritional support is a vital component of holistic client care. However, it is well documented that a significant number of hospitalized clients develop malnutrition because of mismanagement or neglect.[6] Impaired wound healing and susceptibility to infection are well-known consequences of malnutrition, both of which may prolong hospitalization and increase morbidity and mortality. It is the responsibility of the whole health care team to provide optimal nutritional care by ensuring that hospitals do not fail to:

- Record height and weight.
- Provide consistent care despite frequent staff rotation.
- Assign accountability to nutritional care even if responsibility is diffused.
- Discontinue IV glucose therapy as soon as possible.
- Observe clients' food intake.
- Replace meals withheld for diagnostic tests.
- Use tube feedings that are nutritionally adequate, consistent in composition, and prepared under sanitary conditions.
- Know the composition of vitamin and nutritional products.
- Recognize that illness and injury increase nutritional requirements.
- Assess a client's nutritional status before some types of surgery.
- Support clients nutritionally after surgery.
- Realize the importance of nutrition in the prevention of and recovery from infection and to avoid unwarranted reliance on antibiotics.
- Promote communication and interaction between the dietitian and physician.
- Provide nutritional support to prevent malnutrition; once established, malnutrition may be difficult or impossible to reverse.
- Use laboratory tests as part of nutritional assessment because of neglect or limited availability.

Clients who have permanent nonfunctional GI tracts may require TPN indefinitely. In order for home TPN to be successful, clients and their families must be physically and emotionally prepared. Intensive counseling should focus on the preparation and administration of the solution, catheter and equipment care, assessment skills, as well as the psychological impact of permanent TPN.

Client Goals

The client will:

Attain/maintain "healthy" body weight.

Maintain/replenish body protein, as evidenced by normal serum protein levels (*i.e.*, albumin, transferrin).

Receive _____ calories in _____ ml/day of _____ (mixture used), as ordered.

Be free of any signs and symptoms of parenteral nutrition complications (see box, Potential

Complications of Total Parenteral Nutrition).

Aseptically prepare and administer, and monitor TPN as ordered for use at home, if indicated.

Resume enteral or oral intake when and if possible.

Nursing Interventions

Diet Management

Administer TPN as ordered.

Notify the physician if an intolerance or complication develops.

Client Teaching

Instruct the client

On the importance of TPN when oral/enteral intake is inadequate or impossible.

To alert the nurse if any problems arise.

Not to manipulate the flow rate unless otherwise instructed.

When home TPN is indicated, discharge teaching should encompass aseptic preparation and administration techniques, criteria to monitor, signs and symptoms of systems failure, when to call the doctor, when to call the dietitian, and when to call the pharmacist.[11]

Encourage the client to discuss anxiety, anger, or adaptation to TPN and oral deprivation.[11]

Monitor

Ongoing assessment is vital to the success of TPN.

Time	Procedure
Every 30 minutes	Check the flow rate.
Every 4–6 hours	Check urine glucose.
	Monitor vital signs.
	Check urine specific gravity.
Daily	Record the client's weight: A daily weight gain of 1/4 lb to 1/2 lb is expected.
	Monitor intake (including any oral intake) and output.
2–3 times/week or daily if needed	Check serum levels of glucose and electrolytes.
	Check BUN levels.
	Check hemoglobin.
Weekly	Check serum levels of protein, calcium, phosphorus and ammonia.
	Reassess nutritional status.
	Check liver function studies.
PRN	Check white blood cell count and differential count.
	Check cultures.
	Observe for intolerances and signs of complications.
	Chart significant information.

Evaluation

Evaluation is ongoing. Assuming the plan of care has not changed, the client will achieve the goals as stated above.

BIBLIOGRAPHY

1. American Dietetic Association: Manual of Clinical Dietetics. Developed by The Chicago Dietetic Association and The South Suburban Dietetic Association, 1988
2. Anderson BJ: Tube feeding: Is diarrhea inevitable? Am J Nurs 86:704, 1986
3. ASPEN Board of Directors: Guidelines for the use of enteral nutrition in the adult patient. Journal of Parenteral and Enteral Nutrition 11:435, 1987
4. Bower RH, Talamini MA, Sax HC et al: Postoperative enteral vs. parenteral nutrition. Arch Surg 121:1040, 1986
5. Brown CSB, Stegman MR: Nutritional assessment of surgical patients. QRB 14:302, 1988
6. Butterworth CE, The skeleton in the hospital closet. Nutrition Today 9:4, 1974
7. Cataldo CB, Smith L: Tube Feedings: Clinical Applications. Columbus, OH: Ross Laboratories, 1980
8. Chernoff R: Nutritional support: Formulas and delivery of enteral feeding: I. Enteral formulas. J Am Diet Assoc 79:426, 1981
9. Chernoff R: Nutritional support: Formulas and delivery of enteral feeding: II. Delivery systems. J Am Diet Assoc 79:430, 1981
10. Coffey LM, Carey M: Evaluating an enteral nutrition formulary. J Am Diet Assoc 89:64, 1989
11. Escott-Stump S: Nutrition and Diagnosis-Related Care, 2nd ed. Philadelphia: Lea and Febiger, 1988
12. Farley J: About enteral nutrition. Nursing 88 18(8):82, 1988
13. Frankenfield DC, Beyer PL: Dietary fiber and bowel function in tube-fed patients. J Am Diet Assoc 91:590, 1991
14. Maillet JO: Calculating parenteral feedings: A programmed instruction. J Am Diet Assoc 84:1312, 1984
15. McCrae JAD, Hall NH: Current practices for home enteral nutrition. J Am Diet Assoc 89:233, 1989
16. McGee L: Feeding gastrostomy. Part II: Nursing care. Journal of Enterostomal Therapy 14:201, 1987
17. Methany NM: 20 ways to prevent tube-feeding complications. Nursing 85 15(1):47, 1985
18. Skipper A (ed): Dietitian's Handbook of Enteral and Parenteral Nutrition. Rockville, MD: Aspen, 1989
19. Starkey JF, Jefferson PA, Kirby DF: Taking care of percutaneous endoscopic gastrostomy. Am J Nurs 88:42, 1988

14 Stress, Surgery, and Burns

NUTRITION AND STRESS

Stress, including surgery, burns, infectious, traumatic, and febrile conditions, can have a significant impact on nutritional status and nutrient requirements. The response to stress, characterized by neuroendocrine-mediated changes that promote tissue healing and maintain equilibrium and normal organ function, occurs in three distinct phases.

The initial phase after trauma or stress is the "ebb" phase, a more or less latent period in which few changes occur. The acute, catabolic, or "flow" phase begins within about 24 hours. During this phase, the release of stress hormones causes the body to increase its energy expenditure, to break down body protein, and, consequently, to lose body weight and lean body mass. Potassium and nitrogen excretion increase, serum glucose levels rise, and sodium and fluid are retained. Stress also impairs normal gastrointestinal (GI) function by decreasing motility, which can result in anorexia, distention, nausea, vomiting, or constipation.

Within a few days after the initial stress response, catabolism peaks and the anabolic phase of recovery begins. As stress hormone levels subside, serum glucose levels decline and nitrogen balance is gradually achieved.

The actual physiologic response to stress depends on the severity of the stress, the number of stressors, and the individual's ability to adapt to stress. The stress of minor surgery in a well-nourished client may have little impact. Malnutrition is a stress that also requires adaptation. Clients who are burdened with malnutrition plus another form of stress (surgery, burns, trauma, fractures, infection, sepsis) may lack the nutrient reserves needed for adaptation to occur. The result may be multiple-systems organ failure and death.

Calorie and protein requirements increase in response to stress (Table 14-1). The greater the stress, the greater the impact on nutritional needs. Studies show that although protein requirements increase in general, the requirement for branched-chain amino acids in particular may increase during stress.[2]

Table 14-1

Guidelines for Calorie and Protein Intakes During Various Stages of Stress

Stress Level	Total Calories (cal/kg/day)	Amino Acids (g/kg/day)
Starvation (level 0)	28	1.0
Elective general surgery (level 1)	32	1.5
Polytrauma (level 2) (i.e., general surgery with infection)	32–40	1.5–2.0
Early sepsis (level 3)	40	2.0
Late sepsis	50	2.5

(Adapted from Cerra F: Pocket Manual of Surgical Nutrition. St. Louis: CV Mosby, 1984; and from Dietitians in Critical Care Dietetic Practice Group Quality Assurance Committee: Suggested Guidelines for Nutrition Management of the Critically Ill Patient. Chicago: American Dietetic Association, 1984)

Vitamin, mineral, and electrolyte requirements during stress are unclear and undefined.[3] Although much is known about the role of nutrition in stress, much is yet to be learned. The nutritional implications of various types of stress are outlined in Table 14-2; however, nutritional needs always should be determined on an individual basis.

SURGICAL NUTRITION

Ideally, clients should have an optimal nutritional status before surgery to enable them to withstand the stress of surgery and the short-term starvation that follows. Good nutritional status can speed recovery time and shorten the period of hospitalization. Clients who are well nourished before surgery have a lower incidence of infections, complications, and postoperative mortality compared to malnourished clients.

Studies show that approximately 45% to 50% of surgical clients are malnourished. Disease-related symptoms experienced before surgery, such as anorexia, nausea, vomiting, fever, malabsorption, and blood loss, may leave a client nutritionally compromised. After surgery, nutrient requirements increase depending on the degree of hypermetabolism, hypercatabolism, and wound healing. Problems with ingestion, digestion, absorption, metabolism, or excretion resulting from surgery for cancer or disorders of the GI tract, pancreas, liver, or kidneys, increase the risk of malnutrition and complications. To optimize the chance of a successful outcome of surgery, malnourished clients and those at risk for malnutrition should be identified and given preoperative nutritional support (see box, General Surgical Assessment Criteria).

NURSING PROCESS
Assessment

In addition to the general surgical assessment criteria, assess for the following factors:
Age status: Vulnerable age groups include infants, children, and the elderly because they have smaller reserves to sustain themselves through the stress of surgery and the postoperative period.

Table 14-2
Nutritional Implications of Various Types of Stress

Stressor	Nutritional Objectives	Diet Management
AIDS: an infection caused by the human immuno-deficiency virus (HIV). Typical signs and symptoms include fever, chills, fatigue, anemia, diarrhea, viral infections, anorexia, oral lesions, malabsorption, weight loss, and poor nutritional status.	Correct and treat symptoms. Prevent further weight loss. Correct fluid and electrolyte imbalances.	Provide high-calorie, high-protein diet based on individual requirements. Provide adequate fluid. Encourage small frequent meals. Modify the diet, as needed to control GI symptoms (*i.e.,* diarrhea, malabsorption, see Chap. 15.) Provide soft, puréed, or liquid foods if oral or esophageal lesions impair intake. Stress the importance of a well balanced, nutrient-dense diet.
Decubitus ulcers: a pressure sore caused by a lack of oxygen and nutrients to the affected area, usually the bony or cartilaginous prominences of the hip, sacrum, elbow, or heels. Risk is highest among the elderly, bedridden and paralyzed clients, and people with protein–calorie malnutrition.	Attain normal protein status. Promote healing and prevent future sores.	Provide high-calorie, high-protein diet. Supplements of zinc and vitamin C may be indicated. Provide small, frequent meals to maximize intake.
Fever: altered thermoregulation that may occur secondary to infections, neoplasms, connective tissue diseases, or unknown causes.	Meet increased calorie requirements related to the increase in REE: every 1°F increase in temperature above normal increases REE by 7%. Replenish nutrient losses, as needed: nitrogen, electrolytes, CHO stores. Correct and treat any concomitant GI symptoms.	Provide approximately 500 to 600 additional calories for each 1°F rise in temperature. Provide increased fluids: adults may need 10 to 15 cups/day. Modify the diet as needed to control GI symptoms. Small, frequent meals may be indicated. Provide a liquid diet if solids are not tolerated or accepted.
Infection: invasion and growth of pathogenic microorganisms.	Meet increased requirements related to hypermetabolism. Prevent or correct symptoms and complications. Replenish nutrient losses, as needed.	Provide high-calorie, high-protein diet. Provide adequate fluids. Small, frequent meals may be indicated.

Nutritional status, based on nutritional screening criteria (see Fig. 9-1). If a nutritional problem is identified or suspected, a more in-depth nutritional assessment is indicated in order to develop appropriate diet therapy objectives and interventions to meet the client's preoperative and postoperative nutritional needs.

Presurgical symptoms of illness or condition: onset, frequency, causative factors, severity, interventions attempted and the results.

<table>
<tr>
<td>**Assessment Criteria**</td>
<td>

General Surgical Assessment Criteria

Presurgical history: symptoms of acute illness (*i.e.,* nausea, vomiting, diarrhea, anorexia) and existence of chronic illnesses (diabetes mellitus, pulmonary diseases, impaired cardiovascular, hepatic or renal function, GI disorders, alcoholism)

Weight status; recent weight changes

Serum albumin, transferrin

Hydration status, electrolyte status

Blood pressure

Anemia

Nature and extent of anticipated surgery, especially GI surgery

Infections
</td>
</tr>
</table>

Dietary changes made in response to symptoms—foods avoided, foods preferred. Determine foods best and least tolerated.

Weight status. Obesity increases the work load of the heart and increases the risk of infection, pulmonary complications, and delayed wound healing

Past medical history.

Nursing Diagnosis

Altered Nutrition: Less than Body Requirements, related to increased requirements for healing secondary to surgery.

Planning and Implementation

Preoperative Nutrition

Although an optimal nutritional status before surgery can improve the outcome of surgery, intravenous (IV) fluid and electrolytes may be the only form of nutritional rehabilitation possible in clients undergoing emergency surgery.

Clients who are well nourished and who are scheduled for uncomplicated surgery do not need a special preoperative diet and can be maintained on their normal diet.

Deficiencies of vitamins, minerals, fluid, and electrolytes can be corrected quickly and easily, if detected. Adequate protein status and normal weight should be achieved, if time allows. However, it may not be possible to rehabilitate a client nutritionally if emergency surgery is indicated or if the risks of delaying surgery are too great. Clients who are unable to consume an adequate oral intake may need enteral or parenteral nutritional support.

Postoperative Nutrition

Postoperative nutritional support depends on the location, extent, and type of surgery, as well as postsurgical complications, the client's nutritional status, and his ability to eat. Minor surgery may have little affect on nutritional status and nutrient requirements. However, extensive surgery, surgery involving the GI tract, and the development of postoperative complications can increase nutritional requirements and influence the method of feeding.

Simple IV solutions are nutritionally and calorically inadequate and should be discontinued as soon as possible. Increased nutritional requirements combined with short-term starvation (NPO) or an inadequate diet may result in a weight loss of about 0.5 lb/day early in the postoperative period. A greater weight loss may be experienced by clients who have extensive surgery, postoperative complications, or other medical conditions. Weight loss may not be apparent if the client has edema.

The following interventions may help relieve discomfort, irritability, and a preoccupation with eating that can develop in clients who are NPO:

- Apply cold compresses or petroleum jelly to the lips to ease dryness.
- Encourage mouth-rinsing with cold water or a mouthwash.
- Divert the client's attention away from eating with other activities, such as listening to the radio, watching television, talking with other clients, and so forth.

A needle-catheter jejunostomy tube may be inserted during surgery if the client is malnourished, hypermetabolic, or not expected to resume an oral intake within a few days after surgery. Unlike the stomach, which does not regain motility for 24 to 48 hours after surgery, the small intestine resumes peristalsis and the ability to absorb nutrients within several hours after surgery.

The actual postoperative diet depends on the client's prior nutritional status and the type and extent of surgery. Potential nutritional problems and diet interventions for various surgical procedures of the GI tract are listed in the box, Nursing Interventions and Considerations for Potential Nutritional Problems of Various Surgical Procedures of the GI Tract.

To maximize intake, especially in an anorexic client, solicit food preferences, individualize the diet, offer small, frequent meals, and allow food from home if possible.

Encourage ambulation as soon as possible after surgery to prevent postoperative complications, to stimulate the appetite, and to prevent complications of immobility (*i.e.*, increased losses of protein and calcium).

Client Goals

The client will:

Attain/maintain "healthy" weight and optimal nutritional status before (if possible) and after surgery.

Avoid aspiration during anesthesia and recovery.

Maintain normal fluid and electrolyte balance.

Achieve nitrogen balance to promote wound healing.

Describe the principles and rationale for postoperative diet management, as appropriate, and implement the recommended dietary interventions.

Avoid GI complications, if appropriate.

(*Text continued on page 394*)

Nursing Interventions and Considerations for Potential Nutritional Problems of Various Surgical Procedures of the GI Tract

Gastric Surgery

Gastrectomy: Partial or total removal of the stomach or duodenum used in the treatment of gastric or duodenal ulcers, gastric cancer, gastric trauma

Billroth I: Gastroduodenostomy. May cause *dumping syndrome,* anemia, malabsorption, weight loss

Billroth II: Gastrojejunostomy; *dumping syndrome* and other problems are more common than with Billroth I

Partial gastrectomy: Anastomosis between the remaining portion of the stomach and the jejunum

Total gastrectomy: Radical removal of the stomach with anastomosis between the esophagus and jejunum

Vagotomy: Partial or total severance of the vagus nerve; may cause *dumping syndrome,* diarrhea, increased feeling of fullness

POTENTIAL PROBLEMS/RATIONALE

Diarrhea and the *dumping syndrome* related to a decrease in the holding capacity of the stomach; undigested food that is quickly "dumped" into the jejunum causes a rapid increase in the osmolarity of the intestinal contents. Extracellular fluid shifts from the circulating blood volume into the intestine to dilute the high particle concentration, resulting in distention, cramping, pain, and diarrhea, usually within 15 to 30 minutes after eating.

Due to a rapid transit time, fat may not be exposed to bile and pancreatic enzymes long enough to be thoroughly digested. As a result, steatorrhea and other symptoms of fat maldigestion may occur. The etiology of weight loss is multifactorial: diarrhea, steatorrhea, a voluntary restriction of food intake, a restrictive diet, and so forth.

NURSING INTERVENTIONS AND CONSIDERATIONS

Instruct the client to follow the postgastrectomy (*antidumping*) diet (see box, Sample Postgastrectomy ["Antidumping"] Menu that includes the following modifications:

- Eat five to six or more small meals daily.
- Increase fat and protein intake; fat is isotonic and protein is hydrolyzed more slowly than CHO and therefore does not increase osmolarity as readily. Include some fat and protein in each feeding.
- Decrease CHO intake; avoid simple sugars that form a hyperosmolar solution in the jejunum.
- Avoid high-fiber foods that stimulate peristalsis.

(continued)

Nursing Interventions and Considerations for Potential Nutritional Problems of Various Surgical Procedures of the GI Tract (*continued*)

- Adjust total calorie intake to attain and maintain weight.
- Avoid fluid with meals and 1 hour before and after eating.
- Eliminate individual intolerances.
- Lie down for 20 to 30 minutes after eating to delay gastric emptying time.

Clients with steatorrhea may need a low-fat diet, MCT oil, and water-soluble forms of the fat-soluble vitamins.

Lactose intolerance may develop, requiring a low-lactose or lactose-free diet (see Chap. 15).

Foods high in pectin (unripe bananas, raw apple, and white rice) may help prevent symptoms of the *dumping syndrome*.

Eventually the diet can be liberalized as the remaining portion of the stomach or duodenum hypertrophies to hold more food and allow for more normal digestion.

POTENTIAL PROBLEM/RATIONALE

Reactive hypoglycemia (sweating, dizziness, and rapid heart beat), which may occur as a secondary reaction 1 to 3 hours after eating, related to the rapid absorption of CHO from the duodenum → increase in blood glucose levels → oversecretion of insulin → rapid drop in blood glucose levels.

NURSING INTERVENTIONS AND CONSIDERATIONS

Advise the client to follow the modifications outlined above for the *antidumping* diet to avoid hypoglycemia.

Instruct the client to carry a source for concentrated sugar with him to treat reactive hypoglycemia when it occurs, such as hard candy, lumps of sugar, LifeSavers, and so forth.

POTENTIAL PROBLEM/RATIONALE

Anemia may occur as a result of (1) chronic blood loss, (2) impaired iron absorption because of decreased exposure to HCl in the stomach or because the duodenal site of iron absorption is bypassed, or (3) vitamin B_{12} malabsorption related to inadequate secretion of intrinsic factor (IF) or because of bacterial overgrowth in a *blind loop*.

NURSING INTERVENTIONS AND CONSIDERATIONS

Observe for signs and symptoms of anemia (see Chap. 16). Adjust the diet and provide supplements accordingly.

Clients with pernicious anemia require intramusclar injections of vitamin B_{12}.

(*continued*)

Nursing Interventions and Considerations for Potential Nutritional Problems of Various Surgical Procedures of the GI Tract (*continued*)

Intestinal Surgeries

Intestinal bypass: Surgical removal of 50% or more of the small bowel because of inflammatory bowel disease, cancer, obstruction, and so forth.

POTENTIAL PROBLEM/RATIONALE

Short bowel syndrome: Diarrhea, fluid and electrolyte imbalances, severe weight loss, muscle wasting, malabsorption, steatorrhea, anemia, and malnutrition resulting from a decrease in absorptive area of the intestine.

NURSING INTERVENTIONS AND CONSIDERATIONS

The client is usually maintained on total parenteral nutrition for 2 to 3 months after surgery. Oral intake resumes when fecal output is about 1 liter/day with clear liquids or a hydrolyzed (chemically defined) diet.

Monitor fluid and electrolyte balance and correct abnormalities. Antidiarrheals and potassium supplements may be needed for 5 or more months after surgery.

Low-residue foods are introduced as the client's tolerance improves.

Instruct the client
- To eat six to eight small, frequent meals
- To decrease fat intake; MCT oil may be used for additional calories
- To increase protein intake to replace losses
- To increase calorie intake to restore normal weight
- To take supplements as directed
- To avoid high-fiber foods
- To avoid caffeine for at least the first year after surgery, because it stimulates GI motility.

Malabsorption of fat can result in deficiencies of the fat-soluble vitamins, calcium, and magnesium. Observe for signs and symptoms of deficiencies and provide supplements as needed.

Eventually the remaining small bowel can adapt by enlarging and by increasing its ability to absorb nutrients. However, depending on the extent of surgery, adaptation may not be possible and the client may need parenteral nutritional support indefinitely.

Ileostomy

An opening (stoma) in the abdominal wall into the ileum for continuous discharge of the liquid contents of the small intestine.

Colostomy

An opening (stoma) in the abdominal wall into the colon for defecation of liquid to formed stools after removal of the rectum and anus.

(*continued*)

Nursing Interventions and Considerations for Potential Nutritional Problems of Various Surgical Procedures of the GI Tract (*continued*)

Either procedure may be used in the treatment of severe ulcerative colitis or inflammatory bowel disease, intestinal lesions, obstructions, or colonic cancer; ostomies may be temporary or permanent. Ileostomies are more likely to cause nutritional problems than colostomies.

POTENTIAL PROBLEM/RATIONALE

Frequent, watery stools related to a decrease in absorptive surface (large amounts of water and electrolytes are normally absorbed in the colon)

NURSING INTERVENTIONS AND CONSIDERATIONS

Losses of fluid, sodium, and potassium may be considerable, depending on the location of the stoma and whether adaptation has occurred. Monitor fluid and electrolyte balance and correct abnormalities.

Initially, clear liquids are given and progressed to a low-residue diet to prevent irritation and slow GI transit time. As the client improves, gradually and individually add small amounts of foods containing fiber to the diet and assess the client's tolerance. Foods not tolerated initially can be reintroduced in a few months.

Encourage the client to drink a lot of fluid. Excess fluid intake does not contribute to diarrhea, but is excreted through the kidneys. It is important for ileostomy clients to maintain a normal urine output to minimize the risk of renal calculi.

POTENTIAL PROBLEM/RATIONALE

Weight loss related to diarrhea or a fear of eating

NURSING INTERVENTIONS AND CONSIDERATIONS

Provide a high-calorie, high-protein diet to replenish losses and restore normal weight.

Encourage the client to verbalize fears; counsel the client on the importance of eating to attain/maintain wellness

POTENTIAL PROBLEM/RATIONALE

Anemia related to vitamin B_{12} malabsorption (vitamin B_{12} is normally absorbed in the distal ileum)

NURSING INTERVENTIONS AND CONSIDERATIONS

Clients with ileal resections require parenteral vitamin B_{12} injections for the rest of their lives.

POTENTIAL PROBLEM/RATIONALE

Odor related to poor stomal hygiene or to the action of bacteria on food

(*continued*)

Nursing Interventions and Considerations for Potential Nutritional Problems of Various Surgical Procedures of the GI Tract (continued)

NURSING INTERVENTIONS AND CONSIDERATIONS

Encourage good stomal hygiene.

Advise the client to eliminate foods that may produce odorous gas, such as beer and other alcoholic beverages, beans, onions, green pepper, broccoli, cabbage, asparagus, brussel sprouts, turnips, beets, corn, and spicy foods. Individual intolerances should also be eliminated.

POTENTIAL PROBLEM/RATIONALE

Intestinal blockage related to improperly chewed food

NURSING INTERVENTIONS AND CONSIDERATIONS

Advise the client to avoid high-fiber fruits and vegetables and to chew food thoroughly.

POTENTIAL PROBLEM/RATIONALE

Depression and anxiety related to altered body image, altered body function, and dietary restrictions

NURSING INTERVENTIONS AND CONSIDERATIONS

Provide emotional support and allow the client and family to verbalize their feelings.

Advise the client that with time, a more normal diet is possible as adaptation occurs. The stools usually become more firm and less frequent within 7 to 10 days after an ileostomy.

Nursing Interventions

Diet Management

Before Surgery

Provide a high-calorie, high-protein diet.

Promote a liberal intake of nutrients important for wound healing (Table 14-3), especially vitamins C and K.

Withhold all food and liquids (NPO) for at least 8 hours before surgery to avoid aspiration related to anesthesia. To minimize fecal residue and postoperative distention after intestinal surgery, a low-residue, residue-free (see Chap. 15), or hydrolyzed formula diet may be used before surgery for 2 to 3 days (see Chap. 13).

After Surgery

Give IV fluid and electrolytes as ordered to maintain hydration until oral intake is resumed, usually with the return of bowel sounds 24 to 48 hours after surgery.

Table 14-3
Nutrients Important for Wound Healing and Recovery

Nutrient	Rationale for Increased Need	Possible Deficiency Outcome
Protein	To replace the lean body mass lost during the catabolic phase following stress To restore blood volume and plasma proteins lost during exudates, bleeding from the wound, and possible hemorrhage To replace losses resulting from immobility (increased excretion) To meet the increased needs for tissue repair and resistance to infection	Significant weight loss Impaired/delayed wound healing Shock related to decreased blood volume Edema related to decreased serum albumin Diarrhea related to decreased albumin Anemia Increased risk of infection related to decreased antibodies, impaired tissue integrity Decreased lipoprotein synthesis → fatty infiltration of the liver → liver damage Increased mortality
Calories	To replace losses related to NPO, hypermetabolism during catabolic phase following stress To spare protein To restore normal weight	Signs and symptoms of protein deficiency may develop when protein is used to meet energy requirements. Extensive weight loss
Water	To replace losses through vomiting, hemorrhage, exudates, fever, drainage, diuresis To maintain homeostasis	Signs, symptoms, and complications of dehydration such as poor skin turgor, dry mucous membranes, oliguria, anuria, weight loss, increased pulse rate, decreased central venous pressure (CVP)
Vitamin C	Important for tissue synthesis and wound healing through collagen formation	Impaired/delayed wound healing related to impaired collagen formation and increased capillary fragility and permeability
Thiamine, niacin, riboflavin	Requirements based on metabolic rate: increased metabolic rate → increased requirements	Decreased enzymes available for energy metabolism
Folic acid, vitamin B_{12}	Needed for cell proliferation and therefore tissue synthesis Important for maturation of red blood cells Impaired folic acid synthesis related to some antibiotics; impaired vitamin B_{12} absorption related to some antibiotics	Decreased or arrested cell division Megoblastic anemia
Vitamin A	Important for tissue synthesis and wound healing Enhances resistance to infection	Impaired/delayed wound healing related to decreased collagen synthesis Increased risk of infection
Vitamin K	Important for normal blood clotting Impaired intestinal synthesis related to antibiotics	Prolonged prothrombin time
Iron	To replace iron lost through blood loss	Signs, symptoms, and complications of iron deficiency anemia, such as fatigue, weakness, pallor, anorexia, dizziness, headaches, stomatitis, glossitis, cardiovascular and respiratory changes, possible cardiac failure
Zinc	Needed for protein synthesis and wound healing	Impaired/delayed wound healing

Sample Postgastrectomy ("Antidumping") Menu

Breakfast

1 soft-cooked egg
1 slice white toast with butter
One Hour Later
½ cup milk

Midmorning Snack

Firm banana
Graham crackers

Lunch

½ cup cottage cheese with 2 canned
   peach halves
Dinner roll with butter
One Hour Later
½ cup milk

Midafternoon snack

1 oz cheddar cheese
4 saltine crackers

Dinner

2 oz baked chicken
½ cup white rice with butter
¼ cup mashed butternut squash
One Hour Later
½ cup milk

Bedtime Snack

½ plain bagel with cream cheese

Progress oral intake from clear liquids to full liquids to a soft or regular diet as tolerated (see Chap. 13, Table 13-1).

Depending on the extent of surgery and the development of complications:

- Increase protein intake to promote wound healing and replace protein losses (see Table 14-1).
- Increase calorie intake to meet increased energy requirements and spare protein (see Table 14-1).
- Encourage a liberal intake of those nutrients necessary for wound healing and recovery (see Table 14-3).

Modify the diet, as needed, to avoid potential nutritional problems related to GI surgery (see boxes, Nursing Interventions and Consideration for Potential Nutritional Problems of Various Surgical Procedures of the GI Tract; and Sample Postgastrectomy ["Antidumping"] Menu).

Clients who are unable or unwilling to consume an adequate oral intake may require enteral or parenteral nutritional support.

Client Teaching

Instruct the client

On the importance of nutrition in recovery and wound healing.

How to increase protein and calorie intake (see box, Ways to Add Protein and Calories to the Diet).

On the principles and rationale of diet management of post-GI surgery, as appropriate.

To eat small, frequent meals if anorexia or nausea exists.

Ways to Add Protein and Calories to the Diet

For added protein and calories:
- Add skim milk powder to milk to make double-strength milk; chill well before serving
- Use double-strength milk on hot or cold cereals, and in scrambled eggs, soups, gravies, casseroles, milk shakes, milk-based desserts
- Substitute whole milk or evaporated milk for water in recipes
- Add grated cheese to soups, casseroles, vegetables dishes, rice, noodles
- Use peanut butter as a spread on slices of apple, banana, pears, crackers, or waffles; use as a filling for celery
- Add finely chopped, hard-cooked eggs to sauces, soups, and casseroles
- Choose desserts made with eggs or milk, like sponge cake, angel food cake, custard, puddings
- Dip meat, poultry, and fish in eggs or milk and coat with bread or cereal crumbs before baking, broiling, or pan frying
- Use yogurt as a topping for fruit, plain cakes, or other desserts; use in gravies and dips

For added calories:
- Mix cream cheese with butter and spread on hot bread and rolls
- Whenever possible, add butter to hot foods: breads, pancakes, waffles, soups, vegetables, potatoes, cooked cereal, rice, pasta
- Substitute mayonnaise for salad dressing in salads, eggs, casseroles, sandwiches
- Add dried fruit, nuts, or granola to desserts and cereal
- Use whipped cream on pies, fruit, pudding, gelatin, ice cream, and other desserts; to lighten coffee and tea; in hot chocolate
- Use marshmallows in hot chocolate, on fruit, and in desserts
- Top baked potatoes, vegetables, and fruits with sour cream
- Snack frequently on nuts, dried fruit, candy, buttered popcorn, cheese, granola, ice cream
- Use honey on toast, cereal, fruits, and in coffee and tea

Monitor

Monitor for the following signs or symptoms:

Tolerance of oral diet, (*i.e.*, absence of postprandial pain, nausea, vomiting, distention)

Compliance with diet (as appropriate), and the need for follow-up diet counseling

Effectiveness of diet, and the need for further diet modification

Weight, weight changes

Healing, postsurgical course

Intake and output; observe for fluid and electrolyte imbalances

Bowel elimination; alterations in bowel function

Evaluation

Evaluation is ongoing. Assuming the plan of care has not changed, the client will achieve the goals as stated above.

BURNS

Burns are the third leading cause of accidental death in the United States. They may be caused by thermal, electrical, chemical, or radioactive insults. Burns are classified according to degree, based on the extent of damage. Burns over more than 20% of the body may be fatal.

Superficial partial-thickness (first-degree) burns destroy the epidermis. The area appears pink to red, with slight edema but no blisters. Pain may last up to 24 hours and is relieved by cooling. Healing occurs spontaneously within a week.

Deep partial-thickness (second-degree) burns may be superficial or deep. A superficial second-degree burn destroys the epidermis layer of the skin. The area appears red and blistered and is painful; however, healing occurs spontaneously if infection does not develop. Deep second-degree burns destroy all but the deep dermis layer of skin. The area appears mottled white and red; red edematous areas blanch when touched. Healing takes several weeks; scarring may occur.

Full-thickness (third-degree) burns may appear red, white, black, or brown; burned areas do not blanch when touched. Third-degree burns destroy the epidermis and dermis layers of the skin and also the nerve endings; therefore, no pain is felt. Debridement and grafting are necessary; scarring and loss of skin function occur. Fourth-degree burns destroy skin, fat, muscles, and bone. Debridement, formation of granulation tissue, and grafting are necessary.

The client's age and past medical history, the extent, depth, and cause of the burn, the presence of associated injuries, and the development of complications influence the client's prognosis. Sepsis is the most common cause of death among burn victims, followed by pneumonia. Other complications include congestive heart failure, adrenal insufficiency, renal failure, hemorrhaging, and stress ulcers (Curling's ulcer) (see box, Risk Factors for Complications in Burned Clients).

Treatment measures depend on the extent of the burn and postburn phase. The goals of treatment are to maintain fluid and electrolyte balance, relieve pain and anxiety, prevent complications and infection, promote healing, provide physical and emotional support, and meet increased nutritional requirements.

NURSING PROCESS

Assessment

Observe and assess:
The percentage of body surface area (BSA) burned.
Thickness or degree of burn, and percentage of third-degree burn.
The type of burn: thermal, electrical, chemical, radioactive.

Risk Factors for Complications in Burned Clients

Burn surface area greater than 20%

Poor nutritional status prior to burn

Preburn illness or disease

Morbid obesity

History of substance abuse

Associated injuries

Complications: pulmonary, circulatory, infectious, metabolic, GI

Weight loss of more than 10% of preburn weight while hospitalized

Low serum transferrin and anergy (impaired immunocompetence) are strongly
   correlated to a high risk of infectious complications.

(Jensen TG, Long JM, Dudrick SJ, et al: Nutritional assessment indications of postburn complications.
J Am Diet Assoc 85:68, 1985)

The location of the burn; assess the client's ability to self-feed.

The possibility of inhalation injury.

Concomitant injuries.

History of chronic illnesses and drug therapy.

Prior nutritional status, especially usual/ideal preburn weight. Be aware that some nutritional assessment criteria may be difficult to obtain or invalid for burned clients. For instance, triceps skinfold and upper arm circumference measurements are contraindicated in patients with upper body burns, and massive fluid shifts make accurate weights impossible during the initial postburn period.

Nursing Diagnosis

Altered Nutrition: Less than Body Requirements, related to hypermetabolism secondary to thermal injury.

Planning and Implementation

Extensive burns are the most severe form of stress that a person can experience. Due to hormonal responses and extensive evaporative water losses, metabolism may increase 100% above normal (hypermetabolism). Glycogen stores are quickly depleted and the body uses its own lean body tissue for energy needs (hypercatabolism). Large amounts of fluid, electrolytes, protein, and other nutrients leach through the burned area. Nutritional support may be complicated by fluid and electrolyte imbalances, paralytic ileus, anorexia, pain, infection or other complications, emotional trauma, and medical–surgical procedures. Weight loss and malnutrition lead to increased morbidity and mortality unless aggressive nutritional support is initiated as soon as possible after fluid resuscitation. Fluid replacement is the primary concern in the immediate postburn phase, also known as the "ebb" or shock phase. Individualized amounts and combinations of IV electrolytes, colloids (whole blood, plasma, or serum protein albumin), fluid, and dextrose may be given. Average fluid requirements range from 3 to 5 liters daily, although up to 10 liters/day may be needed for extensive burns. Generally, half of the calculated fluid volume needed for the first 24 hours is given in the first 8 hours when fluid loss is greatest; the remaining volume is given over the next 16 hours. Immediate use of IV fluids also helps to prevent gastric distention and paralytic ileus.

The high incidence of impaired immunocompetence and protein depletion among burned clients makes aggressive nutritional support vital in order to decrease the risk of infectious complications. Primary goals during the "flow" or recovery period that begins 48 to 72 hours postburn are to maintain fluid and electrolyte balance and to minimize the loss of lean body tissue and body weight. Oral intake should begin as soon as fluid resuscitation is completed and paralytic ileus is resolved, usually around the 3rd postburn day. If bowel sounds have not returned by the 4th postburn day, peripheral or central vein parenteral nutrition should be given. Although it is easier to meet calorie needs than protein needs, clients should be able to achieve neutral balances of both by the 7th postburn day. Goals of this secondary feeding period are to replace nutritional losses and promote wound healing.

The diet management recommendations listed below are guidelines. A starting level should be selected, implemented, and evaluated for its effectiveness. Periodic diet adjustments should be made according to the client's progress. Nutritional requirements are increased by the development of complications and are decreased as wound healing progresses.

Although preferred, a regular diet with in-between meal supplements of high-calorie, high-protein liquids may not be adequate for some clients. Supplemental or complete enteral (NG, gastrostomy, jejunostomy) or parenteral (central, jugular, femoral, cut-down peripheral) feedings may be necessary for clients with the following conditions:

- Extremely high calorie and protein requirements who cannot consume enough food orally to meet their needs
- Inability to swallow because of facial or neck burns
- Adynamic ileus
- Bleeding related to Curling's ulcer (need TPN)
- Anorexia related to fear, pain, altered body image, and frequent medical or surgical procedures; nutritional requirements are highest when appetite is poorest.

Total parenteral nutrition should be used with extreme caution because of the increased risk of infection and sepsis. Other considerations include the location of the burn and the compatibility of IV medications with the TPN solution.

There are no set guidelines for vitamin and mineral supplementation for burned clients. The need for some nutrients may increase directly to promote wound healing (*i.e.*, vitamin C, zinc) or indirectly because of the increased calorie intake (*i.e.*, requirements for thiamine, riboflavin, and niacin increase in proportion to the increase in calorie requirements) (see Table 14-3). Multivitamin and mineral supplements or megadoses of certain nutrients may be prescribed at the physician's discretion, depending upon the client's prior nutritional status.

Decreased weight bearing during immobility results in increased bone resorption and a negative calcium imbalance, regardless of calcium intake. Encourage ambulation to minimize calcium and nitrogen excretion and to improve appetite and outlook. Once weight-bearing activity resumes, calcium requirement increases to replace calcium lost from the bones.

As the client enters the rehabilitation phase after wound healing, diet becomes less important. However, an adequate intake is needed to rebuild body stores and muscle tissue. Obesity is rare during the first 5 years after burns.

Client Goals

The client will:

Attain/maintain fluid and electrolyte balance within 72 hours postburn.

Avoid renal shutdown from decreased plasma volume and cardiac output.

Have minimal catabolism of protein tissues to avoid protein–calorie malnutrition.

Heal wounds and retain grafts, as appropriate.

Avoid weight loss greater than 10% preburn weight (if preburn weight was within client's "healthy" weight range).

Attain nitrogen balance.

Avoid complications.

Nursing Interventions

Diet Management

After bowel sounds return, initiate an oral diet (*i.e.*, liquids) slowly and observe for signs of intolerance; progress the diet as tolerated. Hydrolyzed (chemically defined) tube feedings may decrease the incidence of GI bleeding and provide a higher and more consistent calorie intake than a mixed oral diet in the early secondary feeding period.

Increase protein intake to facilitate wound healing and to replace the loss of lean body mass. Depending on the severity of the burn, daily protein intake should be 1.5 to 3 g/kg, or approximately two to four times greater than the RDA.

Increase calorie intake to meet increased energy requirements (BEE may be 1.5 to 2 times greater than normal) and spare protein for tissue repair. Daily calorie requirements may range from 40 to 60 cal/kg, a 30% to 100% increase above normal. Although metabolic rate peaks around the 10th postburn day, metabolism (and, therefore, calorie requirements) remains high for several weeks or longer, depending on the extent of the burn. The distribution of calories should be approximately 25% protein, 50% CHO, and 25% fat.

EXAMPLE

A 165-lb man (75 kg) needs approximately:

Protein: 75 kg × 1.5 g protein = 112.5 g protein
75 kg × 3 g protein = 225 g protein
Daily protein requirement = 112.5 to 225 g
Calories: 75 kg × 40 cal/kg = 3000 calories
75 kg × 60 cal/kg = 4500 calories
Daily calorie requirement = 3000 to 4500 calories

Provide adequate fluid intake; water losses may be 10 to 12 times above normal in the first few postburn weeks. Encourage fruit juices high in potassium and vitamin C.
Promote maximum intake:

- Work with the client and family to solicit food preferences. Young children may regress in their eating behaviors; adults may prefer foods associated with recovery as children (*e.g.*, chicken soup).
- Encourage the family to bring food from home.
- Discourage the intake of empty-calorie food and beverages.
- Provide small, frequent meals; assist as needed.
- Provide emotional support and allow the client to verbalize his feelings.
- If possible, schedule debridement and other medical and surgical procedures at a time when they are least likely to interfere with meals.
- Provide pain medication as needed before meals.

Client Teaching

Instruct the client
On the importance of nutrition in wound healing and avoiding complications.
On the rationale and principles of diet management for burns, and how to implement the appropriate dietary modifications, especially ways to add protein and calories to the diet (see box).
That postburn weight loss is to be expected, but that weight eventually should be restored.
To take vitamins/minerals as ordered, to hasten recovery and wound healing.

Monitor

Monitor for the following signs or symptoms:
Fluid and electrolyte balance and observe for signs of dehydration/overhydration
Progress and tolerance of the feeding regimen; progress or discontinue as indicated
The need for follow-up diet counseling and additional diet modifications
After fluid balance is restored and feedings have begun, record body weight and intake of protein and calories daily to assess diet adequacy. Suggested guidelines for weight gain (if complications do not develop) are as follows:

- <20% BSA burned: regain weight in about 5 weeks.
- 20% to 30% BSA burned: lose weight for the first 5 postburn weeks. Thereafter, the client should gain weight slowly. Preburn weight may or may not be achieved before discharge.
- ≥40% BSA burned: may lose weight for about the first 8 postburn weeks. Thereafter, the client should gain weight slowly.

Monitor laboratory studies (albumin, transferrin, total lymphocyte count, creatinine–height index) after the initial stress response and peak period of catabolism subsides to assess nutritional status. Low serum transferrin and anergy are strongly correlated to the development of wound infections.[8]

Monitor for signs and symptoms of sepsis: fever, abdominal distention, ileus, disorientation.

Evaluation

Evaluation is ongoing. Assuming the plan of care has not changed, the client will achieve the goals as stated above.

Nutritional Immunology: Looking for the Magic Bullet

Studies have shown that simple protein–calorie malnutrition negatively affects immune function by impairing the effectiveness of phagocytes, reducing the number and function of T lymphocytes, and decreasing the production of antibodies. Stress (*e.g.,* surgery, trauma, critical illness, infection) superimposed on protein–calorie malnutrition can have devastating effects.

Nutritional immunology has been an area of accelerated research within the last decade. Although advances are being made, there is still much to be learned. Future research will likely focus on specialized formulas and specific immunotherapy for defined groups of clients.[6] Futuristic "magic bullets" may include:

Specific amino acids. In animal and human studies, the amino acid arginine has been shown to stimulate cell-mediated immune response and, in animals, protect against bacterial challenges. Clinical studies have shown improved immune function in cancer patients fed arginine,[6] leading some researchers to propose that arginine comprise 25% of the total protein content of enteral and parenteral formulas, instead of the current level of 5%.

Glutamine has been shown to be beneficial for gut function and intestinal mucosal integrity, and may become a conditionally essential nutrient for preserving mucosal integrity during injury.[1] It is also an important substrate for rapidly proliferating cells, including lymphocytes, and it appears to be the major amino acid lost during muscle protein catabolism in the initial response to injury. Enteral glutamine has been shown to preserve and improve muscle cellularity in the small bowel, which may prevent the translocation of bowel organisms into the lymph nodes, other organs, and the bloodstream. Critically ill clients with impaired gut mucosa would benefit the most from this effect.

Studies have shown that branched-chain amino acids (BCAA) improve whole-body protein and albumin synthesis. Because BCAA are required for the synthesis of acute-phase proteins and for gluconeogenesis, the body breaks down muscle tissue to provide BCAA when exogenous intake of BCAA is inadequate. Enteral and parenteral formulas supplemented with BCAA help to minimize muscle wasting and promote the synthesis of proteins involved in immune reactions.

Nucleotides. Dietary nucleotides appear to increase protein synthesis and also have a vital role in the maintenance of cellular immunity. A nucleotide-fortified diet may have therapeutic applications in patients experiencing infectious complications after adaptation to parenteral or enteral formulas that are typically nucleotide-free.[5]

Lipids. Recent research indicates that the type and amount of lipid present in enteral and parenteral formulas influence immune function. Long-chain fatty acids, used extensively for calories and to prevent essential fatty acid deficiency, have been shown to interfere with macrophage function, which ultimately may allow translocated bacteria from the gut to bypass the

(continued)

Food for Thought
(continued)

Nutritional Immunology:
Looking for the Magic Bullet *(continued)*

liver and become sequestered in the lungs, where secondary inflammation may occur.[6] Omega-3 fatty acids have been shown to improve immune function, probably through an alteration of prostaglandin synthesis or by changes in the phospholipid content of cell membranes.

Micronutrients. Zinc is a cofactor for several enzymes involved in the synthesis of acute phase proteins; a deficiency impairs platelet aggregation, chemotaxis, and delays wound healing. Likewise, an increase in oxidation secondary to inflammation increases the need for antioxidants, such as selenium, vitamin E, and copper. Exact amounts and proportions have yet to be determined.

BIBLIOGRAPHY

1. Andrassy RJ: Practical rewards of enteral feeding for the surgical patient. Contemporary Surgery 35(5A):20, 1989
2. Cerra F: Branch-chain amino acids and stress staging. Current Concepts in Nutritional Support, Monograph 1. Prepared and published by Biomedical Information Corporation, New York, as a service by Norwich Eaton Pharmaceuticals, Inc., 1983
3. Clark NG: Vitamin and mineral requirements in the stressed patient. Current Concepts in Nutritional Support, Monograph 3. Prepared and published by Biomedical Information Corporation, New York, as a service by Norwich Eaton Pharmaceuticals, Inc., 1984
4. Escott-Stump S: Nutrition and Diagnosis-Related Care. 2nd ed. Philadelphia, Lea and Febiger, 1988
5. Fanslow WC, Kulkarni AD, Van Buren CT, et al: Effect of nucleotide restriction and supplementation on resistance to experimental murine candidiasis. Journal of Parenteral and Enteral Nutrition 12(1):49, 1988
6. Haw MP, Bell SJ, Blackburn GL: Potential of parenteral and enteral nutrition in inflammation and immune dysfunction: A new challenge for dietitians. J Am Diet Assoc 91:701, 1991
7. Hunt DR, Maslovitz A, Rowlands BJ, et al: A simple nutrition screening procedure for hospital patients. J Am Diet Assoc 85:332, 1985
8. Jensen TG, Long JM, Dudrick SJ, et al: Nutritional assessment indications of postburn complications. J Am Diet Assoc 85:68, 1985
9. Quality Assurance Committee, Dietitians in Critical Care Dietetic Practice Group: Suggested Guidelines for Nutrition Management of the Critically Ill Patient. Chicago: American Dietetic Association, 1984
10. Ross Laboratories: Dietary Modification in HIV Disease. Columbus, OH: Ross Laboratories, 1990
11. Scherer JC: Introductory Medical–Surgical Nursing. 5th ed. Philadelphia: JB Lippincott, 1991

15 Digestive System Disorders

The digestive system is composed of the alimentary canal (gastrointestinal tract) and the accessory organs (the liver, pancreas, and gallbladder). Its function is to break down food physically and chemically into particles that the body can absorb and use (Fig. 15-1). Digestion begins with the oral phase, where food is chewed and mixed with saliva. The gastric phase follows, in which pepsin, gastric acid, salivary amylase, and lipase work to break down food chemically as the stomach physically churns and mixes its contents. The food then enters the small intestine, the primary site of digestion. Pancreatic amylase and lipase, proteases, and phospholipase characterize the pancreatic phase; the intestinal phase involves disaccharidases (maltase, lactase, sucrose), peptidases, and cholecystokinin for bile salts (Table 15-1).

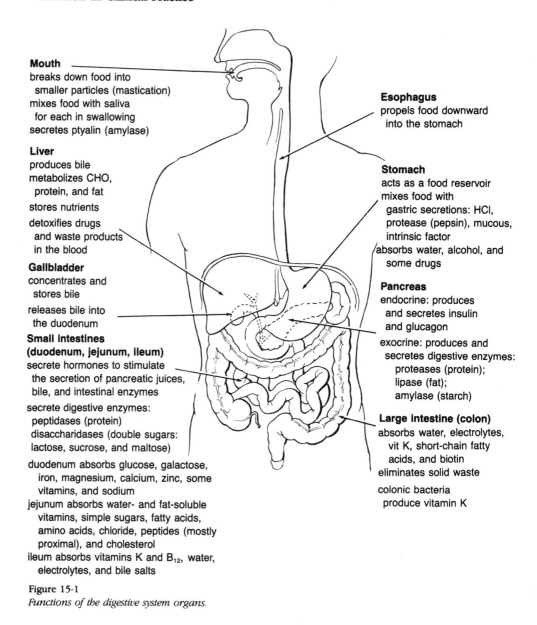

Mouth
breaks down food into
  smaller particles (mastication)
mixes food with saliva
  for each in swallowing
secretes ptyalin (amylase)

Liver
produces bile
metabolizes CHO,
  protein, and fat
stores nutrients
detoxifies drugs
  and waste products
  in the blood

Gallbladder
concentrates and
  stores bile
releases bile into
  the duodenum

**Small intestines
(duodenum, jejunum, ileum)**
secrete hormones to stimulate
  the secretion of pancreatic juices,
  bile, and intestinal enzymes
secrete digestive enzymes:
  peptidases (protein)
  disaccharidases (double sugars:
  lactose, sucrose, and maltose)
duodenum absorbs glucose, galactose,
  iron, magnesium, calcium, zinc, some
  vitamins, and sodium
jejunum absorbs water- and fat-soluble
  vitamins, simple sugars, fatty acids,
  amino acids, chloride, peptides (mostly
  proximal), and cholesterol
ileum absorbs vitamins K and B_{12}, water,
  electrolytes, and bile salts

Esophagus
propels food downward
  into the stomach

Stomach
acts as a food reservoir
mixes food with
  gastric secretions: HCl,
  protease (pepsin), mucous,
  intrinsic factor
absorbs water, alcohol, and
  some drugs

Pancreas
endocrine: produces
  and secretes insulin
  and glucagon
exocrine: produces and
  secretes digestive enzymes:
    proteases (protein);
    lipase (fat);
    amylase (starch)

Large intestine (colon)
absorbs water, electrolytes,
  vit K, short-chain fatty
  acids, and biotin
eliminates solid waste
colonic bacteria
  produce vitamin K

Figure 15-1
Functions of the digestive system organs.

Absorption is the process by which the end products of digestion pass from the gut into the bloodstream, or lymph system, as in the case of fat absorption. Absorption occurs primarily in the small intestine, although water is absorbed from the stomach, small intestine, and large intestine. The large intestine completes the process of absorption and excretes the residue as solid waste.

The entire process of digestion and absorption generally takes 24 hours; however, motility is affected by numerous variables, including food and fluid intake, activity and muscle tone, emotional factors, certain drug therapies, and alterations in digestion or absorption.

Table 15-1
Summary of Chemical Digestion

	CHO (Starch, Lactose, Sucrose, Maltose)	Protein	Fat (Triglycerides: Emulsified, Unemulsified)
Mouth	Starch $\xrightarrow[\substack{(minor) \\ significance}]{amylase}$ dextrin → maltose		
Stomach		Protein $\xrightarrow[HCl]{pepsin}$ polypeptides	Emulsified fat $\xrightarrow{lipase}$ fatty acids and glycerol (minor significance)
Small intestines Gallbladder secretions			Unemulsified fat $\xrightarrow{bile}$ emulsified fat
Pancreatic juices	Starch $\xrightarrow{amylase}$ dextrins → maltose	Protein, polypeptides $\xrightarrow{proteases}$ dipeptides + *amino acids*	Emulsified fat $\xrightarrow{lipase}$ *fatty acids, glycerol, diglycerides, and monoglycerides*
Intestinal villi secretions	Lactose $\xrightarrow{lactase}$ *glucose + galactose* Sucrose $\xrightarrow{sucrase}$ *glucose + fructose* Maltose $\xrightarrow{maltase}$ *glucose + glucose*	Polypeptides, Dipeptides $\xrightarrow{dipeptidases}$ *amino acids*	

Italic denotes end products ready for absorption

ROLE OF DIET THERAPY

Diet intervention is often used to treat/control gastrointestinal (GI) disorders or to alleviate/prevent their symptoms. The reader will note that client goals are often to *lessen* symptoms rather than *eliminate* them; diet is not the sole cause or cure for most altered health states. However, certain therapeutic diets have proved effective in the treatment of GI disorders; the validity of imposing rigid dietary restriction for others is questionable (Table 15-2). Because conservative diet therapy may be unnecessarily restrictive, the trend is toward more liberal dietary approaches. At the very least, diet intervention can help to correct nutritional deficiencies caused by GI disorders and their treatments.

Before the optimal diet intervention can be planned, a general assessment of GI status is indicated (see box, General Gastrointestinal Assessment Criteria). Additional assessment criteria are provided, where applicable.

COMMON GASTROINTESTINAL PROBLEMS

Anorexia, nausea and vomiting, diarrhea, and constipation are common GI disorders that may occur as isolated incidents, as symptoms of underlying GI disorders, as a result of viral or bacterial infections, or secondary to drug therapy or medical treatment. Because they are common symptoms for a variety of disorders, they are covered here in depth. The nursing process for these disorders remains the same whether they are primary or secondary problems, and regardless of the underlying pathology.

Table 15-2
***Effectiveness of Therapeutic Diets
in Gastrointestinal Disorders***

Proven Effective	*Questionable Effectiveness*
Gluten-free for celiac disease	Bland diet for peptic ulcers
Low protein for encephalopathy	High fiber for colon disorders
Restricted CHO for dumping syndrome	Low fat for gallbladder disease
Disaccharide restricted for disaccharide deficiency (*i.e.,* lactose restricted for lactase deficiency)	

Source: *Arvanitakis C: Diet therapy in gastrointestinal disease: A commentary.*
J Am Diet Assoc 75:449, 1979

ANOREXIA

Anorexia is defined as the lack of appetite, and differs from anorexia nervosa, a psychological condition characterized by the denial of appetite. In addition to the contributing factors listed above, anorexia may occur secondary to fear, anxiety, pain, and depression, or from an impaired ability to smell and taste secondary to chronic rhinitis, olfactory and glossopharyngeal damage, laryngectomy, or certain drug therapies. The aim of diet management is to stimulate the appetite and attain/maintain adequate nutritional intake.

Nursing Process

Assessment

In addition to the general GI assessment criteria, assess for the following factors:

Anorexia: onset, frequency, causative factors, severity, interventions attempted and the results.

Dietary changes made in response to anorexia (*i.e.,* foods avoided, foods preferred). Determine foods best tolerated and least tolerated.

Present intake, paying particular attention to meal frequency, food aversions, and fat intake—fat delays gastric emptying and provides a feeling of fullness, which inhibits appetite. Determine how much and how often high-fat foods are eaten: fried foods; fatty meats and luncheon meats; whole milk and milk products; butter, margarine, and oils; and rich desserts.

Intake and output; observe for signs of dehydration.

Weight. Compare actual weight to "healthy" weight. Assess amount and severity of any recent weight loss and observe for signs of malnutrition.

Activity patterns.

Nursing Diagnosis

Altered Nutrition: Less than Body Requirements, related to anorexia.

Assessment Criteria

General Gastrointestinal Assessment Criteria

Appetite

Recent change in appetite

Ability to chew, swallow, and taste; oral and dental health

Activity: frequency, intensity

Feeding modality (oral, enteral, parenteral)

Signs or symptoms of altered GI function (reflux, indigestion, nausea, vomiting, diarrhea, constipation, bloating, cramping); onset, frequency, contributing factors, severity, interventions attempted and results

Weight status

Recent weight change: nature of change, onset, severity, contributing factors

Usual bowel habits: frequency; time of day; description of usual stool characteristics, including amount, consistency, shape, color, odor

Recent changes in bowel elimination

Use of elimination aids: fluids, particular foods, laxatives, stool softeners, enemas

Drug therapies: antacids, stool softeners, diuretics, laxatives, cimetidine, other

Psychological benefits or hazards of diet intervention

Client's attitude and willingness to modify diet

Planning and Implementation

To enhance appetite, serve food attractively and season according to individual taste. If decreased ability to taste is contributing to anorexia, enhance food flavors with tart seasonings (orange juice, lemonade, vinegar, lemon juice) or strong seasonings (basil, oregano, rosemary, tarragon, mint).

If possible, schedule procedures and medications at a time when they are least likely to interfere with appetite. Also, control pain, nausea, or depression with medications, as ordered.

Liquid supplements provided as in-between meal nourishments can significantly improve protein and calorie intake and generally are well accepted. In addition, liquids tend to leave the stomach quickly and are therefore less likely to interfere with meals.

Client Goals

The client will:

Experience less anorexia.

Consume adequate calories and protein to attain/maintain "healthy" weight.

Describe the principles and rationale for dietary management to relieve anorexia, and implement the appropriate dietary interventions.

Identify factors contributing to anorexia, when known.

Nursing Interventions

Diet Management

Provide small, frequent meals or in-between meal supplements, as needed.

Limit fat intake, if fat is contributing to early satiety.

Solicit food preferences and allow food from home if possible. Provide encouragement and a pleasant eating environment.

Client Teaching

Instruct the client

To stay calm, especially at mealtimes, and not to hurry through meals.

On the principles and rationale of diet management to relieve anorexia.

That small, frequent meals may be better tolerated than three large meals.

To eat a varied diet to stimulate appetite.

To avoid high-fat foods, if they are contributing to anorexia.

That an increase in activity, when possible, can help stimulate appetite.

Monitor

Monitor for the following signs or symptoms:

Compliance with the diet, and the need for follow-up diet counseling

Adequacy of intake

Effectiveness of diet interventions and the need for further modifications

Weight, weight changes

Evaluation

Evaluation is ongoing. Assuming the plan of care has not changed, the client will achieve the goals as stated above.

NAUSEA AND VOMITING

Nausea is defined as the sensation of impending vomiting, which may or may not be followed by emesis. Nausea and vomiting may be related to a decrease in gastric acid secretion, a decrease in digestive enzyme activity, a decrease in GI motility, gastric irritation, or acidosis. Other causes include bacterial and viral infections, increased intracranial pressure, equilibrium imbalance, liver, pancreatic, and gallbladder disorders, and pyloric and intestinal obstruction. Drugs and certain medical treatments may also contribute to nausea.

Nursing Process

Assessment

In addition to the general GI assessment criteria, assess for the following factors:

Nausea and vomiting: onset, frequency, causative factors, severity, interventions attempted, and results.

Dietary changes made in response to nausea and vomiting (*i.e.*, foods avoided, foods preferred). Determine foods best and least tolerated.

Fat intake: fat delays gastric emptying and provides a feeling of fullness, which inhibits appetite. Determine how much and how often high-fat foods are eaten: fried foods; fatty meats and luncheon meats; whole milk and milk products; butter, margarine, and oils; and rich desserts.

Fluid intake with meals: fluid can cause a full, bloated feeling.

Intake and output; observe for signs of dehydration and electrolyte imbalances.

Weight, and the severity of any recent weight loss; observe for signs of malnutrition.

Nursing Diagnosis

Altered Nutrition: Less than Body Requirements, related to nausea and vomiting.

Planning and Implementation

Solicit food preferences and observe individual food intolerances. Dry toast, crackers, or other carbohydrates eaten before the client gets out of bed in the morning may help avoid nausea.

Sodium and chloride are lost through emesis and may need to be replaced if vomiting is severe or prolonged.

Client Goals

The client will:

Experience less nausea and vomiting.

Maintain normal fluid and electrolyte balance.

Consume adequate calories and protein to attain/maintain "healthy" weight.

Describe the principles and rationale of diet management to relieve nausea and vomiting, and implement the appropriate dietary interventions.

Identify factors causing nausea and vomiting, when known.

Nursing Interventions

Diet Management

Withhold food until nausea/vomiting subsides.

Progress oral feedings as the client's tolerance improves: clear liquids → full liquids → diet as tolerated. Small, frequent meals of readily digested carbohydrates (toast, crackers, plain rolls, pretzels, angelfood cake, oatmeal, soft, bland fruit) are generally best tolerated.

Elevate the head of the bed.

Encourage the client to eat slowly.

Promote good oral hygiene with mouthwash and ice chips.

Limit liquids with meals because they can cause a full, bloated feeling.

Serve foods at room temperature or chilled; hot foods may contribute to nausea.

Client Teaching

Instruct the client

On the principles and rationale of diet management to relieve nausea and vomiting.

Not to eat when he or she feels nauseated.

To replace fluid and electrolytes with whatever liquids he or she can tolerate: clear soup and juice, gelatin, ginger ale, popsicles.

Monitor

Monitor for the following signs or symptoms:

Compliance with the diet, and the need for follow-up diet counseling

Adequacy of intake

Effectiveness of diet interventions and the need for further diet modifications

Weight, weight changes

Intake and output, and fluid balance (for vomiting)

Evaluation

Evaluation is ongoing. Assuming the plan of care has not changed, the client will achieve the goals as stated above.

DIARRHEA

Diarrhea is characterized by the excretion of frequent, watery stools. It can cause large losses of potassium and fluid, and also reduces the time available for the absorption of all other nutrients. Severe or prolonged diarrhea can quickly lead to nutritional complications.

Emotional or physical stress, GI disorders and malabsorption syndromes, metabolic and endocrine disorders, surgical bowel intervention, certain drug therapies and medical treatments, and bacterial, viral, and parasitic infections are common causes of diarrhea. Nutritionally, food allergies and the use of tube feedings are related to diarrhea. Also, coffee or caffeine stimulates peristalsis in some people, and an excessive intake of foods high in fiber or laxative properties can increase stool frequency.

Nursing Process

Assessment

In addition to the general GI assessment criteria, assess for the following factors:

Diarrhea: onset, frequency, causative factors, severity, interventions attempted and results.

Dietary changes made in response to diarrhea (i.e., foods avoided, foods preferred). Determine foods best and least tolerated.

Intake of high-fiber foods that may be contributing to diarrhea: bran, whole-grain breads and cereals, raw vegetables, fresh fruits, and prunes/prune juice.

Milk intake and whether a relationship exists between milk consumption and diarrhea (i.e., whether the client may have primary or secondary lactose intolerance).

Coffee/caffeine intake, and determine if a relationship exists between caffeine consumption and diarrhea.

Intake and output; observe for signs of dehydration and hypokalemia.

If chronic, client weight and signs of malnutrition.

Nursing Diagnosis

Diarrhea, related to _____ (causative factor).

Planning and Implementation

Because fluid and electrolyte balance is the principal concern with acute diarrhea, a high fluid intake is the primary diet intervention.

Chronic diarrhea can cause not only fluid and electrolyte imbalances, but also weight loss and nutrient inadequacies related to decreased transit time. Any foods suspected of causing or aggravating diarrhea (*e.g.,* milk, coffee, caffeine, high-fiber foods) should be eliminated. Low-residue foods and foods high in pectin (firm bananas, skinless apple, applesauce, white rice) may help firm stools. Clients not responding to traditional medical and dietary treatment may need bowel rest.

Client Goals

The client will:

Have fewer and less frequent stools.

Maintain normal fluid and electrolyte balance.

Consume adequate calories and protein to attain/maintain "healthy" weight.

Describe the principles and rationale of diet management to relieve diarrhea, and implement the appropriate dietary interventions.

Identify causative factors, if known.

Nursing Interventions

Diet Management

Encourage clear fluids for acute diarrhea (usually subsides within 24 to 48 hours); no other diet intervention is necessary.

For chronic diarrhea, withhold food for 24 to 48 hours and provide intravenous fluid and electrolytes to maintain hydration.

Progress oral intake according to individual tolerance: clear liquids → full liquids → low-residue diet (see box, Low-Residue Diet) until diarrhea has completely subsided.

Encourage the intake of foods high in pectin, which helps firm the stools: scraped raw skinless apple, apple sauce, and firm bananas. Increase protein, calorie, and potassium intake, as needed, to replenish losses.

Avoid very hot or cold food and beverages because they stimulate colonic activity. For that reason, caffeine should also be avoided: coffee, strong tea, some sodas, and chocolate (see Appendix 8).

Avoid milk and milk products until diarrhea has completely subsided, because lactose intolerance may be contributing to diarrhea.

Avoid carbonated beverages because their electrolyte content is low and osmolality is high.

Client Teaching

Instruct the client on the principles and rationale of diet management to relieve diarrhea, using these guidelines:

(*Text continued on page 417*)

Low-Residue Diet (Low-Fiber Diet)

Characteristics

Restricts fiber and residue
Restrictions vary considerably among institutions and from mild to severe

Objective

Reduce stool bulk and slow transit time

Indications for Use

Bowel inflammation, as seen in the acute stages of diverticulitis, ulcerative
    colitis, and regional enteritis
Esophageal and intestinal stenosis
Preparation for bowel surgery

Contraindications

Irritable colon
Diverticulosis

Foods Allowed

Meats: Eggs; ground or well-cooked tender meat, fish, and poultry
Dairy: Up to 2 cups of milk/day; mild cheeses
Fruits: Juices without pulp, except prune; canned fruit, and ripe bananas
Vegetables: Vegetable juices without pulp; lettuce, and cooked vegetables
    such as asparagus, beets, green beans, seedless tomatoes, acorn squash,
    spinach, and eggplant
Breads and cereals: Only white bread and refined bread and cereal products:
    crackers, bagels; melba toast, waffles, refined cereals such as Cream of
    Wheat, Cream of Rice, and puffed rice
Miscellaneous: Plain desserts made with allowed foods such as fruit ices, plain
    cakes, puddings (rice, bread, plain), cookies without nuts or coconut,
    sherbet, ice cream (no nuts or coconut); gelatin; candy such as
    butterscotch, jelly beans, marshmallows, plain hard candy; honey,
    molasses, sugar

Foods Not Allowed

Meats: Tough meats
Dairy: More than 2 cups of milk/day

(continued)

Low-Residue Diet (Low-Fiber Diet) *(continued)*

Fruits: All other raw, cooked or dried fruits

Vegetables: All other raw or cooked vegetables

Breads and cereals: Whole-grain breads and cereals, especially those made with bran or cracked wheat

Miscellaneous: Nuts, peanut butter, coconut, anything made with nuts or coconut, olives, pickles, seeds, popcorn, dried peas and beans

Low-Residue Diet

Sample Menu

Breakfast

Strained orange juice

Cream of Rice

Poached egg

White toast with butter and jelly

½ cup milk

Coffee/tea

Salt/pepper/sugar

Lunch

Tomato juice

Sandwich made with white bread, ham, and mayonnaise

Canned peach halves

Sponge cake

½ cup milk

Coffee/tea

Salt/pepper/sugar

Dinner

Roast chicken

White rice

Acorn squash

Italian bread with butter

Gelatin made with bananas

½ cup milk

Coffee/tea

Salt/pepper/sugar

(continued)

Low-Residue Diet (Low-Fiber Diet) *(continued)*

Snack

Saltine crackers

½ cup milk

Potential Problem/Rationale

Nutrient deficiencies, especially of the following:
- Calcium, due to the limited amount of milk and dairy products allowed.
- Iron, because many adults refuse to eat ground meats (meat is the richest source of iron in the diet). In addition, other sources of iron, like dried fruits and many iron-fortified cereals, are prohibited.
- Vitamins, because few kinds of vegetables are allowed on a low-residue diet; those that are allowed may be vitamin-poor because processing techniques used to reduce the fiber content also remove vitamins.

Nursing Interventions and Considerations

Monitor laboratory values and observe for signs of deficiencies. Provide supplements as needed.

Encourage as varied an intake as possible and liberalize the diet as soon as possible.

Potential Problem/Rationale

Inadequate calorie intake related to the highly restrictive nature of the diet. Also, many adults refuse to eat strained food because it resembles baby food.

Nursing Interventions and Considerations

Honor special requests of allowed foods, if possible.

Liberalize the diet as soon as possible.

Potential Problem/Rationale

Constipation related to the low-fiber content of the diet: Insufficient fiber intake causes a decrease in stool bulk and slowing of intestinal transit time.

Nursing Interventions and Considerations

Liberalize the diet to allow more fiber.

(continued)

Low-Residue Diet (Low-Fiber Diet) (*continued*)

Potential Problem/Rationale

Persistent diarrhea related to poor tolerance to even the small amounts of fiber contained in a low-residue diet. Tolerance to fiber varies among clients and conditions.

Nursing Interventions and Considerations

Further reduce the residue content of the diet by eliminating all fruits and vegetables, except strained fruit juice.

Low-Residue Diet Teaching

Instruct the client

That fiber is a component of plants and, therefore, is found in fruits, vegetables, grains, and nuts.

That milk and milk products are limited because they leave a residue after digestion.

That reducing residue intake will slow the passage of food through the bowel.

That the diet will probably be short-term.

On food preparation techniques to reduce residue:
- Skins, seeds, and membranes of fruits and vegetables are high in fiber and should be removed.
- Cook allowed vegetables until very tender.

Follow a low-residue diet until diarrhea subsides.

Replace lost potassium with rich sources that the client can tolerate: bananas, canned apricots and peaches, apricot nectar, tomato juice, fish, potatoes, meat (see Appendix 9).

Eat small, frequent meals.

Avoid foods that may contribute to cramping: carbonated beverages, beer, gassy vegetables (such as broccoli, cauliflower, cabbage, brussels sprouts, onions, legumes, melons), spicy food, excessive sweets.

Drink plenty of liquids, but avoid milk until diarrhea subsides.

Eliminate coffee/caffeine for a trial period to see if any improvement occurs.

Monitor

Monitor for the following signs or symptoms:

Compliance with the diet, and the need for follow-up diet counseling

Effectiveness of diet interventions, and the need for further diet modification

Weight, weight changes

Intake and output, and fluid and electrolyte balance

Evaluation

Evaluation is ongoing. Assuming the plan of care has not changed, the client will achieve the goals as stated above.

CONSTIPATION

Constipation is marked by the difficult or infrequent passage of stools that may be hard and dry. Irregular bowel habits, psychogenic factors, lack of activity, chronic laxative use, inadequate intake of fluid and fiber, metabolic and endocrine disorders, and bowel abnormalities (tumors, hernias, strictures, diverticular disease, irritable colon) are causative factors. Likewise, constipation can occur secondary to certain drug therapies.

Nursing Process

Assessment

In addition to the general GI assessment criteria, assess for the following factors:

Constipation: onset, duration, causative factors, severity, interventions attempted and the results

Dietary changes made in response to constipation, (*i.e.*, foods avoided, foods preferred)

Usual fiber intake, especially foods high in insoluble fiber, which increases stool bulk and stimulates peristalsis (*i.e.*, wheat bran, whole-grain bread and cereals, raw vegetables, and fresh fruits). Assess client's ability to chew high-fiber foods, and his or her willingness to eat a high-fiber diet.

Adequacy of fluid intake: adults need the equivalent of about eight glasses of water a day.

Frequency and intensity of usual activity pattern

Nursing Diagnosis

Constipation, related to an inadequate intake of fluid and fiber.

Planning and Implementation

Elimination patterns vary with diet and activity. Daily bowel movements are not necessary, provided the stools are not hard and dry.

Generally, a high-fiber diet is used to alleviate constipation. This diet is high in both soluble and insoluble fiber, even though only insoluble fiber has been credited with increasing stool bulk and stimulating peristalsis. This diet must be initiated gradually to maximize tolerance; eating too much fiber before tolerance is established may cause gas, distention, or diarrhea. Individual tolerance to fiber varies.

Discourage the use of mineral oil laxatives, which can cause malabsorption of the fat-soluble vitamins. Likewise, discourage the use of fiber "pills," which can cause constipation or even intestinal blockages, especially when taken in large amounts and with inadequate fluid.

In some cases of constipation, adding fat to the diet may have a laxative effect; fat stimulates bile secretion, which draws water into the GI tract (because of high salt content) to produce softer stools and stimulate peristalsis.

Client Goals

The client will:

Have soft bowel movements.

Consume an adequate fiber intake by substituting foods high in fiber for foods low in fiber.

Drink the equivalent of at least eight glasses of water daily.

Describe the principles and rationale of diet management to relieve constipation, and implement the appropriate diet interventions.

Identify causative factors, if known.

Nursing Interventions

Diet Management

Increase fiber intake gradually, until an effective, yet tolerable, level is achieved (see box, High-Fiber Diet).

Promote adequate fluid intake. To help stimulate peristalsis, encourage the client to drink hot coffee, tea, or lemon water after waking.

Encourage the intake of prunes and prune juice, which have laxative effects.

Client Teaching

Instruct the client

On the principles and rationale of diet management to relieve constipation. Explain that diet can produce relief, but does not cure constipation.

To establish a bowel elimination routine.

That physical activity promotes muscle tone and stimulates bowel activity. Encourage the client to exercise regularly.

To avoid the use of over-the-counter laxatives, stool softeners, and fiber "pills" unless recommended by the physician.

Monitor

Monitor for the following signs or symptoms:

Tolerance of increased fiber intake (*i.e.*, absence of excessive flatus, distention, diarrhea)

Compliance with the diet, and the need for follow-up diet counseling

Effectiveness of diet interventions, and the need for further diet modification

Evaluation

The client

Has soft bowel movements.

Consumes an adequate fiber intake by substituting foods high in fiber for foods low in fiber.

Drinks the equivalent of at least eight glasses of water daily.

Describes the principles and rationale of diet management to relieve constipation, and implements the appropriate diet interventions.

Identifies causative factors, if known.

(*Text continued on page 423*)

High-Fiber Diet

Characteristics

Normal diet that substitutes high-fiber foods for foods low in fiber

Unprocessed bran may be added as tolerated.

Includes at least four servings of fruits and vegetables a day, preferably fresh or raw

Objective

Insoluble fiber helps to increase fecal bulk and weight, increase GI motility, and decrease pressure within the bowel. Soluble fibers help lower serum cholesterol levels and improve glucose tolerance in diabetes.

Indications for Use

Constipation, diverticulosis, and irritable bowel syndrome

May be used to improve glucose tolerance in diabetics (see Chap. 17) or to help lower serum cholesterol levels in clients with hypercholesterolemia (see Chap. 16)

May aid weight reduction; may help protect against colon cancer

Contraindications

Intestinal inflammation or stenosis

Excellent Sources of Fiber

Bran

Breads and cereals containing 4.5 g or more fiber/serving

Dried peas and beans

Prunes, apricots, figs

Good Sources of Fiber

Breads and cereals containing 2 g or more fiber/serving

Corn, peas, spinach, sweet potatoes, brussels sprouts

Blueberries, dates, raisins, apples, pears, oranges

High-Fiber Diet

Sample
Menu

Breakfast

Prune juice

Bran cereal

(continued)

High-Fiber Diet (*continued*)

Milk
Whole-wheat toast with butter
Orange
Coffee/tea
Salt/pepper/sugar

Lunch

Split pea soup
Julienne salad made with cheese, egg, lettuce, tomato, carrots, and other
    vegetables as desired
Salad dressing
Whole-wheat crackers
Apple
Milk
Coffee/tea
Salt/pepper/sugar

Dinner

Roast chicken
Brown rice
Buttered peas
Coleslaw
Bran muffin with butter
Fresh strawberries
Coffee/tea
Salt/pepper/sugar

Snack

Oatmeal raisin cookies
Milk

Potential Problem/Rationale

Flatus, distention, cramping, and osmotic diarrhea related to increasing the
fiber content of the diet too much or too quickly.

(*continued*)

High-Fiber Diet (*continued*)

Nursing Interventions and Considerations

Initiate a high-fiber diet slowly to develop the client's tolerance. If symptoms of intolerance persist, reduce the fiber content to the maximum amount tolerated by the client.

Potential Problem/Rationale

Possible malabsorption of calcium, zinc, and iron which may be related to the following situations:
- Increase in GI motility, which allows less time for absorption to occur
- Binding of fiber with nutrients to form compounds that the body cannot absorb
- Added bulk and water content of the intestines, which dilutes the concentration of nutrients
  Actual fiber-induced deficiencies are unlikely, however, possibly because the body adapts to a high-fiber diet.

Nursing Interventions and Considerations

Monitor lab values and observe for signs of deficiencies. Provide supplements if needed.
Encourage the intake of foods rich in calcium, zinc, and iron.

High-Fiber Diet Teaching

Instruct the client
That a high-fiber diet will increase stool bulk and speed the passage of food through the intestines.
On how to increase fiber intake by making subtle changes in eating and cooking habits, such as eating more fresh fruits and vegetables, especially with the skin on.
That switching to high-fiber bread and cereals can significantly increase fiber intake. The first ingredient on the label should be "whole wheat", not just "wheat."
To eat a variety of foods high in fiber; numerous forms of fiber exist and each performs a different action in the body (see Chap. 1).
To serve a meatless main dish made with legumes once a week.
To serve fresh or dried fruit for dessert or snack.
That although nuts and seeds are high in fiber, they are also high in fat and should be used sparingly.

(*continued*)

High-Fiber Diet (*continued*)

That coarse unprocessed wheat bran is most effective as a laxative and generally is cheaper than fresh fruits and vegetables. It can be incorporated into the diet by the following methods:
- Mixing it with juice or milk
- Adding it to muffins, quick breads, casseroles, and meat loaves before baking
- Sprinkling it over cereal, applesauce, eggs, or other foods

To add bran to the diet slowly (up to 3 tablespoons/day) to decrease the likelihood of developing flatus and distention.

That, (in addition to being high in fiber) certain foods have laxative effects: prunes and prune juice, figs, and dates.

To drink at least six to eight glasses of water daily.

IMPAIRED ABILITY TO SWALLOW

Whether the cause is mechanical (*i.e.*, obstruction, inflammation, edema, surgery of the throat) or neurologic (*i.e.*, ALS, myasthenia gravis, post CVA, head injury, Parkinson's disease, multiple sclerosis), alterations in the ability to swallow and chew can have a profound impact on intake and nutritional status, and greatly increase the risk of aspiration.

Swallowing is a complex series of events characterized by four distinct phases. The oral preparatory phase takes place in the mouth, where food (bolus) is chewed in preparation for swallowing. Obviously, liquids need little preparation compared to meat and raw vegetables. Clients who have difficulty with this phase may "pocket" food in the cheek, lose food from the lips, or may be unable to move food toward the back of the mouth.

In the oral phase, the bolus is pushed steadily backward toward the pharynx, which opens to receive the bolus. Impairments in the tongue's muscles or nerves interfere with the oral phase and can cause coughing or choking before the client swallows. Liquids, because they are difficult to control, are especially problematic.

The pharyngeal phase follows; as the food reaches the opening of the pharynx, the swallowing reflex is triggered and the food moves toward and into the esophagus. Food remaining in the throat, prolonged chewing, nasal regurgitation, coughing, choking during or after swallowing, and hoarseness after swallowing are all signs of problems with this phase.[4]

The process of swallowing is completed with the esophageal phase. Peristaltic movements carry the bolus through the esophagus into the stomach. Neurologically impaired clients have less difficulty with this phase than with the other phases. However, obstruction and reduced esophageal peristalsis are concerns. Unfortunately, problems with this phase are less amenable to intervention than problems with the other three phases.

Nursing Process

Assessment

In addition to the general GI assessment criteria, assess for the following factors:

Swallowing dysfunction: signs and symptoms of dysfunction, causative factors, severity, impact on intake. Signs of swallowing problems may not be obvious; observe subtle clues like facial drooping, drooling, and a weak/hoarse voice.

Dietary changes made in response to impaired swallowing (*i.e.,* food avoided and foods preferred).

Foods/liquids that are easiest and hardest to swallow.

Weight. Compare actual weight to "healthy" weight; observe for signs of malnutrition.

Nursing Diagnosis

Altered Nutrition: Less than Body Requirements, related to impaired swallowing secondary to _____ (causative factor).

Planning and Implementation

Encourage dysphagic clients to rest before mealtime, and coordinate meals with peak drug action if the client's motor weakness is dose-related.[5] Give mouth care immediately before meals to enhance the sense of taste.

To stimulate salivation, instruct the client to think of a specific food. A lemon slice, lemon hard candy, or dill pickles may also help trigger salivation.

Reduce or eliminate distractions at mealtime so that the client can focus his attention on swallowing. Limit disruptions, if possible, and do not rush the client. Place the client in an upright or Fowler's position.

Adaptive eating devices, like built-up utensils and mugs with spouts, may be indicated. Syringes should never be used to force liquids in the client's mouth because they may trigger choking or aspiration.[5]

Individualize texture, taste, and temperature. Semisolid or medium-consistency foods with strong flavors (*i.e.,* sweet, sour, and salty) served at room temperature are often best.

Consider tube feedings or parenteral nutrition if the client is unable to consume an adequate oral diet.

Refer clients with actual or potential swallowing impairments to the speech pathology department for a thorough swallowing assessment.

Client Goals

The client will:

Swallow food/liquids without aspirating.

Consume adequate calories and protein to attain/maintain "healthy" weight.

Describe the principles and rationale for the dietary management of swallowing impairments, if appropriate, and implement the appropriate diet interventions.

Nursing Interventions

Diet Management

Provide encouragement during meals.

Position the client in an upright position and tilt his or her head forward to facilitate swallowing. Postpone meals if the client is fatigued.

Individualize texture according to the client's tolerance; semisolid foods (casseroles, custards, scrambled eggs, cheese, yogurt, cottage cheese, cooked cereals) are easiest to swallow.

Serve food at room temperature to avoid overreaction to temperature extremes.

Serve strongly flavored foods to stimulate salivation. Melted butter, gravy, and jelly help moisten foods.

Offer small, frequent meals to maximize intake.

Avoid sticky, mucus-forming foods: peanut butter, white bread, milk, chocolate, ice cream, bananas.

Client Teaching

Instruct the client

On the principles and rationale of diet management to promote swallowing, if appropriate.

To relax and eat slowly, and to avoid eating while fatigued.

Monitor

Monitor for the following factors:

Compliance with the diet, and the need for follow-up diet counseling or swallowing evaluation

Effectiveness of diet intervention and the need for further diet modification

Weight status, weight changes

Evaluation

Evaluation is ongoing. Assuming the plan of care has not changed, the client will achieve the goals as stated above.

DISORDERS OF THE ESOPHAGUS: HIATAL HERNIA AND ESOPHAGITIS

Hiatal hernia and esophagitis are two esophageal disorders whose symptoms can be greatly improved through appropriate diet interventions. Hiatal hernia, characterized by the protrusion of part of the stomach through the esophageal opening of the diaphragm, may be caused by a congenital or acquired weakness of the diaphragm or from increased intra-abdominal pressure related to obesity, pregnancy, ascites, or physical exertion. Reflux esophagitis occurs when the backflow of acidic gastric juices causes irritation and inflammation of the lower esophageal mucosa. It may be caused by viral inflammation, ingestion of an irritant, or intubation. Recurrent reflux is often related to hiatal hernia, reduced lower esophageal sphincter (LES) pressure, and recurrent vomiting. Hiatal hernia and esophagitis can lead to dysphagia and esophageal ulcerations and bleeding.

The presence of a hiatal hernia may not be apparent until the symptoms of reflux esophagitis develop: heartburn, which may radiate to the neck and throat; pain that worsens when the client lies down, bends over after eating, or wears tight-fitting clothing; regurgitation; and possible melena, hematemesis, and dysphagia.

Antacid therapy and diet intervention are the cornerstones of medical treatment of hiatal hernia and esophagitis. If reflux is not relieved by medical treatment, a vagotomy or surgical repair may be necessary.

Nursing Process

Assessment

In addition to the general GI assessment criteria, assess for the following factors:

Symptoms: onset, frequency, relationship to eating, causative factors, severity, interventions attempted and the results

Dietary changes made in response to symptoms (*i.e.*, foods avoided, foods preferred). Determine foods best and least tolerated.

Usual intake of items known to decrease LES pressure, which contributes to "heartburn" (Table 15-3)

Intake of known gastric acid stimulants: coffee (regular and decaffeinated), caffeine (see Appendix 8), and pepper

The frequency of eating, especially if a snack or meal is eaten immediately before bed

Weight, weight status

Nursing Diagnosis

Altered Health Maintenance, related to the lack of knowledge of dietary management of _____ (causative factor).

Planning and Implementation

Low-residue and traditional bland diets, frequently used in the past to treat esophageal disorders, are unnecessarily restrictive and not valid. The most effective interventions are

Table 15-3
Factors that Decrease Lower Esophageal Sphincter (LES) Pressure

Alcohol
Caffeine
Chocolate
Fat
Peppermint and spearmint oils
Cigarette smoke

to lose weight, if overweight, and to avoid items that decrease LES pressure. Encourage a liberal intake of protein, because it increases LES pressure.

For optimal effectiveness, individualize the diet according to the client's tolerance.

Clients avoiding citrus juices because of their acidity should be encouraged to eat other sources of vitamin C: broccoli, brussels sprouts, strawberries, cantaloupe, greens.

Client Goals

The client will:

Be free of symptoms of hiatal hernia/esophagitis.

Lose weight, if overweight.

Describe the principles and rationale for dietary management of hiatal hernia/esophagitis and implement the appropriate diet interventions.

Identify factors contributing to hiatal hernia/esophagitis, when known.

Nursing Interventions

Diet Management

Promote weight loss in overweight clients to decrease intra-abdominal pressure. Eliminate foods known to decrease LES pressure (Table 15-3).

Encourage a liberal protein intake because protein increases LES pressure.

Provide small, frequent meals.

Avoid liquids immediately before and after meals to help prevent gastric distention.

Avoid items that stimulate gastric acid secretion: coffee (regular and decaffeinated), caffeine (see Appendix 8), alcohol, and pepper.

Eliminate foods that may irritate the esophagus, such as acidic juices like orange, grapefruit, and tomato.

Client Teaching

Instruct the client

On the principles and rationale of diet management to relieve symptoms of esophageal disorders.

To avoid foods that decrease LES pressure to help reduce heartburn.

To eliminate any foods not tolerated.

To chew food thoroughly.

To avoid lying down, bending over, and rigorous exercise after eating.

To avoid tight-fitting clothing.

To sleep with the head of the bed elevated.

That small, frequent meals may be better tolerated than three large meals.

Monitor

Monitor for the following signs or symptoms:

Food intolerances; clients who severely limit their food choices and those who eliminate citrus fruits and vegetables may be at risk for vitamin and mineral deficiencies.

Compliance with the diet, and the need for follow-up diet counseling

Effectiveness of diet intervention and the need for further diet modifications

Weight, if appropriate

Evaluation

Evaluation is ongoing. Assuming the plan of care has not changed, the client will achieve the goals as stated above.

DRUG ALERT: **ANTACIDS**

Interfere with iron absorption and may cause iron deficiency anemia.

Produce other side effects, depending on their composition:

Magnesium → diarrhea

Aluminum → constipation

Calcium → hypercalcemia

Sodium → fluid retention (sodium-containing antacids are contraindicated for clients requiring low-sodium diets)

DISORDERS OF THE STOMACH: PEPTIC ULCERS AND GASTRITIS

Peptic ulcer, characterized by erosion of the mucosal layer of the stomach (gastric ulcer) or duodenum (duodenal ulcer), is caused by an excess secretion of or decreased mucosal resistance to hydrochloric acid. Approximately 5% to 15% of American adults develop ulcers, only half of which may be diagnosed. Duodenal ulcers occur 10 times more frequently than gastric ulcers, are 4 times more common in men than in women, and usually are diagnosed around age 50. Gastric ulcers occur twice as frequently among men than women and usually are diagnosed after age 45.

Typically, ulcers produce dull, burning, or piercing pain when the stomach is empty. Heartburn, nausea, vomiting, and melena are possible. Their course usually alternates between periods of exacerbation and remission, with occurrences more common in spring and fall.

The development of ulcers may be related to the presence of one or more of the following risk factors:

- Physiologic and psychological stress
- Cigarette smoking
- Genetic factors
- Use of certain medications, such as aspirin and glucocorticoids
- Excessive coffee and caffeine consumption

Without proper treatment, ulcers can lead to hemorrhage, perforation, pyloric obstruction, and intractable ulcer. Various drug therapies (antacids, anticholinergics, H$_2$-receptor antagonists [cimetidine], antispasmodics, antimotility drugs, sedatives, tranquilizers), bed rest (to reduce environmental stress), and diet intervention are used as treatment. Complications may be treated surgically if medical treatment fails.

Gastritis is an inflammation of the gastric mucosa. Acute gastritis is a temporary irritation, usually self-limiting, caused by the ingestion of corrosive or infectious substances, such as aspirin; food poisoning; acute alcoholism; and uremia. Symptoms vary with the source of the irritation and range from mild (heartburn) to severe (vomiting, bleeding, hematemesis). Chronic gastritis is marked by progressive and irreversible atrophy of the gastric mucosa, which can lead to achlorhydria and pernicious anemia. Symptoms include nausea, vomiting, stomach pain, malaise, anorexia, headache, hematemesis, and hiccupping. Perforation, hemorrhage, and pyloric obstruction related to scar tissue formation may occur. The exact cause of chronic gastritis is unknown, but it may be related to overeating, stress, coffee and alcohol consumption, cigarette smoking, or chronic uremia.

Gastritis is treated by removing the offender and controlling symptoms (*i.e.*, vomiting, pain, blood loss) through drugs and diet. Surgery may be needed to treat complications. The objectives of diet intervention for both peptic ulcers and gastritis are to decrease gastric acid secretion and eliminate gastric irritants.

Nursing Process

Assessment

In addition to the general assessment criteria, assess for the following factors:
Symptoms: nature, onset, frequency, causative factors, severity, interventions attempted and the results. Determine if pain occurs when the stomach is empty or after eating.
Dietary changes made in response to symptoms (*i.e.*, food avoided, foods preferred). Determine foods best and least tolerated.
The client's use of tobacco, alcohol, drugs, and caffeine.

Nursing Diagnosis

Altered Health Maintenance, related to the lack of knowledge of dietary management of _____ (causative factor).

Planning and Implementation

During an attack of acute gastritis, food is withheld and intravenous fluids are provided until symptoms subside. Thereafter, the diet is liberalized according to individual tolerance.

Traditionally, ulcers and gastritis have been treated with progressive bland diets in an attempt to eliminate foods that are chemically and mechanically irritating to the stomach. Bland diets generally consist of three or more stages (see box, Traditional Progressive Bland Diet), and use milk liberally to "soothe" the stomach. Although the protein in milk effectively neutralizes stomach contents and provides immediate pain relief, protein and calcium act as powerful stimulants to acid secretion, and cause irritation and the return of pain within 1 to 3 hours. Another drawback is the possibility of hypercalcemia, especially when milk therapy is used in combination with calcium antacids. Also, there is little agreement as to which foods are actually irritating to the GI mucosa, and there is no proof that a bland diet helps heal or prevent recurrent attacks of ulcers or gastritis. Although bland diets are still used, the trend is toward using a liberal ulcer or liberal bland diet (see box, Liberal Bland Diet).

A liberal bland diet provides four to six small meals a day to help neutralize gastric

Traditional Progressive Bland Diet

General Characteristics

Vary considerably among institutions

Stage 1: 4 to 6 oz of milk every 2 hours for 3 to 4 days, or as determined by the client's progress. Strained cream soup, eggs, cottage cheese, crackers, and refined cereals may be offered.

Stage 2: Six to eight small meals a day of soft, low-residue foods, such as tender meats, fish and poultry, strained fruit juices, bananas, canned fruits, cooked or canned green and yellow beans, sweet potatoes, winter squash

Stage 3: Asymptomatic clients may be progressed to a six small meals/day bland diet

Bland Diet Guidelines

Eat six small meals a day.

Avoid the following foods that are eliminated on a liberal bland diet: pepper, chili powder, coffee (regular and decaffeinated), cocoa, cola beverages, tea, and alcohol.

Also eliminate: fried food, spicy food, whole-grain breads and cereals, meat broth, soups, gravies, most raw fruits and vegetables, nuts, coconut, and seeds.

Bland Diet

Breakfast

½ cup orange juice
Poached egg
1 slice white toast with butter
½ cup milk
Salt/sugar

Midmorning Snack

Graham crackers
½ cup milk
½ banana

Lunch

Sandwich made from two slices white bread, 2 oz chicken, 2 tsp mayonnaise

(continued)

Sample Menu

Traditional Progressive Bland Diet (*continued*)

½ cup canned peaches
½ cup milk

Midafternoon Snack

1 cup vanilla yogurt

Dinner

2 to 3 oz roast beef
½ cup whipped potatoes
½ cup buttered carrots
½ cup vanilla ice cream
Salt/sugar

Evening Snack

2 saltine crackers
½ cup milk

contents. Pepper, chili powder, coffee (regular and decaffeinated), cocoa, cola beverages, tea, and alcohol are eliminated because they are gastric acid stimulants. The only other recommendation is to eliminate any foods not tolerated by the person. Dietary restrictions should be kept to a minimum to help reduce stress in a client who may already be stressed.

Weight loss is experienced by many clients with ulcers or chronic gastritis. Encourage the client to attain and maintain "healthy" weight.

Iron deficiency anemia may result from blood loss and poor iron absorption related to antacid therapy or achlorhydria. Iron supplements may be indicated. Likewise, chronic gastritis can impair the secretion of intrinsic factor and result in pernicious anemia. Vitamin B_{12} status should be evaluated every several years.

Encourage protein and vitamin C intake to facilitate healing.

Discourage late evening snacks that can increase acid secretion and result in loss of sleep.

Be aware of the potential side effects and nutritional problems associated with antacid therapy (see section on Hiatal Hernias).

Client Goals

The client will:
Be free of symptoms of _____.
Consume adequate calories and protein to attain/maintain "healthy" weight.
Avoid foods not tolerated.

Liberal Bland Diet

Eat four to six small meals/day.
Avoid individual intolerances.
Avoid
  Pepper
  Chili powder
  Regular and decaffeinated coffee
  Caffeine
  Alcohol

Describe the principles and rationale of diet management in the treatment of gastric disorders, and implement the appropriate diet interventions.
Identify causative factors, if known.

Nursing Interventions

Diet Management

Promote a liberal bland diet (see box, Liberal Bland Diet) of four to six small meals. Keep dietary restrictions to a minimum.
Encourage adequate calories, protein, and vitamin C.

Client Teaching

Instruct the client
On the principles and rationale of a liberal bland diet to relieve symptoms.
To eat in a relaxed environment and chew food thoroughly.
To avoid rigorous activity immediately before and after eating.
To avoid cigarettes and alcohol. If the client refuses to give up alcohol, it should be consumed with meals or immediately after eating.

Monitor

Monitor for the following signs or symptoms:
Compliance with the diet, and the need for follow-up diet counseling
Effectiveness of the diet and the need for further diet modification
Weight, weight changes

Evaluation

Evaluation is ongoing. Assuming the plan of care has not changed, the client will achieve the goals as stated above.

DISORDERS OF THE INTESTINES

Disorders of the intestines often cause altered bowel elimination; a primary objective of diet therapy is to promote normal bowel elimination by either increasing or decreasing transit time. Additional diet modifications are based on the underlying disease and the clinical manifestations.

Diverticular Disease

Diverticula are pouches that protrude outward from the intestinal wall, usually in the sigmoid colon, that characterize an asymptomatic condition known as diverticulosis. Diverticula are caused by increased pressure within the intestinal lumen, which may be related to chronic constipation and chronic low-fiber diets.

Diverticulitis occurs when the diverticula become inflamed, which may cause cramping, alternating periods of diarrhea and constipation, flatus, abdominal distention, and low-grade fever. Complications include occult blood loss and acute rectal bleeding → iron deficiency anemia; abscesses; bowel perforation → peritonitis; fistula formation → bowel obstruction; and small bowel diverticula → bacterial overgrowth → fat and vitamin B_{12} malabsorption.

In the past, low-residue diets were believed to decrease the likelihood of diverticulitis, based on the idea that particles of fiber could get trapped in the diverticula and cause irritation and inflammation. However, studies suggest that high-fiber diets can decrease the incidence of both diverticulosis and diverticulitis by producing soft, bulky stools that are easily passed, resulting in decreased pressure within the colon and shortened transit time.

The trend is to treat diverticulitis and diverticulosis with a high-fiber diet as tolerated (see box, High-Fiber Diet), although some physicians recommend a low-residue diet until the symptoms of diverticulitis subside. However, diet compliance depends on understanding the rationale and benefits of a high-fiber diet, especially if the client was previously treated with a low-residue diet.

Malabsorption Syndrome

A major clinical manifestation of many intestinal disorders is malabsorption syndrome, characterized by steatorrhea, diarrhea, weight loss, muscle wasting, abdominal cramps and distention, and numerous secondary nutrient deficiencies and metabolic disturbances (see box, Secondary Nutrient Deficiencies and Metabolic Disturbances of Malabsorption Syndrome). Failure of the intestinal mucosa to adequately absorb nutrients can result in serious and sometimes life-threatening malnutrition and metabolic disturbances.

Malabsorption can result from maldigestion related to cystic fibrosis, pancreatitis, gallbladder disease, liver disease, and disaccharidase deficiencies, or from bacterial

Secondary Nutrient Deficiencies and Metabolic Disturbances of Malabsorption Syndrome

Potential Problems/Rationale

Muscle weakness related to hypokalemia

Hypoalbuminemia → edema related to the following problems:
- Protein malabsorption
- Decreased albumin synthesis
- Leakage of albumin into the gut (protein-losing enteropathy)

Iron-deficiency anemia related to iron malabsorption and/or blood loss

Folic acid deficiency anemia related to folic acid malabsorption

Vitamin B_{12} deficiency anemia related to vitamin B_{12} malabsorption

Purpura and easy bleeding related to vitamin K malabsorption

Roughening of the skin and impaired night vision related to vitamin A malabsorption

Osteomalacia → bone pain related to calcium, magnesium, and vitamin D malabsorption

Tetany related to hypocalcemia, hypomagnesemia

Stomatitis, cheilosis, glossitis, and dermatitis related to malabsorption of the B complex vitamins

Lactose intolerance → cramping, distention, flatus, and diarrhea after milk ingestion related to lactase deficiency resulting from intestinal mucosa damage

Kidney stone formation related to increased oxalate absorption (normally, most dietary oxalate binds with calcium in the intestine and is excreted in the feces; calcium malabsorption leads to a secondary increase in oxalate absorption)

Cholesterol gallstone formation related to bile salt malabsorption: bile salt malabsorption → cholesterol-saturated bile → precipitation of cholesterol from bile into gallstones

overgrowth related to blind loop syndrome. Alterations in bowel mucosa, as seen in regional enteritis, ulcerative colitis, celiac disease, radiation enteritis, and malignancy, also cause malabsorption. Other causes include short bowel syndrome related to intestinal surgery, and certain drug therapies.

Malabsorption is treated by correcting the underlying disorder and with nutritional intervention aimed at controlling steatorrhea, reducing bowel stimulation, restoring optimal nutritional status, and promoting healing, where applicable. Selected digestive disorders that may cause malabsorption syndrome are highlighted in Table 15-4.

Table 15-4

Selected Malabsorption Disorders: Description, Symptoms, Diet Management

Disorder	Symptoms	Diet Management for Malabsorption PLUS
Lactose intolerance: Maldigestion of lactose (milk sugar) caused by a deficiency of the digestive enzyme lactase, which is normally found in the intestinal villi. May be congenital, acquired, or occur secondary to bowel disorders, malnutrition, GI surgery, or radiotherapy.	Distention, cramps, flatus, and diarrhea occurring 15 to 30 minutes after lactose ingestion and usually subsiding within 2 hours; undigested lactose increases the osmolality of the intestinal contents and results in a large fluid shift into the intestines to dilute the particle concentration. Individual tolerance to lactose varies considerably.	Reduce lactose to the maximum amount tolerated by the individual (See box, Lactose-Restricted Diet)
Regional enteritis (Crohn's disease): Chronic, progressive, inflammatory disease involving the entire thickness of the bowel wall. Commonly affects the terminal ileum, but it can occur anywhere along the entire GI tract.	Diarrhea with possible melena, weight loss, crampy abdominal pain, fever, fatigue, anorexia, alternating periods of exacerbation and remission. Complications include fistulae and abscesses, hemorrhage, bowel perforations, intestinal obstructions, anemia, malnutrition.	Low lactose. During remission, encourage a well-balanced diet based on individual tolerance.
Ulcerative colitis: Chronic, inflammatory disease involving the mucosal and sometimes submucosal layer of the colon and rectum.	Anorexia, nausea, vomiting, frequent passage of hard or liquid stools containing blood, pus, or mucus; abdominal pain and distention; weight loss, fever, dehydration, alternating periods of exacerbation and remission. Complications include anal fissures, abscesses, bowel perforations, intestinal stenosis from scar tissue, iron deficiency anemia, bleeding tendency re: vitamin K deficiency, malnutrition, colon cancer.	Low lactose. Encourage a well-balanced diet based on individual tolerance during remission.
Celiac disease (gluten-induced enteropathy, nontropical sprue): Sensitivity to gliadin (the protein component of gluten) causes flattened, atrophied intestinal villi, a decreased absorptive surface with a loss of disaccharidases, leading to malabsorption syndrome. Gluten is found in wheat, oats, rye, and barley.	Steatorrhea, malabsorption, weight loss, muscle wasting, disaccharide intolerance, weakness, malnutrition, fatigue.	Gluten-free diet (see box, Gluten-Free Diet). Complete and permanent elimination of gluten causes the villi to return toward normal, usually within a few weeks. Complete regeneration may never occur. A low-lactose diet may be needed temporarily or permanently.
Pancreatitis: inflammation of the pancreas. Retention of pancreatic enzymes within the pancreas leads to autodigestion. Chronic pancreatitis is characterized by scarring and tissue calcification.	Severe abdominal pain, nausea and vomiting, fever, jaundice. Chronic pancreatitis can lead to hyperglycemia, steatorrhea, weight loss, and malnutrition.	Low-fat diet (*i.e.,* 50–70 g), as tolerated. Eliminate gastric acid stimulants: regular and decaf. coffee, tea, alcohol, and pepper. A CHO-controlled diet may be needed if symptoms of diabetes mellitus develop.

Nursing Process

Assessment

In addition to the general GI assessment criteria, assess for the following factors:

Symptoms: onset, frequency, causative factors, severity, interventions attempted and the results

Dietary changes made in response to malabsorption symptoms (*i.e.*, food avoided, foods preferred). Determine foods best and least tolerated.

Fat intake, which can aggravate existing steatorrhea

Intake and output; observe for signs of dehydration and electrolyte imbalance.

Weight status; observe for signs of malnutrition/nutrient deficiencies (see box, Secondary Nutrient Deficiencies and Metabolic Disturbances of Malabsorption Syndrome).

Nursing Diagnosis

Altered Nutrition: Less than Body Requirements, related to malabsorption secondary to _____ (causative factor).

Planning and Implementation

Many factors contribute to malnutrition characteristic of malabsorptive disorders: diarrhea, loss of nutrients through the stool, possible blood loss, decreased food intake, drug therapy, and sometimes surgical intervention. The task of restoring nutritional status without aggravating the bowel in an anorexic client is difficult and frustrating for the health care team and the client.

Some malabsorptive disorders, such as acute regional enteritis, may require complete bowel rest to facilitate healing. The client may either be maintained on total parenteral nutrition or elemental formulas that are completely absorbed without undergoing digestion (see Chap. 13). Likewise, during an acute attack of celiac disease, the client may be ordered NPO (nothing by mouth) and given intravenous fluid and electrolytes to rest the bowel temporarily. Bowel rest has been less effective in treating ulcerative colitis. Food is also withheld initially during an acute attack of pancreatitis. If the client is malnourished, a nasojejunal tube feeding of a hydrolyzed formula diet or total parenteral nutrition may be used until oral intake is resumed (see Chap. 13). Oral intake should progress to a nutrient-rich diet as soon as possible.

Regardless of the underlying disorder, the diet should always be individualized as much as possible to correspond with the client's likes, dislikes, and intolerances. Small, frequent meals are indicated to maximize intake. Clients who are apprehensive about eating need emotional support and encouragement.

Fat intake is limited whenever steatorrhea is present. Because the enzyme activity of lactase may be temporarily impaired during malabsorption syndromes, it is prudent to restrict dietary lactose even when a lactase deficiency has not been objectively diagnosed. Lactase activity may return to normal after malabsorption has been resolved.

Malabsorption can lead to numerous nutrient deficiencies: protein, calcium, magnesium, zinc, iron, vitamin B_{12}, folic acid, vitamin C, potassium, and the fat-soluble vitamins. Multivitamin and mineral supplements and water-soluble supplements of the fat-soluble vitamins are needed not only to replenish losses, but also for the metabolism of a high-calorie, high-protein diet and to facilitate healing.

It is difficult to meet protein and calorie needs with a low-residue diet, especially if the client is lactose-intolerant. If commercial formulas are used to supplement intake,* the following should be taken into consideration:

- Osmolality: hypertonic formulas should be diluted and administered gradually to prevent diarrhea.
- Residue content
- Lactose content
- Client acceptance: to improve palatability, formulas may be served over ice, enhanced with commercial flavor packets, or incorporated into appropriate recipes

The length of time the diet should be followed depends on the underlying disorder and the client's medical status. For instance, during remission of regional enteritis and ulcerative colitis, a well-balanced diet based on individual tolerance is recommended; lactose and residue tolerance varies among individuals. Clients with celiac disease must follow a gluten-free diet permanently.

Client Goals

The client will:

Experience fewer symptoms of malabsorption.

Consume adequate calories and protein to attain/maintain "healthy" weight.

Be free of symptoms of nutrient deficiencies (see box, Secondary Nutrient Deficiencies and Metabolic Disturbances of Malabsorption Syndrome).

Describe the principles and rationale of diet management for malabsorption syndrome and its symptoms, and implement the appropriate diet interventions.

Identify causative factors, if known.

Nursing Interventions

Diet Management

At the very least, clients with malabsorption require a diet low in residue to reduce bowel stimulation. Other diet modifications for malabsorptive disorders depend on the actual underlying disorder and the presenting symptoms. For instance, clients with significant weight loss need a high-calorie, high-protein diet; only clients with celiac disease require a gluten-free diet (see box, Gluten-Free Diet).

General diet interventions for malabsorption are as follows:

Limit residue and fiber to slow transit time and reduce bowel stimulation.

Reduce fat intake to 50 g or less for clients with steatorrhea (see box, Low-Fat Diet). If necessary, use medium-chain triglycerides to increase calorie intake (see Chap. 3).

Increase protein and CHO intake (nonfat calories) to restore weight lost. Clients with increased requirements for healing (i.e., regional enteritis, ulcerative colitis), may need 2000 to 3500 calories/day, and 100 to 150 g/day of protein.

Increase fluid intake to compensate for increased fluid output (i.e., diarrhea, fistula drainage, blood loss, etc).

(*Text continued on page 441*)

---

*Use of commercial supplements is covered in Chapter 13; supplements are outlined in Appendix 7.

Gluten-Free Diet

Characteristics

Eliminates all foods prepared with wheat, rye, oats, and barley

Objective

Prevent intestinal villi changes, steatorrhea, and other symptoms characteristic of celiac disease

Indications for Use

Celiac disease
Dermatitis herpetiformis

Contraindications

None

Foods Allowed

Beverages: Carbonated drinks, cocoa, coffee, tea, fruit juice, milk, decaffeinated coffee containing no wheat flour

Breads and cereals: Products made with arrowroot, cornstarch, cornmeal, potato, rice, soybean, and gluten-free wheat starch flours; pure rice, sago, and tapioca; gluten-free macaroni products; cornbread, muffins, and pone made without wheat flour; corn or rice cereals such as cornflakes, Cream of Rice, hominy, puffed rice, rice flakes, Rice Krispies; rice cakes; grits; popcorn

Desserts: Cakes, cookies, pastries, and other baked products made with allowed flours; custard, gelatin, homemade cornstarch, tapioca, and rice puddings; ice cream and sherbet prepared without gluten stabilizers

Fats: Butter, corn oil, French dressing, pure mayonnaise and olive oil, margarine, other pure animal and vegetable fats and oils

Soups: Broth, bouillon, clear soups, cream soups thickened with allowed flours

Miscellaneous: Pepper, pickles, popcorn, potato chips, sugars and syrups, vinegar, molasses

Plain meats, fruits, and vegetables, or those prepared with allowed foods

Foods Not Allowed

Beverages: Ale, beer, instant coffee containing wheat, Postum, Ovaltine and other cereal beverages, malted milk

(continued)

Gluten-Free Diet (*continued*)

Breads and cereals: All products made from wheat, rye, oats, barley, buck-
wheat, durum, or graham, including the following items:
- All commercial yeast and quick bread mixes
- All-purpose flour
- Baking powder biscuits
- Bran
- Bread crumbs
- Bread flour
- Bulgur
- Crackers and cracker crumbs
- Farina
- Graham flour
- Kasha
- Macaroni
- Malt and malt flavoring
- Matzoh
- Noodles
- Pancakes
- Pastry flour
- Pretzels
- Rye flour
- Self-rising flour
- Semolina
- Vermicelli
- Waffles
- Whole- or cracked-wheat flours
- Wheat germ
- Zwieback

Cooked or ready-to-eat cereals containing malt, bran, rye, wheat, oats, barley
or wheat germ

Desserts: Cakes, cookies, pastries, and other baked products made with flours
not allowed; prepared mixes, prepared pudding thickened with wheat
flour

Fats: Commercial salad dressings that contain gluten stabilizers or homemade
salad dressings thickened with flour

Soups: All soups thickened with wheat products or containing barley, noodles,
or other wheat, rye, and oat products in any form

Meats prepared with wheat, rye, oats, or barley, or gluten stabilizers or fillers

Any thickened or prepared fruits; some pie fillings

Any creamed or breaded vegetables, unless allowed ingredients are used;

(*continued*)

Gluten-Free Diet (*continued*)

canned baked beans; commercially prepared vegetables with cream sauce or cheese sauce

Miscellaneous: Because the following ingredients *may* contain gluten, check with the manufacturer before using products containing the following ingredients:

- Emulsifiers
- Flavorings
- Hydrolyzed vegetable protein (HVP)
- Modified starch and modified food starch
- Stabilizers
- Soy sauce, soy sauce solids
- Vegetable gum
- Vegetable protein or textured vegetable protein (TVP)

Additional Considerations

Clients may be discouraged and overwhelmed when faced with a lifelong restricted diet. Provide support, encouragement, and thorough diet instructions.

The client may be temporarily or permanently lactose-intolerant and may require a lactose-restricted diet.

A celiac crisis may be precipitated by emotional stress.

Potential Problem/Rationale

Difficulty obtaining a variety of allowed foods from grocery stores related to the highly restrictive nature of the diet.

Nursing Interventions and Considerations

Encourage the client to use as many "normal" items as possible, such as corn cereals, cornmeal, rice, and rice cereals. Not only are they easily obtained from any grocery store, but they are also less expensive than special products.

Encourage the client to shop in health food or specialty stores to obtain hard-to-find items such as potato and soybean flours.

Gluten-Free Diet Teaching

Instruct the client

On the importance of adhering to the diet, even when no symptoms are present.

(continued)

Gluten-Free Diet (*continued*)

That "cheating" on the diet will cause the return of symptoms, which will disappear after resumption of the diet.

To eliminate all wheat, oat, rye, and barley flours and products permanently.

To eat an otherwise normal, well-balanced diet adequate in nutrients and calories.

To read labels to identify less obvious sources of wheat, rye, oats, and barley used as extenders and fillers. Clients should check with the manufacturer *before* using products of questionable composition.

To use corn, potato, rice, arrowroot, and soybean flours and their products.

That weight gain may be slowly achieved.

To avoid milk and other sources of lactose if not tolerated.

Provide the client with the following aids:

- A detailed list of foods allowed and not allowed
- Information regarding support groups, such as the American Celiac Society, the Gluten Intolerance Group, and the Midwestern Celiac Sprue Association
- Gluten-free recipes

Modify the diet as needed to alleviate any secondary nutrient deficiencies and metabolic disturbances that develop (see box, Secondary Nutrient Deficiencies and Metabolic Disturbances of Malabsorption Syndrome). Reduce lactose to the maximum amount tolerated by the individual (see box, Lactose-Restricted Diet), as indicated.

Additional diet interventions for selected malabsorptive disorders are summarized in Table 15-4.

Client Teaching

Instruct the client on the principles and rationale of diet management to relieve malabsorption syndrome symptoms, as indicated (see Table 15-4, and the appropriate boxes for specific diet modifications).

Monitor

Monitor for the following signs or symptoms:

Tolerance of fat intake (*i.e.*, decrease or absence of steatorrhea and pain after eating)

Compliance with the diet, and the need for follow-up diet counseling

Effectiveness of the diet, and the need for further diet modification

Fluid and electrolyte balance

Weight, weight changes

Clinical signs of malnutrition

(*Text continued on page 447*)

Low-Fat Diet (50 g)

Characteristics

Limits the total amount of fat, regardless of the type

Foods are baked, broiled, or boiled instead of fried or prepared with added fat.

Visible fat on meats is trimmed and poultry skin removed, preferably before cooking.

Allowed fats can be used as seasonings or in cooking.

Objective

Reduce the symptoms of steatorrhea and pain in clients intolerant of fat

Indications for Use

Chronic pancreatitis

Malabsorption syndromes: celiac disease, radiation enteritis, short bowel syndrome, tropical sprue

Some cases of gallbladder disease

Type I hyperlipoproteinemia (25 to 35 mg fat)

Contraindications

None

Foods Allowed

Meats: Up to 6 oz of lean meat, fish, and skinless poultry daily; up to three egg yolks a week; egg whites and low-fat egg substitutes as desired

Dairy products: Two or more servings/day of skim milk; skim-milk cheeses, yogurt, and puddings

Fruits and vegetables: A total of six servings/day or more of any fruit and vegetable prepared without added fat, except avocado

Bread and cereals: Four or more servings/day of plain cereals, pasta, macaroni, rice, whole grain or enriched breads

Miscellaneous: Sherbet, fruit ices, gelatin, angel food cake, fat-free or skim-milk soups, soft drinks, honey, sugar, seasonings as desired

Fats: Three to five servings of fat daily. Each of the following constitutes one serving:
- 1 teaspoon butter, margarine, shortening, oil, or mayonnaise
- 1 tablespoon diet margarine or diet mayonnaise
- 1 strip crisp bacon

(continued)

Low-Fat Diet (50 g) (*continued*)

- 1 tablespoon heavy cream, Italian or French dressing
- ⅛ avocado
- 2 teaspoons peanut butter
- 2 tablespoons light cream
- 6 small nuts
- 5 small olives

Foods Not Allowed

Meats: Fried, fatty, or heavily marbled meats; sausage, lunch meat, spare ribs, frankfurters, salt pork, tuna and salmon packed in oil

Dairy products: Whole milk; whole-milk cheeses and yogurt, ice cream

Fruits and vegetables: Any buttered, au gratin, creamed, or fried vegetables

Breads and cereals: Products made with added fat such as biscuits, muffins, pancakes, doughnuts, waffles, and sweet rolls; breads made with eggs, cheese, or added fat; buttered popcorn; granola-type cereals; popovers; snack crackers with added fat; snack chips; stuffing

Miscellaneous: Cream sauces, gravy; desserts, candy, and anything made with chocolate or nuts

Low-Fat Diet

Sample Menu

Breakfast

Orange juice
Toast with 1 tsp margarine and jelly
Oatmeal
Skim milk
Coffee/tea
Salt/pepper/sugar

Lunch

Sandwich made with whole-wheat bread, 2 oz skinless chicken breast, lettuce, and 1 tbsp mayonnaise
Tossed salad with 1 tbsp French dressing
Fruit cocktail
Skim milk
Coffee/tea
Salt/pepper/sugar

(*continued*)

Low-Fat Diet (50 g) (*continued*)

Dinner

3 oz broiled fish
Baked potato with 1 tsp butter
Steamed broccoli
Carrot and celery sticks
Dinner roll with 1 tsp butter
Sherbet
Fresh strawberries
Skim milk
Coffee/tea
Salt/pepper/sugar

Snack

Unbuttered popcorn
Fruit juice

Potential Problem/Rationale

Noncompliance related to decreased palatability and satiety from the reduction in fat intake.

Nursing Interventions and Considerations

Encourage the client to eat a variety of the foods allowed. Allow fat exchanges to be substituted for meat and dairy products of a higher fat content than is normally allowed (*e.g.,* decrease the fat allowance by one serving to allow 1 cup of 2% milk instead of skim milk).

Encourage the client to try low-fat or fat-free substitutes of high-fat items, such as fat-free mayonnaise, salad dressings, and frozen desserts.

Encourage the client to use low-calorie butter seasonings to flavor hot vegetables and potatoes. Butter-flavor vegetable sprays can add flavor to unbuttered popcorn.

Potential Problem/Rationale

Persistent symptoms of steatorrhea or pain after eating related to fat intolerance. Fat tolerance varies considerably among clients and conditions.

Nursing Interventions and Considerations

Decrease the fat content of the diet by reducing or eliminating fat exchanges and limiting the amount of low-fat meats allowed.

(*continued*)

Low-Fat Diet (50 g) (*continued*)

Potential Problem/Rationale

Inadequate intake of iron related to the limited allowance of meat (red meat is the best source of iron in the diet).

Nursing Interventions and Considerations

Monitor laboratory values and observe for signs of iron deficiency. Provide supplements as needed.

Encourage a liberal intake of low-fat, high-iron foods, such as dried fruits, fortified cereals and grains, green leafy vegetables, and dried peas and beans. Instruct the client to eat a good source of vitamin C at each meal to enhance iron absorption from plant sources.

Low-Fat Diet Teaching

Instruct the client

That the total amount of dietary fat is reduced, regardless of the source.

That the sources of fat may be visible (butter, margarine, shortening, fat on meat, and salad dressings) or invisible (marbled meat, whole milk and whole-milk products, egg yolks, and nuts).

That substitutions can be made to individualize the diet.

That oil-packed tuna and salmon may be used if thoroughly rinsed.

That fat-free salad dressings may be used as desired.

How to order off a menu while dining out:

- Choose juice instead of soup as an appetizer.
- Use lemon, vinegar, low-calorie dressing (if available) or fresh ground pepper on salad, or request that the dressing be brought on the side.
- Order plain baked or broiled foods.
- Avoid warm bread and rolls that absorb more butter than those at room temperature
- Order fresh fruit, gelatin, or sherbet for dessert.
- Request milk for coffee or tea in place of cream and nondairy creamers.

On food preparation techniques to reduce fat content:

- Trim fat from meat and remove skin from chicken before cooking.
- Place meats to be baked or roasted on a rack to allow the fat to drain.
- Bake, broil, steam, or "sauté" foods in vegetable cooking spray or allowed fats.
- Cook with bouillon, lemon, vinegar, wine, herbs, and spices instead of adding fat.
- Make fat-free soup stock by preparing the stock a day ahead and refrigerating it overnight. The fat will harden and can be easily removed from the surface. Make fat-free gravies by this method also.

To purchase "select" grade meats because they are lower in fat than "choice" and "prime" grades.

Lactose-Restricted Diet

Characteristics

Limits lactose (milk sugar) to the level tolerated by the individual

Indications for Use

Primary, secondary, and acquired lactose intolerance

Contraindications

None

Foods High in Lactose

Milk: whole, 2%, 1%, skim, evaporated, nonfat dry milk, milk solids
Cream; sour cream
All cheese, except aged natural cheeses
Cream soup and sauces
Specialty-flavored instant coffee blends made with creamer
Cocoa and most chocolate beverages
Ice cream, sherbet, ice milk, custard, puddings, commercial desserts and mixes

Food With Less Lactose

Liver, sweetbreads, brain
Products that have milk, butter, margarine, dry milk solids, or whey listed as
    ingredients, including the following foods:
- Breads and cereals, such as Total, Special K, and Cocoa Krispies
- Cookies, cakes, pastries, commercial fruit pie fillings, sherbet
- Cold cuts and hot dogs
- Creamed or breaded meats and vegetables
- Gravy, dried soups, dips, salad dressings
- Commercial french fries, instant potatoes, mashed potatoes
- Butterscotch, caramels, chocolate candy, molasses, peppermints, toffee, chewing gum
- Cordials and liqueurs
- Maraschino cherries
- Powdered soft drinks, powdered coffee creamer
- Some dietetic and diabetic foods
- Sugar substitutes (Sweet 'n Low and Equal tablets)
- Monosodium glutamate (MSG)
- Some vitamin and mineral preparations

(continued)

Lactose-Restricted Diet (*continued*)

Potential Problem/Rationale

Calcium deficiency related to the reduction or elimination of milk and dairy products from the diet.

Nursing Interventions and Considerations

Encourage the client to drink small amounts of milk as tolerated. Some clients may tolerate yogurt, milk with acidophilus added, or milk treated with LactAid. Sometimes chocolate milk is better tolerated because of its higher sucrose content and slower emptying rate from the stomach.[11]

Encourage the intake of calcium from nondairy sources, such as green leafy vegetables, dates, prunes, canned sardines and salmon with bones, oranges, egg yolks, whole grains, nuts, and dried peas and beans.

Provide calcium supplements as needed.

Low-Lactose Diet Teaching

Instruct the client
On the sources of lactose.

To include nondairy sources of calcium in the diet and to take calcium supplements if needed.

To read labels to identify sources of lactose. Lactate, lactalbumin, and calcium compounds are lactic acid salts and are lactose-free. Kosher foods labeled *pareve* are made without milk.

That some amount of milk may be tolerated by those with acquired lactose intolerance, especially if consumed slowly, at room temperature, and after eating.

That nondairy creamer is lactose-free and may be used in beverages, on cereal, and in cooking, if desired.

That acidophilus milk or LactAid milk may be tolerated. The lactose in LactAid has been converted into other absorbable sugars. LactAid is available in supermarkets and can be used as a beverage or in cooking.

Evaluation

Evaluation is ongoing. Assuming the plan of care has not changed, the client will achieve the goals as stated above.

DRUG ALERT: **CORTICOSTEROIDS AND SULFASALAZINE**

Corticosteroids

Can cause calcium and potassium depletion and sodium retention.

Actions

Monitor potassium and sodium status. Encourage intake of potassium-rich and calcium-rich foods. Limit sodium if edema or hypertension develop.

Sulfasalazine

Impairs folic acid absorption, leading to folic acid deficiency anemia. May also lead to crystalluria and renal stone formation.

Actions

Provide folic acid supplements as needed. Encourage a high fluid intake to prevent renal stones.

DISORDERS OF THE LIVER

The liver is a highly active organ involved in the metabolism of almost all nutrients. After absorption, almost all nutrients are transported to the liver, where they are "processed" before being distributed to other tissues. The liver synthesizes plasma proteins, blood clotting factors, and nonessential amino acids, and forms urea from the nitrogenous wastes of protein. Triglycerides, phospholipids, and cholesterol are synthesized in the liver. Glucose is formed (gluconeogenesis), and glycogen is formed, stored, and broken down, as needed. Vitamins and minerals are metabolized and many are stored in the liver. Finally, the liver is vital for detoxifying drugs, alcohol, ammonia, and other poisonous substances.

Liver damage can have profound and devastating effects on the metabolism of almost all nutrients. Liver damage can range from mild and reversible (*i.e.*, fatty liver) to severe and terminal (*i.e.*, hepatic coma).

HEPATITIS AND CIRRHOSIS

Hepatitis is an inflammation of the liver. It can be caused by viral infections (type A, type B, type non-A, non-B), alcohol abuse, and drugs. Early symptoms include anorexia, nausea and vomiting, fever, fatigue, headache, weight loss. Later, dark-colored urine, jaundice, liver tenderness, and possibly liver enlargement may develop. Liver cell damage that occurs from hepatitis is reversible with proper rest and nutrition.

Cirrhosis encompasses all forms of liver disease characterized by extensive loss of liver cells, fibrosis, and fatty infiltration of the liver. Liver function is seriously impaired as liver cells are replaced by functionless scar tissue; normal blood circulation through the liver also is disrupted. During the early stages of cirrhosis, fever, anorexia, weight loss, and fatigue may be evident. Later, portal hypertension, dyspepsia, diarrhea or constipation, jaundice, esophageal varices, hemorrhoids, ascites, edema, bleeding tendencies, anemia, hepatomegaly, and splenomegaly may develop. Cirrhosis can progress to terminal hepatic coma.

The major cause of cirrhosis is alcoholism, with a 10% to 12% incident rate among alcoholics. Other causes include untreated hepatitis, chronic biliary obstruction, and malnutrition.

The objectives of diet intervention for hepatitis and cirrhosis are to avoid/minimize permanent liver damage, promote liver cell regeneration, restore optimal nutritional status, and alleviate symptoms. For clients with cirrhosis, diet intervention may help avoid complications of ascites, esophageal varices, and hepatic coma; however, depending on the extent of liver damage, regeneration may not be possible.

Nursing Process

Assessment

In addition to the general GI assessment criteria, assess for the following factors:

Symptoms: onset, frequency, causative factors, severity, interventions attempted and the results

Dietary changes made in response to symptoms (*i.e.*, foods avoided, foods preferred). Determine foods best and least tolerated.

Protein intake: meat, fish, poultry, milk and milk products, dried peas and beans, grain products.

Fat intake, and determine if the client is experiencing any symptoms of fat intolerance, such as distention, indigestion, or early satiety.

Intake and output; observe for edema.

Weight, weight changes: rapid weight gain signals fluid retention.

Nursing Diagnosis

Altered Nutrition: Less than Body Requirements, related to faulty metabolism secondary to altered liver function.

Planning and Implementation

The importance of optimal nutrition in the management of liver disorders cannot be overestimated. Adequate protein and calories are of paramount importance; protein is needed for liver cell regeneration, calories are used to spare protein. However, depending on the extent of liver cell damage and regenerative capacity, high protein intakes may overburden the liver and precipitate a hepatic coma. In the later stage of cirrhosis, there is a fine line between enough protein and too much protein. Likewise, it may be difficult to provide adequate calories if the client experiences steatorrhea or an intolerance to fat.

Alcohol must be eliminated.

Malnourished, anorexic clients have difficulty consuming an adequate diet, and nausea may worsen as the day progresses. High-calorie, high-protein liquid nourishments may be better tolerated than traditional meals. Solicit individual food preferences and work closely with the family.

Consider tube or intravenous feedings if anorexia, nausea, and vomiting are severe.

A texture-modified diet (*i.e.*, soft, low-residue, or full liquids) may be needed if a regular diet irritates esophageal mucosa. Withhold food if esophageal varices bleed.

For unknown reasons, clients with cirrhosis cannot handle a normal sodium load. If ascites is present, restrict sodium intake to 2 g/day or less. Unfortunately, high-protein foods are also relatively high in sodium. Low-sodium milk is an option; however, it is unpalatable and most clients find its taste offensive.

If sodium restriction alone is not effective, fluid intake also may need to be limited. However, a high fluid intake may be needed to replace losses caused by fever and vomiting. Fluid needs must be assessed on an individual basis.

Clients with severe anorexia, nausea, or vomiting may need enteral or parenteral nutritional support.

Multivitamin and mineral supplements, especially iron, B vitamins, vitamin C, and vitamin K, may be necessary to compensate for alterations in metabolism.

Client Goals

The client will:

Experience fewer and less severe symptoms of _____.

Consume adequate calories and protein to attain/maintain "healthy" weight and regenerate liver cells, if possible.

Describe the principles and rationale of diet management of hepatic disorders, and implement the appropriate diet interventions.

Identify causative factors, if known.

Nursing Interventions

Diet Management

Provide a moderate protein intake of 80 to 100 g/day, emphasizing high-biologic-value sources: milk, meat, and eggs. If hepatic coma is impending, decrease protein to the maximum amount tolerated by the individual.

Increase calories from 2000 to 3000 to spare protein and meet energy needs, with a liberal CHO intake of 300 to 400 g, but moderate amounts of fat. Restrict fat intake if steatorrhea develops.

Provide small, frequent meals and encourage the client to eat all meals and snacks. Offer nutrient-rich morning meals if nausea worsens as the day progresses.

Limit sodium and fluid for clients with ascites. Allowances are determined by the accumulation of fluid as measured by sudden weight gain. Sodium allowance ranges from 250 to 2000 mg (see Chap. 16); fluid allowance ranges from 1500 to 2000 ml/day.

Client Teaching

Instruct the client

On the importance of eating an adequate diet and taking vitamins and minerals as prescribed.

On the principles and rationale of diet management to relieve symptoms of hepatic disorders, and how to implement necessary changes.

To avoid spices, pepper, caffeine, and coarse foods that may irritate esophageal varices.

To chew food thoroughly.

Monitor

Monitor for the following signs or symptoms:

Tolerance to protein intake (*i.e.*, absence of central nervous system manifestations, control/decrease serum ammonia levels)

Compliance with the diet, and the need for follow-up diet counseling
Effectiveness of the diet, and the need for further diet modification
Weight, weight status
Intake and output, and fluid balance

Evaluation

Evaluation is ongoing. Assuming the plan of care has not changed, the client will achieve the goals as stated above.

HEPATIC SYSTEMIC ENCEPHALOPATHY

Hepatic systemic encephalopathy refers to the central nervous system (CNS) manifestations of cirrhosis, and is characterized by mental disturbances or loss of consciousness. Impaired memory and concentration, slow response time, drowsiness, irritability, flapping tremor, and fecal odor to breath may progress to a terminal coma.

The exact cause of hepatic encephalopathy is not known; however, increased serum ammonia levels may be at least partially responsible. Ammonia is a CNS toxin produced by the action of GI flora on protein (dietary sources and protein from GI blood loss). Because the malfunctioning liver cannot convert ammonia to urea, serum ammonia levels increase. Another possible cause is the formation of false neurotransmitters related to an alteration in serum amino acid patterns characteristic of altered liver function.

The primary objective of treatment of hepatic encephalopathy is to decrease intestinal ammonia by limiting dietary protein, controlling GI bleeding, alleviating constipation, and reducing GI flora. Additional goals include correcting fluid and electrolyte imbalances and treating or preventing infection.

Nursing Process

Assessment

In addition to the general GI assessment criteria, assess for the following factors:
Symptoms: onset, frequency, causative factors, severity, interventions attempted and the results
Dietary changes made in response to symptoms (*i.e.*, foods avoided, foods preferred). Determine foods best and least tolerated.
Protein intake and adequacy of calorie intake
Serum ammonia levels, and clinical signs of impending coma
Intake and output; observe for signs of fluid and electrolyte imbalance.
Weight and weight changes

Nursing Diagnosis

Fluid Volume Excess, related to ascites secondary to liver disease.

Planning and Implementation

Sodium intake is restricted to alleviate the fluid accumulation of ascites. Restrictions may be as severe as 250 mg/day, which makes compliance extremely difficult.

Manipulation of dietary protein is critical. Providing protein in excess of what the liver can handle increases serum ammonia levels and worsens CNS symptoms. The same results occur from too little protein; a protein intake inadequate to meet the body's needs stimulates body protein catabolism, which, in effect, is like eating too much protein. Optimal protein allowance is derived by observation of clinical symptoms and serum ammonia levels. Protein intake may need to be adjusted daily, or even more frequently, depending on the course of the disease.

To prevent tissue breakdown, a high calorie intake is indicated.

Texture modification may be necessary to prevent damage to esophageal varices. A soft, puréed, or liquid diet may facilitate swallowing.

Specially defined commercial tube feeding formulas containing altered amino acid patterns may be used to supplement the diet of clients with liver failure (see Appendix 7).

Client Goals

The client will:

Avoid hepatic coma.

Experience a decrease in ascites, avoid complications of esophageal varices.

Consume adequate calories and an optimal amount of protein based on his or her clinical symptoms.

Nursing Interventions

Diet Management

Limit sodium and fluid for clients with ascites. Sodium allowance ranges from 250 to 2000 mg/day; fluid allowance ranges from 1500 to 2000 ml/day.

Reduce protein to 20 to 40 g/day and increase by 10 to 15 g/day as the client improves. Adjust the protein content of the diet according to mental symptoms, and eliminate all protein if the client is comatose. Restrict foods that are sources of preformed ammonia or that contain amino acids that convert readily to ammonia: cheese, chicken, ground beef, ham, salami, buttermilk, gelatin, Idaho potatoes, onions, and peanut butter.

Supply at least 2000 cal/day to prevent tissue breakdown. To increase calorie intake without increasing protein, use the following supplements:

- Butter or margarine on potatoes, bread, vegetables, rice, cereal
- Honey, sugar, glucose in coffee, fruit juice, on toast or cereal
- Hard candy and jelly
- Modular CHO supplements (see Appendix 7)

Client Teaching

Client teaching is not indicated, because of the severity of the condition. Clients who respond to treatment will be maintained on the diet as indicated for cirrhosis; however, protein allowance may be less.

Monitor

Monitor for the following signs or symptoms:
Effectiveness of diet and the need for further diet modification
Intake and output; ascites
Serum ammonia levels
CNS symptoms

Evaluation

Evaluation is ongoing. Assuming the plan of care has not changed, the client will achieve the goals as stated above.

DRUG ALERT: **NEOMYCIN**

Neomycin kills intestinal bacteria → decreased vitamin K synthesis → vitamin K deficiency → easy bleeding and diarrhea.

PANCREATIC DISORDERS: PANCREATITIS

Inflammation of the pancreas, known as pancreatitis, causes the retention of pancreatic enzymes, leading to autodigestion of the pancreas. Symptoms of both acute and chronic pancreatitis include severe abdominal pain, nausea, vomiting, distention, fever, and jaundice. Hyperglycemia, steatorrhea, weight loss, and malnutrition may develop as chronic manifestations.

Acute pancreatitis may develop from unknown causes, alcoholism, biliary tract disease, gastric or biliary tract surgery, pancreatic cancer, or secondary to mumps or a bacterial infection. Chronic pancreatitis, characterized by scarring and tissue calcification, is most often caused by alcohol abuse, although it is also associated with gallstones, hyperparathyroidism, and hyperlipidemia.

Acute pancreatitis is treated by reducing pancreatic stimulation; the client is ordered NPO, and a nasogastric tube is inserted to suction gastric contents. Appropriate measures are taken to correct fluid and electrolyte imbalance, to control pain, and to treat or prevent symptoms. The treatment of chronic pancreatitis focuses on pancreatic enzyme replacements to control maldigestion and diet therapy to reduce steatorrhea, to minimize pain, and to avoid acute attacks. Surgical intervention may be necessary if medical treatment fails.

Nursing Process

Assessment

In addition to the general GI assessment criteria, assess for the following factors:
Symptoms: onset, duration, causative factors, severity, interventions attempted and the
    results

Dietary changes made in response to symptoms (*i.e.*, foods avoided, foods preferred). Determine foods best and least tolerated.

Fat intake and its relationship to the onset of symptoms

Alcohol intake; the intake of other gastric acid stimulants, such as regular and decaffeinated coffee, tea, and pepper

Signs and symptoms of hyperglycemia

Weight, weight changes

Symptoms of malnutrition (see box, Secondary Nutrient Deficiencies and Metabolic Disturbances of Malabsorption Syndrome)

Nursing Diagnosis

Altered Nutrition: Less than Body Requirements, related to faulty digestion secondary to pancreatitis.

Planning and Implementation

Food is withheld initially during an acute attack of pancreatitis. If the client is malnourished, a nasojejunal tube feeding of a defined formula diet or total parenteral nutrition may be used until oral intake is resumed (see Chap. 13). As bowel sounds return, serum amylase levels fall, and pain subsides, clear liquids are given and progressed to a low-fat diet as tolerated (see box, Low-Fat Diet).

A low-fat diet is used to alleviate steatorrhea. Medium-chain triglycerides, which do not require digestion by pancreatic lipase before being absorbed, may be used for calories. However, medium-chain triglycerides do not provide the essential fatty acid and are not capable of sparing protein.

Liberal amounts of protein and carbohydrates are recommended to replace calorie and nutrient losses. However, a CHO-controlled diet may be necessary if signs and symptoms of hyperglycemia develop.

Small, frequent meals may help reduce the amount of pancreatic stimulation at each meal. Known gastric stimulants, such as alcohol, caffeine, coffee, and pepper, should be prohibited.

Steatorrhea may necessitate the use of vitamin C and B-complex vitamin supplements, water-soluble supplements of the fat-soluble vitamins, and vitamin B_{12} injections.

Client Goals

The client will:

Avoid or experience alleviation of symptoms of pancreatitis and chronic complications (*i.e.*, hyperglycemia, steatorrhea, malnutrition).

Describe the principles and rationale of dietary management of pancreatitis, and implement the appropriate dietary changes.

Identify and avoid gastric stimulants.

Nursing Interventions

Diet Management (For Chronic Pancreatitis)

Limit fat to the maximum amount that the client can tolerate without causing steatorrhea or pain, usually 50 to 70 g/day. Encourage a liberal intake of protein and carbohydrates.

Eliminate individual intolerances and gastric acid stimulants: alcohol, regular and decaffeinated coffee, tea, and pepper.

Provide a CHO-controlled diet if signs or symptoms of hyperglycemia develop (see Chap. 17).

Provide six small meals per day.

Client Teaching

Instruct the client

On the principles and rationale of diet management of pancreatitis, and how to implement the appropriate dietary changes.

To eliminate individual intolerances and gastric acid stimulants.

That if pancreatic replacements are prescribed, they must be taken with every meal and snack.

Monitor

Monitor for the following signs or symptoms:

Tolerance to fat intake (*i.e.*, absence of steatorrhea and pain after eating)

Compliance with the diet, and the need for follow-up diet counseling

Effectiveness of the diet and the need for further diet modification

Weight, weight changes

Signs of malnutrition related to malabsorption (see box, Secondary Nutrient Deficiencies and Metabolic Disturbances of Malabsorption Syndrome)

Signs of hyperglycemia

Evaluation

Evaluation is ongoing. Assuming the plan of care has not changed, the client will achieve the goals as stated above.

GALLBLADDER DISORDERS: CHOLELITHIASIS AND CHOLECYSTITIS

Abdominal pain, nausea and vomiting, jaundice, fever, fat intolerance, and flatulence are symptoms of cholecystitis, an inflammation of the gallbladder. Cholecystitis may be caused by gallstones (cholelithiasis) obstructing the cystic duct, trauma, or previous surgery. It occurs mostly in women, especially those who are obese, older than age 40, and multiparous. Cystic duct obstruction can lead to abscess, necrosis, perforation, and peritonitis.

Nursing Process

Assessment

In addition to the general GI assessment criteria, assess for the following factors:

Symptoms: onset, frequency, causative factors, severity, interventions attempted and results.

Dietary changes made in response to symptoms (*i.e.*, foods avoided, foods preferred). Determine foods best and least tolerated.

Fat intake and its relationship with the onset of symptoms.

Weight.

Nursing Diagnosis

Altered Health Maintenance, related to the lack of knowledge of dietary management of cholelithiasis/cholecystitis.

Planning and Implementation

The role of diet in the treatment of cholecystitis is to minimize gallbladder stimulation. During an acute attack of cholecystitis, food is withheld and the client is maintained on intravenous fluid and electrolytes. After 12 to 24 hours, a clear liquid diet may be offered and progressed to a diet as tolerated.

Low-fat diets (varying from 20 to 60 g/day of fat) are frequently used in the management of gallbladder diseases, based on the rationale that limiting fat intake reduces stimulation to the gallbladder and minimizes pain. Although some clients are aggravated by fat, some studies indicate that fat intolerance is no more common among clients with gallbladder disease than it is among the general population. Diet modification, therefore, should be based on individual tolerance.

Coffee, both regular and decaffeinated, has been shown to induce significant increases in plasma cholecystokinin, the hormone released in the upper small bowel that stimulates gallbladder contraction. It is recommended that clients with symptomatic gallstones avoid coffee.[6]

Fat-soluble vitamin deficiencies may develop as a result of impaired bile secretion, making water-soluble forms of vitamins A, D, E, and K necessary.

After gallbladder surgery, some physicians recommend a low-fat diet for 4 to 6 weeks; others believe no diet modification is necessary.

Client Goals

The client will:

Lose weight, if overweight, to reduce intra-abdominal pressure.

Describe the principles and rationale of diet management of cholecystitis, and implement the appropriate diet interventions.

Identify and avoid foods that produce symptoms.

Nursing Interventions

Diet Management

Promote weight loss, if indicated.

Eliminate individual food intolerances.

Some clients may benefit physically or psychologically from a low-fat diet (see box, Low-Fat Diet); otherwise, diet as tolerated.

Food for
Thought

The Fiber Story

Debate continues over the role of fiber in diet and disease. Fiber is a general term used to describe all components of plants that cannot be digested in the small intestine. Some types of fiber, such as gums and pectin found in fruits, vegetables, legumes, oatmeal, and oat bran, are effective for lowering blood cholesterol levels. Celluloses, hemicelluloses, and lignin, fibers abundant in wheat bran and whole grains, increase fecal bulk and GI motility and may be effective against constipation, diverticulosis, and irritable bowel syndrome. They may also be protective against colon cancer, especially when coupled with a low-fat diet.

Even before all the evidence is accumulated on the role of fiber, the American Cancer Society and the United States Department of Agriculture, through its *Dietary Guidelines*,[12] urge the general population to increase its intake of fiber by eating more fruits and vegetables, whole grains, nuts, seeds, and legumes.

Client Teaching

Instruct the client
To lose weight, if overweight.
To avoid any foods not tolerated. Some clients are bothered by highly seasoned food, coffee, eggs, and certain fruits and vegetables such as broccoli, cauliflower, brussels sprouts, cabbage, onions, legumes, and melons.
To limit fat intake, if fat appears to produce symptoms.

Monitor

Monitor for the following signs or symptoms:
Compliance with the diet, and the need for follow-up diet counseling
Effectiveness of the diet, and the need for further diet modification
Weight, if overweight

Evaluation

Evaluation is ongoing. Assuming the plan of care has not changed, the client will achieve the goals as stated above.

BIBLIOGRAPHY

1. American Dietetic Association: Manual of Clinical Dietetics. Developed by The Chicago Dietetic Association and the South Suburban Dietetic Association, 1988
2. Carpenito LJ: Nursing Diagnosis. Application to Clinical Practice, 4th ed. Philadelphia: JB Lippincott, 1991

3. Cerrato PL: Would a new diet help your gallstone patient? RN July:59, 1989
4. DiIorio C, Price ME: Swallowing: An assessment guide. Am J Nurs 90:38, 1990
5. DiIorio C, Price ME: Swallowing: A practice guide. Am J Nurs 90:42, 1990
6. Douglas BR, Jansen JB, Tham RT, et al: Coffee stimulation of cholescystokinin release and gallbladder contraction in humans. Am J Clin Nutr 52:553, 1990
7. Escott-Stump S: Nutrition and Diagnosis-Related Care. 2nd ed. Philadelphia: Lea & Febiger, 1988
8. Kitchin LI, Castell DO: Rationale and efficacy of conservative therapy for gastroesophageal reflux disease. Arch Intern Med 151:448, 1991
9. Porth CM: Pathophysiology: Concepts of Altered Health States, 3rd ed. Philadelphia: JB Lippincott, 1990
10. Scherer JC: Introductory Medical–Surgical Nursing, 5th ed. Philadelphia: JB Lippincott, 1991
11. Slavin JL: Dietary fiber: Classification, chemical analyses, and food sources. J Am Diet Assoc 87:1164, 1987
12. United States Department of Agriculture and United States Department of Health and Human Services: Nutrition and Your Health: Dietary Guidelines for Americans. 3rd ed. Home and Garden Bulletin no. 232, 1990
13. United States Department of Health and Human Services: Eating Hints: Recipes and Tips for Better Nutrition During Cancer Treatment. NIH Publication no. 91-2079. National Cancer Institute, Bethesda, MD. Revised April 1990

16 Cardiovascular Disorders and Nutritional Anemias

THE CARDIOVASCULAR SYSTEM

The cardiovascular system is composed of the heart, arteries, capillaries, and veins. The muscle action of the heart pumps oxygen-depleted blood through veins to the lungs, where carbon dioxide is removed and oxygen is replenished. Arteries carry oxygen-rich blood away from the heart to the capillaries. Oxygen and nutrients are freely exchanged between the blood and body cells through the capillary walls.

Diseases of the heart are the leading cause of death in the United States in people older than 35 years of age, and 90% of those deaths are attributed to atherosclerosis and hypertension. Substantial evidence gathered over the last 2 decades indicates that diet can play a significant role in preventing heart disease.[13] Studies show that although diet modification may not be able to prevent heart disease in all *individuals*, Americans in general can reduce their risk of heart disease by lowering serum cholesterol levels through diet modification.

459

CARDIAC DISORDERS

Atherosclerotic Heart Disease and Coronary Heart Disease

Arteriosclerosis is a condition characterized by thickening and hardening of the arterial walls. Atherosclerosis, a more common yet severe form of arteriosclerosis, is caused by the formation of plaques, which are composed mostly of fats (especially cholesterol), other blood components, and connective tissue.

The process begins asymptomatically with the development of fatty streaks on the lining of the arterial wall. As the streaks enlarge, plaques develop that narrow the artery and restrict the flow of blood. The plaques may become so large as to occlude the artery fully; however, the artery may become blocked before that time with the formation of a blood clot.

Because narrow blood vessels with restricted blood flow have a reduced capacity to deliver oxygen and remove wastes, organs and tissues "serviced" by those arteries can be damaged. The three most common sites affected by atherosclerosis are the legs, brain, and heart. Peripheral vascular disease and cerebral hemorrhage are complications of atherosclerosis of the legs and brain, respectively. Atherosclerosis of the coronary arteries causes coronary heart disease (CHD) (see box, Defining CHD). When the blood supply to the heart is blocked, a myocardial infarction can occur, resulting in further heart damage or sudden death. Atherosclerosis also may be responsible for angina pectoris, aneurysm of the abdominal aorta, and gangrene of the extremities.

The exact cause of CHD is unknown, although numerous risk factors have been identified (see box, CHD Risk Factors). An elevated serum cholesterol level (hypercholesterolemia), particularly of low-density lipoprotein cholesterol, is one of the three major modifiable risk factors (the other two being smoking and hypertension).

Cholesterol and Lipoproteins

Cholesterol, a fat-like substance, is found in all animal cell membranes and is a precursor of bile acids and sex hormones. Because it is insoluble in water (blood), cholesterol is

---

Defining CHD

Definite CHD is indicated when the client has the characteristic clinical picture and objective laboratory findings of either:
- Definite prior myocardial infarction, or
- Definite myocardial ischemia, such as angina pectoris.

Source: Public Health Service, United States Department of Health and Human Services, National Institutes of Health: National Cholesterol Education Program: Report of the Expert Panel on Detection, Evaluation, and Treatment of High Blood Cholesterol in Adults. NIH Publication No. 89-2925. Washington, DC: Government Printing Office, 1989

CHD Risk Factors

Male sex

Family history of premature CHD (definite MI or sudden death before age 55 in a parent or sibling)

Cigarette smoking

Hypertension

Low HDL concentration (below 35 mg/dl confirmed by repeated measurement)

Diabetes mellitus

History of definite cerebrovascular or occlusive peripheral vascular disease

Severe obesity (30% or more overweight)

Source: Public Health Service, United States Department of Health and Human Services, National Institutes of Health: National Cholesterol Education Program: Report of the Expert Panel on Detection, Evaluation, and Treatment of High Blood Cholesterol in Adults. NIH Publication No. 89-2925. Washington, DC: Government Printing Office, 1989

transported through the blood attached to protein in lipoprotein molecules, which also contain triglycerides and phospholipids. The four types of lipoprotein vary in density, composition, and function (Table 16-1). Hyperlipoproteinemia/hyperlipidemia is characterized by elevated levels of one or more of the lipoprotein types. Table 16-2 outlines various types of lipid abnormalities and the nutritional implications of each.

Total serum cholesterol, which is influenced by genetics, diet, various diseases, activity, certain drugs, age, and other variables, is a measure of all cholesterol and does not distinguish between the "good" and "bad" cholesterol.

Table 16-1
Lipoproteins: Types, Composition, and Functions

Type	Composition	Function
Chylomicrons	Mainly triglycerides	Transport triglycerides from the intestines through the lymphatic system to the liver. Severe elevations of chylomicrons induce pancreatitis.
Very-low-density lipoproteins (VLDL)	Mainly endogenously produced triglycerides with a small amount of cholesterol	Transport cholesterol from the liver to the cells. Precursor of LDL. Role in CHD is unclear.
Low-density lipoproteins (LDL)	Mainly cholesterol	Transport cholesterol out of the liver to the cells. Strong positive association between elevated LDL and CHD.
High-density lipoproteins (HDL)	Mainly protein with some cholesterol	Transport cholesterol from the cells to the liver. Elevated HDL are protective against CHD.

Table 16-2
Various Lipid Abnormalities and Their Nutritional Implications

Abnormality	Nutritional Implications
Familial hypercholesterolemia: caused by a defective gene. People with one defective gene usually have LDL levels >200 mg/dl. Two defective genes rarely occur and are characterized by cholesterol levels of 600–1000 mg; severe and often fatal heart disease frequently develops in adolescent years.	Diet intervention rarely is effective as the sole mode of treatment. Step Two diet is recommended to potentiate the action of cholesterol-lowering drugs.
Familial combined hyperlipidemia: characterized by increases in VLDL, LDL, or both VLDL and LDL. Problem appears to be with over-production of lipoproteins by the liver. Represents an increased risk of CHD regardless of the type of lipoprotein actually elevated.	Weight reduction often is effective at lowering lipoproteins, and a low-saturated fat, low-cholesterol diet may further reduce LDL levels. Drug therapy may be needed to completely or adequately control serum lipoproteins.
Severe primary hypercholesterolemia: persistent cholesterol levels over 300 mg/dl with high risk of CHD.	Often diet-resistant; drug therapy usually required.
Familial dysbetalipoproteinemia (type 3 hyperlipoproteinemia): relatively uncommon condition characterized by a high total cholesterol related to an increase in VLDL. Increased risk of premature CHD and peripheral vascular disease; obesity, glucose intolerance, and hyperuricemia are common.	Calorie restriction is indicated for overweight clients. Low-saturated fat, low-cholesterol diet is often helpful; however, drug therapy may be needed.
Hypertriglyceridemia: defined as a fasting plasma triglyceride >500 mg/dl. People with triglyceride levels of 250–750 mg/dl usually have an increase in VLDL. Triglyceride levels >750 mg/dl are associated with increases in both VLDL and chylomicrons. Relationship between elevated triglycerides and heart disease is controversial; levels >1000 mg/dl increase the risk of pancreatitis.	Weight control and restriction of alcohol are recommended. A low-fat diet may help. Drug therapy may be necesssary.
Reduced HDL cholesterol: characterized by HDL levels <35 mg/dl and associated with an increased risk of CHD. Common causes of reduced HDL include cigarette smoking, obesity, lack of exercise, use of androgenic steroids, use of beta-adrenergic blocking agents, hypertriglyceridemia, and genetic factors.	Calorie restriction is indicated for obese clients.
Diabetic dyslipidemia: abnormal lipid and lipoprotein levels are often observed in diabetics, especially hypertriglyceridemia.	Improved glucose control can reduce serum triglycerides.

Source: Public Health Service, United States Department of Health and Human Services, National Institutes of Health: National Cholesterol Education Program: Report of the Expert Panel on Detection, Evaluation, and Treatment of High Blood Cholesterol in Adults. NIH Publication No. 89-2925. Washington, DC: Government Printing Office, 1989

The "good" cholesterol is found in *high-density lipoproteins* (HDL), which are composed mainly of protein, with some cholesterol. High-density lipoproteins are scavengers that act to take cholesterol out of the serum by transporting it from the cells to the liver, where 95% of it is excreted.[9] High-density lipoprotein levels are inversely correlated with the risk of CHD: the higher the HDL levels, the lower the risk of heart disease. Exercise, weight loss if overweight, and moderate alcohol consumption can increase HDL cholesterol levels.

The "bad" cholesterol is in *low-density lipoproteins* (LDL), which contain 60% to 70% of total serum cholesterol and are known as the major atherogenic class of lipoproteins. Low-density lipoproteins transport cholesterol out of the liver to the cells; when cells get too much cholesterol from high levels of LDL, the excess cholesterol accumulates as a waxy deposit that can eventually choke the cells.[9] Numerous clinical, epidemiologic, metabolic, and animal studies strongly indicate that high levels of total and LDL cholesterol, which are increased by diets high in total fat and saturated fat, are a cause of atherosclerosis and increase the risk of CHD. Conversely, findings show that lowering total and LDL cholesterol levels reduces the subsequent incidence of CHD events, and may even help prevent recurrent myocardial infarction and death in clients who have already had a heart attack.[14]

Serum HDL cholesterol can be obtained through a lipoprotein analysis, a procedure that also measures fasting levels of total cholesterol and total triglycerides. Once these values are known, LDL cholesterol can be calculated (see box, Formula for Estimating LDL Cholesterol).

Defining Risk and Intervention Strategies

In 1987, the National Cholesterol Education Program (NCEP) recommended that total serum cholesterol be measured in all adults aged 20 and older, preferably as part of a total physical examination so that other risks can be identified.[14] Total serum cholesterol levels below 200 mg/dl were classified as "desirable blood cholesterol," values of 200 to 239 mg/dl were considered "borderline high blood cholesterol," and values of 240 mg/dl and above were classified as "high blood cholesterol"; at 240 mg/dl, the risk of CHD is double that at 200 mg/dl and is rising steeply. A lipoprotein analysis is indicated for (1) clients with borderline high blood cholesterol levels who have either CHD or two other risk factors; and (2) for all people with high blood cholesterol levels. Table 16-3 lists the classifications of both total serum and LDL cholesterol levels.

Formula for Estimating LDL Cholesterol from a Lipoprotein Analysis Performed After a 12-Hour Fast

LDL cholesterol = total cholesterol − HDL cholesterol − (triglycerides ÷ 5)

Source: Public Health Service, United States Department of Health and Human Services, National Institutes of Health: National Cholesterol Education Program: Report of the Expert Panel on Detection, Evaluation, and Treatment of High Blood Cholesterol in Adults. NIH Publication No. 89-2925. Washington, DC: Government Printing Office, 1989

Table 16-3
Classification of Total Serum and LDL Cholesterol

Classification	Total Serum Cholesterol	LDL Cholesterol
Desirable	<200 mg/dl	<130 mg/dl
Borderline–high risk	200–239 mg/dl	130–159 mg/dl
High	≥240 mg/dl	≥160 mg/dl

Source: Public Health Service, United States Department of Health and Human Services, National Institutes of Health: National Cholesterol Education Program: Report of the Expert Panel on Detection, Evaluation, and Treatment of High Blood Cholesterol in Adults. NIH Publication No. 89-2925. Washington, DC: Government Printing Office, 1989

After a thorough assessment is made, interventions are planned according to the client's serum cholesterol levels and are influenced by the presence of CHD and other risk factors (Fig. 16-1). Minimum goals are to reduce LDL cholesterol to <160 mg/dl for people without CHD or two other risk factors or to <130 mg/dl for people with CHD or two other risk factors; lower levels are desirable. Diet therapy is the cornerstone of treatment. If diet fails to achieve minimum goals within a specified period of time (*i.e.*, 6 months of good adherence), drug therapy may be added.

Diet Therapy

Although the term "diet" is used to describe the nutritional recommendations put forth by the NCEP to treat hypercholesterolemia, "diet" really is a misnomer. Permanent lifestyle changes for both the "well" population and those with high cholesterol levels are urged for both prevention and treatment of hypercholesterolemia.

Generally, the "diet" to lower serum cholesterol is limited in total fat, saturated fat, and cholesterol. Because excessive calorie intake increases LDL cholesterol, calorie intake should be adjusted to attain or maintain "healthy" weight. A high fiber intake, especially soluble fiber, is recommended for its effect in lowering serum cholesterol levels.

The NCEP has outlined the "diet" in two steps (Table 16-4). The Step One diet limits the major and obvious sources of saturated fat and cholesterol; many clients can achieve this diet without a radical alteration in dietary habits.[14] If the Step One diet fails to accomplish its goals after 3 months of good compliance, the diet may need to be progressed to the Step Two diet, which requires more careful attention to the total diet. However, clients with familial hypercholesterolemia may be diet-resistant, necessitating the use of one or more drugs.

Nursing Process

Assessment

In addition to the general cardiovascular assessment criteria, assess for the following factors:

Meal timing and frequency: determine when the client's largest meal is eaten.

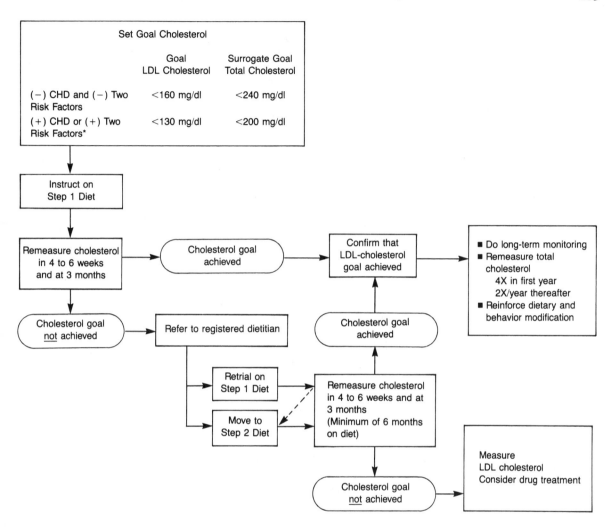

Set Goal Cholesterol

	Goal LDL Cholesterol	Surrogate Goal Total Cholesterol
(−) CHD and (−) Two Risk Factors	<160 mg/dl	<240 mg/dl
(+) CHD or (+) Two Risk Factors*	<130 mg/dl	<200 mg/dl

*One of which can be male sex (see box, CHD Risk Factors).

Figure 16-1

Diet intervention strategy. (National Cholesterol Education Program)

Total fat and cholesterol intake: determine how much and how often butter, whole milk, cheese, ice cream, meat products, bakery goods, eggs, and organ meats are consumed.

Intake of convenience and fast foods.

Fiber intake, especially foods high in soluble fiber: oatmeal, oat bran, dried peas and beans, citrus fruits, apples, and certain vegetables.

Likes and dislikes: determine which foods the client can't live without, and which foods can be easily forfeited.

The impact of lifestyle and work schedule on eating (*i.e.*, are most meals eaten at home, at a restaurant, in a cafeteria?).

Cultural, familial, religious, and ethnic influences on eating habits.

Table 16-4
Characteristics of the Step One and Step Two Diets

Nutrient	Recommended Intake	
	Step One Diet	Step Two Diet
Total fat	Less than 30% of total calories	
Saturated fatty acids	Less than 10% of total calories	Less than 7% of total calories
Polyunsaturated fatty acids	Up to 10% of total calories	
Monounsaturated fatty acids	10 to 15% of total calories	
Carbohydrates	50 to 60% of total calories	
Protein	10 to 20% of total calories	
Cholesterol	Less than 300 mg/day	Less than 200 mg/day
Total calories	To achieve and maintain desirable weight	

Source: Public Health Service, United States Department of Health and Human Services, National Institutes of Health: National Cholesterol Education Program: Report of the Expert Panel on Detection, Evaluation, and Treatment of High Blood Cholesterol in Adults. NIH Publication No. 89-2925. Washington, DC: Government Printing Office, 1989

The client's medical history and any possible effects on intake or nutritional status.
The client's use of alcohol, drugs, and tobacco.
Weight, weight changes.
Dietary changes made in response to diagnosis of atherosclerosis or CHD, if appropriate.
The client's willingness to make dietary changes.
The client's education level, social status, and previous counseling experiences.[1]
Frequency and intensity of exercise.

Nursing Diagnosis

Health Seeking Behaviors, as evidenced by the lack of knowledge of a "heart" healthy diet and a desire to learn.

Planning and Implementation

The goal of diet therapy is to provide a nutritionally adequate diet and reduce serum cholesterol levels; for every 1% drop in serum cholesterol, the risk of CHD decreases by 2%. Diet may also be used to control other medical risk factors that are responsive to diet modification, such as hypertension, obesity, and diabetes mellitus.

    Although diet intervention is considered the first line of treatment for clients with elevated cholesterol levels, "diet" should be viewed as a lifestyle change consistent with good health. All people, regardless of cholesterol level, should be given information on diet and risk reduction for the possible prevention of disease. It has been suggested that it may take 2 to 10 years to make drastic changes in eating habits. Compliance may improve when diet changes are individualized and are instituted gradually. Low-density lipoprotein cholesterol levels should begin to decrease within 3 to 4 weeks after the diet is initiated.

    To implement the Step One diet, foods containing butterfat should be limited (butter, cheese, ice cream, cream, whole and 2% milk). Lean cuts of meat should be chosen and visible fat removed. Skinless chicken and fish should frequently be used in place of red meats, and meatless meals should be served occasionally. Egg yolks should be limited to

| **Assessment Criteria** | ## General Cardiovascular Assessment Criteria |

Age, especially over age 40

Sex

Presence of obesity

Blood pressure

Serum cholesterol

Lipid profiles

Other laboratory results: electrolyte imbalances, LDH and CPK levels

Results of other diagnostic procedures: angiograms, ECGs

Ascites, edema

Chest pain

Xanthomas

Diet high in fat, cholesterol, and calories

Use of alcohol, tobacco

Positive family history of heart disease

Other medical conditions, such as diabetes mellitus, pancreatitis

Medications used

Type A personality, stressful lifestyle

three per week, and organ meats used sparingly. Coconut oil, palm oil, and palm kernel oil are high in saturated fat; products containing these oils should be avoided. See Table 16-5 for specific recommended diet modifications.

Polyunsaturated fats (corn oil, sunflower oil, safflower oil, soybean oil) should be used to replace some of the saturated fats in the diet because they help lower LDL cholesterol. Unfortunately, they may also decrease HDL cholesterol, and in animals, a high-PUFA diet can promote certain cancers. It is recommended that PUFA intake not exceed 10% of total calories.

Omega-3 fatty acids, commonly known as fish oils, are a type of PUFA that have been shown to lower serum triglycerides and decrease platelet aggregation. Population studies indicate that frequent consumption of fish, especially fatty fish, is related to a lower incidence of heart disease. Although increasing consumption of fish is recommended, the use of fish oil capsules has not been demonstrated to be effective or safe; their use should be discouraged.

Monounsaturated fats, like those predominating in olive oil, canola oil, and peanut oil, tend to lower LDL cholesterol without adversely affecting HDL cholesterol. Monounsaturated fats should comprise 10% to 15% of total calorie intake.

Because complex carbohydrates are generally low in fat and rich in fiber and nutrients, a liberal intake is recommended to replace some of the calories lost from a reduced fat intake.

Table 16-5

Recommended Diet Modifications to Lower Blood Cholesterol: The Step One Diet

Choose	Decrease
FISH, CHICKEN, TURKEY, AND LEAN MEATS	
Fish, poultry without skin, lean cuts of beef, lamb, pork or veal, shellfish	Fatty cuts of beef, lamb, pork; spare ribs, organ meats, regular cold cuts, sausage, hot dogs, bacon, sardines, roe
SKIM AND LOW-FAT MILK, CHEESE, YOGURT, AND DAIRY SUBSTITUTES	
Skim or 1% fat milk (liquid, powdered, evaporated)	Whole milk (4% fat): regular, evaporated, condensed; cream, half and half, 2% milk, imitation milk products, most nondairy creamers, whipped toppings
Buttermilk	
Nonfat (0% fat) or low-fat yogurt	Whole-milk yogurt
Low-fat cottage cheese (1% or 2% fat)	Whole-milk cottage cheese (4% fat)
Low-fat cheeses, farmer, or pot cheeses (all of these should be labeled no more than 2–6 g fat/ounce)	All natural cheeses (*e.g.,* bleu, roquefort, camembert, cheddar, swiss)
	Low-fat or "light" cream cheese, low-fat or "light" sour cream
	Cream cheeses, sour cream
Sherbet	Ice cream
Sorbet	
EGGS	
Egg whites (2 whites = 1 whole egg in recipes), cholesterol-free egg substitutes	Egg yolks
FRUITS AND VEGETABLES	
Fresh, frozen, canned, or dried fruits and vegetables	Vegetables prepared in butter, cream, or other sauces
BREADS AND CEREALS	
Homemade baked goods using unsaturated oils sparingly, angel food cake, low-fat crackers, low-fat cookies	Commercial baked goods: pies, cakes, doughnuts, croissants, pastries, muffins, biscuits, high-fat crackers, high-fat cookies
Rice, pasta	Egg noodles
Whole-grain breads and cereals (oatmeal, whole wheat, rye, bran, multigrain, etc.)	Breads in which eggs are major ingredient
FATS AND OILS	
Baking cocoa	Chocolate
Unsaturated vegetable oils: corn, olive, rapeseed (canola oil), safflower, sesame, soybean, sunflower	Butter, coconut oil, palm oil, palm kernel oil, lard, bacon fat
Margarine or shortening made from one of the unsaturated oils listed above	
Diet margarine	
Mayonnaise, salad dressing made with unsaturated oils listed above	Dressings made with egg yolk
Low-fat dressings	
Seeds and nuts	Coconut

Source: Public Health Service, United States Department of Health and Human Services, National Institutes of Health: National Cholesterol Education Program: Report of the Expert Panel on Detection, Evaluation, and Treatment of High Blood Cholesterol in Adults. NIH Publication No. 89-2925. Washington, DC: Government Printing Office, 1989

High-fiber diets, especially those rich in soluble fiber, may help reduce blood cholesterol levels by increasing the excretion of bile salts and acids that contain cholesterol. Oatmeal, oat bran, dried peas and beans, citrus fruits, apples, and some vegetables are rich sources of soluble fiber.

Moderate alcohol consumption has been shown to increase HDL cholesterol. Unfortunately, alcohol can also raise blood pressure and very low-density lipoprotein (VLDL) levels, and impede weight loss.

Claims that various vitamins, minerals, and health foods are protective against atherosclerosis have not been proven. Garlic oil can significantly lower serum triglycerides and cholesterol levels and raise HDL levels. The amount of garlic needed, however, is so large that its use is not practical, and the effectiveness of odorless garlic pills is questionable.

Even though diet can lower serum cholesterol levels, it is not known whether atherosclerosis can be prevented through diet modification or if all Americans should alter their current eating habits. Most experts agree that most Americans have the potential to benefit from a low-fat, low-saturated fat, low-cholesterol diet with calories for "healthy" weight. Possible exceptions include high-risk elderly clients and pregnant women.

A sample menu appears in the box, Sample Step One Diet Menu. Be aware of the potential problems of a Step One diet, and the corresponding nursing interventions and considerations.

Client Goals

The client will:

Experience a decrease in serum cholesterol to the desired level or below (see Fig. 16-1); clients with desirable serum cholesterol levels will maintain those levels.

Explain the principles and rationale of diet management of hypercholesterolemia, implement the appropriate diet changes, and incorporate the changes into his or her lifestyle.

Name foods high in saturated fats, polyunsaturated fats, monounsaturated fats, and cholesterol.

Consume a nutritionally adequate diet with calories to attain/maintain "healthy" weight.

Nursing Interventions

Diet Management

Reduce total fat, saturated fat, and cholesterol to levels recommended in the Step One diet (Tables 16-4 and 16-5).

Adjust calorie intake to attain/maintain "healthy" weight.

Increase intake of carbohydrates, especially complex carbohydrates and soluble fiber.

Allow moderate use of alcohol, if appropriate.

Client Teaching

Instruct the client

That the three most effective dietary modifications to lower serum cholesterol are to (1) decrease total fat intake, especially saturated fat, (2) limit dietary cholesterol, and (3) avoid excessive calorie intake.

(Text continued on page 472)

Step One Diet

Breakfast

Orange juice
Oatmeal with brown sugar
2 slices whole-wheat toast
2 tsp corn oil margarine
Skim milk
Coffee/tea
Salt/pepper/sugar

Lunch

Sandwich made with 2 slices whole-wheat bread, 3 oz turkey breast, 1 tsp
    salad dressing, tomato, and lettuce
Three-bean salad (kidney beans, chick peas, green beans) made with olive
    oil-and-vinegar dressing
Fresh apple
Skim milk
Coffee/tea
Salt/pepper/sugar

Dinner

3 oz baked haddock with lemon
Herbed rice
Steamed broccoli
Coleslaw with canola oil-and-vinegar dressing
Rye bread
2 tsp corn oil margarine
Angel food cake with sliced strawberries
Skim milk
Coffee/tea
Salt/pepper/sugar

Snack

Fruit juice
Popcorn made with canola oil and seasoned with salt

(continued)

Step One Diet *(continued)*

Sample Menu *(continued)*

Potential Problem/Rationale

Inadequate iron intake related to the restriction on the amount of red meat allowed. Red meats are the richest source of iron in the diet.

Nursing Interventions and Considerations

Assess iron status periodically and provide supplements as needed.

Encourage the client to eat other foods high in iron, such as dried fruits, fortified cereals and grains, green leafy vegetables, and dried peas and beans. Instruct the client to consume a good source of vitamin C at each meal to enhance iron absorption from plant sources.

Potential Problem/Rationale

Increased sodium intake related to the use of specially prepared low-cholesterol products, such as imitation cheese, bacon, and eggs.

Nursing Interventions and Considerations

If the client also is following a low-sodium diet, calculate the amount of sodium being consumed from these products. If possible, revise the low-sodium diet to include as many of these products as desired. If necessary, encourage only limited use of high-sodium, cholesterol-free imitation foods.

Potential Problem/Rationale

Difficulty buying a variety of specialty foods related to increased cost. Poly-unsaturated margarines, egg substitutes, and other imitation foods often cost more than the items they are intended to replace.

Nursing Interventions and Considerations

Advise the client that polyunsaturated margarines must be used if the diet is to be followed successfully; for economy, they can be purchased in quantity while on sale and kept frozen until ready to use. Although other imitation products add variety to the diet, they are not essential and need not be used.

Potential Problem/Rationale

Boredom related to the restrictive nature of the diet.

Nursing Interventions and Considerations

Provide a variety of recipes using allowed foods.

Refer the client to the local American Heart Association for additional resources.

That fat present in food is usually a mixture of all three types of fats: saturated, polyunsaturated, and monounsaturated. A food is considered a "saturated" fat or "polyunsaturated" fat based on which type of fat is present in the food in the largest concentration (see Table 3-4).

On the role of saturated fat. Saturated fats tend to raise serum cholesterol levels and are found mostly in animal fats: meats, cheese, lard, butter, suet, salt pork, and bacon drippings. Saturated fat intake should decrease. Coconut oil, palm oil, and palm kernel oil, economical tropical oils used in food processing, are also highly saturated and should be avoided.

On the role of cholesterol. Dietary cholesterol tends to raise serum cholesterol, although the impact is less than that of saturated fat. Cholesterol is produced by the body, so that dietary intake is not essential. Cholesterol is found only in animal products, both in the muscle and the fat; therefore, a low-fat animal product is not necessarily low in cholesterol (*e.g.*, shrimp). The richest sources of cholesterol are organ meats and egg yolks (see Table 3-5); organ meats should be avoided, and egg yolks limited to three per week, including those used in food preparation. Fruits, vegetables, grains, cereals, nuts, and legumes contain no cholesterol. Egg whites are also cholesterol-free and may be used as desired.

On the role of polyunsaturated fats. Polyunsaturated fats, found in highest concentrations in vegetable oils, tend to lower both the "good" and "bad" cholesterol. They should be used in place of some saturated fats; however, their long-term safety at higher-than-recommended levels has not been established.

On the role of monounsaturated fats. Monounsaturated fats, found in highest concentrations in peanut oil, olive oil, and canola oil, tend to lower the "bad" cholesterol without having an adverse effect on the "good" cholesterol. They should provide more calories in the diet than either saturated or polyunsaturated fats.

On the sources of "hidden" fats in the diet: baked goods, cheese, processed meats.

That soluble fiber, abundant in oatmeal, oat bran, dried peas and beans, citrus fruits, apples, and certain vegetables, helps to lower serum cholesterol. Encourage the client to increase fiber intake gradually to reduce the risk of unpleasant side effects (gas, bloating, and diarrhea).

On general diet guidelines:
- Limit egg yolks to three per week, including those used in food preparation.
- Limit meat intake to about 6 oz/day, using mostly chicken, turkey, veal, and fish instead of lean cuts of beef, lamb, pork, and ham.
- Avoid organ meats, bacon, sausage, hot dogs, and luncheon meats.
- Use polyunsaturated oils and margarines in place of butter, solid margarine, shortening, and lard.
- Substitute skim milk and skim-milk products for whole milk and whole-milk products.
- Eat more fruits, vegetables, and whole grains, which are naturally low in fat and are cholesterol-free.

On food preparation techniques and meal planning ideas to reduce saturated fat content:
- Eat occasional meatless meals.
- Trim fat from meat before cooking. Chicken can be cooked with the skin on, but the skin should be removed before eating.
- Tender cuts of meat—sirloin and rib—are higher in fat and calories than less tender cuts such as round, loin, and flank.

- Place meats to be baked or roasted on a rack to allow the fat to drain.
- Bake, broil, steam, or saute foods in vegetable cooking spray or allowed oils.
- Prepare foods from "scratch" instead of purchasing convenience foods and mixes, which tend to be high in saturated fat.
- Use allowed oils to season cooked vegetables and in the preparation of salad dressings, marinades, pie crusts, barbecue sauces, and skim milk cream sauces.
- Reduce fat by one-half or more in casserole and quickbread recipes.
- Substitute low-fat items for high-fat items whenever possible (see box, Low-Fat Cooking).
- Make fat-free soup stock by preparing the stock a day ahead and refrigerating it overnight. The fat will harden and can be removed easily from the surface. Also make fat-free gravies, thickened with cornstarch, by this method.
- Use herbs and spices, lemon juice, and flavored vinegars to flavor foods without fat.

On low-fat snack ideas: low-fat yogurt, fresh fruit and vegetables, dried fruit, unbuttered

Low-Fat Cooking

High-Fat Food	Low-Fat Alternatives	Grams of Fat "Saved"
1 oz hard cheese	1 oz low-fat cheese	4
	1 oz low-fat processed cheese	7
	2 tbsp grated parmesan cheese	6
1 whole egg	¼ cup egg substitute	6
	2 egg whites	6
1 cup whole milk	1 cup 2% milk	5
	1 cup 1% milk	7
	1 cup skim milk	10
1 cup sour cream	1 cup reduced-fat sour cream	32
	1 cup low-fat cottage cheese (puréed)	44
	1 cup plain nonfat yogurt	48
1 cup regular mayonnaise	1 cup reduced-fat mayonnaise	111
	1 cup nonfat mayonnaise	175
1 cup whole-milk ricotta cheese	1 cup part-skim ricotta	12
	1 cup regular cottage cheese	22
	1 cup low-fat cottage cheese	28
1 cup heavy cream, liquid	1 cup half-and-half	61
	1 cup evaporated whole milk	69
	1 cup evaporated skim milk	87
1 cup regular ice cream	1 cup ice milk	8
	1 cup frozen yogurt	10
	1 cup nonfat frozen dessert	14
1 oz cream cheese	1 oz reduced-fat cream cheese	5
	2 tbsp puréed low-fat cream cheese	9.5
1 cup white sauce	1 cup paste-method white sauce made with:	
	2% milk	63
	1% milk	65
	skim milk	67
1 tbsp regular Italian dressing	1 cup low-calorie Italian	8

popcorn, unsalted pretzels, bread sticks, melba toast, frozen juice bars, low-fat crackers.

On how to read labels to identify sources of saturated fats:

- "Hydrogenation" is a process that hardens a liquid vegetable oil, changing it from an unsaturated fat to a more saturated fat. Foods containing hydrogenated or partially hydrogenated oils should be avoided.
- Products claiming to be made from "pure vegetable oil" or containing "no cholesterol" may be high in saturated fat if made from coconut or palm oils. Neither claim assures the product is suitable for a "heart-healthy" diet.
- Nondairy creamers and dessert toppings are cholesterol-free, but are high in saturated fat and should be avoided.

On how to order from a menu while dining out:

- Look for low-fat descriptions, such as "steamed," "in its own juice," "broiled," "roasted," and "poached."
- Avoid high-fat items described as "buttery," "buttered," "in butter sauce," "braised," "creamed," "in cream sauce," "hollandaise," "au gratin," "parmesan," "in cheese sauce," "escalloped," "marinated," "stewed," "basted," and "prime."
- Request margarine instead of butter.
- Request skim milk instead of whole milk, half-and-half, and nondairy creamers.
- Trim visible fat off meat and remove poultry skin.
- Limit portion size to 4 to 6 oz of cooked meat, fish, or poultry.
- Forego gravy and sauces, or ask that they be served "on the side," for portion control.
- Choose fresh fruit for an appetizer or dessert.

Provide the client with appropriate teaching materials, recipes, and information on addition resources.

Monitor

Monitor for the following signs or symptoms:

Compliance with the diet, and the need for follow-up diet counseling

Effectiveness of the diet: LDL cholesterol should begin to decline 2 to 3 weeks after the diet is initiated; if the diet fails to achieve the desired goal after 3 months of good adherence, progress to the Step Two diet

Weight, weight changes

Other risk factors, if appropriate (*i.e.*, hypertension, diabetes, smoking)

Evaluation

Evaluation is ongoing. Assuming the plan of care has not changed, the client will achieve the goals as stated above.

DRUG ALERT　　Bile acid-sequestering resins (such as cholestyramine and colestipol) used to decrease serum cholesterol and LDL levels can cause malabsorption of vitamins A, D, E, K, calcium, and fat. Other common side effects requiring diet modification include constipation (especially among the elderly), nausea, vomiting, and anorexia.

Two drugs frequently used to decrease VLDL levels, clofibrate and nicotinic acid, may cause nausea, vomiting, and gastrointestinal discomfort. Clofibrate may also interfere with carotene, glucose, iron, vitamin B_{12}, and electrolyte absorption. Nicotinic acid commonly causes flushing, a tingling sensation accompanied by a red skin rash.[10] Flushing can be minimized by gradually increasing the dose, taking the drug with meals and not with liquids, and taking an aspirin 30 minutes before the niacin.[10]

Myocardial Infarction

A myocardial infarction (MI) involves the destruction of heart tissue in areas of the heart deprived of blood and oxygen. A MI can occur as a result of atherosclerosis, arterial occlusion from embolus or thrombus, myocardial hypertrophy caused by congestive heart failure and hypertension, or secondary to a temporary reduction in blood flow to the heart related to shock, gastrointestinal (GI) bleeding, severe dehydration, or hypotension. Myocardial infarctions are the most common cause of death in North America; 15% to 20% of white Americans die from myocardial infarctions, with a slightly lower incidence among blacks.

Symptoms of an impending or actual MI include spontaneous, constrictive, prolonged chest pain, which is not relieved by rest or nitrates and may radiate to one or both arms, the neck, and the back. Symptoms of shock, such as hypotension, gray facial color, cold diaphoresis, tachycardia or bradycardia, and weak, irregular pulse, may be observed. The client may experience nausea, vomiting, fever, hypotension, anxiety, and apprehension.

Myocardial infarctions that do not result in sudden death can cause severe and life-threatening complications: arrhythmias, shock, congestive heart failure, rupture of the heart, pulmonary embolism, and recurrent heart attacks.

Treatment of an acute MI seeks to alleviate symptoms and prevent further damage with continual assessment and monitoring, complete rest, sedation, narcotics, oxygen, and intravenous fluids. The diet is also modified to prevent diet-induced arrhythmias and reduce cardiac workload. After the acute phase has passed, treatment focuses on rehabilitation and education of the client and the family. Diet modification is aimed at reducing diet-responsive risk factors, such as hypercholesterolemia, obesity, diabetes mellitus, and hypertension.

Nursing Process

Assessment

In addition to the general cardiovascular assessment criteria, assess for the following factors:

Stage of recovery: acute, subacute, or rehabilitative

The presence of symptoms that interfere with eating, such as shortness of breath, fatigue, anorexia, nausea, apprehension

Other medical conditions that require diet intervention, such as hypertension, diabetes mellitus, or obesity

The use of medications that produce nutritional side effects, such as potassium-depleting diuretics

Nursing Diagnosis

Health Seeking Behaviors, as evidenced by a lack of knowledge of dietary management of heart disease and a desire to learn.

Planning and Implementation

Initially, clients experiencing an MI are ordered NPO (nothing by mouth) and given intravenous fluids; oral intake may resume within 24 to 48 hours post-MI. In an attempt to reduce cardiac workload, total calories and meal size are often restricted. Liquids or soft, bland foods that are easily digested may be given in four to six meals daily. Because they may produce cardiac arrhythmias and slow the heart rate, food and liquids of extreme temperatures are avoided.

When the client enters the rehabilitative phase, usually 5 to 10 days post-MI, the diet is individualized according to the client's weight, serum lipid levels, and medical conditions. A Step One or Step Two diet may be indicated, and calories are adjusted for "healthy" weight. A sodium-restricted diet may be necessary for hypertension, edema, or congestive heart failure. Client education is extremely important to maximize diet compliance. Initiate dietary changes gradually and sequentially.

Client Goals

Acute Phase

The client will:
Avoid diet-induced arrhythmias.
Avoid foods/liquids that increase cardiac workload.

Rehabilitative Phase (Begins 5 to 10 Days Post-MI)

The client will:
Reduce serum lipid levels and control medical risk factors, if appropriate.

Nursing Interventions

Diet Management

Initial diet (begins 24 to 48 hours post-MI until rehabilitative phase begins):
Limit calories and provide small, frequent meals to avoid abdominal distention that could exert pressure on the heart. Calorie intake is increased as the client improves.
Provide liquids or soft, bland foods that are easy to digest; eliminate gassy foods and individual intolerances.
Avoid foods and liquids of temperature extremes, which may produce cardiac arrhythmias.
Eliminate caffeinated beverages, which may stimulate heart rate (see Appendix 8).
Provide complete or partial assistance, depending on the client's strength.
Rehabilitative phase (begins 5 to 10 days post-MI):
Advance the diet to three meals per day; however, small, frequent meals are recommended for clients experiencing persistent angina.
Individualize the diet according to the client's weight, serum lipid levels, and medical conditions. A Step One or Step Two diet may be indicated (see Table 16-5).

Client Teaching

Client teaching is not indicated during the acute and subacute phases. During the rehabilitative phase, the client may be instructed on the Step One or Step Two diet (see above); additional instructions may be necessary to control other diet-responsive risk factors, such as obesity, diabetes mellitus, and hypertension.

Monitor

Monitor for the following signs or symptoms:
Tolerance of the diet (*i.e.*, absence of postprandial cardiac changes such as arrhythmias and
   increased heart rate)
The client's ability to self-feed; as the client moves into the rehabilitative phase, monitor
   the presence of other risk factors and the need for diet counseling

Evaluation

Evaluation is ongoing. Assuming the plan of care has not changed, the client will achieve the goals as stated above.

Congestive Heart Failure

Congestive heart failure (CHF) is a syndrome characterized by the inability of the heart to maintain adequate blood flow through the circulatory system, leading to decreased blood flow to the kidneys, excessive sodium and fluid retention, peripheral and pulmonary edema, and finally, an overworked and enlarged heart. The severity of CHF can vary from mild to severe. Although the heart and circulation are principally affected initially, the entire circulation eventually is affected.

Congestive heart failure develops in 50% to 60% of all cases of organic heart diseases that weaken the muscle action of the heart: MI, hypertension, congenital heart disease, cardiomyopathies, valve disorders, and arrhythmias. Congestive heart failure also may occur secondary to circulatory overload related to excessive intravenous fluids or renal failure. Circulatory deficits, such as hemorrhage and dehydration, as well as pulmonary diseases such as chronic lung disease and pulmonary embolism, may also lead to CHF. In addition, any condition that increases metabolic demands may result in CHF: hyperthyroidism, pregnancy, anemia, fever, infection, and obesity. Frequently, CHF arises from a combination of factors.

Initially, CHF may be classified as left-sided or right-sided failure; eventually, symptoms of both will be present. Symptoms of left-sided heart failure, such as dyspnea, orthopnea, paroxysmal nocturnal dyspnea, pleural effusion, and pulmonary edema, are caused by inefficient oxygenation of the blood related to lung congestion. Right-sided heart failure most commonly causes dependent edema (especially of the feet and ankles), pitting edema, ascites, sudden weight gain related to fluid retention, upper abdominal pain related to liver congestion, anorexia and nausea, nocturia, weakness, and distended neck veins.

The treatment of CHF involves treatment of the underlying cause. Physical and mental rest help decrease cardiac workload. Digitalis may be used to slow the heart rate and strengthen its beat. Diuretic therapy is used to help rid the body of excess fluid. Oxygen therapy may be necessary. Diet intervention is used to reduce sodium and fluid retention, and to minimize cardiac workload.

Nursing Process

Assessment

In addition to the general cardiovascular assessment criteria, assess for the following factors:

Edema: areas affected, severity, interventions attempted and the results

The presence of symptoms that may affect intake (*i.e.*, nausea, anorexia, dyspnea, upper abdominal pain, weakness)

Dietary changes made in response to symptoms (*i.e.*, foods avoided, foods preferred). Determine foods best and least tolerated.

Weight, recent weight changes. Note that sudden weight gain is a symptom of fluid retention.

Usual intake of sodium, which is abundant in table salt, canned soups, meats, and vegetables, processed meats, convenience foods, condiments, and traditional snack foods

Intake of foods high in potassium, such as fresh and dried fruits, fruit juices, many fresh and frozen vegetables, dairy products, whole grains, meats, fish, and poultry

Usual fluid intake—when, what, and how much

The use of diuretics; determine whether they are potassium-sparing or potassium-wasting.

Nursing Diagnosis

Fluid Volume Excess, related to congestive heart failure.

Planning and Implementation

Edema related to congestive heart failure can be relieved by reducing sodium intake, as extracellular fluid retention does not occur in the absence of sodium. Sodium restriction may vary from 250 to 2000 mg, depending on the severity of CHF.

In most cases, sodium restriction alone or used in combination with diuretics (low-sodium diets enhance the sodium-excreting effects of diuretics) effectively reduces fluid volume without the need of a fluid restriction. However, a fluid restriction may be necessary if edema does not respond to a low-sodium diet.

A diet low in calories but otherwise nutritionally adequate is indicated for overweight clients. Attaining ideal or slightly under ideal weight will reduce the cardiac workload.

The diet should be individualized according to the client's tolerance. Emphasize easy-to-digest foods, such as carbohydrates, rather than protein, fat, and gas-forming foods.

It should be noted that malnutrition resulting from poor nutritional intakes and long-term medication use may not be apparent in clients with edema.

Client Goals

The client will

Eliminate or reduce edema.

Consume adequate calories to attain/maintain "healthy" body weight.

Describe the principles and rationale of diet management for CHF and implement the appropriate dietary changes.

Avoid hypokalemia and hyperkalemia by consuming the appropriate potassium intake, based on the type of diuretic used.

Avoid cardiac stimulants.

Avoid gastric distention and pressure on the heart.

Nursing Interventions

Diet Management

Limit sodium intake (range, 250 to 2000 mg; see box, Sodium-Restricted Diets). Initial allowance may be progressed as edema subsides. Some clients may tolerate 4 to 6 g of sodium after their condition is stabilized.

Provide adequate potassium, based on the type of diuretic prescribed. A high-potassium diet may be indicated for clients taking thiazide diuretics (potassium-wasting) and digitalis (see Appendix 9). Spironolactone and triamterene are potassium-sparing diuretics and do not warrant the intake or use of additional potassium.

Provide calories for "healthy" body weight. Decrease calories for weight loss, if overweight, to lessen cardiac workload.

Provide five to six small meals a day of nonirritating and nongas-forming foods to limit gastric distention and pressure on the heart. Fluid may be limited to 3 liters a day or less, depending on the client's response to the sodium restriction.

Initially, eliminate caffeine. After the client is stabilized, coffee intake may be liberalized to 4 to 5 cups a day.

Client Teaching

Instruct the client

On the principles and rationale of diet management for CHF.

On how to implement the changes necessary to comply with a low-sodium diet (see Low-Sodium Diet Teaching section in box, Sodium-Restricted Diets).

Monitor

Monitor for the following signs or symptoms:

Compliance with the diet, and the need for follow-up diet counseling

Effectiveness of the diet (*i.e.*, reduction in edema, weight loss), and evaluate the need for further diet modifications

Serum potassium; observe for signs of hypokalemia and hyperkalemia

Evaluation

Evaluation is ongoing. Assuming the plan of care has not changed, the client will achieve the goals as stated above.

(*Text continued on page 487*)

Sodium-Restricted Diets

The objective of low-sodium diets is to rid the body of excess sodium and fluid accumulation associated with certain disorders, such as liver disease characterized by edema and ascites, congestive heart failure, renal disease characterized by edema and hypertension, and adrenocortical therapy. Low-sodium diets also are used in the treatment, and possible prevention, of hypertension.

Low-sodium diets are contraindicated for sodium-wasting renal diseases, such as pyelonephritis, polycystic renal disease, and bilateral hydronephrosis; pregnancy; clients with ileostomies; and myxedema.

The characteristics of low-sodium diets vary according to the level of restriction; 500-mg and 250-mg sodium diets are unpalatable, are extremely difficult to follow, and are likely to be inadequate in some nutrients. To promote compliance and to allow greater flexibility, exchange lists featuring the sodium content of high- and low-sodium foods may be used.

Levels of Restriction

4000–5000 mg sodium (174–217 mEq)
  Up to ½ teaspoon of salt allowed daily
  Foods high in added sodium limited

2000 mg (87 mEq)
  Up to ½ teaspoon of salt allowed daily, or allow the equivalent amount of
    salt in prepared foods
  Eliminate foods high in added sodium
  Limit milk and milk products to 16 oz/day

1000 mg (45 mEq)
  No salt may be added to food at the table or used in cooking
  Eliminate foods high in added sodium
  Limit milk and milk products to 16 oz/day
  Limit regular bread to four servings daily

500 mg (22 mEq)
  Follow 1000-mg sodium restrictions plus:
    Eliminate vegetables naturally high in sodium: beets, beet greens, carrots,
      kale, spinach, celery, white turnips, rutabagas, mustard greens, chard,
      and dandelion greens
    Use only low-sodium bread in place of regular bread
    Eliminate sherbet and flavored gelatin
    Limit meat to 6 oz/day; one egg may be substituted daily for 1 oz of meat

250 mg (11 mEq)
  Follow 500-mg sodium restrictions plus:
    Use low-sodium milk in place of regular milk

(continued)

Sodium-Restricted Diets (*continued*)

Foods High in Sodium

Food Group	Foods High in Added Sodium	Foods Naturally High in Sodium	Foods Lower in Sodium
Meats	Real and imitation bacon, cold cuts, chipped or corned beef, frankfurters, smoked meats, sausage, salt pork, canned meats, codfish, canned, salted or smoked fish, kosher meats, frozen and powder egg substitutes, regular peanut butter	Brain, kidney, clams, crab, lobster, oysters, scallops, shrimp, and other shellfish	Fresh, frozen, or canned low-sodium meat and poultry; eggs; low-sodium cheeses and peanut butter; fresh bass, bluefish, catfish, cod, eel, flounder, halibut, rockfish, salmon, sole, trout, tuna; canned low-sodium tuna and salmon
Dairy Products	Buttermilk, regular cheeses and cottage cheese; commercial milk products such as ice cream, malted milk, milk mixes, milk shakes, sherbet		Skim, 2% whole, evaporated, and low-sodium milk; low-sodium cheeses, low-sodium cottage cheese
Fruits and Vegetables	Crystallized or glazed fruit, maraschino cherries, dried fruit with sodium preservatives added; canned vegetables and vegetable juices unless low sodium, sauerkraut, frozen vegetables with added salt	Spinach, celery, beets and beet greens, carrots, artichokes, white turnips, Swiss chard, dandelion greens, kale, mustard greens	Fresh, frozen without salt, and low-sodium canned vegetables, except those listed Fresh, frozen, canned or dried fruits without added sodium
Breads and Cereals	Commercial mixes, bread and rolls made from frozen bread dough, graham and all other crackers except low-sodium crackers, instant rice and pasta mixes, commercial casserole		Low-sodium breads, crackers, cereals, and cereal products; baked products made without salt, baking powder containing sodium, and baking soda; low-sodium mixes; unsalted cooked cereals, puffed rice, puffed wheat, shredded wheat,

(*continued*)

Sodium-Restricted Diets (*continued*)

	mixes, commercial stuffing, instant and quick-cooking cereals, most dry cereals (except puffed rice, puffed wheat, and shredded wheat), self-rising flour, self-rising cornmeal, waffles, quick breads, and other baked products containing salt, baking soda, baking powder, or egg white	barley, cornmeal, cornstarch, unsalted matzo; unsalted macaroni, and rice
Fats	Salted butter and margarine, regular commercial salad dressings and mayonnaise	Unsalted butter, margarine, salad dressings, and mayonnaise; cooking oils and shortening
Miscellaneous	Regular canned or frozen soups; soup mixes; salted popcorn, nuts, potato chips, and snack foods; instant cocoa mixes; powdered drink mixes; canned fruit drinks; pastries; commercial candies, cakes, cookies, and gelatin desserts	Alcohol; coffee and coffee substitutes, lemonade, tea, salt-free or low-sodium candy, unflavored gelatin, jam, jelly, maple syrup, honey; unsalted nuts and popcorn
Seasonings and Condiments	Sea salt, rock salt, and kosher salt; barbecue sauce, bouillon cubes, catsup, celery salt, seed, and leaves; chili sauce; tartar sauce; garlic salt; horseradish made with salt; meat extracts, sauces, and tenderizers; Kitchen Bouquet, gravy, and and sauce mixes; monosodium glutamate; prepared mustard, olives, onion salt, pickles, relishes, saccharin, soy sauce,	Allspice, almond extract, anise seed, basil, bay leaf, low-sodium bouillon, caraway seed, cardamon, low-sodium catsup, chili powder, chives, cinnamon, cloves, cocoa (1 to 2 teaspoons), coconut, cumin, curry, dill, fennel, garlic and garlic powder, ginger, horseradish made without salt, juniper, lemon juice, mace, maple extract, marjoram, low-sodium meat extracts, low-sodium meat tenderizers, mint, mustard (dry and seeds),

(*continued*)

Sodium-Restricted Diets (*continued*)

teriyaki sauce, sugar substitutes containing sodium, Worcester-shire sauce

nutmeg, orange extract, oregano, paprika, parsley, pepper, peppermint extract, poppy seed, poultry sea-soning, purslane, rosemary, saffron, sage, salt substitutes (if approved by a physi-cian), savory, sesame seeds, sorrel, sugar, tarragon, thyme, turmeric, vanilla, vinegar, walnut extract, wine

Sample Menu

2000-mg Sodium Diet

Breakfast

½ cup orange juice
½ cup shredded wheat
2 slices toast
2 tsp margarine

1 tbsp strawberry jam
1 cup 1% milk
Sugar
Coffee/tea

Lunch

2 oz slice chicken breast on 2 slices whole-wheat bread with 2 tsp
    mayonnaise, tomato, and lettuce
Tossed salad with oil-and-vinegar dressing
Fresh fruit
4 vanilla wafers
1 cup 1% milk
Coffee/tea
Pepper

Dinner

4 oz broiled halibut
Baked potato
2 tsp margarine
½ cup broccoli
Coleslaw made with oil-
    and-vinegar dressing

1 dinner roll
½ cup sherbet
Coffee/tea
Sugar/pepper

(continued)

Sodium-Restricted Diets (*continued*)

Snack

1 cup unsalted popcorn
Apple juice

Potential Problem/Rationale

Hyponatremia (nausea, malaise, possible confusion, seizures, and coma) related to a sodium intake that is too low, especially when combined with the use of diuretics. For most people, the risk of hyponatremia is insignificant. However, clients with renal disease and the elderly may not be able adequately to reabsorb enough sodium while following a low-sodium diet.

Nursing Interventions and Considerations

To allow homeostatic mechanisms time to adapt in the elderly and clients with renal disease, initiate a low-sodium diet gradually. Observe for signs of sodium deficiency and liberalize the diet if necessary.

Potential Problem/Rationale

Noncompliance, which may be related to the following situations:

Pervasiveness of sodium in the diet

Preference of salt taste

Ethnic or religious customs. For instance, Chinese cooking relies heavily on soy sauce and MSG for seasoning. Kosher meats are bathed in a brine solution for 1 hour after slaughter. Although rinsing does remove some of the salt, kosher meats remain high in sodium.

Reliance on convenience products and canned foods, which are high in sodium. This is especially common among the elderly and people living alone.

Nursing Interventions and Considerations

Assure the client that with time, the taste for salt lessens, and it becomes easier to follow the diet.

Provide thorough and periodic instructions on how to incorporate the diet into the client's lifestyle and budget, information on sources of sodium in food and drugs, and lists of sodium alternatives.

If expense and convenience are a problem, allow the client to continue using regular canned meats and vegetables, if possible. Rinsing canned foods

(continued)

Sodium-Restricted Diets (*continued*)

under running water for at least 1 minute removes much of the sodium content.

Encourage support from the client's family and urge them to follow the diet if possible.

Low-Sodium Diet Teaching

(Be more or less specific depending on the level of sodium allowed.) Instruct the client

That reducing sodium intake will help the body rid itself of excess fluid and help lower high blood pressure.

That the body may need only about 200 mg of sodium a day (less than one-tenth of a teaspoon of salt), although most Americans consume 4000 to 5000 mg/day and can tolerate intakes much higher than this.

That sodium appears in the diet in the form of salt (40% sodium) and to some degree in almost all food and beverages. Most unprocessed, unsalted food generally is low in sodium.

That approximately one third of our sodium intake comes from salt added during cooking and at the table, one quarter to one third from processed foods, and the remainder from food and water naturally high in sodium.

That sodium compounds are used extensively as preservatives (sodium propionate, sodium sulfite, and sodium benzoate), leavening agents (sodium bicarbonate, baking soda, and baking powder), and flavor enhancers (salt, MSG), and are found in foods that may not taste salty.

That many nonprescription drugs (such as aspirin, cough medicines, laxatives, and antacids), toothpastes, toothpowders, and mouthwashes contain large amounts of sodium and should not be used without a physician's approval.

That salt substitutes replace sodium with potassium or other minerals. "Low-sodium" salt substitutes are not sodium-free and may contain half as much sodium as regular table salt. Use neither type without a physician's approval.

That preference for salt taste eventually will decrease.

If he or she "cheats" by eating a high-sodium meal or snack, to compensate by eating less sodium than normally allowed for the rest of the day.

How to order off a menu while dining out:

- Request that food not be salted, if possible.
- Choose fruit juice instead of soup for an appetizer.

(*continued*)

Sodium-Restricted Diets (*continued*)

- Use oil and vinegar or fresh lemon instead of regular salad dressing.
- Order plain meat and vegetables without gravy or sauce.
- Choose plain baked potatoes and season sparingly with sour cream, butter, or just with pepper.
- Select fresh fruit for dessert. If the client is going to splurge, ice cream or sherbet are better choices than pie, cake, cookies, and other desserts.
- Avoid fast-food restaurant meals, which generally are high in sodium.

On food preparation techniques to minimize sodium intake:

- Foods made from "scratch" generally have less sodium than processed foods and mixes.
- Experiment with sodium-free seasoning, such as herbs, spices, lemon juice, vinegar, and wine. Fresh ingredients are more flavorful than dried.
- Commercial "salt alternatives" are sodium-free blends of herbs and spices not intended to taste like salt but to be used as flavor enhancers.
- If permitted by a physician, salt substitutes may be used, although they taste bitter to some people.
- A variety of low-sodium cookbooks are available.

On how to read labels:

- Salt, monosodium glutamate, baking soda, and baking powder contain significant amounts of sodium. Other sodium compounds such as sodium nitrite, benzoate of soda, sodium saccharin, and sodium propionate add less sodium to the diet.
- Products labeled "low-sodium dietetic" do not have added sodium but may not be sodium-free; the sodium naturally occurring in the product remains.
- Products claiming to be "low in sodium" must print the sodium content on the label.
- Numerous low- and reduced-sodium products are available: milk, bread and bread products, cereal, crackers, cakes, cookies, pastries, soups and bouillon, canned vegetables, tomato products, meats, entrées, processed meats, hard and soft cheeses, condiments, nuts and peanut butter, butter, margarine, salad dressings, baking powder, and snack foods.
- The difference in taste between some low-sodium products and their high-sodium counterparts is barely noticeable; others taste flat and may need to have herbs or spices added.

Vascular Disorders

Hypertension

Hypertension is a symptom, not a disease, arbitrarily defined as sustained elevated blood pressure above 140/90 mm Hg. It is estimated that hypertension affects one of every three adults,[8] although only half of these may actually be diagnosed. It is more common among blacks than whites, and more common among women than men.

Ninety percent to 95% of the cases of hypertension occur from unknown causes and are classified as essential hypertension. Obesity and familial tendencies are related to the development of essential hypertension, which can be controlled but not cured. The remaining 5% to 10% of cases of hypertension occur secondary to renal disease, stenosis of the aorta, endocrine imbalances, sodium retention during pregnancy, increased intracranial pressure related to brain tumors, and advanced collagen disease. Eliminating the underlying disorder cures secondary hypertension.

Most hypertensive clients are asymptomatic, although prolonged hypertension can damage small and large vessels throughout the body and cause angina, intermittent claudication, retinal hemorrhages, severe headaches, polyuria, nocturia, dyspnea upon exertion, and edema of the extremities. Untreated, hypertension can lead to myocardial infarction, congestive heart failure, nephrosclerosis, renal failure, cerebrovascular accident, and blindness.

Diet management, designed to reduce cardiac workload, alleviate sodium retention, and help maintain potassium balance, may effectively control essential hypertension in a significant number of clients and preclude the use of drug therapy. Because it has the potential to be completely effective and has no adverse side effects, diet management should be the initial treatment of choice. If diet fails to achieve its goals, drug therapy (*i.e.*, diuretics, vasodilators, adrenergic blocking agents) may be added to diet therapy.

Nursing Process

Assessment

In addition to the general cardiovascular assessment criteria, assess for the following factors:

Weight, weight status

Usual intake of sodium, which is abundant in table salt, canned soups, meats, and vegetables, processed meats, convenience foods, condiments, and traditional snack foods. Investigate the local water supply to determine its sodium content; hard water softened with sodium can contribute large amounts of sodium to the diet.

Usual intake of foods high in potassium, such as fresh and dried fruits, fruit juices, many fresh and frozen vegetables, dairy products, whole grains, meats, fish, and poultry

Usual intake of calcium-rich foods, namely milk and dairy products

The use of diuretics; identify whether they are potassium-sparing or potassium-wasting.

Nursing Diagnosis

Noncompliance, related to poor understanding of the dietary management of hypertension.

Planning and Implementation

The role of diet in the treatment of hypertension has been widely debated since the Kempner "rice diet," in 1904, was found to effectively lower blood pressure. Drastically low in sodium (200 mg) and consisting only of rice, fruit, and sugar, the diet was unpalatable, nutritionally inadequate, and difficult to follow; hence, diet therapy was discounted as a practical means of treating hypertension.

Interest in diet therapy has been renewed. Although it is not known whether decreasing sodium intake can prevent hypertension, most experts agree that sodium restriction always should be part of treatment. Studies have shown that even a mild sodium restriction can modestly lower blood pressure in hypertensives. Approximately 50% of the people who reduce their sodium intake by half will have a significant decrease in blood pressure.[8] Clients with hypertension are advised to follow a low-sodium diet indefinitely. A gradual reduction in intake may be better accepted and easier to comply with than an abrupt withdrawal of sodium.

Losing weight without reducing sodium intake also lowers blood pressure, even if ideal weight is not attained and regardless of the degree of overweight. Weight loss may also reduce or eliminate the need for medication and, thus, the potential for toxicity and unpleasant side effects associated with drug therapy. Because weight control has the potential to control hypertension effectively for a large number of people, it is recommended that weight reduction be used as the initial step in treating overweight clients with mild to modest hypertension.

Other dietary components are being investigated for their influence on blood pressure. Some researchers believe low-potassium diets, or diets low in potassium and high in sodium, may be more significant than total sodium intake in the development of hypertension. Some studies show that doubling potassium intake can lower blood pressure by 3 to 5 mm Hg, and in animals, potassium has been shown to protect against kidney damage and strokes.[8]

Caffeine has been shown to increase blood pressure in some people but not in others. More than two drinks of alcohol causes an increase in blood pressure. The role of polyunsaturated fats is being investigated, but so far, results are inconclusive. One of the most promising areas of research is in the role of calcium. Some studies suggest an inverse relationship between calcium intake and blood pressure, which appears to be independent of age, obesity, and alcohol consumption. Also, clinical trials indicate that calcium supplementation may be protective against hypertension.

Be aware of the potential side effects of antihypertensive and diuretic therapy.

Client Goals

The client will:

Control blood pressure to avoid complications such as CHF and stroke.

Consume adequate calories to attain/maintain "healthy" weight.

Describe the principles and rationale of diet management for the treatment of hypertension, and implement the appropriate dietary changes.

Nursing Interventions

Diet Management

Decrease calories for weight loss, if overweight.

Reduce sodium intake, usually between 2 to 4 g (see box, Sodium-Restricted Diets). To promote a rapid drop in blood pressure, initial sodium allowance may be severely restricted to 200 to 250 mg/day. At this level, the diet is unpalatable and extremely difficult to follow; it is appropriate only for temporary use in an acute care setting.

Adjust potassium intake, depending on drug therapy.

Modify fat intake by increasing polyunsaturated fats and decreasing saturated fats.

Limit caffeine-containing beverages to two to three cups per day, and discourage the use of alcohol.

Client Teaching

Instruct the client

That weight loss in overweight people may be effective in controlling blood pressure without any other dietary or drug therapy.

That although a high sodium intake does not cause hypertension in most people, a low-sodium diet is almost always used in the treatment of hypertension.

On the principles and rationale of diet management of hypertension, and how to implement the appropriate dietary changes (see Low-Sodium Diet Teaching section in box, Sodium-Restricted Diets).

That salt substitutes may contain potassium in place of sodium or may be a combination of sodium and potassium chloride. Neither type should be used without a physician's permission.

That it is important to consume adequate amounts of potassium in the diet, especially when potassium-wasting diuretics are used. Often, clients requiring an increased potassium intake are told to "eat a banana and drink orange juice every day" without any further explanation. Explain the rationale of this oversimplified advice and instruct the client on the many sources of potassium, especially those that are low in sodium and calories (see Appendix 9).

Monitor

Monitor for the following signs or symptoms:

Compliance with the diet and the need for follow-up diet counseling

Effectiveness of the diet (*i.e.*, lowered blood pressure, weight loss if indicated) and evaluate the need for further diet modifications

Fluid and electrolyte balance, if diuretics are used

Evaluation

Evaluation is ongoing. Assuming the plan of care has not changed, the client will achieve the goals as stated above.

DRUG ALERT Potassium-wasting diuretics (thiazide, furosemide) → constipation, diarrhea, nausea, vomiting, GI upset, dry mouth, increased thirst, anorexia, and fluid and electrolyte imbalances. Modify the diet to alleviate unpleasant GI side effects, if possible. Monitor for signs of potassium deficiency and encourage the intake of potassium-rich foods (see Appendix 9). Advise the client to avoid natural licorice, which tends to cause potassium depletion and sodium retention.

Potassium supplements can lead to nausea, vomiting, GI discomfort, and diarrhea, and can produce hyperkalemia when used with salt substitutes containing potassium.

Monitor serum potassium levels and observe for signs of hyperkalemia. Advise against the use of potassium-containing salt substitutes.

NUTRITIONAL ANEMIAS

Anemia is a syndrome characterized by a deficiency in the oxygen-carrying capacity of the blood, related to a decrease in hemoglobin, red blood cell volume, and red blood cell number.

Nutritional anemias occur when one or more of the nutrients necessary for red blood cell production are deficient. Lack of iron, vitamin B_{12}, and folic acid are the most common causes of nutritional anemias. Table 16-6 outlines the role of other nutrients in the production of red blood cells (RBC). For hematologic assessment guidelines, see the box, General Hematologic Assessment Criteria.

Iron Deficiency Anemia

Iron deficiency anemia occurs when total iron stores become depleted, leading to a decrease in hemoglobin. It is classified as microcytic (small red blood cells) and hypochromic (pale red blood cells related to the decrease in hemoglobin pigment).

Iron deficiency anemia is the most common nutritional deficiency disorder in the United States. The incident rate among high-risk populations may be as high as 10% to 50%. Groups most vulnerable include infants under age 2, menstruating women, the elderly, minorities, and people in low-income groups.

Iron deficiency anemia can result from an inadequate intake, such as among low-income groups and vegetarians, or from inadequate absorption secondary to chronic diarrhea, malabsorption syndrome, partial or total gastrectomy, pica, or poor bio-availability of the iron consumed. Chronic blood loss related to bleeding ulcers, gastritis, malignancy, parasites, excessive menstrual losses, or closely spaced pregnancies, may also lead to anemia. Finally, iron deficiency may occur secondary to an increased need for iron due to accelerated growth during pregnancy, infancy, and puberty.

Table 16-6
Role of Various Nutrients in RBC Formation

Nutrient	Role in RBC Formation
Vitamin C	Enhances the absorption of iron and folic acid
Vitamin B_6	Coenzyme in hemoglobin formation
Copper*	Mobilizes iron from storage to plasma
Protein	Necessary for the formation of hemoglobin and enzymes involved in the production of RBC
Vitamin E*	Exact function is unclear; premature infants deficient in vitamin E develop hemolytic anemia.
Vitamin A	Exact function is unclear; may aid in the mobilization of iron from the liver

* Rare incidence of dietary deficiency

Assessment Criteria	**General Hematologic Assessment Criteria**

Hemoglobin, hematocrit, transferrin
Clinical signs of deficiency: beefy red tongue, anorexia, fatigue
General dietary intake
Use of alcohol or tobacco
Concurrent illness, medical history
Recent surgery; history of GI surgery
Infection, sepsis
Family history of anemia
Use of prescription and over-the-counter medications

Signs and symptoms of anemia vary with the degree of severity and chronicity; mild anemia may be asymptomatic. Possible observations include fatigue, weakness, pallor, sensitivity to cold, anorexia, dizziness and headaches, thin, spoon-shaped fingernails, stomatitis, and glossitis. Approximately 50% of people with iron deficiency anemia practice pica (ingestion of nonfood substances such as dirt, clay, laundry starch).[7] Complications of iron deficiency anemia include cardiovascular and respiratory changes that may result in cardiac failure.

The treatment of iron deficiency anemia begins with correcting the underlying disorder, when appropriate. Iron supplements are used; parenteral iron may be given if oral supplements fail or are not tolerated. Although diet therapy is not effective against curing anemia once it is established, it is used adjunctively to increase iron intake and absorption, and to alleviate symptoms, if indicated.

Nursing Process

Assessment

In addition to the general hematologic assessment criteria, assess for the following factors:

Symptoms that may affect intake (*i.e.*, fatigue, anorexia, stomatitis, glossitis); assess onset, severity, interventions attempted and the results.

Dietary changes made in response to symptoms (*i.e.*, foods avoided, foods preferred). Determine foods best and least tolerated.

Usual intake of foods high in iron (Table 16-7)

Vitamin C intake when plant sources of iron (*i.e.*, fortified, enriched, and whole-grain breads and cereal) are consumed. Rich sources of vitamin C include citrus fruits and juices, tomatoes, broccoli, cabbage, baked potatoes, and strawberries.

The intake of tea and coffee when plant sources of iron are consumed; tea and coffee inhibit the absorption of iron.

The quantity and quality of protein usually consumed; determine if the client is a vegetarian.

Table 16-7
Selected Sources of Iron

Heme Iron	Nonheme Iron
Beef: muscle meats, heart, kidney, liver, and tongue	Bran flakes
	Brewer's yeast
	Brown rice
Chicken, especially dark meat	Chocolate, cocoa
	Enriched and whole grain breads, cereals, and flours
Egg yolk	Fortified cereals
Lamb	Dried beans, peas, and soybeans
Liver sausage	Dried fruit: apricots, currants, dates, figs, peaches, prunes, raisins
Pork	
Shellfish	Greens: beet, dandelion, kale, spinach, Swiss chard, turnip
Shrimp	
Tuna	Lentils
Turkey, especially dark meat	Molasses
	Nuts: almonds, brazil nuts, cashews, hazelnuts, pecans, peanuts, walnuts
Veal	
	Oatmeal
	Sweet potatoes

Pica. If the client practices pica, determine what items are eaten and how frequently they are consumed.

Nursing Diagnosis

Altered Nutrition: Less than Body Requirements, related to poor bioavailability of iron consumed.

Planning and Implementation

There are several reasons why an inadequate intake is a common cause of iron deficiency anemia. First, the typical American diet provides 5 to 6 mg of iron/1000 calories. Healthy adult men can easily meet their RDA for iron (10 mg), considering the calorie content of their diets; women of childbearing age, however, require more iron (RDA of 15 mg) than typically can be supplied from the amount of calories that they consume. Also, iron is not widespread in the diet, and has relatively few excellent sources. And, on the average, only 10% of the iron consumed is absorbed. The actual rate of iron absorption depends on need (the rate of absorption increases in response to need) and the form of iron consumed (heme iron, nonheme iron).

Heme iron is the most abundant form of iron in animal sources, such as meat, fish, and poultry; however, it accounts for only 5% to 10% of total iron consumed. The average absorption rate of heme iron, which is influenced only by body need, is 15% to 35%. Heme iron promotes the absorption of nonheme iron from other foods when eaten at the same time.

Table 16-8

Factors That Influence Nonheme Iron Absorption

	Comments
NONHEME IRON ENHANCERS	
Vitamin C	The most potent iron enhancer known; it reduces and binds iron to form a readily absorbable compound. Its enhancing effect is proportional to the amount of vitamin C consumed. To be effective, vitamin C must be eaten at the same time as the iron.
Certain animal proteins	Meat, fish, and poultry enhance nonheme iron absorption when consumed at the same time as nonheme iron.
Gastric acidity	Increases the solubility and availability of iron
NONHEME IRON INHIBITORS	
Tea	Contains tannin, which combines with nonheme iron to form insoluble complexes that cannot be absorbed Can reduce iron absorption by as much as 87% when consumed with meals
Coffee	Exact mechanism is unclear; appears to render iron unabsorbable by changing it from the ferrous to the ferric state. When consumed with meals or up to 1 hour later, can reduce iron absorption by 39%. Does not interfere with iron absorption when consumed 1 hour before eating. Inhibitory effect is dose-related: absorption decreases as the strength of the coffee increases.
Binding agents	Various compounds combine with iron to form insoluble complexes the body cannot absorb. Common binding agents include bran (whole grains), phosphates (dairy products, whole grains, legumes), oxalates (certain fruits and vegetables, soybean products), and phytates (oatmeal, whole grains).
Alkalinity	Antacids decrease iron solubility by increasing gastric pH.
Increased GI motility; steatorrhea	Diarrhea reduces the time available for absorption.
THE FORM OF ELEMENTAL IRON IN SUPPLEMENTS AND ENRICHED PRODUCTS	
Well absorbed	Ferrous sulfate, lactate, fumarate, succinate, glycinesulfate, glutamate
Poorly absorbed	Ferrous citrate, tartrate, pyrophosphate

Nonheme iron is the most abundant form of iron in plant sources: grains, vegetables, legumes, and nuts. It is the most prevalent form of iron in the diet, yet on average, only 3% to 8% of nonheme iron is absorbed. Like heme iron, its rate of absorption is influenced by body need; however, it also is significantly affected by the presence of other dietary factors (Table 16-8). Nonheme iron absorption is enhanced by vitamin C, certain animal proteins, and gastric acidity. Tea, coffee, binding agents, alkalinity, and increased GI motility are factors known to inhibit the absorption of nonheme iron.

Provide small, frequent meals if anorexia is present. Eliminate acidic and salty foods, strong spices, coarse breads, raw vegetables, and hot foods and beverages if the oral mucosa is inflamed. Be aware of the potential side effects of iron supplementation.

Client Goals

The client will:

Experience alleviation of anemia; be free of signs and symptoms.

Replace poor sources of iron in the diet with high sources of iron (*i.e.*, consume iron-fortified cereals, organ meats).

Include a source of vitamin C at every meal to enhance nonheme iron absorption.

Avoid foods known to inhibit iron absorption.

Describe the principles and rationale of diet management for iron deficiency anemia.

Modify the diet, as needed, to alleviate anemia symptoms or side effects of iron therapy.

Nursing Interventions

Diet Management

Increase iron intake (see Table 16-7), especially of heme iron and preferably at every meal.

Include a source of vitamin C at every meal to enhance nonheme iron absorption; avoid foods known to inhibit nonheme iron absorption.

Client Teaching

Instruct the client

On ways to increase the iron content of the diet:

- Add dried fruit to cereals and baked goods.
- Use crushed, iron-fortified cereal as a breading for meat, fish, poultry, and vegetables; mixed with butter or margarine for a casserole topping; as a meat extender in meatloaf, meatballs, and burgers; sprinkled on ice cream; for added crunch to yogurt and pudding.
- Substitute whole-grain products for refined products; brown rice for white rice.
- Cook in iron pots whenever possible, especially acidic foods (*e.g.*, dishes made with tomatoes).

On ways to increase the iron availability of the diet:

- Eat meat at every meal, if possible.
- Consume a rich source of vitamin C at every meal: citrus fruits and their juices, brussels sprouts, strawberries, broccoli, "greens," cabbage, cantaloupe, tomatoes.

Monitor

Monitor for the following signs or symptoms:

Tolerance to oral feedings (*i.e.*, absence of pain), if oral mucosa is inflamed

Compliance with the diet, and the need for follow-up diet counseling

Effectiveness of the diet, and the need for further diet modifications

Hemoglobin and hematocrit

Evaluation

Evaluation is ongoing. Assuming the plan of care has not changed, the client will achieve the goals as stated above.

DRUG ALERT: **ORAL IRON SUPPLEMENTS**

- Are better absorbed if taken between meals; antacids and food in the stomach inhibit absorption.
- Commonly cause GI upset, nausea, heartburn, diarrhea or constipation, and black stools, which are dose-related. Administering a smaller dose, several times a day, for a longer period of treatment or taking the supplements with meals may be necessary to alleviate side effects.
- Can be toxic when taken in excess amounts. Keep this and all medications out of the reach of children.

Vitamin B_{12} Deficiency Anemia

A lack of vitamin B_{12} leads to decreased DNA synthesis, which can result in megaloblastic anemia (red blood cells with delayed and abnormal nuclear maturation). Vitamin B_{12} is absorbed in the ileum and requires intrinsic factor, which is produced and secreted in the stomach. Vitamin B_{12} is found only in animal products.

Vitamin B_{12} deficiency related to an inadequate intake occurs rarely and usually is seen only in strict vegetarians who consume no animal products and do not take vitamin B_{12} supplements. The most common cause of vitamin B_{12} deficiency is impaired absorption, which can result from numerous factors.

Pernicious anemia is vitamin B_{12} deficiency anemia caused by the lack of intrinsic factor production in the stomach, which renders vitamin B_{12} incapable of being absorbed. Pernicious anemia occurs in only 0.1% of the population, most often in people over 50 years old, and may be related to a genetic defect, chronic iron deficiency, an autoimmune disorder, and a total, and sometimes subtotal, gastrectomy.

Absorption of vitamin B_{12} also may be impaired secondary to disorders of the ileum and pancreas, malabsorption syndrome, bacterial overgrowth related to intestinal stasis, or fish tapeworm.

Because normal body stores of vitamin B_{12} are extensive, the onset of deficiency symptoms may be delayed for 5 to 10 years. Symptoms related to anemia include pallor, dyspnea or orthopnea, weakness, fatigue, and palpitations. Gastrointestinal changes may occur: sore mouth with smooth, red, "beefy" tongue, anorexia, indigestion, recurring diarrhea or constipation, and weight loss. Neurologic changes that may be observed include paresthesia of the hands and feet, decreased sense of position, poor muscle coordination, poor memory, irritability, depression, paranoia, delirium, and hallucinations. Prolonged pernicious anemia can lead to permanent neurologic damage; untreated pernicious anemia can result in death. Pernicious anemia also is associated with an increased incidence of benign gastric polyps and gastric carcinoma.

The treatment of pernicious anemia requires lifelong parenteral vitamin B_{12} injections. Vitamin B_{12} deficiency anemia that occurs secondary to GI disorders is treated by correcting the underlying problem and administering vitamin B_{12} as needed. Strict vegetarians who become vitamin B_{12}-deficient because of an inadequate intake can be treated with oral vitamin B_{12} supplements, and should be encouraged to increase their dietary intake, if possible (fortified soybean milk, inclusion of some animal products). Adjunctive diet therapy may also be used to provide nutrients essential for RBC production, help correct any existing nutritional deficiencies, and minimize GI symptoms.

Nursing Process

Assessment

In addition to the general hematologic assessment criteria, assess for the following factors:

Symptoms that may affect eating (*i.e.*, sore mouth, anorexia, indigestion, diarrhea, constipation, weight loss); assess onset, frequency, severity, interventions attempted and the results.

Dietary changes made in response to symptoms (*i.e.*, foods avoided, foods preferred). Determine foods best and least tolerated.

Usual vitamin B_{12} intake; vitamin B_{12} is found only in animal products.

Past and present medical history, especially GI history, to determine if there are any conditions contributing to anemia.

Nursing Diagnosis

Altered Oral Mucous Membrane, related to vitamin B_{12} deficiency as manifested by stomatitis.

Planning and Implementation

A liquid or soft diet may be necessary if glossitis and oral inflammation interfere with eating. Likewise, other dietary changes may be necessary to alleviate anorexia, diarrhea, or constipation (see Chap. 15).

Fat may not be tolerated by clients with achlorhydria due to delayed gastric emptying and a decreased rate of digestion.

Iron deficiency may occur as a result of achlorhydria or may develop secondary to treatment. If iron supplements are prescribed, be aware of the potential side effects (see section on Iron Deficiency Anemia).

Folic acid deficiency can also cause megaloblastic anemia and the same GI symptoms as pernicious anemia. Folic acid given to clients with pernicious anemia reverses the anemia and GI symptoms without affecting the neurologic disturbances, which, if not treated, can be irreversible. It is imperative that the correct cause of megaloblastic anemia be diagnosed before beginning treatment.

Client Goals

The client will:

Experience alleviation of anemia, if possible.

Modify the diet, as needed, to alleviate symptoms.

Describe the principles and rationale of diet management of vitamin B_{12} deficiency anemia, and implement the appropriate dietary changes.

Nursing Interventions

Diet Management

Increase vitamin B_{12}, protein, iron, and folic acid intake by eating more meat (especially liver, beef, and pork), eggs, green leafy vegetables, and milk and milk products.

Provide liquid or soft foods if oral mucosa is inflamed. Modify the diet as need for other GI symptoms (see Chap. 15).

Client Teaching

Instruct the client

On the principles and rationale of diet management of vitamin B_{12} deficiency anemia, and how to implement the appropriate dietary changes.

Monitor

Monitor for the following signs or symptoms:

Tolerance to oral feedings (*i.e.*, absence of pain), if oral mucosa is inflamed

Compliance with the diet, and the need for follow-up diet counseling

Effectiveness of the diet, and the need for additional diet modifications

Anemia and symptoms

Evaluation

The client

Experiences alleviation of anemia, if possible.

Modifies the diet, as needed, to alleviate symptoms (*i.e.*, stomatitis, anorexia, indigestion, diarrhea, constipation, weight loss).

Describes the principles and rationale of diet management of vitamin B_{12} deficiency anemia, and implements the appropriate dietary changes.

Folic Acid Deficiency Anemia

A lack of folic acid leads to decreased DNA synthesis, which can result in megaloblastic anemia. Folic acid deficiency may occur because of an inadequate intake, as in the case of the elderly and alcoholics, or may occur secondary to increased requirements related to growth, such as during pregnancy and infancy. Malabsorption syndromes can also cause folic acid deficiency, as can the use of certain medications, such as anticonvulsants, antimetabolites, and oral contraceptives.

Normal body stores of folate usually become depleted in 2 to 4 months on a folate-deficient diet. Symptoms related to anemia include pallor, dyspnea or orthopnea, weakness, fatigue, and palpitations. Gastrointestinal changes that may be observed include sore mouth with smooth, red, "beefy" tongue, anorexia, indigestion, recurring diarrhea or constipation, and weight loss. Unlike pernicious anemia, no neurologic changes occur.

Folic acid deficiency is treated by correcting the underlying disorder, if appropriate. Oral folate supplements are used; however, intramuscular injections may be necessary if malabsorption is present. Diet therapy may help promote RBC production.

Nursing Process

Assessment

In addition to the general hematologic assessment criteria, assess for the following factors:

Symptoms that may affect intake (*i.e.*, sore mouth, anorexia, indigestion, diarrhea, constipation, weight loss); assess onset, frequency, severity, interventions attempted and the results.

Dietary changes made in response to symptoms (*i.e.*, foods avoided, foods preferred). Determine foods best and least tolerated.

Usual intake of foods rich in folic acid, such as liver, organ meats, broccoli, green leafy vegetables, asparagus, milk, eggs, orange juice, wheat bran, wheat germ, whole-wheat bread, brewer's yeast, dried peas and beans.

Usual intake of vitamin C: vitamin C converts folic acid from its inactive to active form

Nursing Diagnosis

Altered Oral Mucous Membrane, related to folic acid deficiency anemia as manifested by stomatitis.

Planning and Implementation

A liquid or soft diet may be necessary if glossitis and oral inflammation interfere with eating. Likewise, other dietary changes may be needed to alleviate anorexia, diarrhea, or constipation (see Chap. 15).

Encourage the intake of both vitamin C and folic acid at every meal; folic acid supplements may be required.

Because heat destroys folic acid, fruits and vegetables should be eaten raw, or cooked to a minimum.

Folic acid deficiency may be preceded by iron deficiency; iron deficiency → RBC hemolysis → increased need for folate to replenish RBC. Observe for signs of iron deficiency and provide supplements as ordered.

Client Goals

The client will:

Experience alleviation of anemia, if possible.

Modify the diet, as needed, to alleviate symptoms (*i.e.*, stomatitis, anorexia, indigestion, diarrhea, constipation, weight loss).

Describe the principles and rationale of diet management of folic acid deficiency anemia, and implement the appropriate dietary changes.

Nursing Interventions

Diet Management

Increase folic acid intake by eating more foods high in folic acid: liver, organ meats, broccoli, green leafy vegetables, asparagus, milk, eggs, orange juice, wheat bran, wheat germ, whole-wheat bread, brewer's yeast, dried peas and beans.

	## Fish Oil Supplements: Yea or Nay?

Since the mid-1980s, there has been a proliferation of reports and hype that eating fish lowers the risk of coronary heart disease. In the 1970s, Dutch investigators studying the relationship between fish consumption and coronary heart disease found that the greater the intake of fish, the lower the risk of dying from heart disease. The benefit seems to come from the fish oils, known as omega-3 fatty acids. Exactly how they protect against heart disease is not fully understood; although fish oils lower serum triglycerides (which may or may not be protective against heart disease), they may have little effect on serum cholesterol. The benefit appears to be related to the effect fish oils have on blood vessel walls and on platelet aggregation.

Researchers believe that before cholesterol is deposited in an artery, the vessel sustains some sort of microscopic injury, whether from a toxin, infection, oxidized cholesterol, or by some other mechanism. This lesion triggers an immune response: platelets stick to the lesion, increasing the risk of blood clots, and smooth muscle cells migrate from the outside of the artery wall to the inner layer where they rapidly proliferate, creating blockages. Studies suggest that fish oils decrease platelet aggregation and slow the proliferation of smooth muscle cells in the artery wall.

Omega-3 fatty acids are especially abundant in fatty fish such as herring, salmon, mackerel, and trout. Leaner fish also contain omega-3s but in smaller amounts. Some researchers recommend eating one or two servings of fish a week as preventative medicine, but caution is advised; the benefit of eating fish may be negated if the fish is from chemically contaminated water. To be safe, follow any guidelines issued in your area regarding fish consumption, and, as an added measure, remove all fatty tissue, the skin, and dark-colored flesh, and prepare by broiling, grilling, or baking on a rack.

Although leading health authorities advocate that Americans eat more fish, researchers are reluctant to recommend the use of fish-oil supplements, because it is possible that something in addition to the fat content of fish contributes to its protective effect. Other concerns include the potential for vitamin A and D toxicities (if the supplements are produced from cod-liver oil), and false claims on supplement labels, which overstate actual omega-3 content.

While the jury is still out, it's wise to eat more fish.

Provide a rich source of vitamin C with every meal to enhance absorption.
Modify the diet, as needed, to alleviate GI symptoms (see Chap. 15).

Client Teaching

Instruct the client

On the principles and rationale of diet management for folic acid deficiency anemia and
how to implement the appropriate dietary changes.
To modify the diet, as needed, to alleviate GI symptoms.

Monitor

Monitor for the following signs or symptoms:
Tolerance to oral feedings (*i.e.*, absence of pain), if oral mucosa is inflamed
Compliance with the diet, and the need for follow-up diet counseling
Effectiveness of the diet, and the need for further diet modification

Evaluation

The client
Experiences alleviation of anemia, if possible.
Modifies the diet, as needed, to alleviate symptoms.
Describes the principles and rationale of diet management of folic acid deficiency anemia, and implements the appropriate dietary changes.

BIBLIOGRAPHY

1. Allen SS, Froberg D, McCarthy P, et al: Preferences and opinions of consumers vs dietitians on cholesterol education materials. J Am Diet Assoc 91:604, 1991
2. American Dietetic Association: Manual of Clinical Dietetics. Developed by The Chicago Dietetic Association and The South Suburban Dietetic Association, 1988
3. American Heart Association: Dietary Guidelines for Healthy American Adults: A Statement for Physicians and Health Professionals by the Nutrition Committee, American Heart Association. New York: American Heart Association, 1986
4. Becker DM, Larosa JH, Watson JE: Interpreting the new guidelines. Am J Nurs 89:1622, 1989
5. Carpenito LJ: Nursing Diagnosis: Application to Clinical Practice. 4th ed. Philadelphia: JB Lippincott, 1991
6. Ernst ND, et al: The National Cholesterol Education Program: Implications for dietetic practitioners from the Adult Treatment Panel Recommendations. J Am Diet Assoc 88:1401, 1988
7. Escott-Stump S: Nutrition and Diagnosis-Related Care, 2nd ed. Philadelphia: Lea and Febiger, 1988
8. Jacobson M (ed): Tackling high blood pressure. Nutrition Action Health Letter 16(4):1, 1989
9. Leibman B: The HDL/triglycerides trap. Nutrition Action Health Letter 17(7):1, 1990
10. Leibman B: Please adopt this drug. Nutrition Action Health Letter 17(10):8, 1990
11. Leibman B: Fish oil: Fad or find? Nutrition Action Health Letter 16(2):1, 1989
12. Malseed RT: Pharmacology: Drug Therapy and Nursing Considerations. 3rd. ed. Philadelphia: JB Lippincott, 1990
13. Public Health Service, United States Department of Health and Human Services: The Surgeon General's Report on Nutrition and Health: Summary and Recommendations. DHHS (PHS) Publication no. 88-50211. Washington, DC: Government Printing Office, 1988
14. Public Health Service, National Institutes of Health, United States Department of Health and Human Services: National Cholesterol Education Program: Report of the Expert Panel on Detection, Evaluation, and Treatment of High Blood Cholesterol in Adults. NIH Publication no. 89-2925. Washington, DC: Government Printing Office, 1989
15. Scherer JC: Introductory Medical–Surgical Nursing, 5th ed. Philadelphia: JB Lippincott, 1991
16. Shah M, Jeffery RW, Laing B, et al: Hypertension Prevention Trial (HPT): Food pattern changes resulting from intervention on sodium, potassium, and energy intake. J Am Diet Assoc 90:69, 1990
17. Stoy DB: Controlling cholesterol with diet. Am J Nurs 89:1625, 1989

17 Diabetes Mellitus and Other Endocrine Disorders

ENDOCRINE DISORDERS

The endocrine system is composed of ductless glands that secrete hormones into the bloodstream. The endocrine pancreas secretes insulin, the hormone involved not only with glucose metabolism but also with protein and fat metabolism. Diet management is an integral component of treatment for both insulin-dependent diabetes and noninsulin-dependent diabetes. Hormones secreted by other endocrine glands, namely the thyroid gland, parathyroid gland, and adrenal cortex, affect nutritional status by regulating nutrient metabolism (Table 17-1). Alterations in hormone secretion can cause nutrient imbalances, weight changes, and unpleasant symptoms that interfere with eating (*e.g.*, nausea) or nutrient utilization (*e.g.*, diarrhea). Diet management can help alleviate symptoms and may help avoid contributing to nutrient imbalances but cannot fully compensate for hormone secretion abnormalities. For endocrine assessment guidelines, see the box, General Endocrine Assessment Criteria.

501

Table 17-1
Effect of Various Endocrine Secretions on Nutrient Metabolism

Gland	Secretion	Effect on Nutrient Metabolism
Thyroid 2 lobes located in the anterior portion of the neck	Thyroxine (T_4) and Triiodothyronine (T_3)	Regulates basal metabolic rate (BMR) by regulating the rate of CHO, protein, fat, vitamin, and mineral metabolism; stimulates growth and development
Parathyroid 4 small glands embedded in the posterior section of the thyroid gland	Parathormone (PTH)	Regulates blood calcium and phosphorus levels; increases blood calcium levels by increasing GI absorption, decreasing urinary excretion, and promoting bone resorption; lowers blood phosphorus levels
Adrenals 2 small glands located above and in front of the upper end of each kidney. Consists of the cortex (essential for life) and the medulla (nonessential for life)	Cortex *Glucocorticoids* (cortisone and hydrocortisone) *Mineralocorticoids* (aldosterone)	Influences the metabolism of CHO, protein, and fat Promotes sodium retention and potassium excretion

DISORDERS OF THE ENDOCRINE PANCREAS

Diabetes Mellitus

Diabetes mellitus is a chronic heterogeneous disorder characterized by elevated blood glucose levels (hyperglycemia) related to a relative or absolute deficiency of insulin. The two major types of diabetes are type I, or insulin-dependent diabetes mellitus (IDDM), and type II, or noninsulin-dependent diabetes mellitus (NIDDM).

Approximately 10% of the American population has diabetes—only half of whom may be diagnosed. The incidence of diabetes is rising at an annual rate of 6%. The exact cause is unknown and may be multifactorial for each type and each client.

Normal Physiology

Insulin is the major hormone responsible for maintaining blood glucose levels within the normal range of 70 to 110 mg/dl. It is also needed in order for certain amino acids to enter muscle cells, for protein synthesis, and for fatty acids to enter and be stored in fat cells. As such, it is intricately involved in the metabolism of all body fuels.

Insulin is released by the β cells of the islets of Langerhans in response to blood glucose levels. After eating, blood glucose levels rise. The rise in glucose signals the pancreas to secrete insulin, which binds with special insulin receptors on the surface of fat and muscle cells. This allows circulating glucose to leave the bloodstream and enter the cells. It also enhances the transport of amino acids into the cell and promotes glycogen

Assessment Criteria

General Endocrine Assessment Criteria

Weight status, weight changes

Polyphagia

Polydipsia

Abdominal pain

Anorexia, nausea

Headache

Seizures

Syncope

Numbness, tingling, paresthesias

Altered consciousness

Bone pain

Dysuria, polyuria

Frequent infections

Fatigue

Dry, itchy skin

Decreased libido

storage, protein synthesis, and fat formation. As glucose leaves the bloodstream and serum levels drop, insulin secretion falls to keep glucose levels within normal range.

Once inside the cells, glucose can be converted to energy. Glucose that remains after energy needs are met is converted to glycogen (glycogenesis) and stored in the liver and muscles. If glycogen stores are adequate, the remaining glucose is converted to fat (lipogenesis) and stored as adipose.

When serum glucose levels are low, such as during fasting, insulin secretion falls. The fall in insulin causes glycogen stores to release glucose for energy (glycogenolysis) and muscle cells to release amino acids (proteolysis) for their conversion to glucose (gluconeogenesis). This occurs only after glycogen is depleted. If needed, fat stores release fatty acids (lipolysis), which are metabolized to ketone bodies (ketogenesis) and used for energy.

Pathogenesis of Insulin-Dependent Diabetes

Type I diabetes, characterized by a lack of insulin secretion, accounts for only about 10% of all diabetes cases. Although it can occur at any age, it is most often detected in childhood; most type I diabetics are within their normal weight range or slightly below. The exact cause of IDDM is unknown; however, it is possible that an autoimmune response, triggered by a viral infection, causes the destruction of the β cells in genetically susceptible people, resulting in an inability to produce insulin.

Without insulin, serum glucose levels rise and cells are unable to use glucose for energy. Glucose eventually "spills" over into the urine (glycosuria). To some extent, the body compensates for the lack of usable energy by breaking down protein and fat. Unfortunately, ketone bodies accumulate because the body is not able to completely utilize fat for energy. Ketonuria develops; left untreated, ketosis, or ketoacidosis, can lead to coma and death.

Polyuria and polydipsia, classic symptoms of diabetes, develop as the body tries to rid itself of excess glucose and ketones. The third hallmark, polyphagia, occurs because the cells are actually starving for energy despite the high glucose levels. Rapid weight loss, muscle wasting, fatigue, weakness, irritability, itchy skin, and poor wound healing may be observed.

Although the metabolic derangements may be life-threatening (*e.g.*, hyperosmolar coma), the major challenge is to control the progressive vascular damage that occurs over time. Interestingly, the development of complications appears to be more strongly correlated to the duration of the disease rather than the severity; complications are seen in both type I and type II diabetes. Morphologic changes occur in the small vessels, arteries, pancreas, kidneys, retina, nerves, and other tissues. Atherosclerosis is 50% more common among diabetics than the general population, and the death rate from coronary artery disease is two to three times higher among diabetics than among their age- and sex-matched peers. This increased risk may be partly related to a high incidence of other coronary heart disease risk factors, such as hyperlipidemia, hypertension, and clotting abnormalities.[11] Diabetes is the major cause of renal failure, amputations, and all new blindness in the United States. It also leads to neuropathy and neuropathy-induced impotence in men, and is the third leading cause of death in the United States.

Pathogenesis of Noninsulin-Dependent Diabetes

Approximately 90% of the diabetic population has type II diabetes. Because it is a slowly progressive disease, the number of diagnosed and undiagnosed cases may be equal.[5] It is most often diagnosed after age 40 and occurs more frequently in blacks than whites. The incidence of type II diabetes is strongly correlated to obesity (80% to 90% of Type II diabetics are obese) and parental history.

Unlike IDDM, type II diabetes is characterized by normal or above-normal insulin levels; however, there is decreased tissue sensitivity to insulin, primarily in the liver and muscle. The delayed glucose-stimulated insulin response results in ineffective suppression of liver glucose production and decreased glucose uptake by the peripheral tissues. Hyperglycemia results and provides constant stimulation for insulin secretion. Although the amount of insulin secretion may be sufficient, it may take 4 to 5 hours instead of the usual 2 hours for blood glucose levels to return to normal after a meal. Chronic hyperinsulinemia can lead to a decrease in the number of insulin receptors on the cells and a decrease in tissue sensitivity to insulin.

Although not a cause of hyperglycemia, obesity complicates the scenario by contributing to insulin resistance. Another risk factor appears to be the distribution of body fat; obese people with upper body (android) obesity, especially women, are at greater risk for developing diabetes and cardiovascular disease than are obese people with lower body (gynoid) fat distribution.[5] The risk increases in proportion to the degree of obesity.

Because insulin is available, ketoacidosis does not develop, even though blood glucose levels are high. Many people with type II diabetics are asymptomatic and may not know they have diabetes until a complication develops (see above). However, some people display mild cases of the classic symptoms, or experience drowsiness, fatigue, blurred vision, tingling or numbness of the extremities, or frequent infections.

Diabetes Management

The goals of diabetes treatment are to achieve metabolic control as near normal as possible and to prevent or delay the onset of complications. Diet therapy is an essential and lifelong component of treatment for all diabetics, regardless of the client's weight, blood glucose levels, or use of medication. Exercise is another important aspect of treatment for both types of diabetes, regardless of weight status, unless contraindicated for other medical reasons.[5] Exercise lowers serum glucose levels by increasing the uptake of glucose into muscle cells, and can improve glucose tolerance by increasing the numbers of insulin receptors (see box, Potential Benefits of Exercise for Diabetics). Insulin sensitivity also improves with exercise, an important benefit for both lean and obese type II diabetics.

In addition to diet and exercise, type I diabetics require insulin therapy; type II diabetics who do not achieve glycemic control through diet and exercise may need oral hypoglycemic agents, or if that fails, insulin therapy (see Drug Alert).

Diet for Type I Diabetics

The objectives of diet for type I are to maintain "healthy" weight, avoid hypoglycemia, and match calorie intake and expenditure with scheduled insulin therapy. Because most type I diabetics are of normal weight, calorie allowances for weight maintenance should be based on the client's age, sex, and activity patterns (see Appendix 10).

The use of insulin necessitates that, to avoid hypoglycemia, meals and snacks be consistent in number, timing, and calorie composition every day. The actual number of feedings and amount of CHO and calories allowed at each meal and snack should be planned to coincide with peak insulin action (Table 17-2). Consistent meal timing is less important for clients receiving insulin through a pump or by multiple injections.

Potential Benefits of Exercise for Diabetics

Lowered blood glucose levels

Decreased insulin resistance, increased insulin sensitivity

Increased HDL cholesterol, decreased LDL and VLDL cholesterol

Lowered blood pressure

Reduced body fat, when combined with a low-calorie diet

Enhanced weight reduction

Increased work capacity

Improved sense of well-being

Table 17-2
Onset, Peak, and Duration of Insulin Action

Insulin	Onset (hours)	Peak (hours)	Duration (hours)
RAPID-ACTING			
Regular insulin	½–1	5–10	6–8
Prompt insulin suspension (semilente)	1–1½	5–10	12–16
INTERMEDIATE-ACTING			
Isophane insulin suspension (NPH)	1–1½	4–12	24
Insulin zinc suspension (lente)	1–2½	7–15	24
LONG-ACTING			
Protamine zinc insulin suspension (PZI)	4–8	14–24	36
Extended insulin zinc suspension (ultralente)	4–8	10–30	>36

Source: Drug Facts and Comparisons, 1992 ed. St. Louis: Facts and Comparisons, Inc., 1992

Because exercise lowers blood glucose levels, insulin-dependent diabetics may need to consume extra food to avoid hypoglycemia, depending on the duration and intensity of the activity. Although no additional food is indicated for light exercise of short duration, insulin-dependent diabetics may need 10 to 15 g of extra carbohydrate (*i.e.*, approximately one serving of fruit or starch) for each hour of moderate exercise such as hunting or golfing, and 20 to 30 g of extra carbohydrate (*i.e.*, approximately two servings of fruit or two servings of starch) for each hour of vigorous exercise like digging or playing basketball.

Diet for Type II Diabetics

The primary dietary goal for obese type II diabetics is to attain normal blood glucose levels through weight reduction. Clinical symptoms may be immediately improved by a low-calorie diet, and even a moderate reduction in weight (*e.g.*, 5%) can lower blood glucose levels and improve insulin action;[5] other potential benefits include an increase in high-density lipoproteins (the "good" cholesterol) and a decrease in serum triglyceride concentrations.[20] Although attaining "healthy" weight may be the ideal, it often is not a realistic goal and may result in noncompliance in a frustrated and discouraged client.

Because a gradual weight loss is easier to maintain than a large, rapid weight loss, and because weight fluctuations can be detrimental to long-range goals,[5] a modest calorie-restricted diet than allows for a 1- to 2-pound weight loss/week is generally recommended for obese clients. However, severely hyperglycemic obese clients may require medically supervised, drastically low-calorie diets (600 cal/day) until blood sugar levels are controlled. Clients who do not lose weight may eventually need insulin.

For lean type II diabetics, a diet restricted in simple sugars that provides 50% to 60% of total calories from carbohydrates may promote insulin sensitivity and improve blood glucose levels.[20]

After the first priority of attaining normal blood glucose levels is achieved, the diet should be further modified to reduce the risk of cardiac disease by lowering low-density lipoprotein cholesterol. It is recommended that fat provide less than 30% of total calories, saturated fat be limited to less than 10% of total calories, and cholesterol intake not exceed 300 mg/day. Protein should provide 12% to 20% of total calories. The remainder of calories (*i.e.*, 50% to 60% of total calories) should be in the form of carbohydrates, mostly complex CHO. However, it should be noted that some studies indicate that a high-carbohydrate, low-fat diet may not actually decrease the risk of heart disease unless the fiber content is also dramatically increased.[7]

Meal spacing should also be a consideration for NIDDM; eating meals 4 to 5 hours apart allows postprandial glucose levels to return to baseline. Likewise, although meal consistency is especially important for diabetics who take insulin, eating meals of approximately the same composition at approximately the same time every day may help avoid glucose fluctuations, even in NIDDM.

Nursing Process

Assessment

In addition to the general endocrine assessment criteria, assess for the following factors:
Weight, weight status, and recent weight change
Symptoms (*e.g.*, polyphagia, polydipsia): onset, frequency, severity, interventions attempted and the results
Dietary changes made in response to diabetes or its symptoms (*i.e.*, foods avoided, foods preferred)
Meal frequency and timing; consider the impact of shiftwork, if appropriate, and weekend deviations. Determine if mealtimes are relatively consistent or variable from day to day.
Usual overall intake of carbohydrate, protein, and fat
Usual intake of concentrated sweets, such as desserts, candy, and soft drinks
Usual intake of foods high in fiber, especially soluble fiber: oats, oat bran, dried peas and beans, citrus fruits, apples, and certain vegetables
The client's likes and dislikes, nutritional needs, lifestyle and work schedule, religious or ethnic influences, food budget, and other medical disorders that require diet modification (*i.e.*, hypertension, gout, hyperlipidemia)
The client's ability to understand and willingness to make dietary changes
Activity level; determine how energy expenditure can best be increased, given the client's preferences, lifestyle, medical status, and motivation.

Nursing Diagnosis

Altered Health Maintenance, related to the lack of knowledge of diet management of diabetes mellitus.

Planning and Implementation

Before implementing any diet interventions, quality-of-life issues should be addressed.[20] People who are told to make numerous dietary changes may feel overwhelmed and resentful, especially if their diet is already modified for other chronic diseases like hypertension or heart disease. The chance of success may be greatly improved by setting only one goal (*e.g.*, weight loss in obese clients), rather than completely overhauling the diet, especially when weight loss alone can improve other medical problems.[20]

The dietary recommendations listed in the box, Diabetic Diet: American Diabetes Association, are merely guidelines. To maximize compliance, each diet must be individually tailored so that a minimal amount of adjustment is needed. For type II diabetics, calorie restriction takes priority over altering the concentration of carbohydrates, protein, and fat.

Diet modifications should be made sequentially rather than simultaneously.[20] Monitoring and evaluation are ongoing; modify interventions that fail to achieve client goals. After goals are achieved, continue periodic monitoring because of the risk of regaining weight. Also, adjust the diet as needed to meet the client's changing needs related to growth and development (puberty, pregnancy, lactation), significant weight changes, and chronic illnesses.

Many liquid prescription and nonprescription drugs (*e.g.*, cough syrups, expectorants, stool softeners, vitamins, analgesics) contain significant amounts of sugar and should not be used in large amounts without a physician's approval.

Client Goals

The client will:

Consume adequate calories to attain/maintain "healthy" weight.

Maintain blood glucose levels as near normal as possible.

Avoid or delay the onset of complications.

Describe the principles and rationale of diet management of diabetes, and implement the appropriate diet changes.

Nursing Interventions

Diet Management

Adjust calories for "healthy" or reasonable weight, that is, a weight the client can maintain. Clients within their ideal weight range should maintain their weight; obese clients should be encouraged to lose weight. Clients consuming less than 1200 calories may require a multivitamin and mineral supplement.

Individualize the diet as much as possible to correspond with the client's likes, dislikes, and normal eating pattern. Age, physical activity, and medications must also be considered. The "ideal" diet, which may not be appropriate for every *individual*, consists of the following intake:

Three meals plus snacks, if appropriate, eaten at approximately the same time every day and containing approximately the same amount and types of food.

Approximately 50% to 60% CHO, 15% to 20% protein, and 30% or less of fat

Little or no simple sugars, depending on the client's metabolic control and weight status[6]

Less than 10% of total calories from saturated fat, and less than 300 mg/day of cholesterol

Moderate amounts of sodium

Approximately 25 g fiber/1000 calories, with an emphasis on soluble fiber: oat bran, oatmeal, dried peas and beans, apples, citrus fruit, and certain vegetables. Studies show that type II diabetics who consume a high-fiber, high-carbohydrate, low-fat diet have improved serum glucose and lipid levels, as well as improved glucose and insulin responses.[17]

Client Teaching

The goal of diet counseling is to facilitate behavior change, not merely to pass along information. Goals can best be met by providing information in stages, beginning with

(*Text continued on page 515*)

Diabetic Diet: American Diabetes Association

Diet Recommendations[2]	Rationale
Calories	
To attain/maintain "healthy" or desirable body weight	Weight reduction in obese diabetics can help blood glucose levels return toward normal.
Carbohydrates	
Should provide 55% to 60% of total calorie intake	High CHO diets improve glucose tolerance for both types I and II diabetics if sufficient insulin is available.
Emphasize complex CHO (grains, vegetables, legumes).	Compared to simple CHO, complex CHO generally cause less of an increase in blood glucose levels and are better sources of nutrients and fiber.
Restrict simple CHO (pure sugars, foods high in added sugar). Depending on weight status and metabolic control, modest amounts of sucrose and other refined sugars may be used by some individuals.	
Fat	
Restrict to <30% of total calorie intake.	Limiting and modifying the fat content may help prevent or delay the onset of premature and severe atherosclerosis, a prevalent complication of diabetes.
Limit saturated fats to less than 10% of total calories; limit cholesterol to <300 mg/day.	
Protein	
Should provide 12% to 20% of total calorie intake; RDA is 0.8 g/kg/day.	Typical American protein intake is 12% to 15% of total calories; allowance adequately meets RDA recommendations. Excessive protein intake may overburden the kidneys.
Emphasize sources that are low in fat, low in saturated fat and cholesterol.	
Sodium	
Use in moderation; daily intake should not exceed 3000 mg.	Incidence of hypertension among diabetics may be 40% to 80%; hypertension and hyperglycemia occurring together appear to increase the risk of CHD more than the cumulative effect of each.

(continued)

Diabetic Diet: American Diabetes Association (*continued*)

Diet Recommendations[2]	*Rationale*
Fiber	
Increase by substituting high-fiber foods for highly refined CHO that are low in fiber. Up to 40 g of fiber/day is recommended, with an emphasis on soluble fiber.	High-fiber diets have been shown to lower fasting and postprandial blood glucose levels for both types I and II diabetes and may reduce or eliminate the need for insulin therapy.
Alternative Sweeteners	
Use is acceptable.	May add variety and palatability to the diet, and improve client compliance.
Alcohol	
Occasional or no use; limit to 1 to 2 alcohol equivalents 1 to 2 times per week.	Alcohol may aggravate hypoglycemia, neuropathy, glycemic control, obesity, and hyperlipidemia.
Vitamins and Minerals	
Supplements are not indicated.	There is no evidence that diabetes increases vitamin and mineral requirements.
Snacks	
Use is based on individual preferences and glucose patterns; should coordinate with insulin action in IDDM.	IDDM require consistent timing and composition of meals and snacks to coincide with insulin action.

Characteristics

Allowed foods are grouped into six exchange lists according to their composition.

Portion sizes are specified so that each serving within a list contains approximately the same amount of carbohydrates, protein, fat, and calories (see Appendix 11).

The number of servings allowed from each exchange list depends on the calorie content and composition of the diet and should correspond as closely as possible with the client's preferences and food habits.

Meal patterns specify the number of servings from each exchange list allowed for each meal and snack.

Objectives

Attain and maintain ideal body weight.

Maintain near normal blood glucose levels.

(*continued*)

Diabetic Diet: American Diabetes Association (*continued*)

Maintain optimal nutritional status.
Prevent or delay the onset of complications.

Indications

All types of diabetes mellitus.
May also be used for weight reduction in nondiabetics and borderline
   diabetics.

Contraindications

A more liberal diet may be indicated for juvenile type I diabetics because of
growth needs, varying activity patterns, and emotional stress.

Foods Allowed

With the exception of pure sugars and the foods high in sugar listed below,
most foods can be calculated into exchanges and allowed in specified
portions.

Foods to Avoid (high in sugar unless prepared sugar-free; some items
are also high in fat)

Dairy products: chocolate and condensed milk, milkshakes, ice cream,
   puddings.
Fruits and vegetables: fruit canned, frozen, or cooked with sugar; sweetened
   fruit drinks, ices, and juices; cranberry sauce, glazed vegetables.
Breads and cereals: sweet rolls, coffee cakes, sweetened cereals.
Other: cakes, candy, chewing gum, cookies, doughnuts, sweetened gelatin,
   honey, jam and jelly, marmalade, molasses, pastries, pies, popsicles, soft
   drinks, sherbet, sugar, and syrup.

1800-Calorie Diabetic Diet*

Menu	Exchange Equivalents
Breakfast	
½ cup orange juice	1 fruit
½ banana	1 fruit
2 slices whole-wheat toast	2 starch
2 tsp margarine	2 fat
2 tsp sugar-free jelly	free
Coffee/tea	free

Sample Menu

(continued)

Diabetic Diet: American Diabetes Association (*continued*)

Lunch

½ cup vegetable juice	1 vegetable
1 turkey frankfurter	1 meat (high-fat)
1 frankfurter bun	2 starch
Mustard, catsup	free
½ cup baked beans	2 starch
1¼ cup strawberries	1 fruit
Coffee/tea	free

Dinner

2 oz roast turkey	2 meat, lean
½ cup stuffing	2 starch, 2 fat
⅓ cup baked yams	1 starch
½ cup asparagus	1 vegetable
1¼ cup watermelon cubes	1 fruit
1 cup 2% milk	1 milk

Bedtime Snack

1 slice unfrosted raisin toast	1 starch
1 tsp margarine	1 fat
1 cup 2% milk	1 milk

*Actual composition = 1765 calories (55% carbohydrate, 16% protein, 25% fat)

Potential Problem

Noncompliance

Rationale/Nursing Interventions and Considerations

1. Emotional trauma related to the diagnosis of diabetes (denial, anger, and depression)
   - Provide support and encouragement. If possible, withhold diet teaching until the client is emotionally ready.
   - Assure the client that his or her usual diet habits and meal patterns, as well as his or her individual tastes, preferences, and food budget, will all be considered during the formulation of an individualized diet plan.
   - Assure the client that it is not necessary to buy special foods and encourage the family to eat the same food/meals as the client.
2. Lack of motivation
   - Encourage the client to attend group learning sessions, which tend to be more effective than individualized instruction.
   - Provide frequent follow-up and feedback over an extended period of time.

(*continued*)

Diabetic Diet: American Diabetes Association (*continued*)

- Enlist family support and involvement and encourage their participation in group sessions.

3. Unwillingness to follow the diet related to a "sweet tooth"
   - Allow the use of non-nutritive sweeteners (sweeteners that do not contain appreciable amounts of calories), such as saccharin and aspartame.
   - Provide information regarding diabetic cookbooks that include recipes for desserts with the exchange value specified.
   - If the client is not overweight, it may be possible to include some sweets that have traditionally been excluded from diabetic diets (see Food for Thought).

4. Intellectually unable to comprehend the reason for the diet and its strategies
   - Encourage family involvement.
   - Tailor the diet instruction to the client's ability; consider using simplified meal patterns, food models, and pictures. Minimize guidelines and restrictions as much as possible.

5. Lack of knowledge related to oversimplified instructions to eliminate "sugar" from the diet; this is often the only advice given to elderly clients of normal weight
   - Instruct the client that eliminating "sugar" also means eliminating foods high in sugar, such as those listed above.

6. Lack of knowledge related to the misconception that insulin or oral hypoglycemia agents eliminate the need to follow a modified diet
   - Instruct the client that medication and diet work together to control blood sugar levels and that medication is not a substitute for diet therapy.

7. Lack of knowledge related to calculating the amount of exchanges from mixed dishes and other foods not listed on the exchange lists
   - Provide the client with appropriate exchange lists, such as those containing ethnic or regional foods, convenience foods, or fast food and restaurant items.
   - Encourage the client to become familiar with the CHO, protein, fat, and calorie content of each of the exchange lists and to use that information to analyze a recipe or food label for its approximate exchange value.

Potential Problem

Symptoms of hypoglycemia in insulin-dependent diabetics—nervousness, weakness, sweating, shallow breathing, double vision, dizziness, and potential coma. Prolonged hypoglycemia in children can result in permanent neuro-motor damage.

(continued)

Diabetic Diet: American Diabetes Association (*continued*)

Rationale/Nursing Interventions and Considerations

1. Unbalanced meal selection
   - Stress the importance of using the exchange lists correctly. Although all items within an exchange group can be substituted for each other, items from one group cannot be exchanged for items in another.
   - Advise the client to eat a source of protein and/or fat at each meal and snack to slow the rate of CHO digestion and absorption.
   - Stress the importance of eating the prescribed amount of food at each meal and snack. Food should not be "saved" at one meal so that more can be eaten at the next.
2. Inadequate food intake related to too long an interval between feedings
   - Advise the client not to skip meals and snacks. If a delayed meal is anticipated, instruct the client to eat part of the meal allowance as a snack at the usual meal time and eat the remaining exchange as soon as possible.
   - Counsel the client to carry a source of rapidly absorbed sugar (hard candy, sugar cubes, and so forth) with him at all times for unexpectedly delayed meals. The client's normal meal should follow as soon as possible.
   - If neccessary, modify the meal plan to include more snacks.
3. Inadequate food intake related to decreased appetite
   - Determine the cause of the change in appetite. If the client is not under-weight and the change is due to normal causes (decreased activity, decreased metabolic rate related to aging), request a lower calorie allowance and an insulin adjustment from the physician.
   - If the decrease in appetite is related to illness, stress the importance of eating and drinking. Urge the client to attempt to follow the meal plan as closely as possible, using only liquids or soft foods if necessary.
   - Instruct the client to report episodes of vomiting or illnesses lasting more than 2 days to the physician.
4. Decreased insulin requirement related to weight loss
   - Instruct the client to inform the physician of any true weight loss (*i.e.*, loss of body fat, not minor, daily, weight fluctuations).
5. Decreased insulin requirement related to increased fiber intake
   - Obtain a diet history to determine the approximate fiber content and any recent changes in fiber intake. If the increase in fiber intake is expected to be permanent, advise the physician.
6. An increase in exercise
   - Remind the client to eat extra CHO before moderate and vigorous exercise and to eat a source of sugar if symptoms of hypoglycemia develop while exercising. A change in the meal pattern may be necessary if the increase in exercise is expected to be permanent.

basic information and progressing to in-depth details as information is not only understood, but then assimilated.[5] Reinforcement and feedback are also useful. Learning goals should be mutually developed.[16]

Over a period of time, instruct the client

On the appropriate dietary strategies and diet recommendations based on the type of diabetes.

That diet therapy is essential in the treatment of all forms of diabetes and the diet must be followed permanently, even when no symptoms are apparent.

That medication may be used in addition to diet therapy, not as a substitute.

That the calorie level of the diet is determined by the client's health, energy needs, and activity patterns, and may change as needed.

That, generally, sugars, foods high in sugar, and foods prepared with added fat are restricted. For special occasions, regularly sweetened foods can be included in the meal plan (see Appendix 12).

That if alcohol is consumed, it should be used in moderation, that is, not more than two equivalents of alcohol once or twice a week (an equivalent is 1.5 oz of distilled beverage, 12 oz of beer, or 4 oz of wine). Because alcohol can induce hypoglycemia, especially in clients taking insulin or hypoglycemic agents, it should not be consumed in a fasting state. Dry wine and light or "near" beer are preferred because of their reduced calorie and alcohol content.[4] Sugar-free sodas or water are acceptable mixers. Generally, either fat or fat and bread exchanges are deducted from the meal plan for each alcohol equivalent.

That the amounts of CHO, protein, and fat allowed in the diet are controlled because each provides calories and can be converted to sugar in the body.

That eating too much food raises blood sugar levels (hyperglycemia) and can cause excessive urination, increased appetite, increased thirst, confusion, nausea, vomiting, difficulty breathing, and acetone breath.

That not eating enough food while on insulin therapy causes low blood sugar levels (hypoglycemia), which is characterized by nervousness, weakness, sweating, shallow breathing, double vision, and dizziness. To counter hypoglycemic reactions, a readily absorbed form of sugar (hard candy, sugar cubes, and so forth) should be carried at all times.

On the use of exchange lists (see Appendix 11):

- Exchange lists simplify meal planning, eliminate the need for daily calculations, ensure a consistent, nutritionally balanced diet, and add variety. However, the exchange lists may not be appropriate or acceptable for all ethnic and cultural groups; individual adjustments may be vital for compliance.
- There are six exchange lists: all foods within a list have approximately the same CHO, protein, fat, and calorie value per specified serving (see box, Exchange Lists).
- Foods within an exchange list can be substituted for one another, but not from one list to another.
- Portion sizes are important; weigh or measure food until portion sizes can be estimated accurately.
- Certain foods and beverages are considered "free" and may be used as desired.

On the use of sugar substitutes:

- Non-nutritive sugar substitutes and calorie-free products made with sugar substitutes can be used freely.

Exchange Lists

Exchange List	Carbohydrate (g)	Protein (g)	Fat (g)	Calories
Starch/Bread	15	3	Trace	80
Meat				
Lean	—	7	3	55
Medium-fat	—	7	5	75
High-fat	—	7	8	100
Vegetable	5	2	—	25
Fruit	15	—	—	60
Milk				
Skim	12	8	Trace	90
Low-fat	12	8	5	120
Whole	12	8	10	150
Fat	—	—	5	45

Source: American Diabetes Association, American Dietetic Association: Exchange List for Meal Planning. Alexandria, VA: American Diabetes Association; Chicago: American Dietetic Association, 1986

- The use of products made with non-nutritive sugar substitutes but containing other calorie-contributing ingredients must be calculated into the meal plan.
- The nutritive sweeteners fructose, sorbitol, and xylitol should be used only with a physician's approval.

On sick day management:

- Unless otherwise instructed by the physician, clients should maintain their normal medication schedule; blood glucose or urine acetone should be monitored frequently.
- Clients unable to consume a normal diet should rely on liquids to prevent hypoglycemia and replenish losses that may occur from vomiting or diarrhea.
- Because illness can increase serum glucose levels, precise replacement of all carbohydrate calories may not be required.[4] Generally, 15 g of carbohydrate (*i.e.*, one starch equivalent or fruit exchange) should be eaten every half hour and 1.5 cups of fluid every hour. Each of the following have approximately 15 g of carbohydrate and may be acceptable during illness: 6 oz of regular ginger ale, 1/2 cup ice cream, 1/2 cup apple juice, one frozen juice bar, 1/4 cup sherbet, 1/2 cup regular gelatin, 1/2 cup orange juice, 1 cup cream soup.

How to order from a menu when dining out:

- Estimate portion sizes of all foods.
- For foods not included on the exchange lists, figure out the number of bread, meat, and fat exchanges by analyzing the ingredients and categorizing them into the appropriate exchange group.
- Choose tomato juice, unsweetened fruit juice, clear broth, bouillon or consommé as an appetizer instead of sweetened juices, fried vegetables, seafood cocktail (unless meat exchange is deducted from entrée), or cream or thick soups.

- Choose fresh vegetable salads and use oil and vinegar or fresh lemon instead of regular salad dressings, or request that the dressing be put on the side. Avoid coleslaw and other salads with the dressing already added.
- Order plain (without gravy or sauce) roasted, baked, or broiled meat, fish, and poultry instead of fried, sautéed, or breaded entrées. Avoid stews and casseroles. Request a "doggie bag" if the portion exceeds the meal-plan allowance.
- Order steamed, boiled, or broiled vegetables.
- Choose plain, baked, mashed, boiled, or steamed potatoes, rice, or noodles.
- Select fresh fruit for dessert.
- Request a sugar substitute for coffee or tea, if desired.
- Diabetic exchange lists are available for fast-food restaurants.
- Most airlines will provide diabetic meals if requested at the time that flight reservations are made.
- Exchange lists for Special Occasion Foods appear in Appendix 12.

On food preparation ideas:

- Food does not have to be prepared separately from the rest of the family's, as long as extra sugar and fat are not added.
- For variety, use margarine or oil from the fat allowance to sauté meat or vegetables.
- Trim all visible fat from meat after cooking, and remove the skin from chicken.
- Use diabetic cookbooks for variety; their recipes specify portion sizes and the number of exchanges per portion.

On food purchasing and label reading:

- Try to buy only those prepared foods that have nutrition information on the label, so that the exchange value can be calculated, or write to the manufacturer to request nutrition information.
- Compare the nutrition information and ingredient labels of different brands of the same product, which can vary greatly.
- Although ingredients are listed on labels in descending order by weight, it may be difficult to determine the total sugar content because different forms can be listed separately, such as dextrose, glucose, granulated sugar, confectioner's sugar, maltose, fructose, corn syrup, corn sugar, corn sweetener, molasses, brown sugar, sucrose, date sugar, "raw" sugar, invert sugar, lactose, maple syrup, sorghum, and honey. If some form of sugar is listed in the first three ingredients and the food has a high CHO content, do not use it unless approved by the physician or dietitian.
- Buy fresh, frozen without sugar, or water-packed canned fruit, if economically possible; if not, rinse sweetened fruit under running water for 1 minute or more to remove sugary syrup.
- "Dietetic" products are not necessarily calorie-free or specifically intended for diabetics; foods labeled "dietetic" may be made without sugar, without salt, with a particular type of fat, or for special food allergies. Read the ingredient label and check with a diet counselor before adding a dietetic food to the diet, or avoid dietetic foods altogether because they are expensive and usually do not taste as good as the foods they are intended to replace.
- Avoid foods that contain coconut oil, palm oil, palm kernel oil, unspecified vegetable oils, and hydrogenated oils because they are high in saturated fats.

Provide the client with the following, if appropriate:

- An individualized meal pattern

- The exchange lists and supplemental exchange lists, if desired (*i.e.*, for illnesses, special occasions, ethnic foods, fast-food restaurants, alcoholic beverages)
- Diabetic recipes, titles of diabetic cookbooks

Monitor

Monitor for the following signs or symptoms:
Serum glucose, glycosylated hemoglobin, serum lipid levels
Weight, weight changes
Compliance with the diet, and the need for follow-up diet counseling
Effectiveness of the diet, and the need for further diet modifications
The onset of complications

Evaluation

Evaluation is ongoing. Assuming the plan of care has not changed, the client will achieve the goals as stated above.

DRUG ALERT For type II diabetics, treatment with insulin, and to a lesser degree, oral hypoglycemic agents, can hinder weight loss and actually promote weight gain.[5] Before determining that the diet is not effective and drug therapy is necessary, every attempt should be made to achieve metabolic control through diet alone.

Hyperinsulinism

Hyperinsulinism is characterized by an excessive insulin secretion in response to carbohydrate-rich foods, leading to hypoglycemia (blood glucose levels of 40 mg/dl or less). Organic hyperinsulinism, which occurs during fasting, is a rare disorder caused by hyperplasia of the islets of Langerhans or by insulin-secreting pancreatic tumors. It is treated by surgical removal of the insulin-secreting tumor or pancreatic resection of hyperplastic tissue. The exact cause of functional hyperinsulinism, which occurs after eating, is unknown; approximately 15% of the cases result in diabetes mellitus. Functional hyperinsulinism may occur after a gastrectomy. Diet management, designed to avoid stimulating insulin secretion, is used to treat functional hyperinsulinism.

Nursing Process

Assessment

In addition to the general endocrine assessment criteria, assess for the following factors:
The relationship between eating and the onset of hypoglycemic symptoms. Observe for weakness, hunger, nervousness, trembling, sweating, and faintness occurring 2 to 4 hours after eating. Convulsions and loss of consciousness occur in severe cases.
The impact of CHO ingestion on symptoms—eating CHO should reverse symptoms.
Dietary changes made in response to symptoms (*i.e.*, foods avoided, foods preferred).

Nursing Diagnosis

Altered Health Maintenance, related to the lack of knowledge of diet management of functional hyperinsulinism.

Planning and Implementation

The diet for functional hyperinsulinism should be nutritionally sound and provide calories for "healthy" weight; obese clients should be encouraged to lose weight.

To avoid excessive insulin secretion, restrict carbohydrate-rich foods that produce a rapid rise in blood glucose. However, restricting total carbohydrate intake is neither necessary nor practical.[4] Instead, to slow the rise in blood glucose levels, care should be taken to eat protein and/or fat whenever carbohydrates are consumed. A high fiber intake, especially soluble fiber, may be beneficial.

The diet should be liberal in protein, because protein does not stimulate insulin secretion. Fat supplies the remainder of calories.

Small, frequent meals, each containing protein and/or fat, will help slow the rate of CHO absorption, decrease the rise in blood glucose levels, and reduce insulin secretion. The diabetic exchange lists may be used for meal planning.

Client Goals

The client will:

Avoid symptoms of hypoglycemia after eating.

Consume adequate calories and protein to attain/maintain "healthy" weight.

Describe the principles and rationale of diet management of functional hyperinsulinism, and implement the appropriate dietary changes.

Identify foods/meals that cause hypoglycemic symptoms.

Nursing Interventions

Diet Management

Provide calories for "healthy" weight.

Limit simple sugars and dried fruits. Encourage a high fiber intake, especially foods high in soluble fiber.

Increase protein intake to 1.0 to 1.5 g/kg/day.

Provide three meals and two to three snacks daily, each containing protein and/or fat.

Prohibit alcohol and caffeine.

A sample menu appears in the box, Sample Menu for Hyperinsulinism.

Client Teaching

Instruct the client

On the principles and rationale of diet management of functional hyperinsulinism.

On the use of exchange lists (see section on Client Teaching for Diabetes).

That eliminating "sugar" also means eliminating foods high in sugar (see box, Diabetic Diet: American Diabetes Association).

That the use of sugar substitutes is allowed.

Hyperinsulinism Diet

Breakfast

½ banana
½ cup oatmeal
1 slice whole-wheat toast with margarine
½ cup 2% milk
Coffee/tea

Midmorning Snack

1 oz cheddar cheese
6 saltine crackers
½ cup 2% milk

Lunch

Tomato soup
Turkey sandwich
Carrot and celery sticks
1 cup 2% milk
Apple

Midafternoon Snack

Peanuts
Sugar-free carbonated beverage

Dinner

Roast beef
Roasted potatoes
Tossed salad
Winter squash
½ cup 2% milk
½ cup rice pudding

Bedtime Snack

Popcorn
1 cup 2% milk

To carry a source of readily absorbable CHO (such as hard candy or sugar cubes) at all times in case of a hypoglycemic attack.

To avoid alcohol and caffeine, which can aggravate hypoglycemia.

Monitor

Monitor for the following signs or symptoms:

Weight, weight changes

Compliance with the diet, and evaluate the need for further diet counseling

Effectiveness of the diet, and determine whether additional diet modifications are needed

Signs or symptoms of diabetes mellitus

Evaluation

Evaluation is ongoing. Assuming the plan of care has not changed, the client will achieve the goals as stated above.

THYROID DISORDERS

The thyroid gland secretes two active hormones, tetraiodothyronine (thyroxine or T4) and triiodothyronine (T3). Alterations in thyroid hormone secretion cause alterations in the basal metabolic rate, as evidenced by weight changes and changes in bowel elimination.

Hypothyroidism

Hypothyroidism (which may be triggered by idiopathic causes, or occur secondary to surgical removal of the thyroid gland, radioactive iodine therapy, or an autoimmune disorder [Hashimoto's thyroiditis]) is characterized by deficient thyroid hormone secretion leading to decreased basal metabolic rate, possibly by 15% to 30% or more. *Cretinism* refers to a thyroid deficiency present at birth; *myxedema* is the advanced stage of hypothyroidism in adults. Myxedema is five times more common in women than men and usually occurs between 30 to 60 years of age. Early symptoms include fatigue, menstrual changes (menorrhagia or amenorrhea), hair loss, brittle nails, dry skin, paresthesia of the hands and feet, and thick speech. Later, decreased body temperature and pulse rate, weight gain, physical and mental slowness, edematous appearance; enlarged tongue, hands, and feet; constipation, and intolerance to cold may develop. Complications of myxedema include rapid onset of atherosclerosis, coronary heart disease, angina pectoris, myocardial infarction, and congestive heart failure. Increased sensitivity to sedatives, opiates, and anesthetic drugs may develop, as well as acute organic psychosis characterized by paranoia and delusions. Hypoventilation, hypothermia, and respiratory acidosis occur with myxedema coma; only 50% of its victims survive.

Hypothyroidism is treated with thyroid hormone replacement and diet management to prevent and/or alleviate symptoms of weight gain and constipation.

Hyperthyroidism

Hyperthyroidism (Graves' disease, thyrotoxicosis, exophthalmic goiter) is characterized by excessive thyroid hormone secretion leading to increased basal metabolic rate, possibly by 15% to 25% in mild cases, and up to 50% to 75% in severe cases. The exact cause is unknown, but it is believed to be caused by an autoimmune disorder; it may be related to emotional stress or infection. Hyperthyroidism is five times more common in women than men and most often occurs between 30 to 40 years of age.

Symptoms include nervousness, irritability, apprehension, and decreased attention span; increased pulse rate, palpitations, and increased systolic blood pressure; intolerance to heat, profuse perspiration; flushed, warm, soft, moist skin; bulging eyes (exophthalmos); ravenous appetite accompanied by progressive weight loss; muscular weakness; amenorrhea; and diarrhea or constipation. Mild cases may be marked by alternating periods of exacerbation and remission, with possible spontaneous recovery within months or years. Emaciation, intense nervousness, delirium, disorientation, and heart disease (tachycardia, atrial fibrillation, congestive heart failure) are possible complications; death occurs in rare instances.

Drug therapy, radiation, or surgical removal of part or all of the thyroid gland may be used to treat hyperthyroidism. The choice of treatment depends on the client's age, the cause and severity of the disease, and the development of complications. Diet management is used to prevent further weight loss and restore normal body weight, reverse negative nitrogen balance and replenish nutritional losses, and alleviate diarrhea or constipation.

Nursing Process

Assessment of Thyroid Disorders

In addition to the general endocrine assessment criteria, assess for the following factors:
Symptoms of thyroid disorder that directly or indirectly affect nutritional status or intake; assess onset, frequency, severity, interventions attempted and the results.
Dietary changes made in response to thyroid disorder or its symptoms (*i.e.*, foods avoided, foods preferred). Determine foods best and least tolerated.
Bowel elimination and any recent, significant changes
Weight status, recent weight changes

Nursing Diagnosis

Altered Nutrition: More or Less than Body Requirements, related to altered metabolism secondary to hyperthyroidism or hypothyroidism.

Planning and Implementation

Provide a well-balanced, nutritionally adequate diet with calories for "healthy" weight, based on the client's nutritional status, weight status, and symptoms.

Adjust fiber intake to promote normal bowel elimination, as needed.
See Table 17-3 for considerations specific for each thyroid disorder.

Table 17-3

Diet Management Considerations for Hypothyroidism and Hyperthyroidism

Hypothyroidism	Hyperthyroidism
Until normal metabolism is restored, clients with myxedema experience weight gain even if calorie intake is low. However, a low-calorie diet combined with thyroid hormone therapy should enable the client to achieve normal weight. A high-fiber diet will not only help alleviate constipation but is useful in weight reduction; high-fiber foods generally are low in calories and provide feeling of fullness. Low-cholesterol, low-fat, or low-sodium diet modifications may be indicated for complications of atherosclerosis and heart disease.	Calorie requirements may increase to 4500 to 5000 cal or more. A liberal protein intake of 100 g or more combined with a liberal CHO intake is recommended. Vitamin and mineral needs increase related to the accelerated rate of metabolism and nutrient utilization. Clients experiencing steady weight loss despite eating large amounts of food are often frustrated and discouraged. Provide emotional support and a pleasant eating environment. Solicit food preferences and encourage the intake of nutritionally dense foods (*i.e.,* fortified milk shakes, foods with added milk powder, eggs, cheese, butter, or meat). Provide six to eight feedings to maximize intake. Eliminate CNS stimulants, such as caffeine and alcohol. Clients with hyperthyroidism may experience osteoporosis and an increased risk of bone fractures related to an increase in calcium and phosphorus excretion. Encourage the intake of foods high in calcium (Appendix 13) and provide calcium supplements if needed. Hypothyroidism or hypoparathyroidism resulting from a partial or total thyroidectomy may require diet modification.

Client Goals

The client will:

Consume adequate calories and protein to attain/maintain "healthy" body weight and restore/maintain optimal nutritional status.

Have normal bowel elimination (*i.e.,* not have diarrhea or constipation).

Describe the principles and rationale of diet management for hypothyroidism or hyperthyroidism, and implement the appropriate dietary changes.

Nursing Interventions

Diet Management

Provide calories for "healthy" body weight, based on age, sex, and activity.

Modify fiber intake to either promote or reduce bowel stimulation, as indicated.

See Table 17-3 for other diet management considerations.

Client Teaching

Instruct the client

On the principles and rationale of diet management of hypothyroidism or hyperthyroidism.

Monitor

Monitor for the following signs or symptoms:

Compliance with the diet, and the need for follow-up diet counseling

Effectiveness of the diet (*i.e.*, normal weight status, normal bowel elimination), and evaluate the need for further diet modifications

Evaluation

Evaluation is ongoing. Assuming the plan of care has not changed, the client will achieve the goals as stated above.

DRUG ALERT   Replacement thyroid hormones used to treat hypothyroidism can lead to elevated blood glucose levels. It may be necessary to restrict the intake of concentrated sweets or to provide a diabetic diet if insulin therapy is used.

Clients receiving iodine in preparation for thyroid surgery may need to restrict their intake of rich sources of iodine—iodized salt, seafood, and bread made with iodate dough conditioners.

PARATHYROID DISORDERS

The parathyroid glands, tiny organs embedded on each side of the thyroid gland, secrete parathyroid hormone (PTH), which regulates calcium and phosphorus metabolism. Parathyroid disorders cause alterations in the calcium content of bones and in serum and urinary calcium levels. Because calcium and phosphorus have an inverse relationship, serum levels of phosphorus are also altered.

Hypoparathyroidism

Hypoparathyroidism occurs most commonly as a result of a thyroidectomy, parathyroidectomy, or radical neck dissection, related to suppression of the gland or an interference with the blood supply.[18] It may develop immediately after surgery, or within 1 to 2 days, and is usually temporary.

Parathyroid hormone deficiency decreases the mobilization of calcium from the bone; serum phosphorus rises, urinary excretion both of calcium and phosphorus decreases, and hypocalcemia develops. Hypocalcemia increases neuromuscular irritability and can lead to tetany (painful, involuntary muscle spasms); tingling, numbness, and cramping in the extremities; bronchospasms; laryngeal spasms; Trousseau's sign (carpopedal spasm occurring when circulation is occluded in the arm with a blood pressure cuff); and Chvostek's sign (facial muscle spasms occurring when muscles or branches of facial nerves are tapped). Dysphagia, increased sensitivity to light, cardiac arrhythmias, convulsions, anxiety, irritability, depression, and delirium may develop. Other complications include cataracts, psychoses, and permanent brain damage. Heart failure may develop in cases of chronic idiopathic hypoparathyroidism.

In acute hypoparathyroidism (*i.e.*, tetany), intravenous calcium gluconate is given to raise serum calcium levels. Sedatives may be needed to control convulsions. For chronic hypoparathyroidism, treatment involves oral calcium and vitamin D supplements, and aluminum hydroxide gel or aluminum carbonate to bind phosphate and increase its excretion.

Hyperparathyroidism

Excessive parathyroid hormone secretion leads to hyperparathyroidism, which may vary from mild to severe. Primary hyperparathyroidism is caused by hyperactivity of the parathyroid glands related to benign or malignant tumor growth, or tissue hyperplasia and hypertrophy; secondary causes include chronic renal disease, rickets, osteomalacia, and acromegaly.

An increase in PTH secretion causes calcium to leave the bones and enter the bloodstream; the rise in serum calcium causes a corresponding drop in serum phosphorus. Hypercalcemia leads to a decrease in neuromuscular irritability, which may be evidenced by apathy, fatigue, depression, paranoia, muscular weakness, nausea, vomiting, constipation, and anorexia. The increase in urinary calcium can lead to numerous renal complications, such as formation of calcium phosphate renal stones, renal obstruction, calcification of renal parenchyma, pyelonephritis, and renal failure. Gastrointestinal complications include pancreatitis and peptic ulcers, leading to perforation and hemorrhage. Loss of calcium from the bone can lead to back and joint pain, pain on weight-bearing, pathologic fractures, skeletal deformities, and loss of height. Calcium phosphate may precipitate in the lungs, muscles, heart, and eyes.

A hypercalcemic crisis occurs when serum calcium levels exceed 8 to 9 mEq/L. Polyuria, polydipsia, volume depletion, fever, altered consciousness, azotemia, and mental disturbances are common symptoms. Cardiac arrest is responsible for the high mortality rate.

Hyperparathyroidism is treated by surgical removal of abnormal tissue, which may result in hypoparathyroidism.

Nursing Process

Assessment of Parathyroid Disorders

In addition to the general endocrine assessment criteria, assess for the following factors:
Symptoms of parathyroid disorder that directly or indirectly affect nutritional status or intake; assess onset, frequency, severity, interventions attempted and the results.
Dietary changes made in response to parathyroid disorder or its symptoms (*i.e.*, foods avoided, foods preferred). Determine foods best and least tolerated.
Usual calcium intake: milk and dairy products, green leafy vegetables, and canned fish with bones
Usual vitamin D intake, and exposure to sunlight

Nursing Diagnosis

Altered Health Maintenance, related to lack of knowledge of diet management of parathyroid disorders.

Planning and Implementation

For both hypoparathyroidism and hyperparathyroidism, diet management may be used to help restore normal calcium balance. However, although the manipulation of dietary calcium may help, in most cases it does not fully compensate for an imbalance of parathyroid hormone. In addition, it is difficult to increase dietary calcium (*i.e.*, for hypoparathyroidism) *and* avoid a high phosphorus intake because milk and dairy products are rich sources of both calcium and phosphorus.

In addition to adjusting calcium intake, the diet for hyperparathyroidism may also be modified to alleviate vomiting, constipation, anorexia, and GI upset, as needed (see Chap.15), or to help prevent renal complications.

Client Goals

The client will:

Increase or decrease calcium intake to help normalize serum calcium levels in hypoparathyroidism or hyperparathyroidism, respectively.

Modify the diet, as needed, to help prevent or alleviate GI or renal complications.

Identify foods high in calcium, phosphorus, and vitamin D.

Consume a nutritionally adequate diet.

Nursing Interventions

Diet Management

Increase calcium intake for hypoparathyroidism; but use milk and dairy products with caution because they are rich sources of phosphorus. Sources of calcium appear in Appendix 13.

Decrease calcium intake for hyperparathyroidism. After surgery, a high calcium diet may be indicated.

Other considerations for hypoparathyroidism and hyperparathyroidism are outlined in Table 17-4.

Client Teaching

Instruct the client

On the principles and rationale of diet management for hypoparathyroidism or hyperparathyroidism.

On rich sources of dietary calcium, phosphorus, and vitamin D.

On the role of vitamin D in increasing serum calcium, if appropriate, and to increase daily exposure to the sunlight.

To take supplements only as prescribed by the physician.

Monitor

Monitor for the following signs or symptoms:

Serum calcium and phosphorus; restrict milk and dairy products if phosphorus levels are elevated.

Tolerance of and compliance with the diet, and the need for follow-up diet counseling

Effectiveness of the diet, and the need for further diet modification

Evaluation

Evaluation is ongoing. Assuming the plan of care has not changed, the client will achieve the goals as stated above.

Table 17-4
Diet Management Considerations for Hypoparathyroidism and Hyperparathyroidism

Hypoparathyroidism	Hyperparathyroidism
In addition to calcium and vitamin D supplements, a high-calcium, low-phosphorus diet may be prescribed, even though the diet order is not likely to be achieved. Green leafy vegetables are good sources of calcium, but they contain compounds that bind calcium and inhibit its absorption. Milk and dairy products are the best sources of calcium, but they may be allowed only in limited amounts because they are also rich in phosphorus (Appendix 13). Diets lacking in milk and dairy products are not likely to provide the RDA for calcium (800 mg) and certainly cannot meet the needs of clients who may require 1000 to 2000 mg or more of calcium/day.	Increase fluids to 3000 to 4000 ml or more a day to dilute the urine and prevent the precipitation of renal stones. Urge the client to drink large amounts of fluid before bed and periodically through the night to avoid concentrated urine.
Calcium absorption is enhanced by vitamin C and some amino acids because calcium is soluble in an acid medium. More calcium is absorbed when supplements are given in small, divided doses rather than in large individual doses.	Drinking cranberry juice is often recommended to acidify the urine and prevent the precipitation of basic stones, such as calcium. However, it takes at least 1.2 liters of pure cranberry juice (not cranberry juice cocktail, which is a mixture of cranberry juice, water, and sugar) to make a significant change in urinary pH. Modify the diet as needed to alleviate anorexia, constipation, GI upset, or ulcers (see Chap. 15).

ADRENAL CORTEX DISORDERS

The adrenal glands are located above the kidneys. The cortex, or outer portion, secretes corticosteroids, which include glucocorticoids, mineralocorticoids, and small amounts of sex hormones. A deficiency of adrenal cortex hormones primarily affects glucose metabolism and fluid and electrolyte balance.

Primary Adrenocortical Insufficiency (Addison's Disease)

Primary adrenocortical insufficiency is caused by destruction of adrenal cortical tissue, either from idiopathic atrophy or secondary to infections such as tuberculosis. A deficient secretion of glucocorticoid hormones leads to depletion of liver glycogen and hypoglycemia. Mineralocorticoid deficiency (aldosterone) results in increased excretion of sodium, chloride, and water, leading to retention of potassium, acidosis, decreased blood volume, and decreased cardiac output.

With primary adrenocortical insufficiency, adrenal failure occurs over a period of time. Symptoms include muscular weakness, fatigue, weight loss, anorexia, nausea, vomiting, diarrhea, constipation, abdominal pain, hypotension, and symptoms of hypoglycemia, hyponatremia, and hyperkalemia. Diffuse or patchy darkening of the skin is characteristic of Addison's disease; depression, irritability, anxiety, or apprehension may develop. A possible complication of Addison's disease is an Addisonian crisis, a medical emergency characterized by cyanosis, fever, shock, headache, nausea, abdominal pain, diarrhea, confusion, and restlessness. Circulatory collapse can result from mild overexertion, expo-

Glycemic Index—Delight or Dilemma?

Because simple sugars are absorbed quickly and can cause rapid elevations in blood glucose levels, diabetic diets are usually devoid of sweets and limited in natural sugars like fructose (fruit sugar). Most CHO calories are provided by starches, which are digested more slowly than sugars and have less of an impact on blood glucose levels.

Recent studies, however, indicate that a food's glycemic index (the effect of food on blood glucose levels compared to the response of an equivalent amount of glucose) is related to numerous other factors than just whether the food consists of sugar or starch. Fat, fiber (particularly pectin and guar), the action of enzyme inhibitors, protein, protein–starch interactions, and the structure of a food may all influence glycemic index.

Pure sugars, for instance, do raise blood glucose levels; however, high-sugar, high-fat foods like candy bars and ice cream cause less of an increase in blood glucose levels than brown rice or cornflakes. Glycemic indexes vary even among starches; as a group, root vegetables (carrots, parsnips, potatoes) have the highest average glycemic index, 72, compared to the lowest group average of 31 for legumes.

Experts are not concluding that diabetics should eat ice cream instead of brown rice (a high-fat diet may suppress swings in blood glucose levels, but also increases the risk of cardiovascular disease, obesity, and certain types of cancer), or even reduce the amount of CHO in their diets (controlled diabetics experience improved glucose tolerance on high-CHO diets). Instead, the glycemic index, in addition to a food's nutrient density and composition, may become another factor to consider when choosing carbohydrates.

Glycemic Index*

100%
Glucose

80%–90%
Cornflakes
Carrots†
Parsnips†
Potatoes (instant mashed)
Maltose
Honey

70%–79%
Bread (wholemeal)
Millet

Rice (white)
Weetabix
Broad beans (fresh)†
Potatoes (new)
Swede†

60%–69%
Bread (white)
Rice (brown)
Muesli
Shredded wheat
Ryvita
Water biscuits
Beetroot†

(continued)

Glycemic Index—Delight or Dilemma? (*continued*)

Bananas
Raisins
Mars bar

50%–59%

Buckwheat
Spaghetti (white)
Sweet corn
All–bran
Digestive biscuits
Oatmeal biscuits
Rich tea biscuits
Peas (frozen)
Yam
Sucrose
Potato chips

40%–49%

Spaghetti (wholemeal)
Porridge oats
Potatoes (sweet)
Beans (canned navy)
Peas (dried)

Oranges
Orange juice

30%–39%

Butter beans
Haricot beans
Blackeye peas
Chick peas
Apples (golden delicious)
Ice cream
Milk (skim)
Milk (whole)
Yogurt
Tomato soup

20%–29%

Kidney beans
Lentils
Fructose

10%–19%

Soya beans
Soya beans (canned)
Peanuts

*As determined by feeding portion sizes yielding 50 g of CHO. (Jenkins DJ: Lente carbohydrate—a newer approach to the dietary management of diabetes. Diabetes Care 5:634, 1982. Reproduced with permission from the American Diabetes Association, Inc.)

†25 g CHO portion given.

sure to cold, acute infections, or a decrease in salt intake. Death may occur from hypotension and vasomotor collapse.

Addison's disease is treated with hormone replacement: fludrocortisone is a synthetic corticosteroid that has both glucocorticoid and mineralocorticoid properties. Diet management is used to prevent or treat hypoglycemia and promote normal fluid and electrolyte balance.

Nursing Process

Assessment

In addition to the general endocrine assessment criteria, assess for the following factors:
Symptoms: onset, frequency, causative factors (if known), severity, interventions attempted and the results

Dietary changes made in response to symptoms (*i.e.*, foods avoided, foods preferred)

Usual sodium intake: convenience foods, processed meats, canned meat, soups, and vegetables; condiments, traditional snack foods, salt-cured foods

Usual intake of simple sugars

Usual fluid intake

The frequency of meals and snacks. Determine if the client frequently skips meals.

Nursing Diagnosis

Fluid Volume Deficit, related to abnormal fluid loss (increased excretion) secondary to primary adrenocortical insufficiency.

Planning and Implementation

Depending on the client's fluid and electrolyte status and the type of medication used, the requirements for sodium and potassium may be increased or decreased. Clients treated with cortisone may require a high sodium intake of up to 4 to 6 g/day or more of sodium. A high sodium intake is contraindicated for clients receiving fludrocortisone because it is a sodium-retaining hormone. Likewise, potassium requirement is determined on an individual basis; although serum potassium levels are elevated in untreated Addison's disease, hormone therapy tends to deplete potassium. A high fluid intake of up to 3 L/day may be indicated to replace losses.

Because hypoglycemia is a recurrent problem, small, frequent meals high in protein and moderate in carbohydrate are recommended. The client should consume a large meal at bedtime to avoid early morning hypoglycemia. Concentrated sweets should be avoided.

Supplemental B vitamins and vitamin C may be required for increased metabolism.

Client Goals

The client will:

Attain/maintain normal fluid and electrolyte balance.

Avoid hypoglycemia by consuming frequent meals, avoiding concentrated sweets, and eating a large meal at bedtime.

Attain/maintain "healthy" weight.

Describe the principles and rationale of diet management of Addison's disease, and make the appropriate diet changes.

Identify signs and symptoms of hypoglycemia, and carry food at all times.

Nursing Interventions

Diet Management

Adjust sodium and potassium intake according to individual requirements.

Provide a high-protein, moderate-carbohydrate diet with calories for "healthy" weight. Clients who have lost weight should have calories for weight gain. Restrict concentrated sweets.

Increase fluid intake up to 3 L/day, if indicated.

Provide frequent meals and a large meal at bedtime to prevent hypoglycemia.

Client Teaching

Instruct the client

On the principles and rationale of diet management of Addison's disease, and how to make the appropriate diet changes.

On the signs and symptoms of hypoglycemia. Advise the client to eat frequent meals and to carry food at all times (*e.g.*, cheese and crackers).

Monitor

Monitor for the following signs or symptoms:

Compliance with the diet, and the need for follow-up diet counseling

Effectiveness of the diet, and the need for further diet changes

Weight, weight status

Fluid and electrolyte status; observe for signs of fluid and potassium retention

DRUG ALERT Glucocorticoids (*i.e.*, cortisone, prednisone, dexamethasone) are used to treat Addison's disease and numerous inflammatory, allergic, and immunoreactive disorders. Prolonged or excessive use can cause the following changes in metabolism.

	Dietary Intervention
Increased protein catabolism Negative nitrogen balance, muscle wasting, thinning of the skin, poor wound healing, stunted growth in children	Increase protein intake to at least 1 g/kg/day Provide sufficient calories for protein-sparing, especially carbohydrates
Increased gluconeogenesis Persistent hyperglycemia $\rightarrow$ diabetes mellitus	Avoid concentrated sweets Follow diabetic diet if necessary (see Chap. 17)
Increased fat deposition "Moon face," "buffalo hump," truncal obesity with thin limbs	Not amenable to dietary intervention, unless total calorie intake can be restricted
Potassium depletion Hypokalemia, arrhythmias, muscular weakness	Increase potassium intake (Appendix 9)
Sodium and fluid retention Edema, hypertension, complications of hypertension	Restrict sodium intake (see Chap. 16)
Vitamin C depletion from the adrenal glands	Increase vitamin C intake Provide vitamin C supplements
Increased HCl secretion GI upset, ulcers	Eat small frequent meals. Avoid gastric acid stimulants (see Chap. 15)

BIBLIOGRAPHY

1. American Diabetes Association: Clinical practice recommendations of the American Diabetes Association, 1989–1990. Diabetes Care 13:(Suppl 1) 18, 1990
2. American Diabetes Association: Nutritional recommendations and principles for individuals with diabetes mellitus: 1986. Diabetes Care 10:126, 1987
3. American Diabetes Association, American Dietetic Association: Exchange Lists for Meal Planning. Alexandria, VA: American Diabetes Association; Chicago: American Dietetic Association, 1986
4. American Dietetic Association: Manual of Clinical Dietetics. Developed by The Chicago Dietetic Association and The South Suburban Dietetic Association. 1988
5. Beebe CA, Pastors JG, Powers MA, et al: Nutrition management for individuals with noninsulin-dependent diabetes mellitus in the 1990s: A review by the Diabetes Care and Education Dietetic Practice Group. J Am Diet Assoc 91:196, 1991
6. Bertorelli AM, Czarnowski-Hill JV: Review of present and future use of nonnutritive sweeteners. The Diabetes Educator 16:415, 1990
7. Coulston AM: Dietary management of patients with non-insulin-dependent diabetes mellitus: A different perspective. Nutrition Counselor 6(3):4, 1990
8. Crapo P, Vinik AI: Nutrition controversies in diabetes management. J Am Diet Assoc 87:25, 1987
9. Escott-Stump S: Nutrition and Diagnosis-Related Care, 2nd ed. Philadelphia: Lea and Febiger, 1988
10. Franz MJ, Harold H, Powers MA, et al: Exchange lists: Revised 1986. J Am Diet Assoc 87:28, 1987
11. Hagan J, Wylie-Rosett J: Lipids: Impact on dietary prescription in diabetes. J Am Diet Assoc 89:1104, 1989
12. Hauenstein DJ, Schiller MR, Hurley RS: Motivational techniques of dietitians counseling individuals with type II diabetes. J Am Diet Assoc 87:37, 1987
13. Jenkins DJA, Wolever TMS, Jenkins AL: Starchy foods and glycemia index. Diabetes Care 11:198, 1988
14. Krall LP, Beaser RS: Joslin Diabetes Manual, 12th ed. Philadelphia: Lea and Febiger, 1989
15. Leveille GA: The glycemic index: Potential for clinical application in non-insulin-dependent diabetes mellitus. Nutrition Counselor 6(3):3, 1990
16. Marynuik M: Nutrition education: Taking it one step at a time. Diabetes Educator 16:26, 1990
17. O'Dea K, Traianedes K, Ireland P, et al: The effects of diet differing in fat, carbohydrate, and fiber on carbohydrate and lipid metabolism in type II diabetes. J Am Diet Assoc 89:1076, 1989
18. Porth CM: Pathophysiology: Concepts of Altered Health States, 3rd ed. Philadelphia: JB Lippincott, 1990
19. Scherer JC: Introductory Medical–Surgical Nursing, 5th ed. Philadelphia, JB Lippincott, 1991
20. Wheeler ML, Belahanty L, Wylie-Rosett: Diet and exercise in noninsulin-dependent diabetes mellitus: Implications for dietitians from the NIH Consensus Development Conference. J Am Diet Assoc 87:480, 1987

18 Renal and Urinary Disorders

The kidneys are two bean-shaped organs embedded in fatty tissue and located at the back of the abdominal cavity, one on each side of the spinal column. Each kidney consists of more than a million functional units, called nephrons. Nephrons consist of a glomerulus (tufts of capillaries where blood is filtered) attached to a tubule (where reabsorption and secretion occur). About 1.2 liters, or one-fourth of the total cardiac output, is filtered through the kidneys each minute. The kidneys and other organs of the urinary system are depicted in Figure 18-1.

The kidneys perform numerous vital endocrine and exocrine functions. One of their principal functions is to maintain normal blood volume and composition by reabsorbing needed nutrients and excreting wastes through the urine. Urinary excretion is the primary method by which the body rids itself not only of excess water, electrolytes, sulfates, organic acids, toxic substances, and drugs, but also the nitrogenous wastes from exogenous and endogenous protein metabolism such as ammonia, urea, uric acid, and creatinine. Other kidney functions include the regulation of acid–base balance, achieved by secreting hydrogen ions to increase pH or excreting bicarbonate to lower pH. The kidneys also synthesize renin, an enzyme important for blood pressure regulation, and erythropoietin, a hormone that stimulates the bone marrow to produce red blood cells. Vitamin D is converted to its active form (1,25 dihydroxycholecalciferol) in the kidneys; therefore, the kidneys have an important role in maintaining normal calcium and phosphorus metabolism.

Renal damage, and subsequent loss of renal function, profoundly affects metabolism, nutritional requirements, and nutritional status. For instance, nitrogenous wastes, fluid, electrolytes, and other compounds in the blood may accumulate to toxic levels as urine output decreases. Uremia ("urine in the blood") is a toxic systemic syndrome caused by the retention of nitrogenous waste products in the blood (see box, Signs and Symptoms of Uremia). In general, the degree of uremia is related largely to dietary protein intake. Although protein restriction is indicated to reduce uremic symptoms, exactly when protein restriction should be initiated and how severe it should be are controversial.

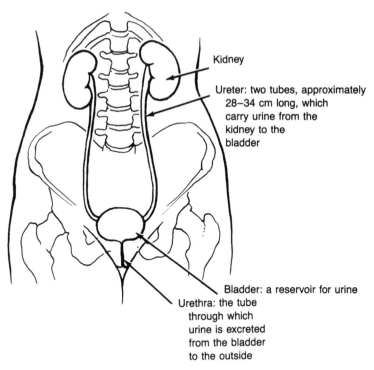

Kidney

Ureter: two tubes, approximately 28–34 cm long, which carry urine from the kidney to the bladder

Bladder: a reservoir for urine

Urethra: the tube through which urine is excreted from the bladder to the outside

Figure 18-1
Organs of the urinary system.

Certainly, protein restriction is contraindicated for clients with protein malnutrition, which often develops with progressive renal failure. Conversely, renal damage can impair the kidney's ability to reabsorb needed nutrients, which are then "wasted" in the urine. Kidney failure also impairs gastrointestinal (GI) absorption of certain minerals, like calcium and iron. Impaired synthesis of renin, erythropoietin, and vitamin D can lead to high blood pressure, anemia, and bone demineralization, respectively. Certain peptide hormones, like insulin, parathyroid hormone, and glucagon are not adequately inactivated and contribute to altered metabolism. Poor intake related to complex, unpalatable dietary restrictions, anorexia, alterations in taste, nausea, vomiting, stomatitis, depression, and anxiety is common. In addition, nutrients may be lost secondary to drug therapy, dialysis, or renal transplantation. For assessment guidelines, see the box, General Renal and Urinary Assessment Criteria.

The objectives of diet intervention for renal diseases are to (1) lessen renal workload to forestall or prevent further kidney damage, (2) restore or maintain optimal nutritional status, and (3) avoid the symptoms or complications of uremia. The optimal interventions needed to meet these objectives vary among individuals and the nature, severity, and stage of the disease. Generally, diet modifications are made in response to symptoms and laboratory values, and therefore require frequent monitoring and adjustments. Nutrients that may be increased *or* decreased for clients with renal disease include protein, fluid, sodium, and potassium. Calorie requirements generally increase to spare protein, and supplemental calcium may be needed because of impaired vitamin D metabolism. Phosphorus intake may need to be restricted, depending on urine output. Multivitamin and

Signs and Symptoms of Uremia

Gastrointestinal

Anorexia

Nausea

Stomatitis

GI ulcerations and bleeding

Metallic taste

Vomiting

Protein-calorie malnutrition

Weight loss

Cardiovascular

Congestive heart failure

Hypertension

Retinopathy

Neurologic

Anxiety

Coma

Convulsions

Decreased mental alertness

Drowsiness

Fatigue

Hallucinations

Headaches

Muscle twitching

Peripheral neuropathy

Personality changes

Metabolic

Hyperglycemia

Hypermagnesemia

Hypertriglyceridemia

Hyperuricemia

Hypo/hypercalcemia

Hypo/hyperkalemia

Hypo/hypernatremia

Hypo/hyperphosphatemia

Hypothermia

Metabolic acidosis

Volume deficit/overload

Respiratory

Pleuritis

Pulmonary edema

Reproductive

Amenorrhea

Impotence

Infertility

Loss of libido

Dermatologic

Decrease perspiration

Dry itchy skin

Skin discoloration

Pallor

(continued)

Signs and Symptoms of Uremia (*continued*)

Hematologic

Anemia (normocytic and normochromic)
Bleeding tendencies
Decreased resistance to infection
Fatigue

Musculoskeletal

Calcium deposits in soft tissues
Fractures related to bone demineralization
Muscular irritability and cramping

Endocrine

Hypothyroidism   Renal osteodystrophy
Impaired growth and development   Secondary hyperparathyroidism

mineral supplements may be indicated. In the acute care setting, clients with renal disease may receive a low-sodium diet, a low-protein diet, or a combination diet that restricts protein, sodium, potassium, and phosphorus.

Chronic renal failure (CRF), acute renal failure (ARF), and urolithiasis are discussed in detail. The principles and rationale of diet management for CRF can be applied to other renal diseases that impair renal function. General diet management recommendations for other selected kidney disorders are outlined in Table 18-1. However, they are only guidelines—actual nutrient requirements are determined by the client's nutritional status, degree of renal functioning, laboratory values, and clinical presentation. Close monitoring and frequent diet adjustments may be necessary, depending on the client's progress and tolerance.

DISORDERS OF THE KIDNEYS AND URINARY TRACT

Chronic Renal Failure

Chronic renal failure is characterized by the progressive loss of renal function related to irreversible nephron deterioration. The clinical course of renal failure can be divided into three phases. *Decreased renal function* is an asymptomatic period in which homeostasis is maintained despite nephron damage and a 50% reduction in the glomerular filtration rate (GFR). *Renal insufficiency* occurs when the GFR decreases by 70% to 75%, serum creatinine and blood urea nitrogen (BUN) levels rise, the urine becomes more dilute, and mild anemia develops. However, the client is asymptomatic because the remaining neph-

Assessment Criteria

General Renal and Urinary Assessment Criteria

Urine output: volume, abnormal characteristics, pain on voiding

Altered blood pressure; presence of edema

Bone pain; loss of height

Presence or history of UTI

Treatment measures: hemodialysis, peritoneal dialysis, renal transplant

Signs and symptoms of uremia

BUN, serum creatinine, serum sodium, serum potassium, Ca^{++}:P ratios, serum triglycerides, cholesterol

rons become hypertrophic to maintain homeostasis. *Renal failure* occurs as serum creatinine and BUN levels steadily increase; overt symptoms develop after 80% to 85% of renal function is lost.

Chronic renal failure may result from chronic glomerulonephritis, polycystic disease, chronic pyelonephritis, or urinary tract obstruction and infection. It may also develop

Protein Content of High- and Low-Biologic-Value Proteins

HBV proteins: complete proteins (generally animal sources) that contain sufficient amounts of all the essential amino acids.

Item	Serving Size	Approximate Protein Content (g)
Egg	1	7
Milk and yogurt	½ cup	4
Meat, fish, poultry, cheese	1 oz	7
Tuna, cottage cheese	¼ cup	7

LBV protein: incomplete proteins (generally plant sources) that lack sufficient amounts of all the essential amino acids.

Bread, regular	1 slice	3
Bread, low protein	1 slice	0.3
Cereals, pasta, rice	½ cup	3
Vegetables*	½ cup	<1–4 g
Fruits*	½ cup	0.5–1 g

*Groups may be divided into three or more subgroups (*i.e.*, vegetable group I, vegetable group II, and so forth) according to the potassium content.

Table 18-1

General Diet Recommendations for Selected Renal Disorders

Disorder	Symptoms/Complications	Diet Management
Acute glomerulonephritis: inflammation of the glomeruli. Most often caused by an allergic or autoimmune reaction to a streptococcal infection of the throat; may also result from impetigo and scarlet fever.	Oliguria Edema, hypertension Nitrogenous waste retention May progress to chronic glomerulonephritis, uremia, and death	Decrease protein to 0.2–0.5 g/kg for clients with uremia. For oliguria, restrict fluid to 500–700 ml, restrict potassium as needed. For edema or high blood pressure, limit sodium to 500–1000 mg. Increase calories to promote protein sparing. Provide supplements as ordered.
Nephritis: kidney inflammation that may be acute or chronic.	Edema, hypertension Uremia; net protein catabolism	Limit sodium to 1–2 g/day. Restrict protein; increase nonprotein calories. Determine fluid allowance: urine output + 500 ml.
Nephrotic syndrome: increased capillary permeability in the glomeruli leads to leakage of serum proteins into the urine, causing proteinuria, hypoalbuminemia, and massive edema. Hypercholesterolemia may develop for some unknown reason.	Proteinuria Edema Hypercholesterolemia, elevated triglycerides	Increase protein to 1.5 g/kg to replace losses; emphasize HBV protein. Increase calories to 40–60 cal/kg to spare protein. Limit sodium to 2–4 g or less; fluid restriction is not necessary unless renal failure develops. Provide adequate potassium, as tolerated, and according to diuretic use. Limit dietary cholesterol and sugar.
Chronic pyelonephritis: bacterial invasion of the kidneys leads to fibrosis, scarring, and dilatation of the tubules, and impaired renal function.	Hypertension; possible sodium depletion if sodium is not adequately reabsorbed Possible hyperkalemia Possible loss of renal function	Adjust sodium intake according to symptoms. Limit potassium. Limit protein, accordingly. Encourage appropriate fluid intake.

secondary to poor circulation related to atherosclerosis or heart failure, or secondary to drugs, nephrotoxic agents, infection, dehydration, diabetic nephropathy, hypertension, lupus erythematosus, and arthritis.

Complications of CRF include anemia, renal osteodystrophy, severe resistant hypertension, edema, congestive heart failure, infection, paresthesia, and alterations in neuromuscular activity. Chronic renal failure results in death unless treated with dialysis or renal transplantation; the underlying cause must also be treated.

Nursing Process

Assessment

In addition to the general renal and urinary assessment criteria, assess for the following factors:

Symptoms of uremia (see box, Signs and Symptoms of Uremia), which develop in response to increasing BUN levels, and vary with the client's individual tolerance. Generally, all symptoms increase in intensity as uremia progresses.

The impact of symptoms on intake or nutritional status: onset, frequency, severity, interventions attempted and the results

Dietary changes made in response to CRF or its symptoms (*i.e.*, foods avoided, foods preferred). Determine foods best and least tolerated.

Usual quantity and quality of protein consumed—whether most of the protein is of high biologic value (generally animal sources) or low biologic value (plant sources)

Adequacy of calorie intake; calorie intake becomes increasingly important when protein is restricted to spare body and dietary protein.

The use of salt and intake of high-sodium foods: cold cuts, bacon, frankfurters, smoked meats, sausage, canned meats, chipped or corned beef, buttermilk, cheese, crackers, canned soups and vegetables, convenience products, pickles, condiments. Determine whether a salt substitute is used, and if so, determine its chemical composition.

Weight, weight status. Be aware that fluid retention masks true weight.

Intake and output; observe for signs of fluid and electrolyte imbalance.

Nursing Diagnosis

Fluid Volume Excess, related to decreased urine output secondary to CRF.

Planning and Implementation

Renal failure produces profound alterations in metabolism, nutrient requirements, and nutritional status. Diet management is a critical component of treatment (see box, Daily Diet Recommendations for Chronic Renal Failure), and daily adjustments in the diet may be necessary to prevent malnutrition and uremic symptoms.

Protein

Although low-protein diets traditionally have been prescribed at the point when dialysis was needed, recent studies have shown that early initiation of a low-protein, low-phosphorus diet, used alone or in combination with ketoacids, slows or stops renal function deterioration.[14] The diet may be more effective when initiated early; dialysis may be postponed, and the symptoms of uremia prevented.

A narrow margin of error exists with regard to the protein intake of clients with renal failure. Too much protein will increase BUN levels and the symptoms of uremia; too little protein will result in protein catabolism (which will increase serum potassium and BUN levels) and a negative nitrogen balance. Protein restriction is rarely necessary until GFR falls below 15 to 20 ml/minute, thereafter, protein allowance decreases accordingly. At GFR rates less than 4 to 5 ml/minute, severe low-protein diets may not effectively control uremic symptoms and are monotonous, unpalatable, and may cause malnutrition and wasting.

Daily Diet Recommendations for Chronic Renal Failure

	Predialysis		Hemodialysis	Continuous Cyclic Peritoneal Dialysis
Protein	GFR ml/min 15–20 10–15 4–10 Not less than 35–40 g/day	g/kg <1.0 0.7 0.55–0.6	1.0–1.2 g/kg	1.2–1.5 g/kg
Calories	35 cal/kg for normal weight; 20–30 cal/kg for obesity; 45 cal/kg for underweight		Same as predialysis	Same as predialysis
Sodium	2.0–3.0 g/day; increase for sodium-wasting nephropathies		2.0–3.0 g/day	Individualized according to blood pressure and weight
Potassium	Restricted only when urine output <1000 ml and serum potassium is elevated		2.0–3.0 g/day; must be individualized	Restricted only if serum potassium is elevated
Phosphorus	600–800 mg/day		800–1200, mg/day	1200–1600 mg/day
Fluid	Balance intake with output		1000 ml + urine output per day	As tolerated

Source: The American Dietetic Association: Manual of Clinical Dietetics. Developed by The Chicago Dietetic Association and The South Suburban Dietetic Association. 1988

However, supplementing very-low-protein diets (30 g or less) with commercial essential amino acid supplements or their keto analogues may promote neutral or positive nitrogen balance, reduce uremic symptoms, and even prevent further kidney damage (see Appendix 7 for specially defined supplements for renal failure).[4]

Whenever the quantity of protein is restricted, the quality becomes more important. Most of the protein consumed should come from animal sources (high biologic value), which provide adequate amounts of all the essential amino acids and are used more efficiently than plant sources (low biologic value). The protein content of high- and low-biologic-value proteins is listed in the box, Protein Content of High- and Low-Biologic-Value Proteins.

Once dialysis is initiated, protein requirements are increased above normal to compensate for the loss of serum proteins and amino acids lost in the dialysate. At least half of the protein consumed should be of high biologic value.

Calories

It is extremely important to provide adequate nonprotein calories to prevent body protein catabolism and to prevent the use of dietary protein for energy. Pure sugars and pure fats are recommended for calories, even though they are not considered "nutritious"

Sources of Protein-Free Calories and Seasonings

Protein-Free Calories

Beverages*
  Alcoholic
  Carbonated
  Fruit drinks and punches
  Kool-Aid
  Lemonade, limeade
Candies
  Butterballs
  Butterscotch drops
  Candy corn, fondant
  Cotton candy
  Hard candy
  Gum
  Gumdrops
  Jelly beans
  LifeSavers
  Lollipops
  Marshmallows
  Mints
Desserts
  Fruit ice*
  Popsicle*
Fats
  Butter and margarine (unsalted)
  Lard
  Mayonnaise, oils
  Shortening

Flour Products
  Arrowroot
  Cornstarch
  Rice starch
  Tapioca, granulated
  Wheat starch
Sweeteners
  Corn syrup
  Honey
  Jams
  Jellies
  Maple syrup
  Marmalade
  Sugar: confectioners', white

Protein-Free Seasonings

Flavoring extracts
Herbs
Spices
Vinegar

*As allowed by fluid restriction.

foods (see box, Sources of Protein-free Calories and Seasonings). Unfortunately, the use of sweets is contraindicated in diabetics, and approximately 50% of CRF clients exhibit glucose intolerance. Also, a low carbohydrate intake may be indicated for 40% to 60% of the clients with chronic renal failure who develop type IV hyperlipidemia (elevated triglycerides and very-low-density lipoproteins).

Sodium and Fluid

Even though clients with renal failure have a decreased ability to reabsorb sodium, they can usually maintain sodium balance on a moderate sodium intake. However, in end-stage renal disease (GFR less then 4–10 ml/minute), the kidneys are unable to excrete normal amounts of sodium and the use of diuretics and restricted sodium and fluid intakes may be necessary. See Chapter 16 for foods high in sodium and sodium restricted diets.

Sources of Fluid

Liquids

Alcoholic beverages
Carbonated beverages
Cereal beverages
Coffee
Cream
Fruit juices, drinks, and punches
Juice and syrup from canned fruit and vegetables
Liquid medications
Milk
Soup, bouillon, consommé, broth
Tea
Vegetable juices
Water

Foods That Liquefy at Room Temperature

Ice (melts to 9/10 initial volume)
Ice cream (melts to ½ initial volume)
Ice milk (melts to ½ initial volume)
Gelatin
Popsicles
Sherbet

Some clients with advanced renal failure are unable to conserve sodium, and a sodium deficit may occur if sodium intake is restricted. If the client does not have edema, hypertension, or signs of heart failure, increasing sodium intake as tolerated may slightly improve GFR.

If blood pressure and serum sodium levels are normal and edema is not present, fluid intake can exceed 24-hour urine output by 500 ml (the amount of fluid lost through skin, lungs, and perspiration; see box, Sources of Fluid). Sodium and fluid restrictions are more severe in oliguric or anuric clients on dialysis.

Potassium

Most clients with renal failure can tolerate a normal potassium intake if urine output is greater than 1 liter. However, an excessive potassium intake, the use of potassium-containing medications, acidosis, oliguria, and catabolic stress can lead to fatal hyperkalemia. Conversely, clients on potassium-wasting diuretics, or those experiencing severe potassium losses from GI fistulas or gastric suctioning, may need more potassium to avoid hypokalemia.

Other Considerations

Exchange lists may be used to eliminate the need for daily diet calculations. Allowed foods are grouped into exchange lists based on their protein, sodium, and potassium content; fluid and phosphorus content also may be considered. Portion sizes are specified so that each serving contains approximately the same amount of protein, sodium, and potassium. Items within an exchange list may be substituted for each other; substitutions from one list to another are not allowed. An individualized meal pattern specifies the number of servings allowed from each exchange list; allowances are based on laboratory data and clinical symptoms and should correspond as closely as possible with the individual's food preferences and habits (see box, Sample Renal Failure Menu). The composition, complexity, and number of exchange lists used in the treatment of renal failure varies considerably among institutions.

Clients with uremia may experience a deterioration of their appetite as the day progresses. Encourage a good breakfast. Uremia may also cause alterations in taste, so that clients may prefer highly seasoned or strongly flavored foods.

Children with renal failure experience growth failure, which may be permanent if not corrected before puberty. An optimal diet may prevent depletion of body protein and fat stores in clients of any age.

Enteral nutritional support may be indicated if the client has a functional GI tract but is unable to consume an adequate oral diet; total parental nutrition is used if the GI tract is nonfunctional. The requirements of clients receiving parenteral nutrition are controversial, especially for amino acids; therefore, total parenteral nutrition solutions should be individualized for each client. High-glucose solutions (hyperosmolar) with lipid emulsions are used to deliver the maximum amount of calories without increasing the volume.

Vitamin D deficiency is caused by the inability of the kidneys to convert the vitamin to its active form. Consequently, the metabolism of calcium, phosphorus, and magnesium is altered and may result in bone demineralization, bone pain, and possible calcification of the soft tissues. Renal osteodystrophy may be prevented by the following measures:

- Limiting phosphorus intake. Low-protein diets are usually low in phosphorus and may control hyperphosphatemia effectively. Otherwise, phosphate binders that decrease GI absorption (*i.e.*, aluminum hydroxide gels) are preferred over a low-phosphorus diet (see Drug Alert).
- Providing vitamin D supplements
- Providing calcium supplements. Unfortunately, high-calcium diets are contraindicated because they rely heavily on dairy products, which are also high in phosphorus.

Iron deficiency anemia is common in clients with renal failure and may be related to decreased iron absorption, frequent blood tests, GI bleeding, blood loss during dialysis, and poor iron intake. Intramuscular or intravenous iron may be given to clients who cannot tolerate oral supplements.

Clients undergoing dialysis may develop a deficiency of zinc, which could contribute to anorexia and taste alterations. Therapeutic doses of zinc may be added to the dialysate. It is recommended that all other trace elements be routinely removed from the dialysate to prevent toxicities. Dialysate contaminated with aluminum has been associated with progressive mental disorders and osteomalacia.

Clients with renal failure have an increased risk of hypermagnesemia and should avoid magnesium-containing over-the-counter drugs such as antacids, laxatives, and enemas.

Water-soluble vitamin deficiencies are common in clients with renal failure and may be caused by an inadequate intake related to anorexia or dietary restrictions, altered

Sample Renal Failure Menu*: Controlled Sodium, Controlled Potassium, 40 g Protein

Breakfast

½ cup grape juice
¾ cup puffed wheat with ½ cup whole milk
1 fried egg
2 slices low-protein bread toasted
2 tsp margarine
2 tablespoons jelly
½ cup coffee

Lunch

Sandwich made with
  1 oz turkey
  2 slices low-protein bread
  2 teaspoons mayonnaise
  Lettuce
½ cup fried fresh cauliflower
1 canned pear half in heavy syrup
1 plain doughnut
½ cup ginger ale

Dinner

1 oz roast beef
½ cup unsalted noodles with 2 teaspoons butter and parsley
½ cup green beans
½ cup beets
2 slices low-protein bread with 2 teaspoons butter
½ cup fruit cocktail
½ cup cola

Snacks

Protein-free calories (see box, Daily Diet Recommendations for Chronic Renal Failure)

*Contains approximately 600 ml of fluid; sodium intake can be decreased by using low-sodium breads and vegetables; calories can be increased with liberal use of nonprotein fats and sweets.

metabolism related to uremia or medications, and increased losses related to dialysis. Although exact requirements are unknown, supplements of the water-soluble vitamins are recommended for both nondialyzed and dialyzed clients.

After a successful renal transplant, the only diet modifications that may be necessary are those to alleviate the side effects of steroids, which are taken to prevent rejection of the new kidney (see Chap. 17, Corticosteroid Drug Alert). However, temporary or permanent rejection of the transplanted kidney may result in uremia and may require the resumption of chronic renal failure dietary restrictions.

Client Goals

The client will:
Attain and maintain adequate nutritional status.
Avoid symptoms and complications of uremia.
Restore and maintain fluid and electrolyte balance.
Retard progression of renal failure and postpone the initiation of dialysis.
Minimize tissue catabolism by consuming adequate nonprotein calories.
Describe the rationale and principles of diet management of CRF and implement the appropriate dietary changes

Nursing Interventions

Diet Management

Adjust and modify protein intake to promote nitrogen balance while maintaining BUN levels below 60 to 90 mg/dl (uremic symptoms usually do not appear until BUN levels exceed 90 mg/dl).[11] Recommended protein intake appears in the box, Daily Diet Recommendations for Chronic Renal Failure. Approximately two thirds of total protein should be from high-biologic-value sources.

Provide adequate nonprotein calories. Although exact requirements are not known, a high intake of nonprotein calories is needed when protein intake is restricted to prevent the use of dietary protein for energy, prevent tissue catabolism, and maintain or restore ideal weight. Obese clients may require fewer calories (see box, Sources of Protein-free Calories and Seasonings).

Limit sodium intake to 2.0 to 3.0 mg/day if signs of sodium retention are present: sudden weight gain, edema, hypertension, and symptoms of heart failure. Liberalize sodium intake if the client has signs of sodium depletion: unexplained weight loss, low blood pressure, and a further reduction in GFR.

Restrict fluid to urine output + 500 ml for insensible losses.

Moderately restrict potassium intake to prevent hyperkalemia to 1.5 to 2.8 g/day. Actual requirements are based on urine and serum levels of potassium. Foods high in potassium are listed in Appendix 9.

Restrict phosphorus intake, if indicated.

Client Teaching

Because diet prescriptions for clients with renal disease are very complex, difficult to fulfill, often unpalatable, and continually changing, thorough diet teaching and periodic evaluations of the client's (and the family's) knowledge and understanding are necessary.
Instruct the client and family

To view the diet as an integral component of treatment and a means of life support. To increase the chance of compliance, clients should be urged to assume more responsibility for the management of their medical problems.[8]

That strict adherence to the diet can improve the quality of life and decrease the workload on the kidneys.

That accurate daily weights are necessary to assess fluid balance and diet adequacy. Instruct the client to weigh himself or herself at approximately the same time every day, with the same scale, and the same amount of clothing. Unexpected weight gain or loss should be reported to the physician.

That a lag time of about 12 hours may exist between when food is eaten and the resultant change in blood chemistries. "Cheating" on the diet is not advised, but if the client chooses to do so, it should be at least 12 hours before dialysis.

That renal diet cookbooks are available to increase variety in the diet.

That the vitamin and mineral supplements prescribed by the physician are needed to meet nutritional requirements.

That although eating out is possible, ordering from a restaurant menu requires special attention and planning to comply with the diet restrictions.

On the importance of a consistent, controlled protein intake:
- Too little or too much protein in the diet can cause BUN levels to increase and uremic symptoms to return, therefore, portion sizes initially should be weighed or measured and thereafter be periodically spot-checked for accuracy.
- To spread the protein allowance over the whole day instead of saving it all for one meal.
- Low-protein breads, cereals, cookies, gelatin, and pastas are available to help boost calorie intake without sacrificing protein restriction, although their taste and texture differ from the products they are intended to replace and they are more costly. Because acceptability varies greatly among low-protein products, clients should be encouraged to try a variety.

On the importance of an adequate calorie intake:
- Too few calories can have the same effect as eating too much protein.
- Nonprotein calories, like butter, oils, and allowed sweets, should be used freely.

On the importance of a fluid restriction, if appropriate:
- Sources of fluid include liquids and foods that liquefy at room temperature.
- An easy way to measure fluid intake is to place a pitcher of water containing a total daily fluid allowance in the refrigerator. As fluids are consumed, the equivalent amount of water should be discarded from the pitcher.
- To relieve thirst try:
  - Hard candies
  - Very cold water instead of tap water
  - Popsicles and ices, as allowed by fluid allowance
  - Petroleum jelly applied to the lips, frequent mouth rinsing, and good oral hygiene

On a sodium-restricted diet, if appropriate (see Chap. 16).

On the importance of a potassium restriction, if appropriate.
- Sources of potassium are listed in Appendix 9.
- To reduce the potassium content of vegetables and potatoes, cut them in small pieces, soak them overnight, and boil them in fresh water.

Monitor

Monitor for the following signs or symptoms:

Compliance with the diet, the need for follow-up diet counseling. It is estimated that only 25% of hemodialysis clients have a good dietary compliance rating.[8]

Effectiveness of diet management, and evaluate the need for further diet modifications.

Weight, weight changes

Intake and output; observe for signs of fluid and electrolyte imbalances and nutritional excesses/deficiencies.

Laboratory values, when available, especially of BUN, serum proteins (*i.e.*, albumin, transferrin), triglycerides, and electrolytes

Evaluation

Evaluation is ongoing. Assuming the plan of care has not changed, the client will achieve the goals as stated above.

DRUG ALERT: **ALUMINUM HYDROXIDE GEL**

Use

Phosphate binder. Should be taken with meals. May be incorporated into cookies or fudge to increase its palatability and client acceptance.

Possible Adverse Side Effects

bloating, constipation, fecal impaction, nausea, vomiting, anorexia, stomach cramps, hypophosphatemia, vitamin A malabsorption, inactivation of thiamine. Prolonged use (>90 days) may lead to osteomalacia, especially when combined with a low-phosphorus diet.

Actions

Monitor serum phosphate levels; increase fiber intake if constipation develops.

Acute Renal Failure

Acute renal failure is characterized by a decrease in renal blood flow or glomerular or tubular damage leading to sudden loss of renal function and oliguria or anuria.

Its clinical course begins with an oliguric phase, characterized by a low urine output of less than 400 to 600 ml/24 hours, which may deteriorate to anuria. Sometimes large amounts of urine are excreted despite the loss of renal function and nitrogenous waste retention (this is called *high-output renal failure*). The oliguric phase may last 10 to 20 days or longer.

The diuretic phase occurs when the kidneys are unable to conserve water. Urine volume may double daily until a fixed amount is reached; losses of fluid, sodium, and potassium are extensive. The diuretic phase usually lasts 14 to 21 days.

The recovery phase is characterized by a gradual improvement in kidney function over a 3- to 12-month period.

Acute renal failure may have *prerenal* causes, such as decreased renal blood flow related to shock, trauma, hemorrhage, surgery, burns, hypotension, severe dehydration, or heart failure. Nephron damage related to nephrotoxins, autoimmune diseases, infections, or acute glomerulonephritis can cause *intrarenal* failure. *Postrenal* etiologies include obstructed urine outflow from the kidney related to benign prostatic hypertrophy, bladder or prostate cancer, calculi, trauma, or medications.

Complications of ARF include infection, hyperkalemia resulting in cardiac arrest, metabolic acidosis, hypercatabolism, circulatory overload (dyspnea, orthopnea, pulmonary congestion, pulmonary edema), hypertension, hypertensive crisis, convulsions, neurologic abnormalities, and permanent loss of some renal function (reduction in glomerular filtration rate, decreased ability to concentrate urine, decreased ability to acidify urine). Acute renal failure may progress to CRF; average prognosis for recovery is slightly greater than 50%.

The primary focus of treatment is to correct the underlying disorder. Dialysis (peritoneal or hemodialysis) may be used during the oliguric phase if the client has azotemia, fluid overload, resistant hyperkalemia, severe acidosis, nephrotoxins, or symptoms of uremia. Diuretics and other measures to restore fluid and electrolyte balance are used. Diet management may help to lessen the workload of the kidneys and restore optimal nutritional status.

Nursing Process

Assessment

In addition to the general renal and urinary assessment criteria, assess for the following factors:

Symptoms of uremia: onset, causative factors, severity

Dietary changes made in response to ARF, if appropriate

Intake and output; observe for signs of fluid and electrolyte imbalances.

Weight, and weight changes. Be aware that sudden weight gain or loss indicates sodium retention and depletion, respectively.

Nursing Diagnosis

Fluid Volume Excess, related to decreased urine output secondary to ARF.

Planning and Implementation

The optimal diet for clients with acute renal failure is more elusive even than the optimal diet for chronic renal failure. Although a high-protein diet is contraindicated because of nitrogenous waste retention, hypercatabolism and infection or sepsis imposed by a major underlying illness increase the need for protein. Exact nutritional requirements are not known, although it is evident that needs vary among individuals and the phases of acute renal failure. Once dialysis is instituted, diet restrictions are liberalized.

Little agreement exists concerning how much protein should be allowed once oral feedings are resumed. Protein may be restricted to 0.2 to 0.5 g/kg or 30 to 40 g/day, of mostly high biologic value, to lessen the workload of the kidneys. As GFR returns to normal or dialysis is instituted, protein allowance is increased to promote nitrogen balance and tissue healing.

For both the oliguric and diuretic phases of acute renal failure, fluid intake should equal total fluid output (volume of urine plus losses through diarrhea and vomiting plus insensible losses through the skin, lungs, and perspiration, which may be increased due to fever and infection). Generally, fluid allowance during the oliguric phase equals 24-hour urine output plus 400 to 500 ml of water or more, depending on the client's hydration status. Up to 3 liters of fluid may be needed daily after diuresis begins.

Life-threatening hyperkalemia seen during the oliguric phase of acute renal failure is related to potassium retention and tissue catabolism, which causes potassium to leave the cells and enter the serum. Diets low in potassium (2 g or less) and exchange resins may be used during the oliguric phase to reduce serum potassium levels (see Drug Alert). Intravenous dextrose and insulin may be given as a temporary measure to lower serum potassium (insulin causes dextrose and potassium to leave the serum and enter the cells). Once diuresis begins, large amounts of potassium are excreted and potassium supplements may be necessary to avoid hypokalemia.

Client Goals

The client will:
Attain/maintain fluid, electrolyte, and mineral balances.
Avoid progression of renal failure.
Avoid symptoms/complications of uremia.
Lessen renal workload.
Control body catabolism and weight loss.

Nursing Interventions

Diet Management

Adjust protein intake according to renal function. Initially, parenteral solutions of amino acids and glucose may be given if the client is unable to eat, although some studies suggest that regular total parenteral nutrition solutions and aggressive dialysis are more effective against uremia and acidosis. Protein allowance may begin at 0.8 g/kg and increase as renal function improves. At least two thirds of the total protein should come from high-biologic-value sources.

Increase calorie intake to approximately 50 cal/kg to promote nitrogen balance and replenish losses. Carbohydrate modules, pure fats, refined sugars, and low-protein starches should be used liberally.

Adjust fluid intake to avoid overhydration and dehydration. Allow urine output + 500 ml/day.

Adjust sodium intake according to urine output, serum sodium level, symptoms of sodium imbalance, and concurrent use of dialysis. Sodium intake may be restricted to 500 to 1000 mg/day during the oliguric phase; sodium requirements increase during the diuretic phase to replace extensive losses.

Adjust potassium intake according to urine output, serum potassium level, and concurrent use of dialysis. Restrict potassium during the anuric phase; liberalize during the diuretic phase.

Provide small, frequent meals and assistance with eating, as needed, for clients receiving an oral diet who are weak or fatigued.

Client Teaching

Instruct the client and family
On the principles and rationale of diet management for ARF.
On the importance of dietary monitoring and restrictions so that the family does not provide the client with inappropriate food and beverages.

Monitor

Monitor for the following signs or symptoms:
Compliance with the diet, and the need for follow-up diet counseling
Effectiveness of the diet and evaluate the need for further diet modifications
Weight, intake, and output, and observe for changes over 24- to 48-hour periods

Evaluation

Evaluation is ongoing. Assuming the plan of care has not changed, the client will achieve the goals as stated above.

DRUG ALERT: **SODIUM POLYSTYRENE SULFONATE**

Use

Oral or rectal ion exchange resin used to lower serum potassium levels by increasing fecal excretion. Powdered form may be mixed with food, but should not be heated. Suspended form contains sorbitol, which acts as a laxative to facilitate GI excretion, prevent constipation, and improve palatability.

Possible Adverse Side Effects

GI irritation, anorexia, nausea, vomiting, constipation, fecal impaction, or diarrhea; possible hypokalemia, sodium retention, hypocalcemia; may cause metabolic acidosis in clients with renal disease if given orally with cation-donating antacids and laxatives such as magnesium hydroxide or calcium carbonate.

Actions

Administer cautiously to clients requiring a low-sodium diet; monitor serum electrolyte levels. Observe for signs of hypokalemia and sodium retention; increase fiber intake if constipation develops.

Urolithiasis

The precipitation of insoluble crystals in the urine leads to the formation of stones (calculi) that vary in size from sandlike "gravel" to large, branching stones. Although they form most often in the kidney, they can occur anywhere in the urinary system. Generally, stones less than 1 cm in diameter are spontaneously voided; larger stones may require removal. Renal stones can lead to infections and obstruction that result in renal damage, which may require a nephrectomy.

Renal calculi occur more frequently in men than women, develop most often between the ages of 30 to 50 years, and tend to recur. The cause of urolithiasis may be idiopathic or related to certain infections, urinary stasis, metabolic abnormalities, hormone imbalances, and concentrated urine related to inadequate fluid intake. The precipitation of stones also depends on urinary pH. Other causes, specific for the stone's composition, are listed in Table 18-2.

The signs and symptoms of renal stones are dependent on the site of the stones and the presence of obstruction, infection, and edema. Nausea, vomiting, diarrhea, and abdominal pain may be present. Bladder stones may produce symptoms of urinary tract infection, such as chills, fever, dysuria. Renal pelvic stones may cause renal colic: severe flank pain that radiates down the urinary tract, accompanied by sweating, pallor, nausea, vomiting, and possible abdominal pain and diarrhea. Large amounts of urine containing blood and pus are voided. An attack may last minutes to several hours. Finally, stones in the ureter may cause ureteral colic: severe, colicky pain that comes in waves and radiates down the thigh and to the genitalia. Although the urge to urinate is frequent, only small amounts of urine, often containing blood, are voided.

The treatment of renal stones involves pain and infection control, drug therapy to alter the absorption or excretion of stone components, and diet intervention to dilute the urine and help prevent future stone formation. Surgical intervention may be necessary if the stone causes progressive renal damage or obstruction, pain, or infection that does not respond medically. Some stones may be dissolved by irrigation through ureteral catheters or percutaneous nephrostomy tubes.

Nursing Process

Assessment

In addition to the general urinary and renal assessment criteria, assess for the following factors:

Symptoms and their impact on nutritional status and intake (*i.e.*, nausea, vomiting, diarrhea, abdominal pain); assess onset, frequency, severity, interventions attempted and the results.

Dietary changes made in response to renal stones or symptoms (*i.e.*, foods avoided, food preferred). Determine foods best and least tolerated.

Usual intake of offender (*i.e.*, calcium for calcium calculi).

Adequacy of fluid intake, especially immediately before bedtime.

Table 18-2
*Possible Causes of Renal Calculi,
Based on Composition*

Composition	Possible Cause
CALCIUM CALCULI	Hypercalcuria may be related to hyperparathyroidism, immobility, excessive use of alkali antacids, renal disease, or excessive intakes of protein, calcium, or vitamin D. Some clients with calcium stones have idiopathic hypercalcuria related to excess GI calcium absorption or altered renal reabsorption of calcium. Calcium oxalate may occur secondary to malabsorption syndrome→GI absorption of dietary oxalate (which normally is excreted in the feces)→hyperoxaluria→ risk of calcium oxalate stone formation. Also, regular megadoses of vitamin C (>4 g/day) increase urinary excretion of oxalate and the risk of stone formation.
MAGNESIUM AMMONIUM PHOSPHATE CALCULI (struvite stones)	Sometimes called "infection stones" because they normally accompany urinary tract infections; bacteria that contain urease (an enzyme that converts urea to ammonia) increase the urinary pH, which favors the precipitation of magnesium ammonium phosphate calculi.
CYSTINE CALCULI	Caused by a rare genetic disorder of cystine (an amino acid) metabolism.
URIC ACID CALCULI	Idiopathic causes are characterized by hyperuricosuria and normal serum uric acid levels. May also occur as a side effect of antigout drugs that increase uric acid excretion (*i.e.,* probenecid). An acidic urine favors the precipitation of uric acid stones.

Nursing Diagnosis

Altered Health Maintenance, related to the lack of knowledge of dietary management of renal calculi.

Planning and Implementation

The most effective diet intervention used in the treatment and prevention of renal calculi is to increase fluids to dilute the urine. A high urine output not only helps the client to pass an existing stone, but it also decreases the likelihood of another stone precipitating out of the urine.

Sometimes acid or basic ash diets are used in conjunction with drugs to alter urine pH (see box, Acid-Forming, Base-Forming, and Neutral Foods). Acid-forming foods (acid ash

Acid-Forming, Base-Forming, and Neutral Foods

Acid-Forming Foods

Meat, fish, poultry, shellfish, cheese, eggs
Grains: bread, cereals, crackers, rice, pasta
Corn and lentils
Cranberries, prunes, plums, and their juices

Base-Forming Foods

All types of milk and milk products
All vegetables (except corn and lentils)
All fruits (except cranberries, prunes, and plums)

Neutral Foods

Butter, margarine, oil, lard
White sugar, honey, syrup
Cornstarch, arrowroot, tapioca
Coffee, tea, Postum

diet) may help lower urine pH and protect against calcium phosphate and magnesium ammonium phosphate stones, which form only in alkaline urine. For instance, cranberry juice is often emphasized as part of an acid ash diet, even though the volume and concentration of juice needed may be too great to be of practical use.[6] A diet rich in base-forming foods (basic ash diet) may help increase urine pH and prevent uric acid and cystine stones, which form only in acidic urine. Drug therapy, however, has largely replaced diet therapy as an easier and more effective and consistent means of altering urine pH.

Also under debate is whether excluding dietary components of the stone is preventative against future stone formation. Often, stones are composed of more than one dietary substance, or from substances produced by the body regardless of dietary intake. In those instances, a restrictive diet may be of little value. However, if dietary excesses do contribute to stone formation, a restricted diet may be helpful.

Client Goals

The client will:
Consume increased fluids to dilute the urine.
Avoid a recurrence.
Describe the principles and rationale of diet management of renal calculi, and make the appropriate dietary changes.
Identify causative factors, if known.

Nursing Interventions

Diet Management

For all types of renal stones
* Increase fluid intake to 3 to 4 liters/day.

Calcium phosphate stones
* Avoid foods high in calcium (see Appendix 13), vitamin D-fortified foods, and vitamin D supplements.
* Avoid excessive protein intake, which increases calcium excretion.
* Increase intake of acid-forming foods.

Calcium oxalate stones
* Avoid foods high in oxalate (Table 18-3; a low-oxalate diet may not be effective if endogenous oxalate production is high).
* Avoid vitamin C supplements, which increase oxalate excretion.

Magnesium ammonium phosphate stones
* Increase intake of acid-forming foods.

Cystine stones
* Increase intake of base-forming foods.
* Diets low in methionine (an amino acid precursor of cystine) or protein (all protein sources contain cystine) have been used in the past, but they are difficult to follow, unpalatable, and may not be effective.

Table 18-3
Foods to Avoid on a Low-Oxalate Diet (Contain >15 mg Oxalate/Serving)

BEVERAGES	VEGETABLES
Draft beer	Baked beans canned in tomato sauce
Cocoa	Beets
Ovaltine and other	Celery
beverage mixes	Chard, Swiss
Tea	Eggplant
	Escarole
FRUITS	Greens: beet, collard, dandelion
Blackberries	Leeks
Blueberries	Okra
Currants, red	Parsley
Green gooseberries	Peppers, green
Grapes, Concord	Pokeweed
Lemon peel	Potatoes, sweet
Lime peel	Rutabagas
Raspberries, black	Spinach
Rhubarb	Summer squash
GRAINS	**OTHER**
Grits (white corn)	Chocolate
Soybean crackers	Nuts: peanuts, pecans
Wheat germ	Peanut butter

(Ney DM, Hofmann AF, Fischer C, Stubblefield N: The Low Oxalate Diet Book for the Prevention of Oxalate Kidney Stones. San Diego: University of California, 1981)

Food for Thought

Protein—Too Much of a Good Thing?

Americans hold protein in high regard, believing it has mystical powers essential for well-being. In fact, some nutrition advocates have promoted the idea that it is impossible to eat too much protein, and the myth that eating protein builds muscles has been around for a long time. Food manufacturers have capitalized on our protein obsession by offering "high-protein" varieties of foods that normally are not known for their protein content, such as cereal, infant cereal, pasta, and flour. It's no wonder that the average American consumes double the RDA for protein.

However, interest in avoiding excess fat and cholesterol, as well as ecologic and economic concerns, have led an increasing number of people to question the necessity and advantage of overdoing protein. Many sources of animal protein also are rich sources of saturated fat and cholesterol, excesses of which increase the risk of heart disease. Some studies suggest that high protein intake also may increase the risk of osteoporosis because protein causes an increase in urinary calcium excretion. And still other studies on animals indicate that high-protein diets may damage the kidney over time, whereas low-protein diets may prevent the mild loss of kidney function that typically occurs with aging. Health concerns aside, animal protein generally is economically and ecologically costly.

Because of the potential dangers from consuming excess protein, Americans would be wise to stick close to the RDA for protein and forget the idea that "more is better."

Uric acid stones
- Increase intake of base-forming foods.
- Low-purine diets (uric acid precursor) may be used, although they are difficult to achieve and are not as effective as drug therapy.

Client Teaching

Instruct the client

On the principles and rationale of diet management of renal calculi, and how to implement the appropriate diet changes.

On the importance of drinking fluid. Clients should be encouraged to drink 8 oz/hour during waking hours. Encourage fluid intake before bed and during the night to maintain a large, dilute urine output.

Monitor

Monitor for the following signs or symptoms:

Compliance with the diet, and the need for follow-up diet counseling

Effectiveness of the diet, and evaluate the need for further diet modifications

Evaluation

Evaluation is ongoing. Assuming the plan of care has not changed, the client will achieve the goals as stated above.

Urinary Tract Infections

The only diet recommendation for urinary tract infections is to increase fluid intake to flush out bacteria. However, an acid ash diet may also be recommended if antibiotics used to treat the infection function better in an acid medium.

BIBLIOGRAPHY

1. Ahmed FE: Effect of diet on progression of chronic renal disease. J Am Diet Assoc 91:1266, 1991
2. American Dietetic Association: Manual of Clinical Dietetics. Developed by The Chicago Dietetic Association and the South Suburban Dietetic Association, 1988
3. Blume E: Overdosing on protein. Nutrition Action Health Letter 14(2):1, 1987
4. DiChiro J: Can nutritional therapy alter the course of renal disease? Dietetic Currents 18(2):1, 1991
5. Edwards MS, Doster S: Renal transplant diet recommendations: Results of a survey of renal dietitians in the United States. J Am Diet Assoc 90:843, 1990
6. Escott-Stump S: Nutrition and Diagnosis-Related Care, 2nd ed. Philadelphia: Lea and Febiger, 1988
7. Goodship THJ, Mitch WE: Nutritional approaches to preserving renal function. Adv Intern Med 33:337, 1988
8. Hoover H: Compliance in hemodialysis patients: A review of the literature. J Am Diet Assoc 89:957, 1989
9. Ihle BU, Becker GJ, Whitworth JA, et al: The effect of protein restriction on the progression of renal insufficiency. N Engl J Med 321:1773, 1989
10. Kopple JD: The role of nutrition in preventing renal failure. Nephrol News Iss 2:6:37, 1988
11. Ney DM, Hofman AF, Fischer C, et al: The Low Oxalate Diet Book for the Prevention of Oxalate Kidney Stones. San Diego: University of California, 1981
12. Porth CM: Pathophysiology: Concepts of Altered Health States, 3rd ed. Philadelphia: JB Lippincott, 1990
13. Scherer J: Introductory Medical–Surgical Nursing, 5th ed. Philadelphia: JB Lippincott, 1991
14. Van Duyn MAS: Acceptability of selected low-protein products for use in a potential diet therapy for chronic renal failure. J Am Diet Assoc 87:909, 1987

19 Musculoskeletal Disorders

SYSTEM COMPONENTS AND FUNCTIONS

Bones support and shape the body, protect vital organs and other soft tissues, store minerals, play a role in red blood cell production, and act as levers to make movement possible. Collagen (connective tissue protein) serves as the bone matrix, which is strengthened and hardened by deposits of mineral salts. Calcium phosphate and calcium carbonate, which together are called *hydroxyapatite*, are the most abundant mineral salts.

Bone formation and maintenance depends on an adequate supply of nutrients and is regulated by hormones (see box, Role of Nutrients and Hormones in Bone Formation and Maintenance). Bone remodeling occurs continuously as new bone is formed and existing bone is resorbed. Before age 30 to 35 years, when peak bone mass is attained, bone formation exceeds bone resorption. Thereafter, bone resorption exceeds bone formation and all people lose bone with age.

The contact point between two or more bones is called a joint (or articulation). Joints usually are formed of fibrous connective tissue and cartilage and are classified as immovable, slightly movable, or freely movable.

ROLE OF DIET THERAPY

Joint disorders often affect nutritional status by interfering with intake, and some disorders may be relieved by diet therapy (weight reduction for osteoarthritis). Diet intervention initiated early in life may help protect against osteoporosis, a prevalent bone disorder

Role of Nutrients and Hormones in Bone Formation and Maintenance

Nutrients

Calcium and phosphorus are components of hydroxyapatite, the organic salt providing strength and rigidity to bones and teeth.

Fluoride, magnesium, sodium, and chloride are components of bone in small amounts.

Vitamin A is necessary for bone growth and development because of its role in bone cell differentiation and protein synthesis.

Vitamin C and protein are necessary for the production and integrity of collagen, the protein matrix of bones.

Hormones

Parathyroid hormone (PTH) prevents serum calcium levels from falling by:
- Stimulating the release of calcium from the bone (resorption)
- Increasing intestinal absorption of calcium
- Enhancing calcium retention by the kidneys
- Reducing serum phosphorus levels

Excessive PTH secretion → bone demineralization

Calcitonin lowers serum calcium levels by:
- Stimulating bone deposition of calcium
- Inhibiting bone resorption of calcium
- Reducing tubular reabsorption of calcium and phosphorus

Vitamin D functions as a hormone to increase the amount of calcium and phosphorus available to mineralize the surface of the bone by:
- Stimulating intestinal calcium absorption
- Increasing resorption of calcium and phosphate from bone

Sex hormones aid in the growth of new bone.

among postmenopausal women; once osteoporosis develops, diet therapy is used routinely in its treatment. Other conditions, such as bone fractures and prolonged immobility, require diet modification because of increased nutritional requirements and altered body metabolism.

Guidelines for musculoskeletal assessment are listed in the box, General Musculoskeletal Assessment Criteria.

JOINT DISORDERS

Rheumatoid Arthritis

Rheumatoid arthritis is a chronic, debilitating, inflammatory disease characterized by progressive joint deformity and destruction, and systemic manifestations such as anemia, Sjögren's syndrome, and bone disease.[12] The cause of rheumatoid arthritis is not known,

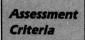

General Musculoskeletal Assessment Criteria

Weight status, weight loss

Loss of height

Pain or edema in muscles, joints, bone

Decreased range of motion; decreased mobility; unsteady gait

Weakness in the extremities

Contractures

Anorexia

Easy fatigue

Insomnia

however, it may be caused by an immunologic response centered in the synovial joints. The onset is insidious and most often occurs between the ages of 25 to 35 years. Women are affected three times more frequently than men. It is estimated that the incidence rate in women over 60 years old may be as high as 15%.

Complications of rheumatoid arthritis include severe weight loss, fever, anemia, muscle atrophy, osteoporosis, dry eyes, dry mouth, and liver or spleen enlargement. In addition, degenerative changes leading to ischemia and thrombosis may occur in the lungs, heart, muscles, blood vessels, pleura, and tendons, and vasculitis may develop in the eyes, nervous system, and skin.

Drug therapy to control the inflammatory process is the cornerstone of treatment. There are several primary drug classifications used to treat rheumatoid arthritis; actual drug choice depends on the client's tolerance, response, and compliance (see Drug Alert). Rest and exercise and application of heat and cold may help relieve pain. Diet intervention may be needed to improve overall nutritional status or to counter the side effects of drug therapy.

Nursing Process

Assessment

In addition to the general musculoskeletal assessment criteria, assess for the following factors:

Affected joints that may appear painful, stiff, swollen, red, warm, and tender; observe for impaired range of motion and strength, and assess the impact on the client's ability to procure, prepare, and eat meals.

Symptoms of fatigue, weakness, anorexia, and low-grade fever; assess onset, frequency, severity, interventions attempted and the results.

Dietary changes made in response to arthritis or its symptoms (*i.e.*, foods avoided, foods preferred). Determine foods best and least tolerated.

The use of unorthodox or unproven dietary remedies to treat arthritis, and the potential impact on nutritional status

Medications used, and their side effects
Weight, weight changes

Nursing Diagnosis

Altered Nutrition: Less than Body Requirements, related to inability to prepare meals adequately secondary to pain and limited motion in the fingers and hands.

Planning and Implementation

There is no specific diet for clients with rheumatoid arthritis; diet management is determined by the symptoms and complications of the disease and side effects of drug therapy.[12] For instance, clients with rheumatoid arthritis often are poorly nourished. The process of inflammation can increase nutritional requirements by increasing metabolic rate, and also may cause malabsorption of nutrients by altering the gastrointestinal mucosa. Intake may be impaired because of gastrointestinal upset and peptic ulcers, which may develop as a result of arthritis or secondary to drug therapy. Pain and medications contribute to anorexia. Dry mouth, a complication of rheumatoid arthritis, may cause difficulty in swallowing and increase the risk of dental decay. Bone and joint deformities and loss of function often hinder physical preparation of meals.

It is estimated that arthritis sufferers spend $8 to $10 billion each year in search of relief.[15] The chronic, debilitating nature of rheumatoid arthritis makes its victims vulnerable to claims of nutritional cures and fad diets. Low-carbohydrate diets, high-protein diets, vegetarian diets, no-dairy-products diets, supplemental B vitamins, vitamin C, vitamin A, and sulfur all have been used unsuccessfully in the treatment of arthritis. Cod-liver oil, alfalfa, apple cider vinegar, pokeberries, and blackstrap molasses all have been touted as "cures" for arthritis. Unfortunately, diet management can restore nutritional status and help alleviate arthritis symptoms, but cannot cure or prevent arthritis.

Clients with Sjögren's syndrome may have chewing and swallowing difficulties and are at increased risk for dental decay. Moist, texture-modified foods and cold liquids may facilitate swallowing; concentrated sweets should be avoided. Unsweetened lemon may be used to help stimulate saliva, and good oral hygiene is encouraged.

Although a multivitamin and mineral supplement may be indicated to help restore optimal nutritional status, clients should be advised not to self-prescribe megadoses of vitamins to "cure" arthritis.

Hypochromic anemia may be an inherent characteristic of arthritis and may not respond to iron supplementation.

Be aware of the potential side effects of drug therapy and the appropriate dietary interventions to relieve those side effects.

Client Goals

The client will:

Experience fewer symptoms of arthritis and its complications, and fewer side effects of arthritis medication, as appropriate.

Consume adequate calories and protein to attain/maintain "healthy" weight and restore/maintain optimal nutritional status.

Describe the principles and rationale of diet management to relieve the symptoms of arthritis and the side effects of medications.

Nursing Interventions

Diet Management

Provide adequate calories and protein to attain/maintain "healthy" weight. Calorie requirements increase in response to inflammation when the disease is active and decline when the disease is in remission; adjust calories accordingly.

Increase protein during active disease to 1.5 to 2.0 g/kg to reverse negative nitrogen balance and restore nutritional status.

Modify the diet as needed to alleviate anorexia, peptic ulcer, and difficulty in swallowing (see Chap. 15) (*i.e.*, eliminate food intolerances if gastric irritation exists, provide soft/thick puréed foods as needed, if the client has dysphagia).

Client Teaching

Instruct the client

On the principles and rationale of diet management to relieve symptoms of arthritis and the side effects of medications, as indicated, and how to implement the appropriate dietary changes.

That there is no dietary cure for arthritis. Advise the client to avoid unproven diets and supplements, which may not only be costly but also may be potentially dangerous.

On joint-saving ideas for food preparation (see box, Joint-Saving Ideas for Food Preparation).

Monitor

Monitor for the following signs or symptoms:

Tolerance to oral feedings (*e.g.*, ability to swallow for clients with Sjögren's syndrome)

Compliance with the diet, and the need for follow-up diet counseling

Effectiveness of diet (*i.e.*, attains "healthy" weight, avoids side effects of medications), and the need for further diet modifications

Evaluation

Evaluation is ongoing. Assuming the plan of care has not changed, the client will achieve the goals as stated above.

DRUG ALERT Aspirin is the treatment of choice for rheumatoid arthritis. Nonsteroidal anti-inflammatory drugs, steroidal anti-inflammatories, and gold compounds have a higher incidence of adverse side effects and are used only after aspirin therapy fails (See box, Rheumatoid Arthritis: Drug Alert).

Degenerative Joint Disease (Osteoarthritis)

Osteoarthritis is a chronic, progressive, noninflammatory joint disorder characterized by destruction of joint cartilage, spur and bone cyst formation, pain, and impaired joint movement. It most commonly affects weight-bearing joints (knees, hips, ankles, and spine) and fingers.

Joint-Saving Ideas for Food Preparation

Kitchen Organization Ideas

Keep utensils that are used most often within easy reach and place duplicates at strategic locations around the kitchen.

Wear an apron with several pockets to keep small utensils handy.

Hang pots and pans on a wall rack to avoid bending and stretching.

Use lazy Susans and pull-out shelves.

Use drawer dividers to create vertical filing so that items can be located easily without moving others.

Training or financial assistance for kitchen remodeling and equipment may be available from the local Division of Vocational Rehabilitation.

Meal Preparation Ideas

Take advantage of "good" days by making double or triple portions and freezing the extras.

Use one-dish meals and convenience foods whenever possible.

Invest in labor-saving appliances such as a food processor, blender, mixer, electric knife, and electric can opener.

Prepare meals while sitting on a moveable swivel stool and use a wheeled cart to move heavy items.

Use lightweight cooking utensils and bowls, such as aluminum and plastic.

Use nonstick cookware and soak dishes and pans immediately after use to reduce clean-up.

Whenever possible, use paper plates, napkins, and tablecloths.

Don't overdo it, and ask for help from family and friends.

Assistance may be available from community resources, such as Meals on Wheels and volunteer shoppers.

Joint Protection Ideas

Tie a looped rope around cabinet, drawer, refrigerator, and oven handles and open by slipping the forearm through the loop and pulling.

Use a rubber gripper to open lids by twisting with the palm or heel of the hand placed flat on the top of the lid.

Build up utensil handles with foam rubber to make them easier to hold.

Open pull-top cans with a knife or screwdriver inserted through the metal ring.

Lay boxes flat on their side and open by cutting with a knife.

(continued)

Joint-Saving Ideas for Food Preparation (*continued*)

Anchor bowls with a rubber mat in the corner of the sink to make stirring easier.

Beat eggs with a whisk instead of a fork or spoon, because whisks offer less resistance.

Tongs release food more easily than a fork.

Use cookware with two handles.

Boil foods in a wire mesh basket inserted in a pot; when the food is done, simply remove the basket rather than lifting the whole pot.

Use an oven shovel or wooden rack jack to reduce bending while retrieving hot items from the oven.

Use a toaster oven or stove-top oven if using the oven is difficult.

For clean-up, use sponge mitts instead of a hand-held sponge.

Select joint protection gadgets, such as open-handled knives and jar openers, suited to meet your needs.

Numerous eating aids, such as utensils with built-up plastic handles, scooper bowls with nonskid bases, plate guards, swivel spoons, and large-handled mugs are available to simplify eating.

(Arthritis Health Professions Section of the Arthritis Foundation: Self-Help Manual for Patients with Arthritis. Atlanta: Arthritis Foundation, 1980)

Osteoarthritis, which affects more than 16 million people, is the most common form of arthritis. As much as 80% of the population over 55 years old may be affected, and it is equally prevalent in men and women. Approximately twice as many obese people have osteoarthritis as do people of normal weight;[10] however, it is not known whether obesity is an etiologic factor or whether it occurs secondary to reduced activity related to osteoarthritis.

Osteoarthritis is believed to result from prolonged mechanical stress, although it probably does not have a single cause. Predisposing factors include aging, congenital abnormalities, trauma, obesity, and systemic diseases.

Drug therapy to control pain and discomfort and physical therapy are used to treat osteoarthritis. Surgical intervention may be used if medical treatment fails to control pain or if joint destruction is severe. Diet intervention is used to promote weight loss in obese clients, thereby reducing strain on weight-bearing joints.

Nursing Process

Assessment

In addition to the general musculoskeletal assessment criteria, assess for the following factors:

Rheumatoid Arthritis: Drug Alert

Drug	Side Effects	Diet Interventions
Salicylates		
Aspirin	High doses or chronic use can cause gastric pain and bleeding, peptic ulcer, heartburn, nausea, vomiting, increased excretion of vitamin C, potassium depletion, iron deficiency anemia, delayed blood clotting	GI problems may be avoided by taking aspirin with food, milk, or a full glass of water, or by using enteric coated types. Buffered compounds containing sodium may be contraindicated for clients on sodium restricted diets. Encourage the intake of foods high in vitamin C and provide supplements if needed.
Nonsteroidal Anti-inflammatories		
Indomethacin Phenylbutazone Ibuprofen Fenoprofen Sulindac Naproxen Tolmetin	Dyspepsia, dizziness, nausea, GI bleeding, epigastric pain, heartburn, diarrhea, stomatitis, duodenal ulcer, constipation, anemia	Administer with food, milk, or a full glass of water.
Steroid Anti-inflammatories: May be taken orally or as local injections		
Prednisone	Sodium retention; edema Increased potassium excretion Protein catabolism, delayed wound healing, muscle wasting; negative nitrogen balance Impaired glucose tolerance GI upset, duodenal ulcer Increased need for vitamin B_6, vitamin C, folic acid, and vitamin D Decreased calcium and phosphorus absorption, decreased bone formation, osteoporosis	Possible modifications: Decrease sodium Increase potassium Increase protein Diabetic diet Small, frequent meals Provide multivitamin and mineral supplements.
Gold Compounds		
Aurothioglucose	Can produce significant dermatologic, mucous membrane, and renal side effects. Signs of gold toxicity include mouth sores, pruritus, GI upset, dermatitis, rash, bleeding gums, petechiae, fever, chills, weakness, sore throat, dysphagia, proteinuria	Modify the diet as needed to alleviate dysphagia and other GI side effects (see Chap. 15).

Limitation of motion, contractures, and muscle spasms, and determine the impact on procuring, preparing, and eating meals

Dietary changes made in response to arthritis or its symptoms (*i.e.*, foods avoided, foods preferred). Determine foods best and least tolerated.

The use of unorthodox or unproven dietary remedies to treat arthritis, and the potential impact on nutritional status

Medications and their side effects

Weight, weight status

Nursing Diagnosis

Altered Health Maintenance, related to lack of knowledge of diet intervention for osteoarthritis.

Planning and Implementation

Clients with osteoarthritis are often obese, which contributes to strain on the weight-bearing joints. For some unexplained reason, weight reduction has been shown to eliminate symptoms of osteoarthritis throughout the body, not just in the weight-bearing joints. However, weight loss may be hindered because of impaired physical mobility and exercise-related pain. Provide emotional support and periodic diet follow-up.

Arthritis affecting finger joints may impair ability to prepare meals.

With the exception of oral steroidal anti-inflammatories, osteoarthritis may be treated with the same drugs as rheumatoid arthritis (see rheumatoid arthritis Drug Alert). Local injections of corticosteroids may be given.

Client Goals

The client will:

Lose weight, if overweight, to lessen the strain on weight-bearing joints.

Consume a well-balanced, nutritionally adequate diet.

Describe the principles and rationale of diet intervention of osteoarthritis, and implement the appropriate dietary changes.

Modify the diet, as needed, to minimize the side effects of drug therapy.

Nursing Interventions

Diet Management

Decrease calories to attain and maintain ideal weight (see Appendix 10).

Modify the diet, as needed, to minimize the side effects of drug therapy.

Client Teaching

Instruct the client

On the principles and rationale of diet management of osteoarthritis, and how to implement the appropriate dietary changes.

To avoid unorthodox dietary "cures" for arthritis, which are unfounded and may be potentially dangerous.

On joint-saving ideas for food preparation (see box, Joint-Saving Ideas for Food Preparation).

Monitor

Monitor for the following signs or symptoms:
Compliance with the diet, and the need for follow-up diet counseling
Effectiveness of the diet (*i.e.*, weight loss, avoids side effects of medication), and the need for additional diet modification

Evaluation

Evaluation is ongoing. Assuming the plan of care has not changed, the client will achieve the goals as stated above.

Gout

Gout is characterized by the overproduction or underexcretion of uric acid (or a combination of both), leading to hyperuricemia, precipitation of uric acid crystals in joints and connective tissue, and inflammation. Tophi, which are relatively painless deposits of urate crystals on the ears, fingers, hands, forearms, or feet, may form, depending on the duration of the disease, the degree of hyperuricemia, and renal function status.

The sudden onset of severe pain in one or more peripheral joints, most commonly the joints of the large toe, the feet, ankles, knees, wrist, and elbow, signals an acute attack. Usually the affected joints return to normal within 1 week. Recurrent attacks occur at irregular intervals and may be precipitated by fasting, weight loss, low CHO intake, alcohol, stress, and the use of aspirin and thiazide diuretics. Attacks become more frequent and last longer as the disease worsens.

Chronic gout leads to bone and joint erosion, which can result in gross deformities, loss of joint function, chronic pain, and progressive renal dysfunction. Left untreated, gout can lead to chronic renal disease secondary to urate kidney stones.

Primary gout is caused by a genetic defect of purine metabolism or by a renal defect causing a decrease in uric acid excretion; it most commonly affects men in their fifth decade and is associated with obesity. Gout may also occur secondary to other disorders, such as polycythemia or leukemia, and may be precipitated by prolonged use of thiazide diuretics and aspirin, trauma, and treatment of myeloproliferative diseases.

Gout is treated with drug therapy: colchicine, analgesics, anti-inflammatory drugs. Rest and elevation of the affected joint may help relieve pain during an acute attack. A high fluid intake is indicated to help flush the kidneys, and high-purine foods may be eliminated from the diet.

Nursing Process

Assessment

In addition to the general musculoskeletal assessment criteria, assess for the following factors:
Symptoms (possible headache, fever, malaise, and anorexia); onset, frequency, severity, interventions attempted and the results

Dietary changes made in response to gout (*i.e.*, foods avoided, foods preferred). Determine if unorthodox dietary practices are followed. Determine if a relationship exists between an acute attack and diet—whether attack was precipitated by fasting, weight loss, a low-carbohydrate diet, or alcohol.

Nursing Diagnosis

Altered Health Maintenance, related to a lack of knowledge of the dietary management of gout.

Planning and Implementation

Uric acid is the end product of purine metabolism; purines are found in nucleoproteins, which are most abundant in high-protein foods but are present to some degree in all foods. The body also synthesizes purines from dietary CHO, protein, and fat, and from endogenous purine breakdown.

The most effective diet intervention in the treatment of gout is to increase fluid intake to dilute the urine and avoid kidney stone formation.

Weight loss also is effective at reducing serum uric acid levels but must be undertaken gradually to avoid precipitating an acute attack of gouty arthritis. Fasting, low CHO diets, and rapid weight loss should be avoided; all favor the formation of ketones, which inhibit uric acid excretion.

Severe purine-restricted diets have been replaced largely by drug therapy. From a practical standpoint, a low-purine diet is difficult to achieve; some foods are rich in purines and all foods contain nucleoproteins, from which purines are derived. Also, restricting purine intake does not affect endogenous uric acid synthesis and has little impact on serum uric acid levels. Instead of following a rigid low-purine diet, clients may benefit from avoiding foods extremely high in purines.

An acidic urine favors the precipitation of uric acid stones and should be avoided. However, it is not likely that the client will consume enough acid-ash foods (cranberries, cranberry juice, prunes, prune juice, meat, fish, and poultry) to produce a significant decrease in urine pH.

Excessive food intake, especially fat, may precipitate an acute gouty attack and should be avoided.

Generally, high-CHO diets tend to increase uric acid excretion, however, a high fructose intake (fruit sugar) may increase uric acid production and should be avoided.

In the past, clients with gout were instructed to avoid coffee, tea, and cocoa based on the rationale that they contain compounds that are readily converted to uric acid. However, there is no scientific evidence to support the elimination of coffee, tea, and cocoa on a purine-restricted diet.

If chronic renal disease develops, additional diet modifications are necessary (see Chap. 18).

Client Goals

The client will:

Consume appropriate calories and protein to attain/maintain "healthy" weight; if weight reduction is indicated, client will lose weight gradually (*i.e.*, 1 to 2 pounds/week) to avoid precipitating an attack.

Increase fluid intake to at least 2 quarts/day to promote the excretion of uric acid.

Modify the diet, as needed, to minimize the side effects of drug therapy.

Describe the principles and rationale of diet management of gout, and implement the appropriate dietary changes.

Identify factors contributing to an acute attack, when known.

Avoid chronic renal failure as a complication of gout.

Nursing Interventions

Diet Management

Increase fluid intake to at least 2 quarts/day.

Decrease calories for gradual weight loss, if overweight.

Eliminate high-purine foods (more than 150 mg of purine/100 g of food): anchovies, dried legumes, lentils, kidney, liver, brains, mackerel, meat extracts (meat drippings, gravy, broth, consommé), sardines, shrimp, sweetbreads.

Moderate protein intake should not exceed 1 g/kg of ideal body weight/day. Limit meat intake to 3 to 4 oz/meal. Cheese, eggs, milk, and vegetables are low in nucleoproteins and should comprise most of the moderate protein allowance. Fish, meat, meat-based soups, poultry, and shellfish are higher in purines and may be restricted during acute attacks.

Client Teaching

Instruct the client

On the principles and rationale of diet management for gout.

To increase fluid intake to at least 2 quarts/day. Encourage fluid intake before bed and during the night to avoid concentrated urine, which is more conducive to stone formation.

To avoid alcohol, or use moderate amounts infrequently and diluted with other liquids or foods, because excessive alcohol consumption increases uric acid production and reduces uric acid excretion.

Monitor

Monitor for the following signs or symptoms:

Compliance with the diet, and the need for follow-up diet counseling

Effectiveness of diet, and evaluate the need for further dietary changes

Weight, weight status

Evaluation

Evaluation is ongoing. Assuming the plan of care has not changed, the client will achieve the goals as stated above.

DRUG ALERT   Drugs used in the treatment of gout are aimed at reducing serum uric acid levels (uricosuric agents) and providing symptomatic relief of acute attacks of gouty arthritis.

Be aware of the potential side effects associated with anti-inflammatory agents

Gout: Drug Alert

Drug	Side Effects	Diet Interventions
Colchicine decreases uric acid deposition	Nausea, vomiting, diarrhea Abdominal pain Malabsorption of sodium, potassium, fat, carotene, and vitamin B_{12} Decreased lactase activity Loss of appetite	Take with water immediately before, with, or after meals to avoid GI upset. Encourage high fluid intake (greater than 2000 ml/day) to reduce risk of urate kidney stone formation.
Allopurinol: controls hyperuricemia from overproduction of uric acid	Skin rash Vomiting, diarrhea, abdominal pain Enhances iron absorption and hepatic iron stores	Encourage high fluid intake (greater than 2000 ml/day) to reduce the risk of urate kidney stone formation.
Uricosuric Agents Used to Promote Urinary Excretion of Uric Acid		
Probenecid	GI irritation and nausea (initially worsens symptoms of acute gouty arthritis)	Encourage high fluid intake (greater than 2000 ml/day) to reduce the risk of urate kidney stone formation.
Sulfinpyrazone	Nausea, epigastric pain, burning, dyspepsia	Take with water immediately before, during, or after meals to avoid GI upset.

(indomethacin, phenylbutazone) used in the treatment of acute attacks of gouty arthritis (see rheumatoid arthritis Drug Alert).

BONE DISORDERS

Osteoporosis

Osteoporosis is a group of disorders characterized by a decrease in total bone mass without a change in its chemical composition. Loss of bone density increases the risk of bone fractures and spinal compressions. Osteoporosis most commonly affects the spine, hips, and forearms.

Osteoporosis is the most common skeletal disorder in the world, estimated to affect 20 million Americans. The incidence of osteoporosis increases with age; approximately half of all 45-year-old women have some degree of osteoporosis and by age 80 bone mass may be decreased by 30% to 60%.

Although primary osteoporosis is complex and multifactorial, low peak bone mass and estrogen deficiency appear to be the most important risk factors in its development. Other risk factors appear in box, Osteoporosis: Risk Factors and include:

Secondary osteoporosis may result from endocrine, gastrointestinal, and renal diseases, neoplasms of the bone marrow, excessive use of corticosteroids, prolonged immobility, radiation therapy, and long-term use of heparin.

Progressive bone loss occurring over a long time may not be detected until a fracture occurs; vertebral, hip, and wrist fractures are the hallmarks of osteoporosis. Each year, about 1.3 million fractures are related to osteoporosis; medical complications may cause as many as 300,000 deaths annually. Other long-term effects of decreased stature and deformity include decreased thoracic and abdominal volume, chronic back pain, early satiety, and decreased tolerance to exercise related to decreased lung capacity.

The treatment of osteoporosis is neither totally effective nor completely safe. Although long-standing calcium deficiency plays a role in the development of osteoporosis, a high calcium intake alone does not adequately halt or restore bone loss. Estrogen replacement is the most effective method of treating osteoporosis, however, it is correlated with an increased risk for endometrial cancer. Weight-bearing exercise is encouraged. Pain resulting from fractures may be treated with bed rest and analgesics. Because prevention is more important and more effective than treatment, an adequate calcium intake and regular weight-bearing exercises should be stressed early in life.

Nursing Process

Assessment

In addition to the general musculoskeletal assessment criteria, assess for the following factors:

Symptoms that may affect intake (*i.e.*, anorexia related to pain, mild ileus related to T10 and L2 fractures); onset, frequency, causative factors, severity, interventions attempted and the results

Dietary changes made in response to osteoporosis (*i.e.*, foods avoided, foods preferred)

Usual calcium intake. Determine if the client is taking supplemental calcium; if so, find out what type, how much, how often, and whether the client experiences any unpleasant side effects.

Frequency and intensity of weight-bearing exercise

Use of tobacco and alcohol

Nursing Diagnosis

Altered Health Maintenance, related to the lack of knowledge of the dietary management of osteoporosis.

Planning and Implementation

Studies suggest a strong relationship between calcium deficiency and the development of osteoporosis. Although bone mass constantly is being gained and lost, net loss exceeds net gain after peak bone mass is attained sometime between the ages 30 to 35 years. The rate of bone loss appears to be accelerated by a calcium deficiency and retarded by a high calcium intake. The optimal amount of calcium needed to slow/prevent the progression of osteoporosis is not known, although studies suggest that calcium requirements for adults increase with age and are higher than the current RDA.

Food consumption surveys indicate a large percentage of the adult population con-

Osteoporosis: Risk Factors

	Rationale
Female sex	Women have 30% less bone mass than men, which may also be influenced by hereditary factors, inactivity, and low calcium intakes. Osteoporosis is four times more common among women than men, and women tend to develop it earlier and more severely.
Natural or surgically induced menopause	After the onset of menopause, bone loss is rapidly accelerated for 3 to 5 years and continues for 20 years. Estrogen deficiency appears to increase calcium requirement by decreasing its absorption and retention. Studies have shown that fair-skinned women have less estrogen than dark-skinned women, which increases their risk of osteoporosis.
Long-standing calcium deficiency	Studies suggest osteoporotics have lower calcium intakes than nonosteoporotics and that an inadequate calcium intake contributes to bone loss. Also, inadequate calcium intake prior to age 30 to 35 may prevent attainment of peak bone mass.
Inactivity	The rate bone resorption exceeds bone formation when normal weight-bearing and muscle tension is impaired.
Positive family history	Although conclusive evidence is lacking, studies on twins suggest osteoporosis may be related to genetic factors.
Smoking and alcohol abuse	Associated with decreased estrogen levels; excessive alcohol promotes calcium excretion.

sumes considerably less calcium than the RDA of 800 mg. According to the Second National Health and Nutrition Examination Survey (NHANES II), the median daily dietary calcium intake for women in the United States is 574 mg, and 826 mg for men.[13] Between the ages of 18 and 30, more than two thirds of all American women consume less than the RDA for calcium; 75% of American women over age 35 do not meet the RDA for calcium on any given day. At all ages, men consume more calcium than women. Also, calcium intake decreases with age, as does calcium absorption for both normal and osteoporotic people.

Some balance studies indicate that diets high in calcium and phosphorus enhance both calcium and phosphorus balance, thus promoting bone mineralization and maintenance.[13] Lactose and vitamin D also promote calcium absorption. However, other dietary factors, such as high intakes of alcohol, caffeine, and fiber, may contribute to a negative calcium balance. Most researchers agree that protein intakes in excess of the RDA increase urinary excretion of calcium. Studies also suggest that a negative calcium balance occurs when calorie intake is inadequate, despite a high calcium intake.

Current research shows that premenopausal women need approximately 1000 mg of calcium daily to maintain normal calcium balance; clients with osteoporosis and postmenopausal women may need 1500 mg/day. Calcium intakes up to 2500 mg/day do not increase the risk of hypercalcemia, calcium kidney stones, or calcification of soft tissues, and are safe for normal people.

Increasing dietary calcium is safe and effective and is preferred over pharmacologic supplements because it is better absorbed and contains the correct proportion of calcium to protein, phosphorus, and vitamin D. Milk and dairy products are the richest sources of calcium; five cups of milk or its equivalent supplies about 1500 mg of calcium. However, clients with lactose intolerance who must restrict their intake of calcium to low-lactose sources (hard cheese, yogurt, buttermilk, lactose-reduced milk, and possibly small, frequent servings of milk [see Chap. 15]) may not be able to consume adequate calcium through diet alone. And unfortunately, many women voluntarily restrict their intake of dairy products in an attempt to control their weight.

Calcium supplements are indicated for clients who cannot or will not consume adequate calcium. Supplements differ significantly in their calcium content (Table 19-1). and rate of absorption. Calcium carbonate generally is recommended because it is the least expensive and contains the largest percentage of calcium by weight. However, one study found that calcium citrate malate, currently available only in fortified orange juice, prevented loss of spine bone, whereas calcium carbonate, the most common calcium supplement, did not.[2]

The effects of long-term calcium supplementation are not known; some researchers are concerned that calcium supplements increase the risk of calcium oxalate stones. A high

Table 19-1
Calcium Supplements

	% of Calcium	Comments
Calcium carbonate (*e.g.,* Tums)	40	High incidence of constipation; can cause hypercalcemia.
Tricalcium phosphate (*e.g.,* Posture)	39	Occasional GI upset.
Calcium chloride	36	Administer with food to reduce GI irritation.
Bone meal	33	Not recommended because of possible lead and mercury contamination.
Dibasic calcium phosphate (dihydrate dicalcium phosphate)	23	Administer with food to reduce GI irritation.
Dolomite	22	Not recommended because of possible lead and mercury contamination.
Calcium citrate	21	Better absorbed than calcium carbonate in people who lack stomach acid and who are fasting. Not better absorbed than calcium carbonate in most people.
Calcium lactate	13	Lactose may enhance absorption. Administer with food to reduce GI irritation.
Calcium gluconate	9	GI irritation is minimal, but may cause constipation.
Calcium glubionate (*e.g.,* Neo–Calglucon)	6.5	Rare incidence of GI disturbances. Administer before meals to enhance absorption.

(Malseed RT: Pharmacology, Drug Therapy, and Nursing Considerations, 3rd ed. Philadelphia: JB Lippincott, 1990.

fluid intake (*i.e.*, 10 to 20 oz of fluid with each calcium dose) is recommended during the first 3 months of supplementation to dilute urinary calcium.[13] Another concern is that calcium supplements may interfere with the absorption of other minerals, particularly iron. To reduce adverse effect on iron absorption, calcium supplements should not be taken with meals. Supplements may be contraindicated for clients predisposed to urinary calculi. Vitamin D supplements generally are not recommended because of the risk of toxicity.

Fluoride supplements have been used in Europe to treat osteoporosis because fluoride has been shown to prevent bone loss and increase bone formation. Unfortunately, the newly formed bone structure is abnormal, which may be why fluoride therapy has not decreased the incidence of fractures. Fluoride supplements have not been approved for use in the United States; studies have shown that up to 40% of the people treated do not respond and as many as 40% have significant adverse side effects. Nausea, vomiting, peptic ulcers, and rheumatic conditions are the most common reasons for discontinuing therapy. Also, the potential for fluoride toxicity exists.

The prolonged or frequent use of aluminum-containing antacids should be discouraged because they may contribute to bone loss by increasing bone resorption, depleting phosphorus and calcium, and impairing fluoride absorption.

Because bone remodeling is a relatively slow process, it may take 2 to 3 years before any improvement is noted.

Client Goals

The client will:

Consume at least 1000 to 1500 mg of calcium daily, preferably from dairy products and other food sources.

Describe the rationale and principles of diet management of osteoporosis, and implement the appropriate dietary changes.

Identify risk factors, if known (*i.e.*, smoking, sedentary lifestyle, low calcium intake, etc.).

Nursing Interventions

Diet Management

Promote a well-balanced diet containing at least 1000 mg calcium before menopause and 1500 mg calcium after menopause (see Appendix 13 for sources of calcium).

Avoid excessive protein intake, which may increase calcium requirement by reducing calcium retention.

Avoid excessive caffeine and alcohol intake because they promote calcium excretion and can contribute to negative calcium balance.

Client Teaching

Instruct the client

On the principles and rationale of diet management of osteoporosis, and how to implement the appropriate dietary changes.

That calcium supplements may be necessary if fewer than three servings of dairy products are consumed daily. Advise the client to drink at least 10 to 20 oz of water with each supplement, unless the client also is taking thiazide, and to take the supplements between meals. Explain that calcium supplements may not be effective at protecting against calcium loss in all types of bone, and that they are not a panacea against osteoporosis.

To modify the diet, as needed, to minimize the side effects of calcium supplements, if appropriate.

To practice other preventative measures, as appropriate: increase weight-bearing exercise, quit smoking, avoid excessive alcohol intake.

Monitor

Monitor for the following signs or symptoms:

Tolerance to increased intake of dairy products, if appropriate (*i.e.*, absence of gas, distention, cramping, and diarrhea after consuming milk and milk products)

Compliance with the diet, and the need for follow-up diet counseling

Effectiveness of the diet in minimizing side effects of calcium supplements, if appropriate, and evaluate the need for further diet modification

Evaluation

Evaluation is ongoing. Assuming the plan of care has not changed, the client will achieve the goals as stated above.

Prolonged Immobilization

Diet Recommendations	Rationale
Increase protein intake by approximately 15 g/day to 20 g/day	Both prolonged bed rest and stress increase nitrogen excretion and result in a negative nitrogen balance. A high protein intake is needed to prevent skin breakdown, decubitus ulcers, infection, and to restore nitrogen balance.
Adjust calorie intake periodically according to need	In the acute phase following trauma, calorie requirements are high due to the effect of stress hormones and the need for protein-sparing calories. Calorie requirements level off in the chronic phase and should be adjusted to prevent excessive weight gain. Clients with paraplegia, hemiplegia, and paralysis have decreased energy requirements.
Maintain normal calcium intake, despite increased bone resorption, hypercalcemia, and hypercalcuria	Decreased activity→ increased calcium resorption and bone loss (osteopenia)→ elevated levels of serum and urinary calcium. Calcium kidney stones and calcification of the kidney and other soft tissues may also occur. Altered calcium metabolism is not nutritionally related and cannot be prevented or treated by diet intervention.
Calcium requirements may increase after mobility is resumed	Normal calcium metabolism is restored only after remobilization, and bone losses are replenished only if sufficient calcium is available.
Increase fluid intake	High fluid intake is necessary to dilute urine and prevent the formation of calcium kidney stones.

<table>
<tr><td>

Food For Thought

</td><td>

Can Rheumatoid Arthritis Sufferers Benefit From Fish-Oil Supplements?

</td></tr>
</table>

A double-blind, placebo-controlled, crossover study was conducted to study the effects of fish-oil supplements on rheumatoid arthritis sufferers.[6] Participants received either 15 MAX-EPA supplements or a placebo over 14-week treatment periods, followed by 4-week washout periods; their usual drug therapy and diet remained unchanged. Results showed that participants experienced less fatigue and fewer tender joints while using fish-oil supplements compared to the placebo. In addition, the effect from the fish oil persisted beyond the 4-week washout period. Until further research proves or disproves the benefit of fish oils on rheumatoid arthritis symptoms, sufferers may be wise to hedge their bets and eat more fish—eating more fish is virtually risk-free and may confer numerous health benefits.

DRUG ALERT Although estrogen therapy has been shown to reduce bone loss, especially during the 5 to 10 years after menopause, its use is still controversial, since estrogen therapy increases the risk of endometrial cancer. Common side effects include nausea, fluid retention, and breast fullness or tenderness.

It is estimated that an increased intake of 500 mg of calcium/day will produce the same effect on calcium balance as moderate doses of estrogen, without the associated risks.

Prolonged Immobilization

Prolonged immobilization resulting from bone fractures and other types of trauma can lead to numerous nutritional problems. The objectives of diet therapy are to promote healing and avoid complications related to altered body metabolism.

Nursing Considerations

During the acute phase following trauma, clients often are anorexic and may benefit from small, frequent meals.

Thirst may not be a valid indicator of fluid need in clients who are immobilized; monitor intake and output. If bladder training is indicated, give fluids at regular, specified intervals.

Cranberry juice often is recommended to help acidify the urine and prevent the formation of calcium kidney stones. However, large volumes of concentrated juice (80% cranberry juice) may be needed to produce a significant change in urine pH, making it therapeutically impractical.

Decreased physical activity may lead to constipation. Encourage the intake of high-fiber foods (see Chap. 15) and fluids.

Observe for signs and symptoms of hypercalcemia, which may develop insidiously or rapidly: anorexia, nausea, vomiting, abdominal cramps, constipation, headache, malaise, lethargy, and possible polydipsia and polyuria. Untreated hypercalcemia can result in renal insufficiency, hypertension, seizures, and hearing loss.

BIBLIOGRAPHY

1. American Dietetic Association: Manual of Clinical Dietetics. Developed by The Chicago Dietetic Association and The South Suburban Dietetic Association, 1988
2. American Dietetic Association: Extra calcium slows bone loss in women getting less than half the RDA. J Am Diet Assoc 90:1692, 1990
3. Dawson-Hughes B, Dallal GE, Krall EA, et al: A controlled trial of the effect of calcium supplementation on bone density in postmenopausal women. N Engl J Med 323:878, 1990
4. Escott-Stump S: Nutrition and Diagnosis-Related Care, 2nd ed. Philadelphia: Lea and Febiger, 1988
5. Howat PM, Carbo ML, Mills, GQ, et al: The influence of diet, body fat, menstrual cycling, and activity upon the bone density of females. J Am Diet Assoc 89:1305, 1989
6. Kremer JM, Jubik W, Michalek A, et al: Fish-oil fatty acid supplementation in active rheumatoid arthritis: A double-blinded, placebo-controlled, crossover study. Ann Intern Med 106:497, 1987
7. Liebman B: Brittle bones. Nutrition Action Health Letter 12(3):1, 1985
8. Malseed RT: Pharmacology: Drug Therapy and Nursing Considerations, 3rd ed. Philadelphia: JB Lippincott, 1990
9. National Dairy Council: Calcium: A Summary of Current Research for the Health Professional. Rosemont, IL: National Dairy Council, 1987
10. O'Connor BW, Sobal J, Muncie HL: Dietary habits, weight history, and vitamin supplement use in elderly osteoarthritis patients. J Am Diet Assoc 89:378, 1989
11. Porth CM: Pathophysiology: Concepts of Altered Health States. 3rd ed. Philadelphia: JB Lippincott, 1990
12. Touger-Decker R: Nutritional considerations in rheumatoid arthritis. J Am Diet Assoc 88:327, 1988
13. Walden O: The relationship of dietary and supplemental calcium intake to bone loss and osteoporosis. J Am Diet Assoc 89:397, 1989
14. Wardlow G: The effects of diet and lifestyle on bone mass in women. J Am Diet Assoc 88:17, 1988
15. Wolman PG: Management of patients using unproven regimens for arthritis. J Am Diet Assoc 87:1211, 1987

20 Oncology

CANCER
Incidence and Etiology
Treatment

CANCER CACHEXIA

Incidence and Etiology
Prevention and Treatment
Nursing Process

The relationship between diet, nutritional status, and cancer is complex and multifaceted. Nutrition education in the well population should focus on cancer prevention. For clients being aggressively treated for cancer, diet intervention plays a vital role in maintaining nutritional status and optimizing the chance of successful cancer treatment, and also may decrease morbidity and mortality. Palliative nutritional support for the terminally ill may improve the quality of life and enhance the client's sense of well-being.

CANCER

Cancer, neoplasm, and malignant tumor are used interchangeably to describe a group of diseases characterized by the uncontrolled growth and spread of abnormal cells. Cancer develops when an *initiating* event (*i.e.*, repeated or prolonged exposure to carcinogens or radiation) changes the DNA structure or reproductive code of normal cells. Exactly why this change in normal cell structure occurs is not known. After a latent period of usually 5 to 30 years, a *promoting* event (*i.e.*, a favorable hormonal environment) transforms initiated cells into cancer cells, which autonomously proliferate and invade, infiltrate, and destroy surrounding tissues. Eventually cancer cells detach from the tumor mass and migrate or are transported to a distant site, where they lodge and grow (metastasize) in the new location to form a secondary tumor mass. Left unchecked, cancer ends in death.

In addition to its destructive invasive nature, cancer alters the metabolism of carbohydrates, protein, and fat. The net effect of these alterations—increased energy expenditure, increased protein catabolism and whole-body protein turnover, tumor-induced nitrogen "trapping," increased lipolysis, and preferential use of fat as an energy source—is to affect nutritional status negatively and contribute to cancer cachexia. Unless aggressive nutritional support is initiated early, cancer and its treatments can have profound and devastating effects on nutritional status, often resulting in cachexia and death. Although the general course of the disease and its metabolic effects are predictable, cancer is not a single disease with one cause but represents a group of distinct diseases with different causes, manifestations, treatments, and prognoses.

Incidence and Etiology

Cancer strikes one of three Americans and does not discriminate against age, sex, race, or any body organ. Today, 40% of Americans who get cancer will be alive 5 years after diagnosis; however, cancer causes approximately 430,000 deaths annually and ranks second as the leading cause of death in the United States.[1]

There is no single etiology of cancer in humans. Fortunately, many cancers are curable if detected early, and the risk of getting cancer can be greatly reduced by lifestyle changes. As many as 80% of all cases of cancer may be related to environmental causes and may potentially be preventable[13] (Table 20-1). Numerous animal, clinical, and epidemiologic studies suggest that diet may cause or prevent the development of certain types of cancer; it

Table 20-1
Non-dietary Cancer Risk Factors

Factor	Risk	Risk Reduction
Smoking: cigarettes, cigars, pipes	Cigarette smokers have a 10 times greater chance of getting lung cancer than nonsmokers. Smoking is also associated with an increased risk of cancer of the mouth, pharynx, esophagus, proximal end of the stomach, and bladder, especially when combined with heavy alcohol consumption.	Don't smoke.
Chewing tobacco, snuff	Increases the risk of oral cancer	Don't use tobacco in any form.
Estrogen therapy	Long-term, high-dose usage increases the risk of endometrial cancer.	Take estrogen only as long as necessary and in the smallest dose possible.
Exposure to various chemical compounds: nickel, chromate, uranium, asbestos, petroleum, vinyl chloride, agricultural insecticides, herbicides, fertilizers, and preservatives	Occupational or environmental exposure to one or more carcinogens increases the risk of several cancers.	Follow safety precautions in the workplace to avoid unnecessary exposure to harmful chemicals.
Repeated or prolonged exposure to x-rays	Increases the risk of many types of cancer	Avoid unnecessary x-rays; wear a protective shield to cover other parts of the body, if possible.
Excessive exposure to sunlight	Increases the risk of squamous cell carcinoma, basal cell carcinoma, and melanoma, especially in fair-skinned people	Avoid excessive exposure to the sun, especially from 10 AM to 3 PM when sunlight is most direct; use a sunscreen; wear protective clothing.
Alcohol	Alcohol, especially when combined with smoking, increases the risk of cancer of the mouth, larynx, liver, and esophagus.	Drink alcohol only in moderation.

is estimated that 30% to 35% of all cancers may be diet-related and therefore potentially preventable by changes in eating habits.[1]

Dietary Factors

Food may contain carcinogens or procarcinogens that can be converted to cancer-causing agents under the proper conditions. Nitrates, nitrites, some naturally occurring compounds, and intentional and accidental additives all may be carcinogenic. Aflatoxin B, a substance produced by mold that grows on improperly stored grains and nuts, has been implicated as the cause of liver cell cancer.

Other diet-related cancers may be due to nutritional excesses or deficiencies that alter the body's ability to defend against cancer (altered immunocompetence), or may alter enzymes, gastrointestinal (GI) flora, and hormone levels to create an environment favorable to cancer promotion. Epidemiologic and animal studies indicate a strong correlation between high-fat diets and a high incidence of colon and breast cancers. High intakes of calories, cholesterol, and animal protein may also be involved in promoting some cancers.

Vitamin A, especially beta-carotene, the vegetable form of vitamin A, helps to maintain the body's immune system and its ability to defend against cancer, and also may be protective against epithelial cancers. Vitamin C may decrease the risk of gastric and esophageal cancers. Fiber, folic acid, compounds found in cruciferous vegetables (broccoli, cabbage, Brussels sprouts, etc.), selenium and other trace minerals may also protect against certain types of cancer.

Current evidence suggests that the risk of cancer can be reduced by changing eating habits. A varied diet and moderation in all things seems prudent. Although not guaranteed to prevent cancer in all people, the American Cancer Society's dietary guidelines for reducing the risk of cancer appear in Table 20-2.

Other Etiologic Factors

In addition to environmental causes, genetic factors also may be involved in cancer incidence; a familial tendency exists for breast, stomach, colon, ovarian, and lung cancers. Familial-linked cancers appear to have a younger age of onset and an increased incidence of bilateral development.

Viral factors, such as Epstein-Barr Virus, also have been linked to the development of certain cancers, such as Burkitt's lymphoma. Although evidence is lacking, viruses are suspected of being able to invade cells and alter their genetic code for reproduction.

Treatment

Because the chance of curing cancer lessens with each advancing stage ("staging" may classify cancer from stage 1 through stage 4, with ascending degrees of size, involvement, and metastasis), health teaching should emphasize prevention and early detection. General cancer assessment criteria, including cancer's seven warning signals, are also useful for screening and early detection (see box, General Cancer Assessment Criteria).

Cancer may be treated with chemotherapy, radiation, surgery, or a combination of therapies. Some hematologic cancers are treated with bone marrow transplants. Each of

Table 20-2
Dietary Guidelines for Reducing the Risk of Cancer

Recommendation	Rationale
Avoid obesity.	Obesity is correlated to cancers of the uterus, gallbladder, breast, and colon, possibly due to an alteration in hormone levels.
Cut fat intake to 30% of total calories or less.	High-fat diets generally are high-calorie diets, which increase the risk of obesity.
	A high-fat diet may promote breast, colon, and prostate cancers. Although the exact mechanism is unknown, fat may promote cancer by stimulating the secretion of bile acids into the intestines; bile acids and their byproducts are structurally similar to certain carcinogens.
Eat more high-fiber foods.	Fiber may help protect against colon cancer, possibly by diluting the intestinal contents and decreasing transit time.
Include foods rich in vitamins A and C in your daily diet.	Vitamin A, or possibly beta-carotene, may reduce the risk of cancers of the lung, esophagus, larynx, and bladder, possibly through its function as an antioxidant.
	Vitamin C prevents nitrites from combining with amines to form nitrosamines, which are carcinogens that increase the risk of stomach, and esophageal cancers.
Include cruciferous (cabbage family) vegetables in your diet.	Cruciferous vegetables produce powerful enzymes in the liver, which may break down cancer-promoting chemicals. They may reduce the risk of cancers of the stomach, colon, rectum, and lung.
Cut down on salt-cured, smoked, and nitrite-cured foods.	Salt-cured, smoked, and nitrite-cured foods are considered cancer promoters, and they also tend to be high in fat.
Keep alcohol consumption moderate, if you do drink.	Heavy drinking increases the risk of liver cancer; smoking and drinking greatly increases the risk of cancers of the mouth, larynx, throat, and esophagus.

Source: American Cancer Society: Eating Smart. 87-250M No. 2042. Atlanta, GA: American Cancer Society, revised 1989

General Cancer Assessment Criteria

Weight, weight changes

Anorexia, nausea, vomiting, dysphagia

Seven warning signals:
- **C** hange in bowel or bladder habits
- **A** sore that does not heal
- **U** nusual bleeding or discharge
- **T** hickening or lump on the breast or elsewhere
- **I** ndigestion or difficulty swallowing
- **O** bvious change in the size or color of a wart or mole
- **N** agging cough or hoarseness

these treatment modalities can cause significant nutritional problems related to systemic or localized side effects that interfere with intake, increase nutrient losses, or alter metabolism. Actual response to each of these therapies depends on the individual and the type, location, and extent of treatment (Table 20-3).

Nutritional support used as an adjuvant to effective cancer therapy helps sustain the client through adverse side effects and reduces morbidity and mortality. Studies show that improved nutritional status can reverse weight loss, restore or maintain immunocompetence, help restore normal metabolism, enhance tolerance for antineoplastic therapy, maintain body composition during nutritional repletion, and reduce postoperative morbidity.[3] However, for nutritional support to improve the results of cancer therapy, the therapy itself must have a reasonable chance of success. Evidence suggests that aggressive nutritional support may be of little value, or even detrimental, when used in conjunction with ineffective cancer treatment.

Chemotherapy

Chemotherapy damages the reproductive ability of both malignant and normal cells, especially rapidly dividing cells, such as well-nourished cancer cells and normal cells of the GI tract, respiratory system, bone marrow, skin, and gonadal tissue.

The side effects of chemotherapy vary with the type of drug or combination of drugs used. The most common side effects are nausea and vomiting, anorexia, taste changes, sore mouth or throat, diarrhea and constipation. They occur within minutes or hours of drug administration and usually subside within 24 to 48 hours; antiemetics may help relieve nausea. Some combinations of chemotherapeutic drugs may produce severe and long-lasting GI complications.

Radiation

Radiation causes cell death as particles of radioactive energy break chemical bonds, disrupting reproductive ability. Although radiation injures all rapidly dividing cells, it is

Table 20-3
Potential Side Effects of Cancer Treatments

Chemotherapy		Surgery	
General Category	*Potential Side Effects*	*Type*	*Potential Complications*
Adrenocorticosteroids	Potassium depletion Sodium and fluid retention Negative nitrogen and calcium balances Hyperglycemia and symptoms of diabetes mellitus Hyperphagia	Head and neck resection	Difficulty chewing and swallowing Tube feeding dependency
Antimetabolites, alkylating agents	Anorexia Nausea/Vomiting Taste alterations Oral lesions Intestinal lesions Abdominal pain Diarrhea Malabsorption	Esophagectomy or esophogeal resection	Decreased stomach motility Decreased HCl production Diarrhea Steatorrhea
Antibiotics	Nausea/Vomiting Mucositis Stomatitis GI upset Possible decreased calcium and iron absorption	Gastrectomy	"Dumping syndrome": crampy diarrhea that develops quickly after eating accompanied by flushing, dizziness, weakness, pain, distention, and vomiting Hypoglycemia Malabsorption Achlorhydria Vitamin B_{12} malabsorption related to a lack of intrinsic factor
Estrogens	Nausea/Vomiting Anorexia Hypercalcemia	Removal of part of the small intestine	
Vinka alkaloids	Nausea/Vomiting Constipation Obstipation	Jejunum	Malnutrition related to generalized malabsorption
		Ileum	Vitamin B_{12} malabsorption Decreased absorption of bile salts → fat malabsorption and steatorrhea Fluid and electrolyte imbalance Diarrhea Hyperoxaluria → increased risk of renal oxalate stone formation and increased excretion of calcium
Radiation		Massive bowel resection	Steatorrhea Malnutrition related to severe generalized malabsorption Metabolic acidosis
Area	*Potential Complications*	Ileostomy or colostomy	Fluid and electrolyte imbalance Blind loop syndrome
Head and neck	Altered or loss of taste ("mouth blindness") Decreased salivary secretions → dry mouth Thick salivary secretions Difficulty swallowing and chewing Loss of teeth	Pancreatectomy	Generalized malabsorption Diabetes mellitus
Lower neck and midchest	Acute: esophagitis Delayed: fibrosis → esophageal stricture → difficulty swallowing		
Abdomen and pelvis	Extensive radiation to the upper or mid-abdomen → nausea and vomiting Acute or chronic bowel damage → cramps, steatorrhea, malabsorption, disaccharidase deficiency, protein-losing enteropathy; bowel constriction, obstruction, or fistula formation Chronic blood loss from intestine and bladder Pelvic radiation → increased urinary frequency, urgency, and dysuria		

most lethal on the poorly differentiated and rapidly proliferating cells of cancer tissue.[9] Recovery from sublethal doses of radiation occurs in the interval between the first dose and subsequent doses. Fortunately, normal tissue appears to recover more quickly from radiation damage than cancerous tissues.

The side effects of radiation depend on the site of radiation, the volume of tissue irradiated, the dose of radiation, and duration of therapy. The rapidly growing cells of the GI mucosa, skin, and bone marrow are particularly vulnerable. General weakness, fatigue, and anorexia are common side effects, regardless of the site, amount, and duration of therapy.

Radiation to the abdomen may produce acute side effects of nausea, vomiting, and diarrhea that resolve shortly after radiation is discontinued. However, delayed side effects can develop years after radiation is completed. Surgical and nutritional intervention may be required to alleviate progressive diarrhea, malabsorption, and malnutrition.

Radiation to the head, neck, or chest may cause dry mouth, sore mouth, sore throat, taste changes, and dental problems.

Surgery

Surgery may be better tolerated (shorter postoperative hospital stay and fewer complications) by people who have good nutritional status before treatment. Postsurgical requirements increase for protein, calories, vitamin C, B vitamins, and iron to replenish losses and promote healing (see Chap. 14). Actual side effects incurred depend on the location and extent of surgery.

Bone Marrow Transplants

Bone marrow transplants are used primarily to treat hematologic cancers and also are used experimentally to treat solid tumors such as breast cancer. Bone marrow transplants are preceded by high-dose chemotherapy and total-body irradiation, used to suppress immune function and destroy cancer cells; nausea, vomiting, and diarrhea are common side effects, which may last 24 to 48 hours. Other complications include delayed mucositis, stomatitis, esophagitis, taste alterations, and intestinal damage that prevents oral intake; total parenteral nutrition may be needed for 1 to 2 months after bone marrow transplants.

CANCER CACHEXIA

Cancer cachexia is a syndrome characterized by early satiety, anorexia, severe weight loss, anemia, muscle weakness, and loss of immunocompetence, leading to a decreased sense of well-being and quality of life, and increased risks of infection, morbidity, and mortality. Alterations in metabolism, fluid and electrolyte balance, enzyme and endocrine functions, and immune system integrity distinguish cancer cachexia from malnutrition related to other causes.

Incidence and Etiology

Cachexia affects approximately two-thirds of all cancer clients and is responsible for more deaths than cancer itself. Anorexia, altered metabolism, and increased nutrient losses can contribute to the development of cachexia; each of these factors can result from cancer or cancer treatments and may be multifactorial in origin (Fig. 20-1).

Neither the incidence nor the severity of cachexia can be related directly to the site of involvement, calorie intake (cachexia can develop even if calorie intake is high), tumor weight, or tumor cell type. Cachexia has developed in clients whose tumors weighed less than 500 g. The type of tumor does not necessarily determine the severity of cachexia but may influence the time of onset.

Prevention and Treatment

Malnutrition and cachexia are not inevitable results of cancer and cancer therapy; they may be prevented by early and aggressive nutritional support (complete or supplemental enteral or parenteral nutrition). The increased risks of morbidity and mortality associated with cachexia make preventative nutrition imperative; early and ongoing nutritional assessment, planning, implementation, and evaluation are vital.

Used as an adjunct to cancer treatment, aggressive nutritional support can improve cachexia and reduce morbidity and mortality by stimulating weight gain, reversing negative nitrogen balance, improving immunocompetence, and increasing the sense of well-being. However, it is likely that some characteristics of cachexia are not caused simply by an inadequate intake; therefore, it is possible that some cachectic clients may not respond to aggressive nutritional support.

In clients whose prognosis is terminal, the value of nutritional support is a controversial ethical issue. No benefit is derived from "force-feeding" a client whose cancer is not being treated, because both body weight gain and tumor growth are stimulated. Instead, enteral nutrition should be maintained as an integral component of palliative care aimed at providing comfort and improving the quality of life.

Nursing Process

Assessment

In addition to general cancer assessment criteria, assess for the following factors:

Side effects that interfere with intake or metabolism, such as nausea, vomiting, diarrhea, alterations in taste, dry or sore mouth, pain, and so forth; onset, frequency, duration, severity, interventions attempted and results

Dietary changes made in response to symptoms or side effects of cancer or cancer treatment (*i.e.*, foods avoided, foods preferred). Determine foods best and least tolerated.

The use of unorthodox products, diets, or supplements with unproven nutritional benefits

Weight changes. Severe weight loss, defined as a loss of 10% or more of body weight within 6 months, or an unintentional weight loss of 2 lb per week, is associated with an

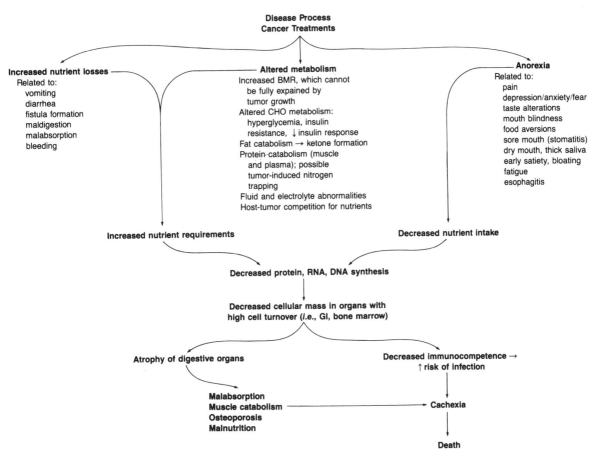

Figure 20-1
The causes of cachexia.

increase in morbidity and mortality. Total parenteral nutrition may be used when weight loss exceeds 20% of body weight and prognosis is good. Loss of 30% of body weight usually is fatal. Note that fluid retention and dehydration can mask true weight status.

Signs of malnutrition, such as skin changes, edema, easy fatigability, and tissue wasting

Intake and output, and observe for signs of fluid and electrolyte balance

Presence of preexisting conditions that require diet intervention, such as endocrine, cardiac, renal, or liver disorders

The client's emotional state and presence of outside support systems

Protein status (serum albumin, serum transferrin) and immune function (total lymphocyte count, skin reactivity to PPD [purified protein derivative of tuberculin]), if available

Nursing Diagnosis

Altered Nutrition: Less than Body Requirements, related to anorexia, dysphagia, and nausea secondary to cancer/cancer therapy.

Planning and Implementation

An overall goal of diet intervention for all cancer clients is to keep the client out of the hospital whenever possible. Because cachexia is easier to prevent than to treat, nutritional support should be initiated before the downhill spiral of malnutrition develops.

For clients with cancer, nutritional needs increase as appetite decreases. However, because a "typical" cancer client does not exist, the diet must be individualized and continually evaluated and revised according to the client's needs and ability to eat. General diet management objectives and interventions are based on the client's treatment goals; diet for clients receiving aggressive treatment to arrest or cure the disease differs from diet for clients receiving palliative care for comfort and improved quality of life.

Nutritional support is one area of treatment in which the client can be an active participant. The client and health care team may "contract" for an acceptable amount of weight loss. As long as the client does not lose more weight than was agreed on, the client is in charge of his own nutritional care.

It is more effective and practical to teach the client how to increase the nutrient density of his diet (increase the protein and calorie content of his diet without increasing the volume of food eaten) and alleviate eating problems than to provide a therapeutic diet specifying exact amounts and rigid guidelines.

Loss of dignity and control, change in sexuality and body image, and loss of appetite can create a frustrating, seemingly hopeless situation for the client, and food may be used to express anger and frustration. Allow the client and family to verbalize feelings, and emphasize a positive, supportive, team-effort approach. The client's rights and preferences should be respected at all times.

Although the client may need the encouragement and support of family and friends, putting them in a position of "force-feeding" the client may add tension to an already stressful situation.

Decreased intake and increased requirements may necessitate the use of multivitamin and mineral supplements.

Client Goals

Clients receiving aggressive nutritional support will:

Modify the diet as needed to lessen the side effects of cancer/cancer therapies.

Consume adequate calories and protein to prevent or correct significant weight loss and prevent or correct nutritional deficiencies.

Describe the principles and rationale of diet management during aggressive cancer treatment and nutritional support.

Clients receiving palliative nutritional support will:

Maintain activity level, if possible.

Experience less discomfort.

Nursing Interventions

Diet Management

Aggressive nutritional support:

Increase protein intake to 1.0 to 2.0 g/kg to prevent body protein catabolism.

Increase calorie intake to meet increased metabolic demands and replace nutritional losses related to cancer or its treatment. At least 25 to 35 cal/kg are needed to maintain

Ways to Increase Nutrient Density With Protein and Calories

Skim milk powder
  Add to milk and milk-based drinks for a fortified beverage.
  Use on hot or cold cereals.
  Add to scrambled eggs, soups, gravies, casseroles, desserts, and baked products.
Milk
  Substitute milk, evaporated milk, or heavy cream for water in recipes.
  Dip meat, poultry, and fish in eggs or milk and coat with bread or cereal crumbs before baking, broiling, or pan frying.
  Choose desserts made with eggs or milk: sponge cake, angel food cake, custard, puddings.
Cheese
  Add grated or cubed cheese, or diced or ground meats, fish, or poultry to soups, omelets, casseroles, vegetable dishes, and sauces.
  Melt on sandwiches, bread, muffins, rice, meats, vegetables, and eggs.
Cream cheese
  Mix with butter and spread on hot bread, rolls, biscuits, and muffins.
  Add to vegetables.
Peanut butter
  Use as a spread on slices of apple, banana, pears, crackers, and waffles.
  Stuff celery with it.
  Combine with cream cheese and use as a sandwich filling.
  Add to milk drinks and milk shakes.
  Blend into soft ice cream or yogurt.
Eggs
  Add chopped, hard-cooked eggs to salads and dressings, vegetables, casseroles, and creamed meats.
  Beat eggs into mashed potatoes, vegetables purees, and sauces.
  Add extra egg yolks to quiches, scrambles, custards, puddings, pancakes, French toast batter, and milkshakes.
  Dip meat, fish, and poultry into eggs and coat with bread or cereal crumbs before baking, broiling, or pan frying.
Butter
  Whenever possible, add butter to hot foods: bread, rolls, pancakes, waffles, soups, vegetables, potatoes, cooked cereal, rice, pasta.
Mayonnaise
  Use in place of salad dressing in salads, eggs, casseroles, sandwiches.
Honey
  Use on toast and cereal.
  Add to coffee and tea.

(continued)

Ways to Increase Nutrient Density
With Protein and Calories (*continued*)

Sour cream or yogurt
  Sweeten with sugar or honey and use as a sauce for desserts and fruit.
  Use as a sauce on vegetables.
  Use in gravies and dips.

Nuts, seeds, and wheat germ
  Sprinkle on fruit, cereal, ice cream, yogurt, vegetables, salads, and toast.
  Use in place of bread crumbs.
  Add to casseroles, breads, muffins, pancakes, cookies, and waffles.

Whipped cream
  Use as a topping on hot chocolate, pies, fruit, pudding, gelatin, ice cream,
  and other desserts.
  Add to coffee and tea.

Marshmallows
  Use in hot chocolate, on fruit, and in desserts.

Food preparation
  Bread meat and vegetables before cooking.
  Sauté and fry foods when possible, to add more calories.
  Add sauces or gravies.

Snack frequently on nuts, dried fruit, candy, buttered popcorn, cheese and
crackers, granola, ice cream.

(United States Department of Health and Human Services: Eating Hints: Tips and Recipes for Better
Nutrition During Cancer Treatment. NIH Publication No. 91-2079. Washington, DC: Government
Printing Office, revised April 1990)

weight and 40 to 50 cal/kg are required to replenish body stores (see box, Ways to
Increase Nutrient Density With Protein and Calories).

Modify the diet as needed to alleviate problems that interfere with appetite and intake
(Table 20-4; see Chap. 15 for diet recommendations, nursing considerations, and client
teaching for general GI problems such as nausea, vomiting, diarrhea, constipation,
esophagitis and heartburn, malabsorption, and lactose intolerance).

If oral intake is inadequate or contraindicated, use enteral tube feedings or total parenteral
nutrition as a supplemental or complete feeding (see Chap. 13).

Palliative nutritional support:

Encourage eating as a source of pleasure. The client's requests and preferences are more
important than the nutritional quality of the diet.

Modify the diet as needed to alleviate problems that interfere with appetite and intake
(Table 20-4; see Chap. 15 for diet recommendations and nursing considerations for
general GI problems).

Use tube feedings only if client is unable to eat; total parenteral nutrition rarely is indicated.

(*Text continued on page 592*)

Table 20-4
*Nursing Interventions and Considerations for Problems
that Interfere with Appetite and Intake*

Potential Problem	Nursing Interventions and Considerations
Anorexia (total lack of appetite)	Anorexia may be continuous or sporadic.
	Encourage the client to overeat during "good" days and to eat whenever hungry.
	Provide small frequent meals seasoned according to individual taste. Snacks of nutrient-dense liquids (instant breakfast, milk shakes, commercial supplements) can provide significant amounts of protein and calories, are easily consumed, and tend to leave the stomach quickly.
	The appearance and aroma of food are more important when appetite is lacking. Attractive food, a bright, cheerful environment, soft music, and company can help make eating a pleasant experience.
	Clients with anorexia should not be expected to order food for the following day. If possible, allow spontaneous meal selections and honor day-to-day requests.
	Provide emotional support and encouragement to the client and family.
	Encourage the family to bring food from home.
	Appetite is often best in the morning and deteriorates gradually throughout the day. Encourage a high-protein, high-calorie, nutrient-dense breakfast.
	Use appropriate medications to control pain, nausea, and depression. If tolerated, a small amount of alcohol before mealtime may stimulate appetite.
Nausea	Provide small, frequent meals; provide liquids between meals to avoid bloating at mealtime.
	Foods served cold or at room temperature may be better tolerated; hot foods may contribute to nausea.
	Try high-carbohydrate, low-fat foods, like toast, crackers, yogurt, sherbet, cooked cereal, soft or canned fruits, watermelon, banana, fruit juices, and angel food cake.
	Advise the client to avoid foods that are fatty, greasy, fried, or strongly seasoned.
	Encourage the client to keep track of foods that cause nausea so that they can be avoided.
	Advise the client to avoid eating 1–2 hours before chemotherapy or radiotherapy to decrease the likelihood of nausea.
	Request an antiemetic be ordered to control nausea.
Pain	Administer analgesics or appropriate pain medication prior to mealtime.
	Relaxation techniques, distraction, and biofeedback may help control pain.
Depression/anxiety/fear	Provide emotional support and give the client a reason to eat: tolerance to treatments and the effectiveness of therapy may be increased if nutritional status is maintained.
	Use appropriate medications to control depression and anxiety.
Taste alterations	Taste changes may be due to cancer or cancer treatments. Radiation-induced taste alterations usually develop by the third week of therapy and return to normal within one year.
	Clients who experience taste changes are more likely to lose

(*continued*)

Table 20-4 (*continued*)

Potential Problem	Nursing Interventions and Considerations
	weight. Conversely, clients who lose weight may be more likely to develop taste alterations.
	Elemental zinc has been shown to correct taste abnormalities. If prescribed, zinc should be taken with food or milk to decrease the risk of GI irritation.
	Clients may experience a decreased threshold for urea (bitter), increased threshold for sucrose (sweet), or both.
	Chemotherapy may cause a metallic taste. Clients who complain of a bitter taste while receiving chemotherapy should be advised to suck on hard candy during therapy.
	Encourage good oral hygiene before eating to eliminate unpleasant tastes.
	Encourage the client to experiment with a variety of seasonings, especially if oral mucosa is not impaired.
	Advise the client to avoid anything that tastes unpleasant.
	Reassure the client that taste changes are not uncommon and encourage him or her to verbalize feelings.
Decreased threshold for urea → *bitter taste*	Red meats, particularly beef and pork, are frequently said to have a "bad," "rotten," or fecal taste. Aversions may also include poultry, fish, coffee, and chocolate.
	Meats may be better tolerated if served cold or at room temperature, or if highly flavored with strong seasonings, sweet marinades, or sauces.
	Assure the client that red meat is not essential in the diet. Encourage the intake of other high-protein foods, such as eggs, cheese, mild fish, nuts, and dried peas and beans. If those sources are not tolerated, milk shakes, eggnogs, puddings, ice cream, and commercial supplements can provide sufficient protein and calories.
Increased threshold for sucrose	Season foods according to individual taste.
Lack of taste (mouth blindness)	Appearance and aroma become more important when taste is absent: Serve attractively presented, steaming food in a bright, cheerful environment.
Food aversions	Food aversions may be intermittent or may worsen as the day progresses.
	To avoid learned aversions, instruct the client to avoid his or her favorite foods or fast completely before receiving radiation or chemotherapy. If nausea and vomiting tend to occur around the same time each day, withholding food beforehand may help avoid learned aversions.
Sore mouth (stomatitis)	Good oral hygiene (thorough cleaning with a soft bristle tooth brush or cotton swabs plus frequent mouth rinses with normal saline and water or baking soda and water) may help prevent or minimize stomatitis. Commercial mouthwashes containing alcohol may burn the oral mucosa.
	Stomatitis may produce taste alterations, mouth blindness, or the association between eating and pain. Topical anesthetics may help relieve discomfort.
	Cut food into small portions
	Clients with stomatitis are more susceptible to *Candida albicans* infections, which may cause ulcerated white or yellow patches on the oral mucosa and further diminish taste sensation.

(*continued*)

Table 20-4 (*continued*)

Potential Problem	Nursing Interventions and Considerations
	Instruct the client to avoid spices, acidic foods, coarse foods, alcohol, and smoking, which can aggravate an already irritated oral mucosa.
	Encourage the client to eat a soft or liquid bland diet, drink plenty of fluids, and avoid hot food and beverages. Cold items may help numb the oral mucosa. Try bananas, applesauce, canned fruit, watermelon, cottage cheese, yogurt, mashed potatoes, macaroni and cheese, custards, pudding, scrambled eggs, cooked cereals, and liquids.
	Straws may ease swallowing.
	Caution the client against wearing ill-fitting dentures.
Dry mouth/thick saliva	Clients with decreased saliva production are susceptible to dental caries. Encourage good oral hygiene, frequent mouth rinsing, and the avoidance of concentrated sweets.
	Artificial saliva and the use of straws may facilitate swallowing. Petroleum jelly applied to the lips may help prevent drying.
	Provide mouth care immediately before mealtime for added moisture.
	Advise the client to avoid dry coarse foods, and to use gravies, sauces, and sugar-free jellies liberally. Some clients may require a liquid diet.
	Offer high-calorie liquids in between meals.
	Encourage the client to use ice chips and sugar-free hard candies and gum between meals to relieve dryness.
Early satiety/bloating	Instruct the client to avoid
	High-fat foods (gravies, rich sauces, greasy foods, excessive butter)
	Gas-forming foods such as onions, garlic, and vegetables in the cabbage family
	Liquids with meals
	Empty-calorie foods and beverages
	Encourage the client to chew foods thoroughly and to eat small frequent meals.
	Recommend moderate exercise before and after eating.
Fatigue	Encourage the client to rest before meals.
	Position the client so that all food and utensils are within easy reach.
	Provide easy-to-eat foods that can be prepared with a minimal amount of effort.
	Commercial prepared oral supplements, like Ensure and Sustacal, may boost protein and calorie intake with a minimum of effort.
	Enlist the help of family and friends to help with meal preparation at home.
	Encourage the use of convenience foods and labor-saving appliances (blender, crockpot, toaster oven, microwave oven, dishwasher).
	Assistance may be available from Meals On Wheels or other community services.
	Encourage a good breakfast, since fatigue may worsen as the day progresses.
Hiccups	If hiccups cannot be managed medically, provide small, frequent meals when the client is hiccup-free.

Anticancer Diet

Food For Thought

Diet's role in the prevention of cancer is the subject of much research. Although epidemiologic and animal studies suggest that high intakes of certain vitamins and minerals act as anticarcinogens to alter the incidence and growth of certain cancers, no one is suggesting that particular nutrients alone, or combined with an "ideal" diet, can prevent or cure cancer. Almost all researchers agree that since it is not known exactly what chemicals or components in foods actually protect against cancer, it is prudent to rely on food, not supplements, to provide an optimal diet. That translates into eating more fruits, vegetables, and whole grains and less high-fat foods, alcohol, and salt-cured, smoked, and nitrite-cured foods.

Eat more fruits, vegetables, and whole grains.

- Eat a variety of fruits and vegetables, preferably with minimal preparation and little or no cooking, to retain vitamin and fiber content.
- Foods high in beta-carotene (vitamin A precursor) include broccoli, cantaloupe, carrots, spinach, squash, and sweet potatoes. Apricots, beet greens, nectarines, peaches, tomatoes, and watermelon are good sources.
- Excellent sources of vitamin C include broccoli, brussels sprouts, citrus fruits and juices, green and red peppers, and strawberries. Good sources include cabbage, cauliflower, potatoes, rutabaga. and tomatoes.
- Eat cruciferous vegetables several times a week: broccoli, cabbage, cauliflower, spinach, brussels sprouts, kale, collards, rutabagas, and bok choy.
- Eat more dried peas and beans. They are good sources of fiber, iron, and B vitamins, and are very low in fat.
- Use whole-grain breads, cereals, and flour to increase fiber, iron, and B vitamin intake.

Eat less fat.

- Reduce total fat intake to approximately 30% of total calories or less.
- Trim all visible fat from meat and remove poultry skin; limit portion size to 2–3 ounces.
- Prepare foods by baking, broiling, steaming, or stewing instead of frying.
- Use poultry, veal, and fish more often; use red meats and high-fat meats sparingly.
- Use low-fat milk and dairy products.
- Avoid high-fat desserts and limit the use of fats and oils.

Minimize the consumption of salt-cured, smoked, and nitrite-cured foods.

- Limit the intake of bacon, ham, hot dogs, and salt-cured fish.

Drink alcohol only in moderation.

Client Teaching

Instruct the client and family

That the client is in charge of his or her nutritional care.

To view food as a medicine, rather than a social pleasure, that must be "taken" even when the desire to eat is lacking.

To eat frequently and as much as possible.

On how to add protein and calories to his or her diet to increase the nutrient density (see box, Ways to Increase Nutrient Density With Protein and Calories).

On how to alleviate eating problems that may develop from the disease process or cancer treatments (see Table 20-4).

That it is necessary to drink ample fluids 1 to 2 days before and after chemotherapy to enhance the excretion of the drugs and decrease the risk of renal toxicity.

That no diets or nutritional supplements can cure cancer and that starving the tumor will also starve the body.

Monitor

Monitor for the following signs or symptoms:

Tolerance to oral feedings (*i.e.*, absence of mouth pain, ability to swallow, absence of nausea, vomiting, and indigestion)

Compliance with the diet and the need for follow-up diet counseling

Effectiveness of diet, and evaluate the need for further diet modification

Weight, weight changes, as appropriate. Unless weight status is needed to adjust drug doses, observing steady weight decline in a terminal client is pointless.[4]

For the development of complications related to disease progression or the side effects of cancer therapy

Protein status, when available

Evaluation

Evaluation is ongoing. Assuming the plan of care has not changed, the client will achieve the goals as stated above.

BIBLIOGRAPHY

1. American Cancer Society: Cancer Facts and Figures—1991. Atlanta, GA: American Cancer Society, 1991
2. American Cancer Society: Eating Smart. 87-250M, no. 2042. Atlanta, GA: American Cancer Society, revised 1989
3. Charuhas PM: Nutrition support of the cancer patient. RD 10(2):1, 1990
4. D'Agostino NS: Managing nutrition problems in advanced cancer. Am J Nurs 89(1):50, 1989
5. Escott-Stump S: Nutrition and Diagnosis-Related Care, 2nd ed. Philadelphia: Lea and Febiger, 1988
6. Lefferts LY: Carcinogens au naturel? Nutrition Action Health Letter 17(6):1, 1990
7. Leibman B: Carrots against cancer? Nutrition Action Health Letter 15(10):1, 1988
8. Leibman B: Clues to colon cancer. Nutrition Action Health Letter 17(2):1, 1990

9. Porth CM: Pathophysiology: Concepts of Altered Health States, 3rd ed. Philadelphia: JB Lippincott, 1990

10. Public Health Service, United States Department of Health and Human Services, National Institutes of Health: Diet, Nutrition and Cancer Prevention: The Good News. Bethesda, MD: National Cancer Institute, Office of Cancer Communications, 1987

11. Rivers JM, Collins KK: Planning Meals that Lower Cancer Risk: A Reference Guide. Washington, DC: American Institute for Cancer Research, 1984

12. United States Department of Health and Human Services: Eating Hints: Tips and Recipes for Better Nutrition During Cancer Treatment. NIH Publication No. 91-2079. Bethesda, MD: Office of Cancer Communications, National Cancer Institute, revised April 1990

13. Watson RR, Leonard TK: Selenium and vitamins A, E, and C: Nutrients with cancer prevention properties. J Am Diet Assoc 86:505, 1986

Abbreviations

< less than

> greater than

ACTH adrenocorticotropic hormone

ADA American Diabetes Association or American Dietetic Association

ADD attention deficit disorder

ADH antidiuretic hormone

AICR American Institute for Cancer Research

ANAD Anorexia Nervosa and Associated Disorders

ASHD arteriosclerotic heart disease

BCAA branched-chain amino acids

BMI body mass index

BMR basal metabolic rate

BSA body surface area

BUN blood urea nitrogen

c cup

CAD coronary artery disease

cal calorie

CF cystic fibrosis

CHF congestive heart failure

CHO carbohydrate

CNS central nervous system

CoA coenzyme A

CVA cerebrovascular accident

CVP central venous pressure

dl deciliter

DNA deoxyribonucleic acid

ECF extracellular fluid

EDTA ethylenediaminetetraacetate

EFA essential fatty acid

F Fahrenheit

FAD flavin adenine dinucleotide

FAO Food and Agriculture Organization

FAS fetal alcohol syndrome

FDA Food and Drug Administration

FIGLU formiminoglutamic acid

FMN flavin mononucleotide

FPC fish protein concentrate

ft foot

GABA gamma-aminobutyric acid

GDM gestational diabetes mellitus

GFR glomerular filtration rate

GH growth hormone

GI gastrointestinal

HBV   high biologic value

HCl   hydrochloric acid

HDL   high-density lipoproteins

HFCS   high fructose corn syrup

HS   hour of sleep

IBW   ideal body weight

ICF   intracellular fluid

IDDM   insulin-dependent diabetes mellitus

IF   intrinsic factor

IGT   impaired glucose tolerance

IM   intramuscular

INQ   index of nutritional quality

IU   international unit

IV   intravenous

l   liter

lb   pound

LBW   low birth weight

LDL   low-density lipoproteins

LES   lower esophageal sphincter

MAC   mid-arm circumference

MAMC   mid-arm muscle circumference

MAO   monoamine oxidase

MAOI   monoamine oxidase inhibitor

MCT   medium chain triglycerides

mEq   milliequivalents

mEq/l   milliequivalents per liter

mg   milligram

MI   myocardial infarction

ml   milliliter

mOsm   milliosmole

MSG   monosodium glutamate

μg   microgram

NAAS   National Anorexic Aid Society

NAD   nicotinamide adenine dinucleotide

NADP   nicotinamide adenine dinucleotide phosphate

NCEP   National Cholesterol Education Program

NCHS   National Center for Health Statistics

ND   nasoduodenal

NE   niacin equivalents

NG   nasogastric

NIA   National Institute on Aging

NIDDM   noninsulin-dependent diabetes mellitus

NJ   nasojejunal

NPO   nothing by mouth

NPU   net protein utilization

oz   ounce

PA   pernicious anemia

PBI   protein bound iodine

PEM   protein-energy malnutrition

PER   protein efficiency ratio

peripheral TPN   peripheral total parenteral nutrition

PIH   pregnancy-induced hypertension

PKU   phenylketonuria

PLP   pyridoxal phosphate

PPD   purified protein derivative of tuberculin

P:S   ratio of polyunsaturated fatty acids to saturated fatty acids

PTH   parathyroid hormone

PUFA   polyunsaturated fatty acid

PZI   protamine zinc insulin

RAI   radioactive iodine uptake

RBC   red blood cells

RDA   recommended dietary allowance

RE   retinol equivalents

RNA   ribonucleic acid

SCP   single-cell protein

SDA   specific dynamic action

SKSD   streptokinase streptodornase

SPE   sucrose polyester

tbsp   tablespoon

TE   alpha-tocopherol equivalents

TG   triglyceride

TLC   total lymphocyte count

TOPS   Take Off Pounds Sensibly

TPN   total parenteral nutrition

TPP   thiamine pyrophosphate

TSF   triceps skinfold

tsp   teaspoon

UBW   usual body weight

UPC   universal product code

USDA   United States Drug Administration

USDHEW   United States Department of Health, Education, and Welfare

USDHHS   United States Department of Health and Human Services

USRDA   United States Recommended Dietary Allowance

UTI   urinary tract infection

UUN   urinary urea nitrogen

VLCD   very-low-calorie diet

VLDL   very-low-density lipoprotein

WBC   white blood cells

WHO   World Health Organization

WIC   Women, Infants, and Children

Appendices

APPENDIX 1. Nutritive Values of the Edible Part of Foods*

| | | | | | | | Fatty Acids | | | | | | | | | | | | |
| | | | | | | | | Unsaturated | | | | | | | | | | | |
Item No. (A)	Foods, Approximate Measures, Units, and Weight (Edible Part Unless Footnotes Indicate Otherwise) (B)		Water (C)	Food Energy (D)	Protein (E)	Fat (F)	Saturated (Total) (G)	Oleic (H)	Linoleic (I)	Carbohydrate (J)	Calcium (K)	Phosphorus (L)	Iron (M)	Potassium (N)	Vitamin A Value (O)	Thiamine (P)	Riboflavin (Q)	Niacin (R)	Ascorbic Acid (S)
		g	Per-cent	Cal-ories	g	g	g	g	g	g	mg	mg	mg	mg	IU	mg	mg	mg	mg

DAIRY PRODUCTS (CHEESE, CREAM, IMITATION CREAM, MILK; RELATED PRODUCTS)

Butter (see Fats, Oils, and Related Products, items 103–108)

Item No.	Food		C	D	E	F	G	H	I	J	K	L	M	N	O	P	Q	R	S
	Cheese																		
	Natural																		
1	Blue..........1 oz.........	28	42	100	6	8	5.3	1.9	0.2	1	150	110	0.1	73	200	0.01	0.11	0.3	0
2	Camembert (3 wedges per 4-oz container)........1 wedge.....	38	52	115	8	9	5.8	2.2	0.2	tr	147	132	0.1	71	350	0.01	0.19	0.2	0
	Cheddar																		
3	Cut pieces........1 oz........	28	37	115	7	9	6.1	2.1	0.2	tr	204	145	0.2	28	300	0.01	0.11	tr	0
4	1 cu in......	17.2	37	70	4	6	3.7	1.3	0.1	tr	124	88	0.1	17	180	tr	0.06	tr	0
5	Shredded.....1 c........	113	37	455	28	37	24.2	8.5	0.7	1	815	579	0.8	111	1200	0.03	0.42	0.1	0
	Cottage (curd not pressed down)																		
	Creamed (cottage cheese, 4% fat)																		
6	Large curd.....1 c..........	225	79	235	28	10	6.4	2.4	0.2	6	135	297	0.3	190	370	0.05	0.37	0.3	tr
7	Small curd.....1 c..........	210	79	220	26	9	6.0	2.2	0.2	6	126	277	0.3	177	340	0.04	0.34	0.3	tr
8	Low fat (2%)....1 c..........	226	79	205	31	4	2.8	1.0	0.1	8	155	340	0.4	217	160	0.05	0.42	0.3	tr
9	Low fat (1%)....1 c..........	226	82	165	28	2	1.5	0.5	0.1	6	138	302	0.3	193	80	0.05	0.37	0.3	tr
10	Uncreamed (cottage cheese dry curd, less than ½% fat)....1 c..........	145	80	125	25	1	0.4	0.1	tr	3	46	151	0.3	47	40	0.04	0.21	0.2	0
11	Cream..........1 oz.........	28	54	100	2	10	6.2	2.4	0.2	1	23	30	0.3	34	400	tr	0.06	tr	0
	Mozzarella, made with—																		
12	Whole milk........1 oz......	28	48	90	6	7	4.4	1.7	0.2	1	163	117	0.1	21	260	tr	0.08	tr	0
13	Part skim milk......1 oz......	28	49	80	8	5	3.1	1.2	0.1	1	207	149	0.1	27	180	0.01	0.10	tr	0
	Parmesan, grated																		

No.	Food, approximate measure	Measure	Grams	Water (%)	Food energy	Protein	Fat	Saturated	Oleic	Linoleic	Carbohydrate	Calcium	Phosphorus	Iron	Potassium	Vit. A	Thiamin	Riboflavin	Niacin	Ascorbic acid
14	Cup, not pressed down	1 c	100	18	455	42	30	19.1	7.7	0.3	4	1376	807	1.0	107	700	0.05	0.39	0.3	0
15	Tablespoon	1 tbsp	5	18	25	2	2	1.0	0.4	tr	tr	69	40	tr	5	40	tr	0.02	tr	0
16	Ounce	1 oz	28	18	130	12	9	5.4	2.2	0.1	1	390	229	0.3	30	200	0.01	0.11	0.1	0
17	Provolone	1 oz	28	41	100	7	8	4.8	1.7	0.1	1	214	141	0.1	39	230	0.01	0.09	tr	0
	Ricotta, made with—																			
18	Whole milk	1 c	246	72	430	28	32	20.4	7.1	0.7	7	509	389	0.9	257	1210	0.03	0.48	0.3	0
19	Part skim milk	1 c	246	74	340	28	19	12.1	4.7	0.5	13	669	449	1.1	308	1060	0.05	0.46	0.2	0
20	Romano	1 oz	28	31	110	9	8	—	—	—	1	302	215	—	—	160	—	0.11	tr	0
21	Swiss	1 oz	28	37	105	8	8	5.0	1.7	0.2	1	272	171	tr	31	240	0.01	0.10	tr	0
	Pasteurized process cheese																			
22	American	1 oz	28	39	105	6	9	5.6	2.1	0.2	tr	174	211	0.1	46	340	0.01	0.10	tr	0
23	Swiss	1 oz	28	42	95	7	7	4.5	1.7	0.1	1	219	216	0.2	61	230	tr	0.08	tr	0
24	Pasteurized process cheese food, American	1 oz	28	43	95	6	7	4.4	1.7	0.1	2	163	130	0.2	79	260	0.01	0.13	tr	0
25	Pasteurized process cheese spread, American	1 oz	28	48	80	5	6	3.8	1.5	0.1	2	159	202	0.1	69	220	0.01	0.12	tr	0
	Cream, sweet																			
26	Half-and-half (cream and milk)	1 c	242	81	315	7	28	17.3	7.0	0.6	10	254	230	0.2	314	260	0.08	0.36	0.2	2
27		1 tbsp	15	81	20	tr	2	1.1	0.4	tr	1	16	14	tr	19	20	0.01	0.02	tr	tr
28	Light, coffee, or table	1 c	240	74	470	6	46	28.8	11.7	1.0	9	231	192	0.1	292	1730	0.08	0.36	0.1	2
29		1 tbsp	15	74	30	tr	3	1.8	0.7	0.1	1	14	12	tr	18	110	tr	0.02	tr	tr
	Whipping, unwhipped (volume about double when whipped)																			
30	Light	1 c	239	64	700	5	74	46.2	18.3	1.5	7	166	146	0.1	231	2690	0.06	0.30	0.1	1
31		1 tbsp	15	64	45	tr	5	2.9	1.1	0.1	tr	10	9	tr	15	170	tr	0.02	tr	tr
32	Heavy	1 c	238	58	820	5	88	54.8	22.2	2.0	7	154	149	0.1	179	3500	0.05	0.26	0.1	1
33		1 tbsp	15	58	80	tr	6	3.5	1.4	0.1	tr	10	9	tr	11	220	tr	0.02	tr	tr
34	Whipped topping, (pressurized)	1 c	60	61	155	2	13	8.3	3.4	0.3	7	61	54	tr	88	550	0.02	0.04	tr	0
35		1 tbsp	3	61	10	tr	1	0.4	0.2	tr	tr	3	3	tr	4	30	tr	tr	tr	0
36	Cream, sour	1 c	230	71	495	7	48	30.0	12.1	1.1	10	268	195	0.1	331	1820	0.08	0.34	0.2	2
37		1 tbsp	12	71	25	tr	3	1.6	0.6	0.1	1	14	10	tr	17	90	tr	0.02	tr	tr
	Cream products, imitation (made with vegetable fat) Sweet — Creamers																			
38	Liquid (frozen)	1 c	245	77	335	2	24	22.8	0.3	tr	28	23	157	0.1	467	220[1]	0	0	0.1	0
39		1 tbsp	15	77	20	tr	1	1.4	tr	0	2	1	10	tr	29	10[1]	0	0	tr	0
40	Powdered	1 c	94	2	515	5	33	30.6	0.9	tr	52	21	397	0.1	763	190[1]	0	0.16[1]	0.1	0
41		1 tsp	2	2	10	tr	1	0.7	tr	0	1	tr	8	tr	16	tr	0	tr	tr	0
	Whipped topping																			
42	Frozen	1 c	75	50	240	1	19	16.3	1.0	0.2	17	5	6	0.1	14	650[1]	0	0	0.2	0
43		1 tbsp	4	50	15	tr	1	0.9	0.1	tr	1	tr	tr	tr	1	30[1]	0	0	tr	0

(continued)

*Dashes (—) denote lack of reliable data for a constituent believed to be present in a measurable amount.

APPENDIX 1. (continued)

Item No. (A)	Foods, Approximate Measures, Units, and Weight (Edible Part Unless Footnotes Indicate Otherwise) (B)	Weight	Water (C) Per cent	Food Energy (D) Calories	Protein (E)	Fat (F)	Fatty Acids — Saturated (Total) (G)	Unsaturated — Oleic (H)	Unsaturated — Linoleic (I)	Carbohydrate (J)	Calcium (K)	Phosphorus (L)	Iron (M)	Potassium (N)	Vitamin A Value (O)	Thiamine (P)	Riboflavin (Q)	Niacin (R)	Ascorbic Acid (S)
		g	Per cent	Cal-ories	g	g	g	g	g	g	mg	mg	mg	mg	IU	mg	mg	mg	mg
44	Powdered, made with whole milk....1 c.	80	67	150	3	10	8.5	0.6	0.1	13	72	69	tr	121	290[1]	0.02	0.09	tr	1
45	....1 tbsp	4	67	10	tr	1	0.4	tr	tr	1	4	3	tr	6	10[1]	tr	tr	tr	tr
46	Pressurized....1 c.	70	60	185	1	16	13.2	1.4	0.2	11	4	13	tr	13	330[1]	0	0	0	0
47	....1 tbsp	4	60	10	tr	1	0.8	0.1	tr	1	tr	1	tr	1	20[1]	0	0	0	0
48	Sour dressing (imitation sour cream) made with nonfat dry milk....1 c.	235	75	415	8	39	31.2	4.4	1.1	11	266	205	0.1	380	20[1]	0.09	0.38	0.2	2
49	....1 tbsp	12	75	20	tr	2	1.6	0.2	0.1	1	14	10	tr	19	tr	0.01	0.02	tr	tr
	Ice cream (see Milk desserts, frozen, items 75–80).																		
	Ice milk (see Milk desserts, frozen items 81–83).																		
	Milk Fluid																		
50	Whole (3.3% fat)....1 c.	244	88	150	8	8	5.1	2.1	0.2	11	291	228	0.1	370	310[2]	0.09	0.40	0.2	2
51	Low fat (2%) No milk solids added....1 c.	244	89	120	8	5	2.9	1.2	0.1	12	297	232	0.1	377	500	0.10	0.40	0.2	2
52	Milk solids added Label claims less than 10 g protein per cup....1 c.	245	89	125	9	5	2.9	1.2	0.1	12	313	245	0.1	397	500	0.10	0.42	0.2	2
53	Label claims 10 or more g protein per cup (protein fortified)....1 c.	246	88	135	10	5	3.0	1.2	0.1	14	352	276	0.1	447	500	0.11	0.48	0.2	3
54	Low fat (1%) No milk solids added....1 c.	244	90	100	8	3	1.6	0.7	0.1	12	300	235	0.1	381	500	0.10	0.41	0.2	2
	Milk solids added																		

No.	Food (measure)	Grams	Water (%)	Food energy (cal)	Protein (g)	Fat (g)	Saturated (g)	Oleic (g)	Linoleic (g)	Carbohydrate (g)	Calcium (mg)	Phosphorus (mg)	Iron (mg)	Potassium (mg)	Vitamin A (IU)	Thiamin (mg)	Riboflavin (mg)	Niacin (mg)	Ascorbic acid (mg)
55	Label claims less than 10 g protein per cup . . 1 c	245	90	105	9	2	1.5	0.6	0.1	12	313	245	0.1	397	500	0.10	0.42	0.2	2
56	Label claims 10 or more g protein per cup (protein fortified) . . 1 c	246	89	120	10	3	1.8	0.7	0.1	14	349	273	0.1	444	500	0.11	0.47	0.2	3
57	Nonfat (skim) No milk solids added . . 1 c	245	91	85	8	tr	0.3	0.1	tr	12	302	247	0.1	406	500	0.09	0.34	0.2	2
58	Milk solids added Label claims less than 10 g protein per cup . . 1 c	245	90	90	9	1	0.4	0.1	tr	12	316	255	0.1	418	500	0.10	0.43	0.2	2
59	Label claims 10 or more g protein per cup (protein fortified) . . 1 c	246	89	100	10	1	0.4	0.1	tr	14	352	275	0.1	446	500	0.11	0.48	0.2	3
60	Buttermilk . . 1 c	245	90	100	8	2	1.3	0.5	tr	12	285	219	0.1	371	80[3]	0.08	0.38	0.1	2
61	Canned Evaporated, unsweetened Whole milk . . 1 c	252	74	340	17	19	11.6	5.3	0.4	25	657	510	0.5	764	610[3]	0.12	0.80	0.5	5
62	Skim milk . . 1 c	255	79	200	19	1	.3	0.1	tr	29	738	497	0.7	845	1000[4]	0.11	0.79	0.4	3
63	Sweetened, condensed . . 1 c	306	27	980	24	27	16.8	6.7	0.7	166	868	775	0.6	1136	1000[3]	0.28	1.27	0.6	8
64	Dried Buttermilk . . 1 c	120	3	465	41	7	4.3	1.7	0.2	59	1421	1119	0.4	1910	260[3]	0.47	1.90	1.1	7
65	Nonfat instant Envelope, net wt 3.2 oz[5] . . 1 envelope	91	4	325	32	1	0.4	0.1	tr	47	1120	896	0.3	1552	2160[6]	0.38	1.59	0.8	5
66	Cup[7] . . 1 c	68	4	245	24	tr	0.3	0.1	tr	35	837	670	0.2	1160	1610[6]	0.28	1.19	0.6	4
67	Milk beverages Chocolate milk (commercial) Regular . . 1 c	250	82	210	8	8	5.3	2.2	0.2	26	280	251	0.6	417	300[3]	0.09	0.41	0.3	2
68	Low fat (2%) . . 1 c	250	84	180	8	5	3.1	1.3	0.1	26	284	254	0.6	422	500	0.10	0.42	0.3	2
69	Low fat (1%) . . 1 c	250	85	160	8	3	1.5	0.7	0.1	26	287	257	0.6	426	500	0.10	0.40	0.2	2
70	Eggnog (commercial) . . 1 c	254	74	340	10	19	11.3	5.0	0.6	34	330	278	0.5	420	890	0.09	0.48	0.3	4
71	Malted milk, home-prepared with 1 c whole milk and 2 to 3 heaping tsp malted milk powder about 3/4 oz) Chocolate . . 1 c milk plus 3/4 oz powder	265	81	235	9	9	5.5	—	—	29	304	265	0.5	500	330	0.14	0.43	0.7	2
72	Natural . . 1 c milk plus 3/4 oz powder	265	81	235	11	10	6.0	—	—	27	347	307	0.3	529	380	0.20	0.54	1.3	2
73	Shakes, thick[8] Chocolate, container, net wt 10.6 oz . . 1 container	300	72	355	9	8	5.0	2.0	0.2	63	396	378	0.9	672	260	0.14	0.67	0.4	0
74	Vanilla, container, net wt 11 oz . . 1 container	313	74	350	12	9	5.9	2.4	0.2	56	457	361	0.3	572	360	0.09	0.61	0.5	0

(continued)

APPENDIX 1. (continued)

Milk desserts, frozen
- Ice cream
  - Regular (about 11% fat)

Item No. (A)	Foods, Approximate Measures, Units, and Weight (Edible Part Unless Footnotes Indicate Otherwise) (B)	Water Per-cent (C)	Food Energy Cal-ories (D)	Protein (E)	Fat (F)	Fatty Acids Saturated (Total) (G)	Unsaturated Oleic (H)	Unsaturated Linoleic (I)	Carbohydrate (J)	Calcium (K)	Phosphorus (L)	Iron (M)	Potassium (N)	Vitamin A Value (O)	Thiamine (P)	Riboflavin (Q)	Niacin (R)	Ascorbic Acid (S)
		g		g	g	g	g	g	g	mg	mg	mg	mg	IU	mg	mg	mg	mg
75	Hardened .... ½ gal	1064	61	2155	38	115	71.3	28.8	2.6	254	1406	1075	1.0	2052	4340	0.42	2.63	1.1	6
76	1 c.	133	61	270	5	14	8.9	3.6	0.3	32	176	134	0.1	257	540	0.05	0.33	0.1	1
77	3 fl oz container	50	61	100	2	5	3.4	1.4	0.1	12	66	51	tr	96	200	0.02	0.12	0.1	tr
78	Soft serve (frozen custard) ..1 c	173	60	375	7	23	13.5	5.9	0.6	38	236	199	0.4	338	790	0.08	0.45	0.2	1
79	Rich (about 16% fat), Hardened ½ gal	1188	59	2805	33	190	118.3	47.8	4.3	256	1213	927	0.8	1771	7200	0.36	2.27	0.9	5
80	1 c.	148	59	350	4	24	14.7	6.0	0.5	32	151	115	0.1	221	900	0.04	0.28	0.1	1
81	Ice milk Hardened (about 4.3% fat) ½ gal	1048	69	1470	41	45	28.1	11.3	1.0	232	1409	1035	1.5	2117	1710	0.61	2.78	0.9	6
82	1 c.	131	69	185	5	6	3.5	1.4	0.1	29	176	129	0.1	265	210	0.08	0.35	0.1	1
83	Soft serve (about 2.6% fat) 1 c.	175	70	225	8	5	2.9	1.2	0.1	38	274	202	0.3	412	180	0.12	0.54	0.2	1
84	Sherbet (about 2% fat) ½ gal	1542	66	2160	17	31	19.0	7.7	0.7	469	827	594	2.5	1585	1480	0.26	0.71	1.0	31
85	1 c.	193	66	270	2	4	2.4	1.0	0.1	59	103	74	0.3	198	190	0.03	0.09	0.1	4
86	Milk desserts, other Custard, baked ...1 c.	265	77	305	14	15	6.8	5.4	0.7	29	297	310	1.1	387	930	0.11	0.50	0.3	1
87	Chocolate 1 c.	260	66	385	8	12	7.6	3.3	0.3	67	250	255	1.3	445	390	0.05	0.36	0.3	1
88	Vanilla (blancmange) 1 c.	255	76	285	9	10	6.2	2.5	0.2	41	298	232	tr	352	410	0.08	0.41	0.3	2
89	Tapioca cream 1 c.	165	72	220	8	8	4.1	2.5	0.5	28	173	180	0.7	223	480	0.07	0.30	0.2	2

Puddings
- From home recipe
  - Starch base
    - Chocolate [87]
    - Vanilla (blancmange) [88]
- Tapioca cream [89]
- From mix (chocolate) and milk

90	Regular (cooked)	1 c.	260	70	320	9	8	4.3	2.6	0.2	59	265	247	0.8	354	340	0.05	0.39	0.3	2
91	Instant	1 c.	260	69	325	8	7	3.6	2.2	0.3	63	374	237	1.3	335	340	0.08	0.39	0.3	2
	Yogurt																			
	With added milk solids																			
	Made with low-fat milk																			
92	Fruit-flavored[9]	1 container, net wt 8 oz	227	75	230	10	3	1.8	0.6	0.1	42	343	269	0.2	439	120[10]	0.08	0.40	0.2	1
93	Plain	1 container, net wt 8 oz	227	85	145	12	4	2.3	0.8	0.1	16	415	326	0.2	531	150[10]	0.10	0.49	0.3	2
94	Made with nonfat milk	1 container, net wt 8 oz	227	85	125	13	tr	0.3	0.1	tr	17	452	355	0.2	579	20[10]	0.11	0.53	0.3	2
	Without added milk solids																			
95	Made with whole milk	1 container, net wt 8 oz	227	88	140	8	7	4.8	1.7	0.1	11	274	215	0.1	351	280	0.07	0.32	0.2	1
	EGGS																			
	Eggs, large (24 oz per dozen)																			
	Raw																			
96	Whole, without shell	1 egg	50	75	80	6	6	1.7	2.0	0.6	1	28	90	1.0	65	260	0.04	0.15	tr	0
97	White	1 white	33	88	15	3	tr	0	0	0	tr	4	4	tr	45	0	tr	0.09	tr	0
98	Yolk	1 yolk	17	49	65	3	6	1.7	2.1	0.6	tr	26	86	0.9	15	310	0.04	0.07	tr	0
	Cooked																			
99	Fried in butter	1 egg	46	72	85	5	6	2.4	2.2	0.6	1	26	80	0.9	58	290	0.03	0.13	tr	0
100	Hard-cooked, shell removed	1 egg	50	75	80	6	6	1.7	2.0	0.6	1	28	90	1.0	65	260	0.04	0.14	tr	0
101	Poached	1 egg	50	74	80	6	6	1.7	2.0	0.6	1	28	90	1.0	65	260	0.04	0.13	tr	0
102	Scrambled (milk added) in butter. Also omelet	1 egg	64	76	95	6	7	2.8	2.3	0.6	1	47	97	0.9	85	310	0.04	0.16	tr	0
	FATS, OILS, AND RELATED PRODUCTS																			
	Butter																			
	Regular (1 brick or 4 sticks per lb)																			
103	Stick (½ cup)	1 stick	113	16	815	1	92	57.3	23.1	2.1	tr	27	26	0.2	29	3470[11]	0.01	0.04	tr	0
104	Tablespoon (about ⅛ stick)	1 tbsp	14	16	100	tr	12	7.2	2.9	0.3	tr	3	3	tr	4	430[11]	tr	tr	tr	0
105	Pat (1″ square, ⅓″ high; 90 per lb)	1 pat	5	16	35	tr	4	2.5	1.0	0.1	tr	1	1	tr	1	150[11]	tr	tr	tr	0
	Whipped (6 sticks or two 8-oz containers per lb)																			
106	Stick (½ cup)	1 stick	76	16	540	1	61	38.2	15.4	1.4	tr	18	17	0.1	20	2310[11]	tr	0.03	tr	0
107	Tablespoon (about ⅛ stick)	1 tbsp	9	16	65	tr	8	4.7	1.9	0.2	tr	2	2	tr	2	290[11]	tr	tr	tr	0

(continued)

APPENDIX 1. (continued)

Item No. (A)	Foods, Approximate Measures, Units, and Weight (Edible Part Unless Footnotes Indicate Otherwise) (B)	(g)	Water Per‑cent (C)	Food Energy Cal‑ories (D)	Protein g (E)	Fat g (F)	Saturated (Total) g (G)	Unsaturated Oleic g (H)	Unsaturated Linoleic g (I)	Carbohydrate g (J)	Calcium mg (K)	Phosphorus mg (L)	Iron mg (M)	Potassium mg (N)	Vitamin A Value IU (O)	Thiamine mg (P)	Riboflavin mg (Q)	Niacin mg (R)	Ascorbic Acid mg (S)
108	Pat (1¼" square, ⅓" high; 120 per lb) ....1 pat	4	16	25	tr	3	1.9	0.8	0.1	tr	1	1	tr	1	120[11]	0	tr	tr	0
109	Fats, cooking (vegetable shortenings) ....1 c	200	0	1770	0	200	48.8	88.2	48.4	0	0	0	0	0	0	0	0	0	0
110	....1 tbsp	13	0	110	0	13	3.2	5.7	3.1	0	0	0	0	0	—	0	0	0	0
111	Lard ....1 c	205	0	1850	0	205	81.0	83.8	20.5	0	0	0	0	0	—	0	0	0	0
112	....1 tbsp	13	0	115	0	13	5.1	5.3	1.3	0	0	0	0	0	0	0	0	0	0
	Margarine																		
	Regular (1 brick or 4 sticks per lb)																		
113	Stick (½ cup) ....1 stick	113	16	815	1	92	16.7	42.9	24.9	tr	27	26	0.2	29	3750[12]	0.01	0.04	tr	0
114	Tablespoon (about ⅛ stick) ....1 tbsp	14	16	100	tr	12	2.1	5.3	3.1	tr	3	3	tr	4	470[12]	tr	tr	tr	0
115	Pat (1" square, ⅓" high; 90 per lb) ....1 pat	5	16	35	tr	4	0.7	1.9	1.1	tr	1	1	tr	1	170[12]	tr	tr	tr	0
116	Soft, two 8‑oz containers per lb ....1 container	227	16	1635	1	184	32.5	71.5	65.4	tr	53	52	0.4	59	7500[12]	0.01	0.08	tr	0
117	....1 tbsp	14	16	100	tr	12	2.0	4.5	4.1	tr	3	3	tr	4	470[12]	tr	tr	tr	0
	Whipped (6 sticks per lb)																		
118	Stick (½ cup) ....1 stick	76	16	545	tr	61	11.2	28.7	16.7	tr	18	17	0.1	20	2500[12]	tr	0.03	tr	0
119	Tablespoon (about ⅛ stick) ....1 tbsp	9	16	70	tr	8	1.4	3.6	2.1	tr	2	2	tr	2	310[12]	tr	tr	tr	0
	Oils, salad or cooking																		
120	Corn ....1 c	218	0	1925	0	218	27.7	53.6	125.1	0	0	0	0	0	—	0	0	0	0
121	....1 tbsp	14	0	120	0	14	1.7	3.3	7.8	0	0	0	0	0	—	0	0	0	0
122	Olive ....1 c	216	0	1910	0	216	30.7	154.4	17.7	0	0	0	0	0	—	0	0	0	0
123	....1 tbsp	14	0	120	0	14	1.9	9.7	1.1	0	0	0	0	0	—	0	0	0	0
124	Peanut ....1 c	216	0	1910	0	216	37.4	98.5	67.0	0	0	0	0	0	—	0	0	0	0
125	....1 tbsp	14	0	120	0	14	2.3	6.2	4.2	0	0	0	0	0	—	0	0	0	0

Fatty Acids: columns (G) Saturated (Total), (H) Unsaturated Oleic, (I) Unsaturated Linoleic.

No.	Food (measure)	Grams	Water (%)	Food energy	Protein (g)	Fat (g)	Saturated (g)	Oleic (g)	Linoleic (g)	Carbohydrate (g)	Calcium (mg)	Phosphorus (mg)	Iron (mg)	Potassium (mg)	Vitamin A (IU)	Thiamin (mg)	Riboflavin (mg)	Niacin (mg)	Ascorbic acid (mg)
126	Safflower . . . . 1 c.	218	0	1925	0	218	20.5	25.9	159.8	0	0	0	0	0	—	0	0	0	0
127	1 tbsp	14	0	120	0	14	1.3	1.6	10.0	0	0	0	0	0	—	0	0	0	0
128	Soybean oil, hydrogenated (partially hardened) . . . 1 c.	218	0	1925	0	218	31.8	93.1	75.6	0	0	0	0	0	—	0	0	0	0
129	1 tbsp	14	0	120	0	14	2.0	5.8	4.7	0	0	0	0	0	—	0	0	0	0
130	Soybean-cottonseed oil blend, hydrogenated . . . 1 c.	218	0	1925	0	218	38.2	63.0	99.6	0	0	0	0	0	—	0	0	0	0
131	1 tbsp	14	0	120	0	14	2.4	3.9	6.2	0	0	0	0	0	—	0	0	0	0
	Salad dressings																		
	Commercial																		
	Blue cheese																		
132	Regular . . . . 1 tbsp	15	32	75	1	8	1.6	1.7	3.8	1	12	11	tr	6	30	tr	0.02	tr	tr
133	Low calorie (5 cal per tsp) . . 1 tbsp	16	84	10	tr	1	0.5	0.3	tr	1	10	8	tr	5	30	tr	0.01	tr	tr
	French																		
134	Regular . . . . . . 1 tbsp	16	39	65	tr	6	1.1	1.3	3.2	3	2	2	0.1	13	—	—	—	—	—
135	Low calorie (5 cal per tsp) . . 1 tbsp	16	77	15	tr	1	0.1	0.1	0.4	2	2	2	0.1	13	—	—	—	—	—
	Italian																		
136	Regular . . . . . . 1 tbsp	15	28	85	tr	9	1.6	1.9	4.7	1	2	1	tr	2	tr	tr	tr	tr	—
137	Low calorie (2 cal per tsp) . . 1 tbsp	15	90	10	tr	1	0.1	0.1	0.4	tr	tr	1	tr	2	tr	tr	tr	tr	—
138	Mayonnaise . . . . . 1 tbsp	14	15	100	tr	11	2.0	2.4	5.6	tr	3	4	0.1	5	40	tr	0.01	tr	—
	Mayonnaise type																		
139	Regular . . . . . . 1 tbsp	15	41	65	tr	6	1.1	1.4	3.2	2	2	4	tr	1	30	tr	tr	tr	tr
140	Low calorie (8 cal per tsp) . . 1 tbsp	16	81	20	tr	2	0.4	0.4	1.0	3	3	4	tr	1	40	tr	tr	tr	tr
141	Tartar sauce, regular . . 1 tbsp	14	34	75	tr	8	1.5	1.8	4.1	1	3	4	0.1	11	30	tr	tr	tr	tr
	Thousand Island																		
142	Regular . . . . . . 1 tbsp	16	32	80	tr	8	1.4	1.7	4.0	2	2	3	0.1	18	50	tr	tr	tr	tr
143	Low calorie (10 cal per tsp) . . 1 tbsp	15	68	25	tr	2	0.4	0.4	1.0	2	2	3	0.1	17	50	tr	tr	tr	tr
	From home recipe																		
144	Cooked type[13] . . . . 1 tbsp	16	68	25	1	2	0.5	0.6	0.3	2	14	15	0.1	19	80	0.01	0.03	tr	tr

FISH, SHELLFISH, MEAT, POULTRY, AND RELATED PRODUCTS

No.	Food (measure)	Grams	Water (%)	Food energy	Protein (g)	Fat (g)	Saturated (g)	Oleic (g)	Linoleic (g)	Carbohydrate (g)	Calcium (mg)	Phosphorus (mg)	Iron (mg)	Potassium (mg)	Vitamin A (IU)	Thiamin (mg)	Riboflavin (mg)	Niacin (mg)	Ascorbic acid (mg)
	Fish and shellfish																		
145	Bluefish, baked with butter or margarine . . . 3 oz	85	68	135	22	4	—	—	—	0	25	244	0.6	—	40	0.09	0.08	1.6	—
	Clams																		
146	Raw, meat only . . . 3 oz	85	82	65	11	1	—	—	tr	2	59	138	5.2	154	90	0.08	0.15	1.1	8
147	Canned, solids and liquid . . . 3 oz	85	86	45	7	1	0.2	tr	tr	2	47	116	3.5	119	—	0.01	0.09	0.9	—

(continued)

APPENDIX 1. (continued)

Fatty Acids — Unsaturated columns comprise Oleic (H) and Linoleic (I); Saturated (Total) (G), Oleic (H), and Linoleic (I) make up the Fatty Acids group.

Item No. (A)	Foods, Approximate Measures, Units, and Weight (Edible Part Unless Footnotes Indicate Otherwise) (B)	g	Water Per-cent (C)	Food Energy Cal-ories (D)	Protein g (E)	Fat g (F)	Saturated (Total) g (G)	Oleic g (H)	Linoleic g (I)	Carbohydrate g (J)	Calcium mg (K)	Phosphorus mg (L)	Iron mg (M)	Potassium mg (N)	Vitamin A Value IU (O)	Thiamine mg (P)	Riboflavin mg (Q)	Niacin mg (R)	Ascorbic Acid mg (S)
148	Crabmeat (white or king), canned, not pressed down ...1 c	135	77	135	24	3	0.6	0.4	0.1	1	61	246	1.1	149	—	0.11	0.11	2.6	—
149	Fish sticks, breaded, cooked, frozen (stick, 4" × 1" × 1/2") ...1 fish stick or 1 oz	28	66	50	5	3	—	—	—	2	3	47	0.1	—	0	0.01	0.02	—	—
150	Haddock, breaded, fried[14] ...3 oz	85	66	140	17	5	1.4	2.2	1.2	5	34	210	1.0	296	—	0.03	0.06	2.7	2
151	Ocean perch, breaded, fried[14] ...1 fillet	85	59	195	16	11	2.7	4.4	2.3	6	28	192	1.1	242	—	0.10	0.10	1.6	—
152	Oysters, raw, meat only (13–19 medium Selects) ...1 c	240	85	160	20	4	1.3	0.2	0.1	8	226	343	13.2	290	740	0.34	0.43	6.0	—
153	Salmon, pink, canned, solids and liquid ...3 oz	85	71	120	17	5	0.9	0.8	0.1	0	167[15]	243	0.7	307	60	0.03	0.16	6.8	—
154	Sardines, Atlantic, canned in oil, drained solids ...3 oz	85	62	175	20	9	3.0	2.5	0.5	0	372	424	2.5	502	190	0.02	0.17	4.6	—
155	Scallops, frozen, breaded, fried, reheated ...6 scallops	90	60	175	20	9	—	—	—	9	—	—	—	—	—	—	—	—	—
156	Shad, baked with butter or margarine, bacon ...3 oz	85	64	170	20	10	—	—	—	0	20	266	0.5	320	30	0.11	0.22	7.3	—
	Shrimp																		
157	Canned meat ...3 oz	85	70	100	21	1	0.1	tr	1	1	98	224	2.6	104	50	0.01	0.03	1.5	—
158	French fried[16] ...3 oz	85	57	190	17	9	2.3	3.7	2.0	9	61	162	1.7	195	—	0.03	0.07	2.3	—
159	Tuna, canned in oil, drained solids ...3 oz	85	61	170	24	7	1.7	1.7	0.7	0	7	199	1.6	—	70	0.04	0.10	10.1	—
160	Tuna salad[17] ...1 c	205	70	350	30	22	4.3	6.3	6.7	7	41	291	2.7	—	590	0.08	0.23	10.3	2
	Meat and meat products																		
161	Bacon (20 slices per lb, raw), broiled or fried, crisp ...2 slices	15	8	85	4	8	2.5	3.7	0.7	tr	2	34	0.5	35	0	0.08	0.05	0.8	—

Item	Food, approximate measure, and weight (g)	Grams	Water (%)	Food energy	Protein (g)	Fat (g)	Saturated (g)	Oleic (g)	Linoleic (g)	Carbohydrate (g)	Calcium (mg)	Phosphorus (mg)	Iron (mg)	Vitamin A (IU)	Thiamin (mg)	Riboflavin (mg)	Niacin (mg)	Ascorbic acid (mg)
	Beef,[18] cooked																	
	Cuts braised, simmered, or pot roasted																	
162	Lean and fat (piece, 2½" × 2½" × ¾") ..... 3 oz	85	53	245	23	16	6.8	6.5	0.4	0	10	114	2.9	30	0.04	0.18	3.6	—
163	Lean only from item 162 ... 2.5 oz.	72	62	140	22	5	2.1	1.8	0.2	0	10	108	2.7	10	0.04	0.17	3.3	—
	Ground beef, broiled																	
164	Lean with 10% fat .... 3 oz or patty 3" × ⅝" ...	85	60	185	23	10	4.0	3.9	0.3	0	10	196	3.0	20	0.08	0.20	5.1	—
165	Lean with 21% fat .... 2.9 oz or patty 3" × ⅝" ...	82	54	235	20	17	7.0	6.7	0.4	0	9	159	2.6	30	0.07	0.17	4.4	—
	Roast, oven-cooked, no liquid added																	
	Relatively fat, such as rib																	
166	Lean and fat (2 pieces, 4⅛" × 2¼" × ¼") ..... 3 oz ...	85	40	375	17	33	14.0	13.6	0.8	0	8	158	2.2	70	0.05	0.13	3.1	—
167	Lean only from item 166 .... 1.8 oz ...	51	57	125	14	7	3.0	2.5	0.3	0	6	131	1.8	10	0.04	0.11	2.6	—
	Relatively lean, such as Heel of round																	
168	Lean and fat (2 pieces, 4⅛" × 2¼" × ¼") ..... 3 oz ...	85	62	165	25	7	2.8	2.7	0.2	0	11	208	3.2	10	0.06	0.19	4.5	—
169	Lean only from item 168 .... 2.8 oz ...	78	65	125	24	3	1.2	1.0	0.1	0	10	199	3.0	tr	0.06	0.18	4.3	—
	Steak																	
	Relatively fat-sirloin, broiled																	
170	Lean and fat (piece, 2½" × 2½" × ¾") ..... 3 oz ...	85	44	330	20	27	11.3	11.1	0.6	0	9	162	2.5	50	0.05	0.15	4.0	—
171	Lean only from item 170 .... 2.0 oz ...	56	59	115	18	4	1.8	1.6	0.2	0	7	146	2.2	10	0.05	0.14	3.6	—
	Relatively lean-round, braised																	
172	Lean and fat (piece, 4⅛" × 2¼" × ½") ..... 3 oz ...	85	55	220	24	13	5.5	5.2	0.4	0	10	213	3.0	20	0.07	0.19	4.8	—
173	Lean only from item 172 .... 2.4 oz ...	68	61	130	21	4	1.7	1.5	0.2	0	9	182	2.5	10	0.05	0.16	4.1	—
	Beef, canned																	
174	Corned beef .... 3 oz	85	59	185	22	10	4.9	4.5	0.2	0	17	90	3.7	—	0.01	0.20	2.9	—
175	Corned beef hash......... 1 c ...	220	67	400	19	25	11.9	10.9	0.5	24	29	147	4.4	—	0.02	0.20	4.6	—
176	Beef, dried, chipped ... 2½ oz jar ...	71	48	145	24	4	2.1	2.0	0.1	0	14	287	3.6	—	0.05	0.23	2.7	0
177	Beef and vegetable stew ...... 1 c ...	245	82	220	16	11	4.9	4.5	0.2	15	29	184	2.9	2400	0.15	0.17	4.7	17

(continued)

609

APPENDIX 1. (continued)

Item No. (A)	Foods, Approximate Measures, Units, and Weight (Edible Part Unless Footnotes Indicate Otherwise) (B)	(g)	Water Per-cent (C)	Food Energy Cal-ories (D)	Protein g (E)	Fat g (F)	Saturated (Total) g (G)	Unsaturated Oleic g (H)	Unsaturated Linoleic g (I)	Carbohydrate g (J)	Calcium mg (K)	Phosphorus mg (L)	Iron mg (M)	Potassium mg (N)	Vitamin A Value IU (O)	Thiamine mg (P)	Riboflavin mg (Q)	Niacin mg (R)	Ascorbic Acid mg (S)
178	Beef potpie (home recipe), baked[19] (piece, 1/3 of 9" diam pie) ..... 1 piece	210	55	515	21	30	7.9	12.8	6.7	39	29	149	3.8	334	1720	0.30	0.30	5.5	6
179	Chili con carne with beans, canned ..... 1 c.	255	72	340	19	16	7.5	6.8	0.3	31	82	321	4.3	594	150	0.08	0.18	3.3	—
180	Chop suey with beef and pork (home recipe) ..... 1 c.	250	75	300	26	17	8.5	6.2	0.7	13	60	248	4.8	425	600	0.28	0.38	5.0	33
181	Heart, beef, lean, braised ..... 3 oz	85	61	160	27	5	1.5	1.1	0.6	1	5	154	5.0	197	20	0.21	1.04	6.5	1
	Lamb, cooked																		
	Chop, rib (cut 3 per lb with bone), broiled																		
182	Lean and fat ..... 3.1 oz	89	43	360	18	32	14.8	12.1	1.2	0	8	139	1.0	200	—	0.11	0.19	4.1	—
183	Lean only from item 182 ..... 2 oz	57	60	120	16	6	2.5	2.1	0.2	0	6	121	1.1	174	—	0.09	0.15	3.4	—
	Leg, roasted																		
184	Lean and fat (2 pieces, 4⅛" × 2¼" × ¼") ..... 3 oz	85	54	235	22	16	7.3	6.0	0.6	0	9	177	1.4	241	—	0.13	0.23	4.7	—
185	Lean only from item 184 ..... 2.5 oz	71	62	130	20	5	2.1	1.8	0.2	0	9	169	1.4	227	—	0.12	0.21	4.4	—
	Shoulder, roasted																		
186	Lean and fat (3 pieces, 2½" × 2½" × ¼") ..... 3 oz	85	50	285	18	23	10.8	8.8	0.9	0	9	146	1.0	206	—	0.11	0.20	4.0	—
187	Lean only from item 186 ..... 2.3 oz	64	61	130	17	6	3.6	2.3	0.2	0	8	140	1.0	193	—	0.10	0.18	3.7	—
188	Liver, beef, fried[20] (slice, 6½" × 2⅜" × ⅜") ..... 3 oz	85	56	195	22	9	2.5	3.5	0.9	5	9	405	7.5	323	45390[21]	0.22	3.56	14.0	23
	Pork, cured, cooked																		

Item	Food		Grams	Water %	Cal.	Protein	Fat	Sat.	Oleic	Lino.	Carb.	Ca	P	Fe	K	Vit. A	Thiamin	Ribo.	Niacin	Asc.
189	Ham, light cure, lean and fat, roasted (2 pieces, 4⅛″ × 2¼″ × ¼″)[22]	3 oz	85	54	245	18	19	6.8	7.9	1.7	0	8	146	2.2	199	0	0.40	0.15	3.1	—
	Luncheon meat																			
190	Boiled ham, slice (8 per 8-oz pkg)	1 oz	28	59	65	5	5	1.7	2.0	0.4	0	3	47	0.8	—	0	0.12	0.04	0.7	—
	Canned, spiced or unspiced:																			
191	Slice, approximately 3″ × 2″ × ½″	1 slice	60	55	175	9	15	5.4	6.7	1.0	1	5	65	1.3	133	0	0.19	0.13	1.8	—
	Pork, fresh,[18]																			
	Chop, loin (cut 3 per lb with bone), broiled:																			
192	Lean and fat	2.7 oz	78	42	305	19	25	8.9	10.4	2.2	0	9	209	2.7	216	0	0.75	0.22	4.5	—
193	Lean only from item 192	2 oz	56	53	150	17	9	3.1	3.6	0.8	0	7	181	2.2	192	0	0.63	0.18	3.8	—
	Roast, oven-cooked, no liquid added:																			
194	Lean and fat (piece, 2½″ × 2½″ × ¾″)	3 oz	85	46	310	21	24	8.7	10.2	2.2	0	9	218	2.7	233	0	0.78	0.22	4.8	—
195	Lean only from item 194	2.4 oz	68	55	175	20	10	3.5	4.1	0.8	0	9	211	2.6	224	0	0.73	0.21	4.4	—
	Shoulder cut, simmered:																			
196	Lean and fat (3 pieces, 2½″ × 2½″ × ¼″)	3 oz	85	46	320	20	26	9.3	10.9	2.3	0	9	118	2.6	158	0	0.46	0.21	4.1	—
197	Lean only from item 196	2.2 oz	63	60	135	18	6	2.2	2.6	0.6	0	8	111	2.3	146	0	0.42	0.19	3.7	—
	Sausages (see also Luncheon meat, items 190–191):																			
198	Bologna, slice (8 per 8-oz pkg)	1 slice	28	56	85	3	8	3.0	3.4	0.5	tr	2	36	0.5	65	—	0.05	0.06	0.7	—
199	Braunschweiger, slice (6 per 6-oz pkg)	1 slice	28	53	90	4	8	2.6	3.4	0.8	1	3	69	1.7	—	1850	0.05	0.41	2.3	—
200	Brown and serve (10–11 per 8-oz pkg), browned	1 link	17	40	70	3	6	2.3	2.8	0.7	tr	—	—	—	—	—	—	—	—	—
201	Deviled ham, canned	1 tbsp	13	51	45	2	4	1.5	1.8	0.4	0	1	12	0.3	—	0	0.02	0.01	0.2	—
202	Frankfurter (8 per 1-lb pkg), cooked (reheated)	1 frankfurter	56	57	170	7	15	5.6	6.5	1.2	1	3	57	0.8	—	—	0.08	0.11	1.4	—
203	Meat, potted (beef, chicken, turkey), canned	1 tbsp	13	61	30	2	2	—	—	—	0	—	—	—	—	—	tr	0.03	0.2	—
204	Pork link (16 per 1-lb pkg), cooked	1 link	13	35	60	2	6	2.1	2.4	0.5	tr	1	21	0.3	35	0	0.10	0.04	0.5	—
	Salami																			
205	Dry type, slice (12 per 4-oz pkg)	1 slice	10	30	45	2	4	1.6	1.6	0.1	tr	1	28	0.4	—	—	0.04	0.03	0.5	—

(continued)

APPENDIX 1. (continued)

Item No. (A)	Foods, Approximate Measures, Units, and Weight (Edible Part Unless Footnotes Indicate Otherwise) (B)	Water (C) Per-cent	Food Energy (D) Calories	Protein (E) g	Fat (F) g	Fatty Acids Saturated (Total) (G) g	Unsaturated Oleic (H) g	Unsaturated Linoleic (I) g	Carbohydrate (K) g	Calcium (L) mg	Phosphorus (M) mg	Iron (N) mg	Potassium (O) mg	Vitamin A Value (P) IU	Thiamine (Q) mg	Riboflavin (R) mg	Niacin (S) mg	Ascorbic Acid mg
206	Cooked type, slice (8 per 8-oz pkg) ....1 slice (28 g)	51	90	5	7	3.1	3.0	0.2	tr	3	57	0.7	—	—	0.07	0.07	1.2	—
207	Vienna sausage (7 per 4-oz can) ....1 sausage (16 g)	63	40	2	3	1.2	1.4	0.2	tr	1	24	0.3	—	—	0.01	0.02	0.4	—
	Veal, medium fat, cooked, bone removed																	
208	Cutlet (4⅛″ × 2¼″ × ½″), braised or broiled ....3 oz (85 g)	60	185	23	9	4.0	3.4	0.4	0	9	196	2.7	258	—	0.06	0.21	4.6	—
209	Rib (2 pieces, 4⅛″ × 2¼″ × ¼″), roasted ....3 oz (85 g)	55	230	23	14	6.1	5.1	0.6	0	10	211	2.9	259	—	0.11	0.26	6.6	—
	Poultry and poultry products Chicken, cooked																	
210	Breast, fried,[23] bones removed, ½ breast (3.3 oz with bones) ....2.8 oz (79 g)	58	160	26	5	1.4	1.8	1.1	1	9	218	1.3	—	70	0.04	0.17	11.6	—
211	Drumstick, fried,[23] bones removed (2 oz with bones) ....1.3 oz (38 g)	55	90	12	4	1.1	1.3	0.9	tr	6	89	0.9	—	50	0.03	0.15	2.7	—
212	Half broiler, broiled, bones removed (10.4 oz with bones) ....6.2 oz (176 g)	71	240	42	7	2.2	2.5	1.3	0	16	355	3.0	483	160	0.09	0.34	15.5	—
213	Chicken, canned, boneless ....3 oz (85 g)	65	170	18	10	3.2	3.8	2.0	0	18	210	1.3	117	200	0.03	0.11	3.7	3
214	Chicken à la king (home recipe) ....1 c (245 g)	68	470	27	34	12.7	14.3	3.3	12	127	358	2.5	404	1130	0.10	0.42	5.4	12
215	Chicken and noodles, cooked (home recipe) ....1 c (240 g)	71	365	22	18	5.9	7.1	3.5	26	26	247	2.2	149	430	0.05	0.17	4.3	tr

FRUITS AND FRUIT PRODUCTS

No.	Food	Measure	g	%	Cal	Pro	Fat	Sat	Oleic	Lin	Carb	Ca	P	Fe	K	Vit A	Thia	Ribo	Niac	Asc
	Chicken chow mein																			
216	Canned	1 c	250	89	95	7	tr	—	—	—	18	45	85	1.3	418	150	0.05	0.10	1.0	13
217	From home recipe	1 c	250	78	255	31	10	2.4	3.4	3.1	10	58	293	2.5	473	280	0.08	0.23	4.3	10
218	Chicken potpie (home recipe), baked,[19] piece (⅓ or 9″ diam pie)	1 piece	232	57	545	23	31	11.3	10.9	5.6	42	70	232	3.0	343	3090	0.34	0.31	5.5	5
	Turkey, roasted, flesh without skin																			
219	Dark meat, piece, 2½″ × 1⅝″ × ¼″	4 pieces	85	61	175	26	7	2.1	1.5	1.5	0	—	—	2.0	338	—	0.03	0.20	3.6	—
220	Light meat, piece, 4″ × 2″ × ¼″	2 pieces	85	62	150	28	3	0.9	0.6	0.7	0	—	—	1.0	349	—	0.04	0.12	9.4	—
	Light and dark meat																			
221	Chopped or diced	1 c	140	61	265	44	9	2.5	1.7	1.8	0	11	351	2.5	514	—	0.07	0.25	10.8	—
222	Pieces (1 slice white meat, 4″ × 2″ × ¼″ with 2 slices dark meat, 2½″ × 1⅝″ × ¼″)	3 pieces	85	61	160	27	5	1.5	1.0	1.1	0	7	213	1.5	312	—	0.04	0.15	6.5	—
	FRUITS AND FRUIT PRODUCTS																			
	Apples, raw, unpeeled, without cores																			
223	2¾″ diam (about 3 per lb with cores)	1 apple	138	84	80	tr	1	—	—	—	20	10	14	0.4	152	120	0.04	0.03	0.1	6
224	3¼″ diam (about 2 per lb with cores)	1 apple	212	84	125	tr	1	—	—	—	31	15	21	0.6	233	190	0.06	0.04	0.2	8
225	Apple juice, bottled or canned[24]	1 c	248	88	120	tr	tr	—	—	—	30	15	22	1.5	250	—	0.02	0.05	0.2	2[25]
	Applesauce, canned																			
226	Sweetened	1 c	255	76	230	1	tr	—	—	—	61	10	13	1.3	166	100	0.05	0.03	0.1	3[25]
227	Unsweetened	1 c	244	89	100	tr	tr	—	—	—	26	10	12	1.2	190	100	0.05	0.02	0.1	2[25]
	Apricots																			
228	Raw, without pits (about 12 per lb with pits)	3 apricots	107	85	55	1	tr	—	—	—	14	18	25	0.5	301	2890	0.03	0.04	0.6	11
229	Canned in heavy syrup (halves and syrup)	1 c	258	77	220	2	tr	—	—	—	57	28	39	0.8	604	4490	0.05	0.05	1.0	10
	Dried																			
230	Uncooked (28 large or 37 medium halves per cup)	1 c	130	25	340	7	1	—	—	—	86	87	140	7.2	1273	14,170	0.01	0.21	4.3	16
231	Cooked, unsweetened, fruit and liquid	1 c	250	76	215	4	1	—	—	—	54	55	88	4.5	795	7500	0.01	0.13	2.5	8
232	Apricot nectar, canned	1 c	251	85	145	1	tr	—	—	—	37	23	30	0.5	379	2380	0.03	0.03	0.5	36[26]
	Avocados, raw, whole, without skins and seeds																			
233	California, mid- and late-winter (with skin and seed, 3⅛″ diam; wt, 10 oz)	1 avocado	216	74	370	5	37	5.5	22.0	3.7	13	22	91	1.3	1303	630	0.24	0.43	3.5	30

(continued)

APPENDIX 1. (continued)

Item No. (A)	Foods, Approximate Measures, Units, and Weight (Edible Part Unless Footnotes Indicate Otherwise) (B)	Water Per-cent (C)	Food Energy Cal-ories (D)	Protein g (E)	Fat g (F)	Fatty Acids Saturated (Total) g (G)	Unsaturated Oleic g (H)	Unsaturated Linoleic g (I)	Carbo-hydrate g (J)	Calcium mg (K)	Phos-phorus mg (L)	Iron mg (M)	Potassium mg (N)	Vitamin A Value IU (O)	Thiamine mg (P)	Riboflavin mg (Q)	Niacin mg (R)	Ascorbic Acid mg (S)
234	Florida, late summer and fall (with skin and seed, 3⅛″ diam; wt, 1 lb)........1 avocado... 304	78	390	4	33	6.7	15.7	5.3	27	30	128	1.8	1836	880	0.33	0.61	4.9	43
235	Banana without peel (about 2.6 per lb with peel).........1 banana ... 119	76	100	1	tr	—	—	—	26	10	31	0.8	440	230	0.06	0.07	0.8	12
236	Banana flakes.........1 tbsp... 6	3	20	tr	tr	—	—	—	5	2	6	0.2	92	50	0.01	0.01	0.2	tr
237	Blackberries, raw.........1 c... 144	85	85	2	1	—	—	—	19	46	27	1.3	245	290	0.04	0.06	0.6	30
238	Blueberries, raw.........1 c... 145	83	90	1	1	—	—	—	22	22	19	1.5	117	150	0.04	0.09	0.7	20
	Cantaloupe. See Muskmelons (item 271)																	
	Cherries																		
239	Sour (tart), red, pitted, canned, water pack.........1 c... 244	88	105	2	tr	—	—	—	26	37	32	0.7	317	1660	0.07	0.05	0.5	12
240	Sweet, raw, without pits and stems.........10 cherries... 68	80	45	1	tr	—	—	—	12	15	13	0.3	129	70	0.03	0.04	0.3	7
241	Cranberry juice cocktail, bottled, sweetened.........1 c... 253	83	165	tr	tr	—	—	—	42	13	8	0.8	25	tr	0.03	0.03	0.1	81[27]
242	Cranberry sauce, sweetened, canned, strained.........1 c... 277	62	405	tr	1	—	—	—	104	13	11	0.6	83	60	0.03	0.03	0.1	6
	Dates																		
243	Whole, without pits.........10 dates... 80	23	220	2	tr	—	—	—	58	47	50	2.4	518	40	0.07	0.08	1.8	0
244	Chopped.........1 c... 178	23	490	4	1	—	—	—	130	105	112	5.3	1153	90	0.16	0.18	3.9	0
245	Fruit cocktail, canned, in heavy syrup.........1 c... 255	80	195	1	tr	—	—	—	50	23	31	1.0	411	360	0.05	0.03	1.0	5
	Grapefruit																		
	Raw, medium, 3¾″ diam (about 1 lb 1 oz)																		

No.	Food, approximate measure	Measure	Grams	%	Cal.			tr												
246	Pink or red ... ½ grapefruit with peel[28]		241	89	50	1	tr	—	—	—	13	20	20	0.5	166	540	0.05	0.02	0.2	44
247	White ... ½ grapefruit with peel[28]		241	89	45	1	tr	—	—	—	12	19	19	0.5	159	10	0.05	0.02	0.2	44
248	Canned, sections with syrup	1 c.	254	81	180	2	tr	—	—	—	45	33	36	0.8	343	30	0.08	0.05	0.5	76
	Grapefruit juice																			
249	Raw, pink, red or white	1 c.	246	90	95	1	tr	—	—	—	23	22	37	0.5	399	(29)	0.10	0.05	0.5	93
	Canned, white																			
250	Unsweetened	1 c.	247	89	100	1	tr	—	—	—	24	20	35	1.0	400	20	0.07	0.05	0.5	84
251	Sweetened	1 c.	250	86	135	1	tr	—	—	—	32	20	35	1.0	405	30	0.08	0.05	0.5	78
	Frozen, concentrate, unsweetened																			
252	Undiluted, 6-fl oz can		207	62	300	4	1	—	—	—	72	70	124	0.8	1250	60	0.29	0.12	1.4	286
253	Diluted with 3 parts water by volume	1 c.	247	89	100	1	tr	—	—	—	24	25	42	0.2	420	20	0.10	0.04	0.5	96
254	Dehydrated crystals, prepared with water (1 lb yields about 1 gal)	1 c.	247	90	100	1	tr	—	—	—	24	22	40	0.2	412	20	0.10	0.05	0.5	91
	Grapes, European type (adherent skin), raw																			
255	Thompson Seedless	10 grapes	50	81	35	tr	tr	—	—	—	9	6	10	0.2	87	50	0.03	0.02	0.2	2
256	Tokay and Emperor, seeded types	10 grapes[30]	60	81	40	tr	tr	—	—	—	10	7	11	0.2	99	60	0.03	0.02	0.2	2
	Grape juice																			
257	Canned or bottled	1 c.	253	83	165	1	tr	—	—	—	42	28	30	0.8	293	—	0.10	0.05	0.5	tr[25]
	Frozen concentrate, sweetened																			
258	Undiluted, 6-fl oz can	1 can.	216	53	395	1	tr	—	—	—	100	22	32	0.9	255	40	0.13	0.22	1.5	32[31]
259	Diluted with 3 parts water by volume	1 c.	250	86	135	1	tr	—	—	—	33	8	10	0.3	85	10	0.05	0.08	0.5	10[31]
260	Grape drink, canned	1 c.	250	86	135	tr	tr	—	—	—	35	8	8	0.3	88	—	0.03[32]	0.03[32]	0.3	(32)
261	Lemon, raw, size 165, without peel and seeds (about 4 per lb with peels and seeds)	1 lemon	74	90	20	1	tr	—	—	—	6	19	12	0.4	102	10	0.03	0.01	0.1	39
	Lemon juice																			
262	Raw	1 c.	244	91	60	1	tr	—	—	—	20	17	24	0.5	344	50	0.07	0.02	0.2	112
263	Canned, or bottled, unsweetened	1 c.	244	92	55	1	tr	—	—	—	19	17	24	0.5	344	50	0.07	0.02	0.2	102
264	Frozen, single-strength, unsweetened, 6-fl oz can	1 c.	183	92	40	1	tr	—	—	—	13	13	16	0.5	258	40	0.05	0.02	0.2	81
	Lemonade concentrate, frozen																			
265	Undiluted, 6-fl oz can	1 can.	219	49	425	tr	tr	—	—	—	112	9	13	0.4	153	40	0.05	0.06	0.7	66
266	Diluted with 4⅓ parts water by volume	1 c.	248	89	105	tr	tr	—	—	—	28	2	3	0.1	40	10	0.01	0.02	0.2	17

(continued)

APPENDIX 1. (continued)

Item No. (A)	Foods, Approximate Measures, Units, and Weight (Edible Part Unless Footnotes Indicate Otherwise) (B)	Water per cent (C) g	Water per cent (C)	Food Energy Cal-ories (D)	Protein (E) g	Fat (F) g	Fatty Acids Saturated (Total) (G) g	Unsaturated Oleic (H) g	Unsaturated Linoleic (I) g	Carbohydrate (J) g	Calcium (K) mg	Phosphorus (L) mg	Iron (M) mg	Potassium (N) mg	Vitamin A Value (O) IU	Thiamine (P) mg	Riboflavin (Q) mg	Niacin (R) mg	Ascorbic Acid (S) mg
	Limeade concentrate, frozen																		
267	Undiluted, 6-fl oz can .... 1 can	218	50	410	tr	tr	—	—	—	108	11	13	0.2	129	tr	0.02	0.02	0.2	26
268	Diluted with 4⅓ parts water by volume .... 1 c	247	89	100	tr	tr	—	—	—	27	3	3	tr	32	tr	tr	tr	tr	6
	Lime juice																		
269	Raw .... 1 c	246	90	65	1	tr	—	—	—	22	22	27	0.5	256	20	0.05	0.02	0.2	79
270	Canned, unsweetened ...... 1 c	246	90	65	1	tr	—	—	—	22	22	27	0.5	256	20	0.05	0.02	0.2	52
	Muskmelons, raw, with rind, without seed cavity																		
271	Cantaloupe, orange-fleshed (with rind and seed cavity, 5" diam, 2⅓ lb) .. ½ melon with rind[33]	477	91	80	2	tr	—	—	—	20	38	44	1.1	682	9240	0.11	0.08	1.6	90
272	Honeydew (with rind and seed cavity, 6½" diam, 5¼ lb) .... 1/10 melon with rind[33]	226	91	50	1	tr	—	—	—	11	21	24	0.6	374	60	0.06	0.04	0.9	34
	Oranges, all commercial varieties, raw																		
273	Whole, 2⅝" diam, without peel and seeds (about 2½ per lb with peel and seeds) .... 1 orange	131	86	65	1	tr	—	—	—	16	54	26	0.5	263	260	0.13	0.05	0.5	66
274	Sections without membranes .. 1 c	180	86	90	2	tr	—	—	—	22	74	36	0.7	360	360	0.18	0.07	0.7	90
	Orange juice																		
275	Raw, all varieties .... 1 c	248	88	110	2	tr	—	—	—	26	27	42	0.5	496	500	0.22	0.07	1.0	124

No.	Food, approximate measure, and weight (in grams)		Water (%)	Food energy	Protein	Fat	Saturated	Oleic	Linoleic	Carbohydrate	Calcium	Phosphorus	Iron	Potassium	Vitamin A	Thiamin	Riboflavin	Niacin	Ascorbic acid
276	Canned, unsweetened ...1 c	249	87	120	2	tr	—	—	—	28	25	45	1.0	496	500	0.17	0.05	0.7	100
	Frozen concentrate																		
277	Undiluted, 6-fl oz can ...1 can	213	55	360	5	tr	—	—	—	87	75	126	0.9	1500	1620	0.68	0.11	2.8	360
278	Diluted with 3 parts water by volume ...1 c	249	87	120	2	tr	—	—	—	29	25	42	0.2	503	540	0.23	0.03	0.9	120
279	Dehydrated crystals, prepared with water (1 lb yields about 1 gal) ...1 c	248	88	115	1	tr	—	—	—	27	25	40	0.5	518	500	0.20	0.07	1.0	109
	Orange and grapefruit juice																		
	Frozen concentrate																		
280	Undiluted, 6-fl oz can ...1 can	210	59	330	4	1	—	—	—	78	61	99	0.8	1308	800	0.48	0.06	2.3	302
281	Diluted with 3 parts water by volume ...1 c	248	88	110	1	tr	—	—	—	26	20	32	0.2	439	270	0.15	0.02	0.7	102
282	Papayas, raw, ½" cubes ...1 c	140	89	55	1	tr	—	—	—	14	28	22	0.4	328	2450	0.06	0.06	0.4	78
	Peaches																		
	Raw																		
283	Whole, 2½" diam, peeled, pitted (about 4 per lb with peels and pits) ...1 peach	100	89	40	1	tr	—	—	—	10	9	19	0.5	202	1330[34]	0.02	0.05	1.0	7
284	Sliced ...1 c	170	89	65	1	tr	—	—	—	16	15	32	0.9	343	2260[34]	0.03	0.09	1.7	12
	Canned, yellow-fleshed, solids and liquid (halves or slices)																		
285	Syrup pack ...1 c	256	79	200	1	tr	—	—	—	51	10	31	0.8	333	1100	0.03	0.05	1.5	8
286	Water pack ...1 c	244	91	75	1	tr	—	—	—	20	10	32	0.7	334	1100	0.02	0.07	1.5	7
	Dried																		
287	Uncooked ...1 c	160	25	420	5	1	—	—	—	109	77	187	9.6	1520	6240	0.02	0.30	8.5	29
288	Cooked, unsweetened, halves and juice ...1 c	250	77	205	3	1	—	—	—	54	38	93	4.8	743	3050	0.01	0.15	3.8	5
	Frozen, sliced, sweetened																		
289	10-oz container ...1 container	284	77	250	1	tr	—	—	—	64	11	37	1.4	352	1850	0.03	0.11	2.0	116[35]
290	Cup ...1 c	250	77	220	1	tr	—	—	—	57	10	33	1.3	310	1630	0.03	0.10	1.8	103[35]
	Pears																		
	Raw, with skin, cored																		
291	Bartlett, 2½" diam (about 2½ per lb with cores and stems) ...1 pear	164	83	100	1	1	—	—	—	25	13	18	0.5	213	30	0.03	0.07	0.2	7
292	Bosc, 2½" diam (about 3 per lb with cores and stems) ...1 pear	141	83	85	1	1	—	—	—	22	11	16	0.4	83	30	0.03	0.06	0.1	6
293	D'Anjou, 3" diam (about 2 per lb with cores and stems) ...1 pear	200	83	120	1	1	—	—	—	31	16	22	0.6	260	40	0.04	0.08	0.2	8
294	Canned, solids and liquid, syrup pack, heavy (halves or slices) ...1 c	255	80	195	1	1	—	—	—	50	13	18	0.5	214	10	0.03	0.05	0.3	3

(*continued*)

APPENDIX 1. (continued)

Item No. (A)	Foods, Approximate Measures, Units, and Weight (Edible Part Unless Footnotes Indicate Otherwise) (B)	Water Per-cent (C)	Food Energy Cal-ories (D)	Protein (E)	Fat (F)	Fatty Acids Saturated (Total) (G)	Unsaturated Oleic (H)	Unsaturated Linoleic (I)	Carbohydrate (J)	Calcium (K)	Phosphorus (L)	Iron (M)	Potassium (N)	Vitamin A Value (O)	Thiamine (P)	Riboflavin (Q)	Niacin (R)	Ascorbic Acid (S)
		g / Per-cent	Cal-ories	g	g	g	g	g	g	mg	mg	mg	mg	IU	mg	mg	mg	mg
	Pineapple																	
295	Raw, diced ... 1 c.	155 / 85	80	1	tr	—	—	—	21	26	12	0.8	226	110	0.14	0.05	0.3	26
	Canned, heavy syrup pack, solids and liquid																	
296	Crushed, chunks, tidbits ... 1 c.	255 / 80	190	1	tr	—	—	—	49	28	13	0.8	245	130	0.20	0.05	0.5	18
	Slices and liquid																	
297	Large ... 1 slice; 2¼ tbsp liquid	105 / 80	80	tr	tr	—	—	—	20	12	5	0.3	101	50	0.08	0.02	0.2	7
298	Medium ... 1 slice; 1¼ tbsp liquid	58 / 80	45	tr	tr	—	—	—	11	6	3	0.2	56	30	0.05	0.01	0.1	4
299	Pineapple juice, unsweetened, canned ... 1 c.	250 / 86	140	1	tr	—	—	—	34	38	23	0.8	373	130	0.13	0.05	0.5	80[27]
	Plums																	
	Raw, without pits																	
300	Japanese and hybrid (2⅛″ diam, about 6½ per lb with pits) ... 1 plum	66 / 87	30	tr	tr	—	—	—	8	8	12	0.3	112	160	0.02	0.02	0.3	4
301	Prune-type (1½″ diam, about 15 per lb with pits) ... 1 plum	28 / 79	20	tr	tr	—	—	—	6	3	5	0.1	48	80	0.01	0.01	0.1	1
	Canned, heavy syrup pack (Italian prunes), with pits and liquid																	
302	Cup ... 1 c[36]	272 / 77	215	1	tr	—	—	—	56	23	26	2.3	367	3130	0.05	0.05	1.0	5
303	Portion ... 3 plums; 2¾ tbsp liquid[36]	140 / 77	110	1	tr	—	—	—	29	12	13	1.2	189	1610	0.03	0.03	0.5	3

(*continued*)

	Prunes, dried "softenized," with pits																		
304	Uncooked	4 extra large or 5 large prunes[36]	49	28	110	1	tr	—	—	—	29	22	34	1.7	298	690	0.04	0.07	0.7	1
305	Cooked, unsweetened, all sizes, fruit and liquid	1 c[36]	250	66	255	2	1	—	—	—	67	51	79	3.8	695	1590	0.07	0.15	1.5	2
306	Prune juice, canned or bottled	1 c	256	80	195	1	tr	—	—	—	49	36	51	1.8	602	—	0.03	0.03	1.0	5
	Raisins, seedless:																			
307	Cup, not pressed down	1 c	145	18	420	4	tr	—	—	—	112	90	146	5.1	1106	30	0.16	0.12	0.7	1
308	Packet, ½ oz (1½ tbsp)	1 packet	14	18	40	tr	tr	—	—	—	11	9	14	0.5	107	tr	0.02	0.01	0.1	tr
	Raspberries, red:																			
309	Raw, capped, whole	1 c	123	84	70	1	1	—	—	—	17	27	27	1.1	207	160	0.04	0.11	1.1	31
310	Frozen, sweetened, 10-oz container	1 container	284	74	280	2	1	—	—	—	70	37	48	1.7	284	200	0.06	0.17	1.7	60
	Rhubarb, cooked, added sugar:																			
311	From raw	1 c	270	63	380	1	tr	—	—	—	97	211	41	1.6	548	220	0.05	0.14	0.8	16
312	From frozen, sweetened	1 c	270	63	385	1	1	—	—	—	98	211	32	1.9	475	190	0.05	0.11	0.5	16
	Strawberries:																			
313	Raw, whole berries, capped	1 c	149	90	55	1	1	—	—	—	13	31	31	1.5	244	90	0.04	0.10	0.9	88
	Frozen, sweetened:																			
314	Sliced, 10-oz container	1 container	284	71	310	1	1	—	—	—	79	40	48	2.0	318	90	0.06	0.17	1.4	151
315	Whole, 1-lb container (about 1¾ cups)	1 container	454	76	415	2	1	—	—	—	107	59	73	2.7	472	140	0.09	0.27	2.3	249
316	Tangerine, raw, 2⅜" diam, size 176, without peel (about 4 per lb with peels and seeds)	1 tangerine	86	87	40	1	tr	—	—	—	10	34	15	0.3	108	360	0.05	0.02	0.1	27
317	Tangerine juice, canned, sweetened	1 c	249	87	125	1	tr	—	—	—	30	44	35	0.5	440	1040	0.15	0.05	0.2	54
318	Watermelon, raw, 4" × 8" wedge with rind and seeds (1/16 of 32⅔-lb melon, 10" × 16")	1 wedge with rind and seeds[37]	926	93	110	2	1	—	—	—	27	30	43	2.1	426	2510	0.13	0.13	0.9	30
	GRAIN PRODUCTS																			
	Bagel, 3" diam:																			
319	Egg	1 bagel	55	32	165	6	2	0.5	0.9	0.8	28	9	43	1.2	41	30	0.14	0.10	1.2	0
320	Water	1 bagel	55	29	165	6	1	0.2	0.4	0.6	30	8	41	1.2	42	0	0.15	0.11	1.4	0
321	Barley, pearled, light, uncooked	1 c	200	11	700	16	2	0.3	0.2	0.8	158	32	378	4.0	320	0	0.24	0.10	6.2	0
	Biscuits, baking powder, 2" diam (enriched flour, vegetable shortening)																			

APPENDIX 1. (continued)

Item No. (A)	Foods, Approximate Measures, Units, and Weight (Edible Part Unless Footnotes Indicate Otherwise) (B)	Water Per-cent (C)	Food Energy Calories (D)	Protein g (E)	Fat g (F)	Saturated (Total) g (G)	Unsaturated Oleic g (H)	Unsaturated Linoleic g (I)	Carbohydrate g (J)	Calcium mg (K)	Phosphorus mg (L)	Iron mg (M)	Potassium mg (N)	Vitamin A Value IU (O)	Thiamine mg (P)	Riboflavin mg (Q)	Niacin mg (R)	Ascorbic Acid mg (S)
322	From home recipe......1 biscuit	28	27	105	2	5	1.2	2.0	1.2	13	34	49	0.4	33	tr	0.08	0.08	0.7	tr
323	From mix......1 biscuit	28	29	90	2	3	0.6	1.1	0.7	15	19	65	0.6	32	tr	0.09	0.08	0.8	tr
	Breadcrumbs (enriched)[38]																		
324	Dry, grated......1 c.	100	7	390	13	5	1.0	1.6	1.4	73	122	141	3.6	152	tr	0.35	0.35	4.8	tr
	Soft (see White bread, items 349–350)																		
	Breads																		
325	Boston brown bread, canned, slice (3¼" × ½")[38]......1 slice	45	45	95	2	1	0.1	0.2	0.2	21	41	72	0.9	131	0[39]	0.06	0.04	0.7	0
	Cracked-wheat bread (¾ enriched wheat flour, ¼ cracked wheat)[38]																		
326	Loaf, 1 lb......1 loaf	454	35	1195	39	10	2.2	3.0	3.9	236	399	581	9.5	608	tr	1.52	1.13	14.4	tr
327	Slice (18 per loaf)......1 slice	25	35	65	2	1	0.1	0.2	0.2	13	22	32	0.5	34	tr	0.08	0.06	0.8	tr
	French or vienna bread, enriched[38]																		
328	Loaf, 1 lb......1 loaf	454	31	1315	41	14	3.2	4.7	4.6	251	195	386	10.0	408	tr	1.80	1.10	15.0	tr
	Slice																		
329	French (5"×2½"×1")......1 slice	35	31	100	3	1	0.2	0.4	0.4	19	15	30	0.8	32	tr	0.14	0.08	1.2	tr
330	Vienna (4¾"×4"×½")......1 slice	25	31	75	2	1	0.2	0.3	0.3	14	11	21	0.6	23	tr	0.10	0.06	0.8	tr
	Italian bread, enriched																		
331	Loaf, 1 lb......1 loaf	454	32	1250	41	4	0.6	0.3	1.5	256	77	349	10.0	336	0	1.80	1.10	15.0	0
332	Slice (4½"×3¼"×¾")......1 slice	30	32	85	3	tr	tr	tr	0.1	17	5	23	0.7	22	0	0.12	0.07	1.0	0
	Raisin bread, enriched[38]																		
333	Loaf, 1 lb......1 loaf	454	35	1190	30	13	3.0	4.7	3.9	243	322	395	10.0	1057	tr	1.70	1.07	10.7	tr
334	Slice (18 per loaf)......1 slice	25	35	65	2	1	0.2	0.3	0.2	13	18	22	0.6	58	tr	0.09	0.06	0.6	tr
	Rye bread																		

No.	Food	Measure	Grams	Water (%)	Food energy	Protein (g)	Fat (g)	Saturated (g)	Oleic (g)	Linoleic (g)	Carbohydrate (g)	Calcium (mg)	Phosphorus (mg)	Iron (mg)	Potassium (mg)	Vitamin A	Thiamin (mg)	Riboflavin (mg)	Niacin (mg)	Ascorbic acid
	American, light (⅔ enriched wheat flour, ⅓ rye flour)																			
335	Loaf, 1 lb	1 loaf	454	36	1100	41	5	0.7	0.5	2.2	236	340	667	9.1	658	0	1.35	0.98	12.9	0
336	Slice (4¾″ × 3¾″ × 7⁄16″)	1 slice	25	36	60	2	tr	tr	tr	0.1	13	19	37	0.5	36	0	0.07	0.05	0.7	0
	Pumpernickel (⅔ rye flour, ⅓ enriched wheat flour)																			
337	Loaf, 1 lb	1 loaf	454	34	1115	41	5	0.7	0.5	2.4	241	381	1039	11.8	2059	0	1.30	0.93	8.5	0
338	Slice (5″×4″×3⁄8″)	1 slice	32	34	80	3	tr	0.1	tr	0.2	17	27	73	0.8	145	0	0.09	0.07	0.6	0
	White bread, enriched[38]																			
	Soft-crumb type																			
339	Loaf, 1 lb	1 loaf	454	36	1225	39	15	3.4	5.3	4.6	229	381	440	11.3	476	tr	1.80	1.10	15.0	tr
340	Slice (18 per loaf)	1 slice	25	36	70	2	1	0.2	0.3	0.3	13	21	24	0.6	26	tr	0.10	0.06	0.8	tr
341	Slice, toasted	1 slice	22	25	70	2	1	0.2	0.3	0.3	13	21	24	0.6	26	tr	0.08	0.06	0.8	tr
342	Slice (22 per loaf)	1 slice	20	36	55	2	1	0.2	0.2	0.2	10	17	19	0.5	21	tr	0.08	0.05	0.7	tr
343	Slice, toasted	1 slice	17	25	55	2	1	0.2	0.2	0.2	10	17	19	0.5	21	tr	0.06	0.05	0.7	tr
344	Loaf, 1½ lb	1 loaf	680	36	1835	59	22	5.2	7.9	6.9	343	571	660	17.0	714	tr	2.70	1.65	22.5	tr
345	Slice (24 per loaf)	1 slice	28	36	75	2	1	0.2	0.3	0.3	14	24	27	0.7	29	tr	0.11	0.07	0.9	tr
346	Slice, toasted	1 slice	24	25	75	2	1	0.2	0.3	0.3	14	24	27	0.7	29	tr	0.09	0.07	0.9	tr
347	Slice (28 per loaf)	1 slice	24	36	65	2	1	0.2	0.3	0.2	12	20	23	0.6	25	tr	0.10	0.06	0.8	tr
348	Slice, toasted	1 slice	21	25	65	2	1	0.2	0.3	0.2	12	20	23	0.6	25	tr	0.08	0.06	0.8	tr
349	Cubes	1 c.	30	36	80	3	1	0.2	0.3	0.3	15	25	29	0.8	32	tr	0.12	0.07	1.0	tr
350	Crumbs	1 c.	45	36	120	4	1	0.3	0.5	0.5	23	38	44	1.1	47	tr	0.18	0.11	1.5	tr
	Firm-crumb type																			
351	Loaf, 1 lb	1 loaf	454	35	1245	41	17	3.9	5.9	5.2	228	435	463	11.3	549	tr	1.80	1.10	15.0	tr
352	Slice (20 per loaf)	1 slice	23	35	65	2	1	0.2	0.3	0.3	12	22	23	0.6	28	tr	0.09	0.06	0.8	tr
353	Slice, toasted	1 slice	20	24	65	2	1	0.2	0.3	0.3	12	22	23	0.6	28	tr	0.07	0.06	0.8	tr
354	Loaf, 2 lb	1 loaf	907	35	2495	82	34	7.7	11.8	10.4	455	871	925	22.7	1097	tr	3.60	2.20	30.0	tr
355	Slice (34 per loaf)	1 slice	27	35	75	2	1	0.2	0.3	0.3	14	26	28	0.7	33	tr	0.11	0.06	0.9	tr
356	Slice, toasted	1 slice	23	24	75	2	1	0.2	0.3	0.3	14	26	28	0.7	33	tr	0.09	0.06	0.9	tr
	Whole-wheat bread																			
	Soft-crumb type[38]																			
357	Loaf, 1 lb	1 loaf	454	36	1095	41	12	2.2	2.9	4.2	224	381	1152	13.6	1161	tr	1.37	0.45	12.7	tr
358	Slice (16 per loaf)	1 slice	28	36	65	3	1	0.1	0.2	0.2	14	24	71	0.8	72	tr	0.09	0.03	0.8	tr
359	Slice, toasted	1 slice	24	24	65	3	1	0.1	0.2	0.2	14	24	71	0.8	72	tr	0.07	0.03	0.8	tr
	Firm-crumb type[38]																			
360	Loaf, 1 lb	1 loaf	454	36	1100	48	14	2.5	3.3	4.9	216	449	1034	13.6	1238	tr	1.17	0.54	12.7	tr
361	Slice (18 per loaf)	1 slice	25	36	60	3	1	0.1	0.2	0.3	12	25	57	0.8	68	tr	0.06	0.03	0.7	tr
362	Slice, toasted	1 slice	21	24	60	3	1	0.1	0.2	0.3	12	25	57	0.8	68	tr	0.05	0.03	0.7	tr
	Breakfast cereals																			
	Hot type, cooked																			
	Corn (hominy) grits, degermed																			
363	Enriched	1 c.	245	87	125	3	tr	tr	tr	0.1	27	2	25	0.7	27	tr[40]	0.10	0.07	1.0	0
364	Unenriched	1 c.	245	87	125	3	tr	tr	tr	0.1	27	2	25	0.2	27	tr[40]	0.05	0.02	0.5	0

(continued)

APPENDIX 1. (continued)

Item No. (A)	Foods, Approximate Measures, Units, and Weight (Edible Part Unless Footnotes Indicate Otherwise) (B)	Water (C) Per-cent	Food Energy (D) Cal-ories	Protein (E) g	Fat (F) g	Saturated (Total) (G) g	Oleic (H) g	Linoleic (I) g	Carbohydrate (J) g	Calcium (K) mg	Phosphorus (L) mg	Iron (M) mg	Potassium (N) mg	Vitamin A Value (O) IU	Thiamine (P) mg	Riboflavin (Q) mg	Niacin (R) mg	Ascorbic Acid (S) mg
365	Farina, quick-cooking, enriched .... 1 c .... 245 g	89	105	3	tr	tr	tr	0.1	22	147	113[41]	(42)	25	0	0.12	0.07	1.0	0
366	Oatmeal or rolled oats .... 1 c .... 240 g	87	130	5	2	0.4	0.8	0.9	23	22	137	1.4	146	0	0.19	0.05	0.2	0
367	Wheat, rolled .... 1 c .... 240 g	80	180	5	1	—	—	—	41	19	182	1.7	202	0	0.17	0.07	2.2	0
368	Wheat, whole-meal .... 1 c .... 245 g	88	110	4	1	—	—	—	23	17	127	1.2	118	0	0.15	0.05	1.5	0
	Ready-to-eat																	
369	Bran flakes (40% bran), added sugar, salt, iron, vitamins .... 1 c .... 35 g	3	105	4	1	—	—	—	28	19	125	5.6	137	1540	0.46	0.52	6.2	0
370	Bran flakes with raisins, added sugar, salt, iron, vitamins .... 1 c .... 50 g	7	145	4	1	—	—	—	40	28	146	7.9	154	2200[43]	(44)	(44)	(44)	0
	Corn flakes																	
371	Plain, added sugar, salt, iron, vitamins .... 1 c .... 25 g	4	95	2	tr	—	—	—	21	(44)	9	(44)	30	(44)	(44)	(44)	(44)	13[45]
372	Sugar-coated, added salt, iron, vitamins .... 1 c .... 40 g	2	155	2	tr	—	—	—	37	1	10	(44)	27	1760	0.53	0.60	7.1	21[45]
373	Corn, oat flour, puffed, added sugar, salt, iron, vitamins .... 1 c .... 20 g	4	80	2	1	—	—	—	16	4	18	5.7	—	880	0.26	0.30	3.5	11
374	Corn, shredded, added sugar, salt, iron, thiamin, niacin .... 1 c .... 25 g	3	95	2	tr	—	—	—	22	1	10	0.6	—	0	0.33	0.05	4.4	13
375	Oats, puffed, added sugar, salt, minerals, vitamins .... 1 c .... 25 g	3	100	3	1	—	—	—	19	44	102	4.0	—	1100	0.33	0.38	4.4	13
	Rice, puffed																	

No.	Food	Measure	Grams	Water (%)	Food energy (cal)	Protein (g)	Fat (g)	Saturated (g)	Unsaturated Oleic (g)	Unsaturated Linoleic (g)	Carbohydrate (g)	Calcium (mg)	Phosphorus (mg)	Iron (mg)	Potassium (mg)	Vitamin A (IU)	Thiamin (mg)	Riboflavin (mg)	Niacin (mg)	Ascorbic acid (mg)
376	Plain, added iron, thiamin, niacin	1 c	15	4	60	1	tr	—	—	—	13	3	14	0.3	15	0	0.07	0.01	0.7	0
377	Presweetened, added salt, iron, vitamins	1 c	28	3	115	1	0	—	—	—	26	3	14	[44]	43	1240[45]	[44]	[44]	[44]	15[45]
378	Wheat flakes, added sugar, salt, iron, vitamins	1 c	30	4	105	3	tr	—	—	—	24	12	83	4.8	81	1320	0.40	0.45	5.3	16
	Wheat, puffed																			
379	Plain, added iron, thiamin, niacin	1 c	15	3	55	2	tr	—	—	—	12	4	48	0.6	51	0	0.08	0.03	1.2	0
380	Presweetened, added salt, iron, vitamins	1 c	38	3	140	3	tr	—	—	—	33	7	52	[44]	63	1680	0.50	0.57	6.7	20[45]
381	Wheat, shredded, plain	1 oblong biscuit or ½ cup spoon-size biscuits	25	7	90	2	1	—	—	—	20	11	97	0.9	87	0	0.06	0.03	1.1	0
382	Wheat germ, without salt and sugar, toasted	1 tbsp	6	4	25	2	1	—	—	—	3	3	70	0.5	57	10	0.11	0.05	0.3	1
383	Buckwheat flour, light, sifted	1 c	98	12	340	6	1	0.2	0.4	0.4	78	11	86	1.0	314	0	0.08	0.04	0.4	0
384	Bulgur, canned, seasoned	1 c	135	56	245	8	4	—	—	—	44	27	263	1.9	151	0	0.08	0.05	4.1	0
	Cake icings (see Sugars and Sweets, items 532–536)																			
	Cakes made from cake mixes with enriched flour[46]																			
	Angelfood																			
385	Whole cake (9¾" diam tube cake)	1 cake	635	34	1645	36	1	—	—	—	377	603	756	2.5	381	0	0.37	0.95	3.6	0
386	Piece, 1/12 of cake	1 piece	53	34	135	3	tr	—	—	—	32	50	63	0.2	32	0	0.03	0.08	0.3	0
	Coffeecake																			
387	Whole cake (7¾"×5⅝"×1¼")	1 cake	430	30	1385	27	41	11.7	16.3	8.8	225	262	748	6.9	469	690	0.82	0.91	7.7	1
388	Piece, 1/6 of cake	1 piece	72	30	230	5	7	2.0	2.7	1.5	38	44	125	1.2	78	120	0.14	0.15	1.3	tr
	Cupcakes, made with egg, milk, 2½" diam																			
389	Without icing	1 cupcake	25	26	90	1	3	0.8	1.2	0.7	14	40	59	0.3	21	40	0.05	0.05	0.4	tr
390	With chocolate icing	1 cupcake	36	22	130	2	5	2.0	1.6	0.6	21	47	71	0.4	42	60	0.05	0.06	0.4	tr
	Devil's food with chocolate icing																			
391	Whole, 2-layer cake (8" or 9" diam)	1 cake	1107	24	3755	49	136	50.0	44.9	17.0	645	653	1162	16.6	1439	1660	1.06	1.65	10.1	1
392	Piece, 1/16 of cake	1 piece	69	24	235	3	8	3.1	2.8	1.1	40	41	72	1.0	90	100	0.07	0.10	0.6	tr
393	Cupcake (2½" diam)	1 cupcake	35	24	120	2	4	1.6	1.4	0.5	20	21	37	0.5	46	50	0.03	0.05	0.3	tr

(continued)

APPENDIX 1. (continued)

Item No. (A)	Foods, Approximate Measures, Units, and Weight (Edible Part Unless Footnotes Indicate Otherwise) (B)	g	Water Per-cent (C)	Food Energy Cal-ories (D)	Protein g (E)	Fat g (F)	Fatty Acids Saturated (Total) g (G)	Unsaturated Oleic g (H)	Unsaturated Linoleic g (I)	Carbohydrate g (J)	Calcium mg (K)	Phosphorus mg (L)	Iron mg (M)	Potassium mg (N)	Vitamin A Value IU (O)	Thiamine mg (P)	Riboflavin mg (Q)	Niacin mg (R)	Ascorbic Acid mg (S)
	Gingerbread																		
	Whole cake																		
394	(8" square) .... 1 cake	570	37	1575	18	39	9.7	16.6	10.0	291	513	570	8.6	1562	tr	0.84	1.00	7.4	tr
395	Piece, 1/9 of cake ...... 1 piece	63	37	175	2	4	1.1	1.8	1.1	32	57	63	0.9	173	tr	0.09	0.11	0.8	tr
	White, 2-layer with chocolate icing																		
396	Whole cake (8" or 9" diam) .. 1 cake	1140	21	4000	44	122	48.2	46.4	20.0	716	1129	2041	11.4	1322	680	1.50	1.77	12.5	2
397	Piece, 1/16 of cake ...... 1 piece	71	21	250	3	8	3.0	2.9	1.2	45	70	127	0.7	82	40	0.09	0.11	0.8	tr
	Yellow, 2-layer with chocolate icing																		
398	Whole cake (8" or 9" diam) .. 1 cake	1108	26	3735	45	125	47.8	47.8	20.3	638	1008	2017	12.2	1208	1550	1.24	1.67	10.6	2
399	Piece, 1/16 of cake ...... 1 piece	69	26	235	3	8	3.0	3.0	1.3	40	63	126	0.8	75	100	0.08	0.10	0.7	tr
	Cakes made from home recipes using enriched flour[47]																		
	Boston cream pie with custard filling																		
400	Whole cake (8" diam) ...... 1 cake	825	35	2490	41	78	23.0	30.1	15.2	412	553	833	8.2	734[48]	1730	1.04	1.27	9.6	2
401	Piece, 1/12 of cake ...... 1 piece	69	35	210	3	6	1.9	2.5	1.3	34	46	70	0.7	61[48]	140	0.09	0.11	0.8	tr
	Fruitcake, dark																		
402	Loaf, 1-lb (7½"×2"×1½") ... 1 loaf	454	18	1720	22	69	14.4	33.5	14.8	271	327	513	11.8	2250	540	0.72	0.73	4.9	2
403	Slice, 1/30 of loaf .... 1 slice	15	18	55	1	2	0.5	1.1	0.5	9	11	17	0.4	74	20	0.02	0.02	0.2	tr
	Plain, sheet cake																		
	Without icing																		
	Whole cake																		
404	(9" square) .... 1 cake	777	25	2830	35	108	29.5	44.4	23.9	434	497	793	8.5	614[48]	1320	1.21	1.40	10.2	2
405	Piece, 1/9 of cake ...... 1 piece	86	25	315	4	12	3.3	4.9	2.6	48	55	88	0.9	68[48]	150	0.13	0.15	1.1	tr
	With uncooked white icing																		

No.	Food	Measure																		
406	Whole cake (9" square)	1 cake	1096	21	4020	37	129	42.2	49.5	24.4	694	548	822	8.2	669[48]	2190	1.22	1.47	10.2	2
407	Piece, 1/9 of cake[49]	1 piece	121	21	445	4	14	4.7	5.5	2.7	77	61	91	0.8	74[48]	240	0.14	0.16	1.1	tr
	Pound[49]																			
408	Loaf, 8½"×3½"×3¼"	1 loaf	565	16	2725	31	170	42.9	73.1	39.6	273	107	418	7.9	345	1410	0.90	0.99	7.3	0
409	Slice, 1/17 of loaf	1 slice	33	16	160	2	10	2.5	4.3	2.3	16	6	24	0.5	20	80	0.05	0.06	0.4	0
	Spongecake																			
410	Whole cake (9¾" diam tube cake)	1 cake	790	32	2345	60	45	13.1	15.8	5.7	427	237	885	13.4	687	3560	1.10	1.64	7.4	tr
411	Piece, 1/12 of cake	1 piece	66	32	195	5	4	1.1	1.3	0.5	36	20	74	1.1	57	300	0.09	0.14	0.6	tr
	Cookies made with enriched flour[50,51]																			
	Brownies with nuts																			
	Home-prepared, 1¾"×¾"×⅞"																			
412	From home recipe	1 brownie	20	10	95	1	6	1.5	3.0	1.2	10	8	30	0.4	38	40	0.04	0.03	0.2	tr
413	From commercial recipe	1 brownie	20	11	85	1	4	0.9	1.4	1.3	13	9	27	0.4	34	20	0.03	0.02	0.2	tr
414	Frozen, with chocolate icing[52] (1½"×1¾"×⅞")	1 brownie	25	13	105	1	5	2.0	2.2	0.7	15	10	31	0.4	44	50	0.03	0.03	0.2	tr
	Chocolate chip																			
415	Commercial (2¼" diam, ⅜" thick)	4 cookies	42	3	200	2	9	2.8	2.9	2.2	29	16	48	1.0	56	50	0.10	0.17	0.9	tr
416	From home recipe, 2⅓" diam	4 cookies	40	3	205	2	12	3.5	4.5	2.9	24	14	40	0.8	47	40	0.06	0.06	0.5	tr
417	Fig bars, square (1⅝"×1⅝"×⅜") or rectangular (1½"×1¾"×½")	4 cookies	56	14	200	2	3	0.8	1.2	0.7	42	44	34	1.0	111	60	0.04	0.14	0.9	tr
418	Gingersnaps (2" diam, ¼" thick)	4 cookies	28	3	90	2	2	0.7	1.0	0.6	22	20	13	0.7	129	20	0.08	0.06	0.7	0
419	Macaroons (2¾" diam, ¼" thick)	2 cookies	38	4	180	2	9	—	—	—	25	10	32	0.3	176	0	0.02	0.06	0.2	0
420	Oatmeal with raisins (2⅝" diam, ¼" thick)	4 cookies	52	3	235	3	8	2.0	3.3	2.0	38	11	53	1.4	192	30	0.15	0.10	1.0	tr
421	Plain, prepared from commercial chilled dough (2½" diam, ¼" thick)	4 cookies	48	5	240	2	12	3.0	5.2	2.9	31	17	35	0.6	23	30	0.10	0.08	0.9	0
422	Sandwich type chocolate or vanilla (1¾" diam, ⅜" thick)	4 cookies	40	2	200	2	9	2.2	3.9	2.2	28	10	96	0.7	15	0	0.06	0.10	0.7	0
423	Vanilla wafers, 1¾" diam, ¼" thick	10 cookies	40	3	185	2	6	—	—	—	30	16	25	0.6	29	50	0.10	0.09	0.8	0
	Cornmeal																			
424	Whole-ground, unbolted, dry form	1 c.	122	12	435	11	5	0.5	1.0	2.5	90	24	312	2.9	346	620[53]	0.46	0.13	2.4	0

(continued)

APPENDIX 1. (continued)

Item No. (A)	Foods, Approximate Measures, Units, and Weight (Edible Part Unless Footnotes Indicate Otherwise) (B)	Water (C) Per-cent	Food Energy (D) Calories	Protein (E) g	Fat (F) g	Fatty Acids Saturated (Total) (G) g	Unsaturated Oleic (H) g	Unsaturated Linoleic (I) g	Carbohydrate (J) g	Calcium (K) mg	Phosphorus (L) mg	Iron (M) mg	Potassium (N) mg	Vitamin A Value (O) IU	Thiamine (P) mg	Riboflavin (Q) mg	Niacin (R) mg	Ascorbic Acid (S) mg
425	Bolted (nearly whole-grain), dry form . . . 1 c . . .	122	12	440	11	4	0.5	0.9	2.1	91	21	272	2.2	303	590[53]	0.37	0.10	2.3	0
	Degermed, enriched																		
426	Dry form . . . 1 c . . .	138	12	500	11	2	0.2	0.4	0.9	108	8	137	4.0	166	610[53]	0.61	0.36	4.8	0
427	Cooked . . . 1 c . . .	240	88	120	3	tr	tr	0.1	0.2	26	2	34	1.0	38	140[53]	0.14	0.10	1.2	0
	Degermed, unenriched																		
428	Dry form . . . 1 c . . .	138	12	500	11	2	0.2	0.4	0.9	108	8	137	1.5	166	610[53]	0.19	0.07	1.4	0
429	Cooked . . . 1 c . . .	240	88	120	3	tr	tr	0.1	0.2	26	2	34	0.5	38	140[53]	0.05	0.02	0.2	0
	Crackers[38]																		
430	Graham, plain (2½" square) . . . 2 crackers . . .	14	6	55	1	1	0.3	0.5	0.3	10	6	21	0.5	55	0	0.02	0.08	0.5	0
431	Rye wafers, whole-grain (1⅞" × 3½") . . . 2 wafers . . .	13	6	45	2	tr	—	—	—	10	7	50	0.5	78	0	0.04	0.03	0.2	0
432	Saltines, made with enriched flour . . . 4 crackers or 1 packet . . .	11	4	50	1	1	0.3	0.5	0.4	8	2	10	0.5	13	0	0.05	0.05	0.4	0
433	Danish pastry (enriched flour), plain without fruit or nuts[54] Packaged ring, 12 oz . . . 1 ring . . .	340	22	1435	25	80	24.3	31.7	16.5	155	170	371	6.1	381	1050	0.97	1.01	8.6	tr
434	Round piece (about 4¼" diam × 1") . . . 1 pastry . . .	65	22	275	5	15	4.7	6.1	3.2	30	33	71	1.2	73	200	0.18	0.19	1.7	tr
435	Ounce . . . 1 oz . . .	28	22	120	2	7	2.0	2.7	1.4	13	14	31	0.5	32	90	0.08	0.08	0.7	tr
	Doughnuts, made with enriched flour[38]																		
436	Cake type, plain (2½" diam, 1" high) . . . 1 doughnut . . .	25	24	100	1	5	1.2	2.0	1.1	13	10	48	0.4	23	20	0.05	0.05	0.4	tr
437	Yeast-leavened, glazed (3¾" diam, 1¼" high) . . . 1 doughnut . . .	50	26	205	3	11	3.3	5.8	3.3	22	16	33	0.6	34	25	0.10	0.10	0.8	0

Macaroni, enriched, cooked (cut lengths, elbows, shells)

No.	Food	Measure	Grams	Water %	Cal	Protein	Fat	Sat.	Oleic	Lino.	Carb.	Calcium	Phos.	Iron	Potas.	Vit A	Thiamin	Ribo.	Niacin	Asc.
438	Firm stage (hot)	1 c	130	64	190	7	1	—	—	—	39	14	85	1.4	103	0	0.23	0.13	1.8	0
	Tender stage																			
439	Cold macaroni	1 c	105	73	115	4	tr	—	—	—	24	8	53	0.9	64	0	0.15	0.08	1.2	0
440	Hot macaroni	1 c	140	73	155	5	1	—	—	—	32	11	70	1.3	85	0	0.20	0.11	1.5	0
	Macaroni (enriched) and cheese																			
441	Canned[55]	1 c	240	80	230	9	10	4.2	3.1	1.4	26	199	182	1.0	139	260	0.12	0.24	1.0	tr
442	From home recipe (served hot)[56]	1 c	200	58	430	17	22	8.9	8.8	2.9	40	362	322	1.8	240	860	0.20	0.40	1.8	tr
	Muffins made with enriched flour[38]																			
	From home recipe																			
443	Blueberry (2⅜″ diam, 1½″ high)	1 muffin	40	39	110	3	4	1.1	1.4	0.7	17	34	53	0.6	46	90	0.09	0.10	0.7	tr
444	Bran	1 muffin	40	35	105	3	4	1.2	1.4	0.8	17	57	162	1.5	172	90	0.07	0.10	1.7	tr
445	Corn, enriched degermed cornmeal and flour (2⅜″ diam, 1½″ high)	1 muffin	40	33	125	3	4	1.2	1.6	0.9	19	42	68	0.7	54	120[57]	0.10	0.10	0.7	tr
446	Plain (3″ diam, 1½″ high)	1 muffin	40	38	120	3	4	1.0	1.7	1.0	17	42	60	0.6	50	40	0.09	0.12	0.9	tr
	From mix, egg, milk																			
447	Corn (2⅜″ diam, 1½″ high)[58]	1 muffin	40	30	130	3	4	1.2	1.7	0.9	20	96	152	0.6	44	100[57]	0.08	0.09	0.7	tr
448	Noodles (egg noodles), enriched, cooked	1 c	160	71	200	7	2	—	—	—	37	16	94	1.4	70	110	0.22	0.13	1.9	0
449	Noodles, chow mein, canned	1 c	45	1	220	6	11	—	—	—	26	—	—	—	—	—	—	—	—	—
	Pancakes (4″ diam)[38]																			
450	Buckwheat, made from mix (with buckwheat and enriched flours), egg and milk added	1 cake	27	58	55	2	2	0.8	0.9	0.4	6	59	91	0.4	66	60	0.04	0.05	0.2	tr
	Plain																			
451	Made from home recipe using enriched flour	1 cake	27	50	60	2	2	0.5	0.8	0.5	9	27	38	0.4	33	30	0.06	0.07	0.5	tr
452	Made from mix with enriched flour, egg and milk added	1 cake	27	51	60	2	2	0.7	0.7	0.3	9	58	70	0.3	42	70	0.04	0.06	0.2	tr
	Pies, piecrust made with enriched flour, vegetable shortening (9″ diam)																			
	Apple																			
453	Whole	1 pie	945	48	2420	21	105	27.0	44.5	25.2	360	76	208	6.6	756	280	1.06	0.79	9.3	9

(continued)

APPENDIX 1. (continued)

Item No. (A)	Foods, Approximate Measures, Units, and Weight (Edible Part Unless Footnotes Indicate Otherwise) (B)	g	Water Per-cent (C)	Food Energy Cal-ories (D)	Protein g (E)	Fat g (F)	Saturated (Total) g (G)	Oleic g (H)	Linoleic g (I)	Carbohydrate g (J)	Calcium mg (K)	Phosphorus mg (L)	Iron mg (M)	Potassium mg (N)	Vitamin A Value IU (O)	Thiamine mg (P)	Riboflavin mg (Q)	Niacin mg (R)	Ascorbic Acid mg (S)
454	Sector, ⅐ of pie ... 1 sector	135	48	345	3	15	3.9	6.4	3.6	51	11	30	0.9	108	40	0.15	0.11	1.3	2
	Banana cream																		
455	Whole ... 1 pie	910	54	2010	41	85	26.7	33.2	16.2	279	601	746	7.3	1847	2280	0.77	1.51	7.0	9
456	Sector, ⅐ of pie ... 1 sector	130	54	285	6	12	3.8	4.7	2.3	40	86	107	1.0	264	330	0.11	0.22	1.0	1
	Blueberry																		
457	Whole ... 1 pie	945	51	2285	23	102	24.8	43.7	25.1	330	104	217	9.5	614	280	1.03	0.80	10.0	28
458	Sector, ⅐ of pie ... 1 sector	135	51	325	3	15	3.5	6.2	3.6	47	15	31	1.4	88	40	0.15	0.11	1.4	4
	Cherry																		
459	Whole ... 1 pie	945	47	2465	25	107	28.2	45.0	25.3	363	132	236	6.6	992	4160	1.09	0.84	9.8	tr
460	Sector, ⅐ of pie ... 1 sector	135	47	350	4	15	4.0	6.4	3.6	52	19	34	0.9	142	590	0.16	0.12	1.4	tr
	Custard																		
461	Whole ... 1 pie	910	58	1985	56	101	33.9	38.5	17.5	213	874	1028	8.2	1247	2090	0.79	1.92	5.6	0
462	Sector, ⅐ of pie ... 1 sector	130	58	285	8	14	4.8	5.5	2.5	30	125	147	1.2	178	300	0.11	0.27	0.8	0
	Lemon meringue																		
463	Whole ... 1 pie	840	47	2140	31	86	26.1	33.8	16.4	317	118	412	6.7	420	1430	0.61	0.84	5.2	25
464	Sector, ⅐ of pie ... 1 sector	120	47	305	4	12	3.7	4.8	2.3	45	17	59	1.0	60	200	0.09	0.12	0.7	4
	Mince																		
465	Whole ... 1 pie	945	43	2560	24	109	28.0	45.9	25.2	389	265	359	13.3	1682	20	0.96	0.86	9.8	9
466	Sector, ⅐ of pie ... 1 sector	135	43	365	3	16	4.0	6.6	3.6	56	38	51	1.9	240	tr	0.14	0.12	1.4	1
	Peach																		
467	Whole ... 1 pie	945	48	2410	24	101	24.8	43.7	25.1	361	95	274	8.5	1408	6900	1.04	0.97	14.0	28
468	Sector, ⅐ of pie ... 1 sector	135	48	345	3	14	3.5	6.2	3.6	52	14	39	1.2	201	990	0.15	0.14	2.0	4
	Pecan																		
469	Whole ... 1 pie	825	20	3450	42	189	27.8	101.0	44.2	423	388	850	25.6	1015	1320	1.80	0.95	6.9	tr
470	Sector, ⅐ of pie ... 1 sector	118	20	495	6	27	4.0	14.4	6.3	61	55	122	3.7	145	190	0.26	0.14	1.0	tr
	Pumpkin																		
471	Whole ... 1 pie	910	59	1920	36	102	37.4	37.5	16.6	223	464	628	7.3	1456	22,480	0.78	1.27	7.0	tr
472	Sector, ⅐ of pie ... 1 sector	130	59	275	5	15	5.4	5.4	2.4	32	66	90	1.0	208	3210	0.11	0.18	1.0	tr

Fatty Acids — Unsaturated (columns H, I)

No.	Foods, approximate measures, units, and weight	Grams	Water (%)	Food energy (cal)	Protein (g)	Fat (g)	Saturated (g)	Oleic (g)	Linoleic (g)	Carbohydrate (g)	Calcium (mg)	Phosphorus (mg)	Iron (mg)	Potassium (mg)	Vitamin A (IU)	Thiamin (mg)	Riboflavin (mg)	Niacin (mg)	Ascorbic acid (mg)
473	Piecrust (home recipe) made with enriched flour and vegetable shortening, baked....1 pie shell, 9" diam	180	15	900	11	60	14.8	26.1	14.9	79	25	90	3.1	89	0	0.47	0.40	5.0	0
474	Piecrust mix with enriched flour and vegetable shortening, 10-oz pkg prepared and baked......Piecrust for 2-crust pie, 9" diam	320	19	1485	20	93	22.7	39.7	23.4	141	131	272	6.1	179	0	1.07	0.79	9.9	0
475	Pizza (cheese) baked (4¾" sector; ⅛ of 12" diam pie)[19]....1 sector	60	45	145	6	4	1.7	1.5	0.6	22	86	89	1.1	67	230	0.16	0.18	1.6	4
476	Popcorn, popped / Plain, large kernel....1 c	6	4	25	1	tr	tr	0.1	0.2	5	1	17	0.2	—	—	—	0.01	0.1	0
477	With oil (coconut) and salt added, large kernel....1 c	9	3	40	1	2	1.5	0.2	0.2	5	1	19	0.2	—	—	0.01	0.01	0.2	0
478	Sugar coated....1 c	35	4	135	2	1	0.5	0.2	0.4	30	2	47	0.5	—	—	0.02	0.02	0.4	0
479	Pretzels, made with enriched flour / Dutch, twisted (2¾" × 2⅝")....1 pretzel	16	5	60	2	1	—	—	—	12	4	21	0.2	21	0	0.05	0.04	0.7	0
480	Thin, twisted (3¼" × 2¼" × ¼")....10 pretzels	60	5	235	6	3	—	—	—	46	13	79	0.9	78	0	0.20	0.15	2.5	0
481	Stick (2¼" long)....10 pretzels	3	5	10	tr	tr	—	—	—	2	1	4	tr	4	0	0.01	0.01	0.1	0
482	Rice, white, enriched / Instant, ready-to-serve, hot....1 c	165	73	180	4	tr	tr	tr	tr	40	5	31	1.3	—	0	0.21	[59]	1.7	0
483	Long grain / Raw....1 c	185	12	670	12	1	0.2	0.2	0.2	149	44	174	5.4	170	0	0.81	0.06	6.5	0
484	Cooked, served hot....1 c	205	73	225	4	tr	0.1	0.1	0.1	50	21	57	1.8	57	0	0.23	0.02	2.1	0
485	Parboiled / Raw....1 c	185	10	685	14	1	0.2	0.1	0.2	150	111	370	5.4	278	0	0.81	0.07	6.5	0
486	Cooked, served hot....1 c	175	73	185	4	tr	0.1	0.1	0.1	41	33	100	1.4	75	0	0.19	0.02	2.1	0
487	Rolls, enriched[38] / Commercial / Brown-and-serve (12 per 12-oz pkg), browned....1 roll	26	27	85	2	2	0.4	0.7	0.5	14	20	23	0.5	25	tr	0.10	0.06	0.9	tr
488	Cloverleaf or pan (2½" diam, 2" high)....1 roll	28	31	85	2	2	0.4	0.6	0.4	15	21	24	0.5	27	tr	0.11	0.07	0.9	tr
489	Frankfurter and hamburger (8 per 11½-oz pkg)....1 roll	40	31	120	3	2	0.5	0.8	0.6	21	30	34	0.8	38	tr	0.16	0.10	1.3	tr
490	Hard (3¾" diam, 2" high)....1 roll	50	25	155	5	2	0.4	0.6	0.5	30	24	46	1.2	49	tr	0.20	0.12	1.7	tr
491	Hoagie or submarine (11½" × 3" × 2½")....1 roll	135	31	390	12	4	0.9	1.4	1.4	75	58	115	3.0	122	tr	0.54	0.32	4.5	tr
492	From home recipe / Cloverleaf (2½" diam, 2" high)....1 roll	35	26	120	3	3	0.8	1.1	0.7	20	16	36	0.7	41	30	0.12	0.12	1.2	tr

(continued)

APPENDIX 1. (continued)

Item No. (A)	Foods, Approximate Measures, Units, and Weight (Edible Part Unless Footnotes Indicate Otherwise) (B)	Water (C)	Food Energy (D)	Protein (E)	Fat (F)	Fatty Acids Saturated (Total) (G)	Unsaturated Oleic (H)	Unsaturated Linoleic (I)	Carbohydrate (J)	Calcium (K)	Phosphorus (L)	Iron (M)	Potassium (N)	Vitamin A Value (O)	Thiamine (P)	Riboflavin (Q)	Niacin (R)	Ascorbic Acid (S)
		g Per-cent	Cal-ories	g	g	g	g	g	g	mg	mg	mg	mg	IU	mg	mg	mg	mg
	Spaghetti, enriched, cooked																	
493	Firm stage, "al dente," served hot......1 c.........	130 64	190	7	1	—	—	—	39	14	85	1.4	103	0	0.23	0.13	1.8	0
494	Tender stage, served hot......1 c......	140 73	155	5	1	—	—	—	32	11	70	1.3	85	0	0.20	0.11	1.5	0
	Spaghetti (enriched) in tomato sauce with cheese																	
495	From home recipe......1 c.........	250 77	260	9	9	2.0	5.4	0.7	37	80	135	2.3	408	1080	0.25	0.18	2.3	13
496	Canned......1 c.........	250 80	190	6	2	0.5	0.3	0.4	39	40	88	2.8	303	930	0.35	0.28	4.5	10
	Spaghetti (enriched) with meat balls and tomato sauce																	
497	From home recipe......1 c......	248 70	330	19	12	3.3	6.3	0.9	39	124	236	3.7	665	1590	0.25	0.30	4.0	22
498	Canned......1 c......	250 78	260	12	10	2.2	3.3	3.9	29	53	113	3.3	245	1000	0.15	0.18	2.3	5
499	Toaster pastries......1 pastry	50 12	200	3	6	—	—	—	36	54[60]	67[60]	1.9	74[60]	500	0.16	0.17	2.1	[60]
	Waffles, made with enriched flour, 7" diam[38]																	
500	From home recipe......1 waffle......	75 41	210	7	7	2.3	2.8	1.4	28	85	130	1.3	109	250	0.17	0.23	1.4	tr
501	From mix, egg and milk added......1 waffle......	75 42	205	7	8	2.8	2.9	1.2	27	179	257	1.0	146	170	0.14	0.22	0.9	tr
	Wheat flours All-purpose or family flour, enriched																	
502	Sifted, spooned......1 c......	115 12	420	12	1	0.2	0.1	0.5	88	18	100	3.3	109	0	0.74	0.46	6.1	0
503	Unsifted, spooned......1 c......	125 12	455	13	1	0.2	0.1	0.5	95	20	109	3.6	119	0	0.80	0.50	6.6	0
504	Cake or pastry flour, enriched, sifted, spooned......1 c......	96 12	350	7	1	0.1	0.1	0.3	76	16	70	2.8	191	0	0.61	0.38	5.1	0
505	Self-rising, enriched, unsifted, spooned......1 c......	125 12	440	12	1	0.2	0.1	0.5	93	331	583	3.6	—	0	0.80	0.50	6.6	0
506	Whole-wheat, from hard wheats, stirred......1 c......	120 12	400	16	2	0.4	0.2	1.0	85	49	446	4.0	444	0	0.66	0.14	5.2	0

LEGUMES (DRY), NUTS, SEEDS, AND RELATED PRODUCTS

No.	Food	Measure																	
	Almonds, shelled																		
507	Chopped (about 130 almonds)	1 c.	130	5	775	24	70	5.6	47.7	12.8	25	304	655	6.1	1005	0	0.31	1.20	4.6	tr
508	Slivered, not pressed down (about 115 almonds)	1 c.	115	5	690	21	62	5.0	42.2	11.3	22	269	580	5.4	889	0	0.28	1.06	4.0	tr
	Beans, dry																		
	Common varieties as Great Northern, navy, and others																		
	Cooked, drained																		
509	Great Northern	1 c.	180	69	210	14	1	—	—	—	38	90	266	4.9	749	0	0.25	0.13	1.3	0
510	Pea (navy)	1 c.	190	69	225	15	1	—	—	—	40	95	281	5.1	790	0	0.27	0.13	1.3	0
	Canned, solids and liquid																		
	White with—																		
511	Frankfurters (sliced)	1 c.	255	71	365	19	18	—	—	—	32	94	303	4.8	668	330	0.18	0.15	3.3	tr
512	Pork and tomato sauce	1 c.	255	71	310	16	7	2.4	2.8	0.6	48	138	235	4.6	536	330	0.20	0.08	1.5	5
513	Pork and sweet sauce	1 c.	255	66	385	16	12	4.3	5.0	1.1	54	161	291	5.9	—	—	0.15	0.10	1.3	—
514	Red kidney	1 c.	255	76	230	15	1	—	—	—	42	74	278	4.6	673	10	0.13	0.10	1.5	—
515	Lima, cooked, drained	1 c.	190	64	260	16	1	—	—	—	49	55	293	5.9	1163	—	0.25	0.11	1.3	—
516	Blackeye peas, dry, cooked (with residual cooking liquid)	1 c.	250	80	190	13	1	—	—	—	35	43	238	3.3	573	30	0.40	0.10	1.0	—
517	Brazil nuts, shelled (6–8 large kernels)	1 oz	28	5	185	4	19	4.8	6.2	7.1	3	53	196	1.0	203	tr	0.27	0.03	0.5	—
518	Cashew nuts, roasted in oil	1 c.	140	5	785	24	64	12.9	36.8	10.2	41	53	522	5.3	650	140	0.60	0.35	2.5	—
	Coconut meat, fresh																		
519	Piece (about 2″ × 2″ × ½″)	1 piece	45	51	155	2	16	14.0	0.9	0.3	4	6	43	0.8	115	0	0.02	0.01	0.2	1
520	Shredded or grated, not pressed down	1 c.	80	51	275	3	28	24.8	1.6	0.5	8	10	76	1.4	205	0	0.04	0.02	0.4	2
521	Filberts (hazelnuts), chopped (about 80 kernels)	1 c.	115	6	730	14	72	5.1	55.2	7.3	19	240	388	3.9	810	—	0.53	—	1.0	tr
522	Lentils, whole, cooked	1 c.	200	72	210	16	tr	—	—	—	39	50	238	4.2	498	40	0.14	0.12	1.2	0
	Peanuts, roasted in oil, salted																		
523	(whole, halves, chopped)	1 c.	144	2	840	37	72	13.7	33.0	20.7	27	107	577	3.0	971	—	0.46	0.19	24.8	0
524	Peanut butter	1 tbsp	16	2	95	4	8	1.5	3.7	2.3	3	9	61	0.3	100	—	0.02	0.02	2.4	0
525	Peas, split, dry, cooked	1 c.	200	70	230	16	1	—	—	—	42	22	178	3.4	592	80	0.30	0.18	1.8	—
526	Pecans, chopped or pieces (about 120 large halves)	1 c.	118	3	810	11	84	7.2	50.5	20.0	17	86	341	2.8	712	150	1.01	0.15	1.1	2
527	Pumpkin and squash kernels, dry, hulled	1 c.	140	4	775	41	65	11.8	23.5	27.5	21	71	1602	15.7	1386	100	0.34	0.27	3.4	—
528	Sunflower seeds, dry, hulled	1 c.	145	5	810	35	69	8.2	13.7	43.2	29	174	1214	10.3	1334	70	2.84	0.33	7.8	—
	Walnuts																		
	Black																		
529	Chopped or broken kernels	1 c.	125	3	785	26	74	6.3	13.3	45.7	19	tr	713	7.5	575	380	0.28	0.14	0.9	—
530	Ground (finely)	1 c.	80	3	500	16	47	4.0	8.5	29.2	12	tr	456	4.8	368	240	0.18	0.09	0.6	—

(continued)

APPENDIX 1. (continued)

Item No. (A)	Foods, Approximate Measures, Units, and Weight (Edible Part Unless Footnotes Indicate Otherwise) (B)	Grams	Water Per-cent (C)	Food Energy Cal-ories (D)	Protein g (E)	Fat g (F)	Saturated (Total) g (G)	Oleic g (H)	Linoleic g (I)	Carbohydrate g (J)	Calcium mg (K)	Phosphorus mg (L)	Iron mg (M)	Potassium mg (N)	Vitamin A Value IU (O)	Thiamine mg (P)	Riboflavin mg (Q)	Niacin mg (R)	Ascorbic Acid mg (S)
531	Persian or English, chopped (about 60 halves)...1 c	120	4	780	18	77	8.4	11.8	42.2	19	119	456	3.7	540	40	0.40	0.16	1.1	2
SUGARS AND SWEETS																			
	Cake icings																		
	Boiled, white																		
532	Plain...1 c	94	18	295	1	0	0	0	0	75	2	2	tr	17	0	tr	0.03	tr	0
533	With coconut...1 c	166	15	605	3	13	11.0	0.9	tr	124	10	50	0.8	277	0	0.02	0.07	0.3	0
	Uncooked																		
534	Chocolate made with milk and butter...1 c	275	14	1035	9	38	23.4	11.7	1.0	185	165	305	3.3	536	580	0.06	0.28	0.6	1
535	Creamy fudge from mix and water...1 c	245	15	830	7	16	5.1	6.7	3.1	183	96	218	2.7	238	tr	0.05	0.20	0.7	tr
536	White...1 c	319	11	1200	2	21	12.7	5.1	0.5	260	48	38	tr	57	860	tr	0.06	tr	tr
	Candy																		
537	Caramels, plain or chocolate...1 oz	28	8	115	1	3	1.6	1.1	0.1	22	42	35	0.4	54	tr	0.01	0.05	tr	tr
	Chocolate																		
538	Milk, plain...1 oz	28	1	145	2	9	5.5	3.0	0.3	16	65	65	0.3	109	80	0.02	0.10	0.1	tr
539	Semisweet, small pieces (60 per oz)...1 c or 6-oz pkg	170	1	860	7	61	36.2	19.8	1.7	97	51	255	4.4	553	30	0.02	0.14	0.9	0
540	Chocolate-coated peanuts...1 oz	28	1	160	5	12	4.0	4.7	2.1	11	33	84	0.4	143	tr	0.10	0.05	2.1	tr
541	Fondant, uncoated (mints, candy corn, other)...1 oz	28	8	105	tr	1	0.1	0.3	0.1	25	4	2	0.3	1	0	tr	tr	tr	0
542	Fudge, chocolate, plain...1 oz	28	8	115	1	3	1.3	1.4	0.6	21	22	24	0.3	42	tr	0.01	0.03	0.1	tr
543	Gum drops...1 oz	28	12	100	tr	tr	—	—	—	25	2	tr	0.1	1	0	0	tr	0	0
544	Hard...1 oz	28	1	110	0	tr	—	—	—	28	6	2	0.5	1	0	0	0	0	0
545	Marshmallows...1 oz	28	17	90	1	tr	—	—	—	23	5	2	0.5	2	0	tr	tr	tr	0
	Chocolate-flavored beverage powders (about 4 heaping tsp per oz)																		

No.	Food	Measure	Grams	Water (%)	Food energy	Protein	Fat	Saturated	Oleic	Linoleic	Carbohydrate	Calcium	Phosphorus	Iron	Potassium	Vitamin A	Thiamin	Riboflavin	Niacin	Ascorbic acid
546	With non-fat dry milk	1 oz	28	2	100	5	1	0.5	0.3	tr	20	167	155	0.5	227	10	0.04	0.21	0.2	1
547	Without milk	1 oz	28	1	100	1	1	0.4	0.2	tr	25	9	48	0.6	142	—	0.01	0.03	0.1	0
548	Honey, strained or extracted	1 tbsp	21	17	65	tr	0	0	0	0	17	4	1	0.1	11	tr	tr	0.01	0.1	tr
549	Jams and preserves	1 tbsp	20	29	55	tr	tr	—	—	—	14	4	2	0.2	18	tr	tr	0.01	tr	tr
550		1 packet	14	29	40	tr	tr	—	—	—	10	3	1	0.1	12	tr	tr	tr	tr	tr
551	Jellies	1 tbsp	18	29	50	tr	tr	—	—	—	13	4	1	0.3	14	tr	tr	0.01	tr	1
552		1 packet	14	29	40	tr	tr	—	—	—	10	3	1	0.2	11	tr	tr	tr	tr	1
	Syrups																			
	Chocolate-flavored syrup or topping																			
553	Thin type	1 fl oz or 2 tbsp	38	32	90	1	1	0.5	0.3	tr	24	6	35	0.6	106	tr	0.01	0.03	0.2	0
554	Fudge type	1 fl oz or 2 tbsp	38	25	125	2	5	3.1	1.6	0.1	20	48	60	0.5	107	60	0.02	0.08	0.2	tr
	Molasses, cane																			
555	Light (first extraction)	1 tbsp	20	24	50	—	—	—	—	—	13	33	9	0.9	183	—	0.01	0.01	tr	—
556	Blackstrap (third extraction)	1 tbsp	20	24	45	—	—	—	—	—	11	137	17	3.2	585	—	0.02	0.04	0.4	—
557	Sorghum	1 tbsp	21	23	55	—	—	—	—	—	14	35	5	2.6	—	—	—	0.02	tr	—
558	Table blends, chiefly corn, light and dark	1 tbsp	21	24	60	0	0	0	0	0	15	9	3	0.8	1	0	0	0	0	0
	Sugars																			
559	Brown, pressed down	1 c	220	2	820	0	0	0	0	0	212	187	42	7.5	757	0	0.02	0.07	0.4	0
	White																			
560	Granulated	1 c	200	1	770	0	0	0	0	0	199	0	0	0.2	6	0	0	0	0	0
561	Granulated	1 tbsp	12	1	45	0	0	0	0	0	12	0	0	tr	tr	0	0	0	0	0
562	Granulated	1 packet	6	1	23	0	0	0	0	0	6	0	0	tr	tr	0	0	0	0	0
563	Powdered, sifted, spooned into cup	1 c	100	1	385	0	0	0	0	0	100	0	0	0.1	3	0	0	0	0	0

VEGETABLE AND VEGETABLE PRODUCTS

No.	Food	Measure	Grams	Water (%)	Food energy	Protein	Fat	Saturated	Oleic	Linoleic	Carbohydrate	Calcium	Phosphorus	Iron	Potassium	Vitamin A	Thiamin	Riboflavin	Niacin	Ascorbic acid
	Asparagus, green																			
	Cooked, drained																			
	Cuts and tips (1½"–2" lengths)																			
564	From raw	1 c	145	94	30	3	tr	—	—	—	5	30	73	0.9	265	1310	0.23	0.26	2.0	38
565	From frozen	1 c	180	93	40	6	tr	—	—	—	6	40	115	2.2	396	1530	0.25	0.23	1.8	41
	Spears (½" diam at base)																			
566	From raw	4 spears	60	94	10	1	tr	—	—	—	2	13	30	0.4	110	540	0.10	0.11	0.8	16
567	From frozen	4 spears	60	92	15	2	tr	—	—	—	2	13	40	0.7	143	470	0.10	0.08	0.7	16
568	Canned, spears (½" diam at base)	4 spears	80	93	15	2	tr	—	—	—	3	15	42	1.5	133	640	0.05	0.08	0.6	12
	Beans																			
	Lima, immature seeds, frozen cooked, drained																			
	Thick-seeded types (Fordhooks)																			
569		1 c	170	74	170	10	tr	—	—	—	32	34	153	2.9	724	390	0.12	0.09	1.7	29

(continued)

APPENDIX 1. (continued)

Item No. (A)	Foods, Approximate Measures, Units, and Weight (Edible Part Unless Footnotes Indicate Otherwise) (B)	Water Per-cent (C)	Food Energy Cal-ories (D)	Protein g (E)	Fat g (F)	Saturated (Total) g (G)	Unsaturated Oleic g (H)	Unsaturated Linoleic g (I)	Carbohydrate g (J)	Calcium mg (K)	Phosphorus mg (L)	Iron mg (M)	Potassium mg (N)	Vitamin A Value IU (O)	Thiamine mg (P)	Riboflavin mg (Q)	Niacin mg (R)	Ascorbic Acid mg (S)
570	Thin-seeded types (baby limas) ....1 c.........	180	69	210	13	tr	—	—	—	40	63	227	4.7	709	400	0.16	0.09	2.2	22
	Snap																		
	Green																		
	Cooked, drained																		
	From raw (cuts and																		
571	French style).......1 c.........	125	92	30	2	tr	—	—	—	7	63	46	0.8	189	680	0.09	0.11	0.6	15
	From frozen																		
572	Cuts...........1 c...	135	92	35	2	tr	—	—	—	8	54	43	0.9	205	780	0.09	0.12	0.5	7
573	French style ......1 c...	130	92	35	2	tr	—	—	—	8	49	39	1.2	177	690	0.08	0.10	0.4	9
574	Canned, drained solids (cuts).......1 c...	135	92	30	2	tr	—	—	—	7	61	34	2.0	128	630	0.04	0.07	0.4	5
	Yellow or wax																		
	Cooked, drained																		
	From raw (cuts and																		
575	French style ......1 c.........	125	93	30	2	tr	—	—	—	6	63	46	0.8	189	290	0.09	0.11	0.6	16
576	From frozen (cuts).......1 c...	135	92	35	2	tr	—	—	—	8	47	42	0.9	221	140	0.09	0.11	0.5	8
577	Canned, drained solids (cuts).......1 c...	135	92	30	2	tr	—	—	—	7	61	34	2.0	128	140	0.04	0.07	0.4	7
	Beans, mature (see Beans, dry, items 509–515, and Blackeye peas, dry, item 516)																		
	Bean sprouts (mung)																		
578	Raw ....1 c...	105	89	35	4	tr	—	—	—	7	20	67	1.4	234	20	0.14	0.14	0.8	20
579	Cooked, drained ......1 c...	125	91	35	4	tr	—	—	—	7	21	60	1.1	195	30	0.11	0.13	0.9	8
	Beets																		
	Cooked, drained, peeled																		

No.	Food	Measure	Grams	Water %	Cal.	Protein	Fat												
580	Whole beets (2″ diam)	2 beets	100	91	30	1	tr	—	—	7	14	23	0.5	208	20	0.03	0.04	0.3	6
581	Diced or sliced	1 c	170	91	55	2	tr	—	—	12	24	39	0.9	354	30	0.05	0.07	0.5	10
	Canned, drained solids																		
582	Whole beets, small	1 c	160	89	60	2	tr	—	—	14	30	29	1.1	267	30	0.02	0.05	0.2	5
583	Diced or sliced	1 c	170	89	65	2	tr	—	—	15	32	31	1.2	284	30	0.02	0.05	0.2	5
584	Beet greens, leaves and stems, cooked, drained	1 c	145	94	25	2	tr	—	—	5	144	36	2.8	481	7400	0.10	0.22	0.4	22
	Blackeye peas, immature seeds, cooked and drained																		
585	From raw	1 c	165	72	180	13	1	—	—	30	40	241	3.5	625	580	0.50	0.18	2.3	28
586	From frozen	1 c	170	66	220	15	1	—	—	40	43	286	4.8	573	290	0.68	0.19	2.4	15
	Broccoli, cooked, drained																		
	From raw																		
587	Stalk, medium size	1 stalk	180	91	45	6	1	—	—	8	158	112	1.4	481	4500	0.16	0.36	1.4	162
588	Stalks cut into ½″ pieces	1 c	155	91	40	5	tr	—	—	7	136	96	1.2	414	3880	0.14	0.31	1.2	140
	From frozen																		
589	Stalk (4½″–5″ long)	1 stalk	30	91	10	1	tr	—	—	1	12	17	0.2	66	570	0.02	0.03	0.2	22
590	Chopped	1 c	185	92	50	5	1	—	—	9	100	104	1.3	392	4810	0.11	0.22	0.9	105
	Brussel sprouts, cooked, drained																		
591	From raw, 7–8 sprouts (1¼″–1½″ diam)	1 c	155	88	55	7	1	—	—	10	50	112	1.7	423	810	0.12	0.22	1.2	135
592	From frozen	1 c	155	89	50	5	tr	—	—	10	33	95	1.2	457	880	0.12	0.16	0.9	126
	Cabbage																		
	Common varieties																		
	Raw																		
593	Coarsely shredded or sliced	1 c	70	92	15	1	tr	—	—	4	34	20	0.3	163	90	0.04	0.04	0.2	33
594	Finely shredded or chopped	1 c	90	92	20	1	tr	—	—	5	44	26	0.4	210	120	0.05	0.05	0.3	42
595	Cooked, drained	1 c	145	94	30	2	tr	—	—	6	64	29	0.4	236	190	0.06	0.06	0.4	48
596	Red, raw, coarsely shredded or sliced	1 c	70	90	20	1	tr	—	—	5	29	25	0.6	188	30	0.06	0.04	0.3	43
597	Savoy, raw, coarsely shredded or sliced	1 c	70	92	15	2	tr	—	—	3	47	38	0.6	188	140	0.04	0.06	0.2	39
598	Cabbage, celery (also called pe-tsai or wongbok), raw, 1″ pieces	1 c	75	95	10	1	tr	—	—	2	32	30	0.5	190	110	0.04	0.03	0.5	19
599	Cabbage, white mustard (also called bokchoy or pakchoy), cooked, drained	1 c	170	95	25	2	tr	—	—	4	252	56	1.0	364	5270	0.07	0.14	1.2	26
	Carrots																		
	Raw, without crowns and tips, scraped																		
600	Whole (7½″ × 1⅛″), or strips, 2½″–3″ long	1 carrot or 18 strips	72	88	30	1	tr	—	—	7	27	26	0.5	246	7930	0.04	0.04	0.4	6

(continued)

635

APPENDIX 1. (continued)

Item No. (A)	Foods, Approximate Measures, Units, and Weight (Edible Part Unless Footnotes Indicate Otherwise) (B)	(g)	Water Per-cent (C)	Food Energy Cal-ories (D)	Protein (E)	Fat (F)	Fatty Acids Saturated (Total) (G)	Unsaturated Oleic (H)	Unsaturated Linoleic (I)	Carbohydrate (J)	Calcium (K)	Phosphorus (L)	Iron (M)	Potassium (N)	Vitamin A Value (O)	Thiamine (P)	Riboflavin (Q)	Niacin (R)	Ascorbic Acid (S)
		g	Per-cent	Cal-ories	g	g	g	g	g	g	mg	mg	mg	mg	IU	mg	mg	mg	mg
601	Grated..........1 c.	110	88	45	1	tr	—	—	—	11	41	40	0.8	375	12,100	0.07	0.06	0.7	9
602	Cooked (crosswise cuts), drained..........1 c.	155	91	50	1	tr	—	—	—	11	51	48	0.9	344	16,280	0.08	0.08	0.8	9
603	Canned, Sliced, drained solids.......1 c.	155	91	45	1	tr	—	—	—	10	47	34	1.1	186	23,250	0.03	0.05	0.6	3
604	Strained or junior (baby food)..........1 oz (1¾–2 tbsp)	28	92	10	tr	tr	—	—	—	2	7	6	0.1	51	3690	0.01	0.01	0.1	1
	Cauliflower																		
605	Raw, chopped..........1 c.	115	91	31	3	tr	—	—	—	6	29	64	1.3	339	70	0.13	0.12	0.8	90
606	Cooked, drained From raw (flower buds) .....1 c.	125	93	30	3	tr	—	—	—	5	26	53	0.9	258	80	0.11	0.10	0.8	69
607	From frozen (flowerets) .....1 c.	180	94	30	3	tr	—	—	—	6	31	68	0.9	373	50	0.07	0.09	0.7	74
	Celery, Pascal type, raw																		
608	Stalk, large outer (8″ × 1½″ at root end).......1 stalk.	40	94	5	tr	tr	—	—	—	2	16	11	0.1	136	110	0.01	0.01	0.1	4
609	Pieces, diced..........1 c.	120	94	20	1	tr	—	—	—	5	47	34	0.4	409	320	0.04	0.04	0.4	11
610	Collards, cooked, drained From raw (leaves without stems)..........1 c.	190	90	65	7	1	—	—	—	10	357	99	1.5	498	14,820	0.21	0.38	2.3	144
611	From frozen (chopped)..........1 c.	170	90	50	5	1	—	—	—	10	299	87	1.7	401	11,560	0.10	0.24	1.0	56
	Corn, sweet Cooked, drained																		
612	From raw, ear (5″ × 1¾″)....1 ear[61]	140	74	70	2	1	—	—	—	16	2	69	0.5	151	310[62]	0.09	0.08	1.1	7
613	From frozen Ear (5″ long)..........1 ear[61]	229	73	120	4	1	—	—	—	27	4	121	1.0	291	440[62]	0.18	0.10	2.1	9
614	Kernels..........1 c.	165	77	130	5	1	—	—	—	31	5	120	1.3	304	580[62]	0.15	0.10	2.5	8

(*continued*)

Item No.	Food and approximate measure	Measure	Weight (g)	Water (%)	Food energy (cal)	Protein (g)	Fat (g)	Saturated (g)	Oleic (g)	Linoleic (g)	Carbohydrate (g)	Calcium (mg)	Phosphorus (mg)	Iron (mg)	Potassium (mg)	Vitamin A (IU)	Thiamin (mg)	Riboflavin (mg)	Niacin (mg)	Ascorbic acid (mg)
	Canned																			
615	Cream style	1 c	256	76	210	5	2	—	—	—	51	8	143	1.5	248	840[62]	0.08	0.13	2.6	13
	Whole kernel																			
616	Vacuum pack	1 c	210	76	175	5	1	—	—	—	43	6	153	1.1	204	740[62]	0.06	0.13	2.3	11
617	Wet pack, drained solids	1 c	165	76	140	4	1	—	—	—	33	8	81	0.8	160	580[62]	0.05	0.08	1.5	7
	Cowpeas (see Blackeye peas, Items 585–586)																			
	Cucumber slices, ⅛" thick (large, 2⅛" diam; small, 1¾" diam)																			
618	With peel	6 large or 8 small slices	28	95	5	tr	tr	—	—	—	1	7	8	0.3	45	70	0.01	0.01	0.1	3
619	Without peel	6½ large or 9 small pieces	28	96	5	tr	tr	—	—	—	1	5	5	0.1	45	tr	tr	0.01	0.1	3
620	Dandelion greens, cooked, drained	1 c	105	90	35	2	1	—	—	—	7	147	44	1.9	244	12,290	0.14	0.17	—	19
621	Endive, curly (including escarole), raw, small pieces	1 c	50	93	10	1	tr	—	—	—	2	41	27	0.9	147	1650	0.04	0.07	0.3	5
	Kale, cooked, drained																			
622	From raw (leaves without stems and midribs)	1 c	110	88	45	5	1	—	—	—	7	206	64	1.8	243	9130	0.11	0.20	1.8	102
623	From frozen (leaf style)	1 c	130	91	40	4	1	—	—	—	7	157	62	1.3	251	10,660	0.08	0.20	0.9	49
	Lettuce, raw																			
	Butterhead, as Boston types																			
624	Head, 5" diam	1 head[63]	220	95	25	2	tr	—	—	—	4	57	42	3.3	430	1580	0.10	0.10	0.5	13
625	Leaves	1 outer, 2 inner, or 3 heart leaves	15	95	tr	tr	tr	—	—	—	tr	5	4	0.3	40	150	0.01	0.01	tr	1
	Crisphead, as Iceberg																			
626	Head, 6" diam	1 head[64]	567	96	70	5	1	—	—	—	16	108	118	2.7	943	1780	0.32	0.32	1.6	32
627	Wedge, ¼ of head	1 wedge	135	96	20	1	tr	—	—	—	4	27	30	0.7	236	450	0.08	0.08	0.4	8
628	Pieces, chopped or shredded	1 c	55	96	5	tr	tr	—	—	—	2	11	12	0.3	96	180	0.03	0.03	0.2	3
	Looseleaf (bunching varieties including romaine or cos)																			
629	chopped or shredded pieces	1 c	55	94	10	1	tr	—	—	—	2	37	14	0.8	145	1050	0.03	0.04	0.2	10
630	Mushrooms, raw, sliced or chopped	1 c	70	90	20	2	tr	—	—	—	3	4	81	0.6	290	tr	0.07	0.32	2.9	2
631	Mustard greens, without stems and midribs, cooked, drained	1 c	140	93	30	3	1	—	—	—	6	193	45	2.5	308	8120	0.11	0.20	0.8	67
632	Okra pods (3" × ⅝"), cooked	10 pods	106	91	30	2	tr	—	—	—	6	98	43	0.5	184	520	0.14	0.19	1.0	21

APPENDIX 1. (continued)

Item No. (A)	Foods, Approximate Measures, Units, and Weight (Edible Part Unless Footnotes Indicate Otherwise) (B)	Water (C) Per-cent	Food Energy (D) Cal-ories	Protein (E) g	Fat (F) g	Saturated (Total) (G) g	Oleic (H) g	Linoleic (I) g	Carbohydrate (J) g	Calcium (K) mg	Phosphorus (L) mg	Iron (M) mg	Potassium (N) mg	Vitamin A Value (O) IU	Thiamine (P) mg	Riboflavin (Q) mg	Niacin (R) mg	Ascorbic Acid (S) mg
		g		g	g	g	g	g	g	mg	mg	mg	mg	IU	mg	mg	mg	mg
	Onions																	
	Mature																	
	Raw																	
633	Chopped . . . . 1 c . . . . (170)	89	65	3	tr	—	—	—	15	46	61	0.9	267	tr[65]	0.05	0.07	0.3	17
634	Sliced . . . . 1 c . . . . (115)	89	45	2	tr	—	—	—	10	31	41	0.6	181	tr[65]	0.03	0.05	0.2	12
635	Cooked (whole or sliced), drained . . . . 1 c . . . . (210)	92	60	3	tr	—	—	—	14	50	61	0.8	231	tr[65]	0.06	0.06	0.4	15
636	Young green, bulb (3/8" diam and white portion of top . . . . . . 6 onions . . . (30)	88	15	tr	tr	—	—	—	3	12	12	0.2	69	tr	0.02	0.01	0.1	8
637	Parsley, raw, chopped . . . . 1 tbsp . . . . (4)	85	tr	tr	tr	—	—	—	tr	7	2	0.2	25	300	tr	0.01	tr	6
638	Parsnips, cooked (diced or 2" lengths) . . . . 1 c . . . . (155)	82	100	2	1	—	—	—	23	70	96	0.9	587	50	0.11	0.12	0.2	16
	Peas, green																	
	Canned																	
639	Whole, drained solids . . . . 1 c . . . . (170)	77	150	8	1	—	—	—	29	44	129	3.2	163	1170	0.15	0.10	1.4	14
640	Strained (baby food) . . . . . . 1 oz (1¾ to 2 tbsp) . . . . (28)	86	15	1	tr	—	—	—	3	3	18	0.3	28	140	0.02	0.03	0.3	3
641	Frozen, cooked, drained . . . . 1 c . . . . (160)	82	110	8	tr	—	—	—	19	30	138	3.0	216	960	0.14	0.43	2.7	21
642	Peppers, hot, red, without seeds, dried (ground chili powder, added seasonings) . . . . 1 tsp . . . . (2)	9	5	tr	tr	—	—	—	1	5	4	0.3	20	1300	tr	0.02	0.2	tr
	Peppers, sweet (about 5 per lb, whole), stem and seeds removed																	
643	Raw . . . . 1 pod . . . . (74)	93	15	1	tr	—	—	—	4	7	16	0.5	157	310	0.06	0.06	0.4	94
644	Cooked, boiled, drained . . . . 1 pod . . . . (73)	95	15	1	tr	—	—	—	3	7	12	0.4	109	310	0.05	0.05	0.4	70

No.	Food, approximate measure, and weight (in grams)		Grams	Water (%)	Food energy (cal.)	Protein (g)	Fat (g)	Saturated fat (g)	Oleic (g)	Linoleic (g)	Carbohydrate (g)	Calcium (mg)	Iron (mg)	Potassium (mg)	Vit. A (IU)	Thiamin (mg)	Riboflavin (mg)	Niacin (mg)	Ascorbic acid (mg)
645	Baked, peeled after baking (about 2 per lb, raw)	1 potato	156	75	145	4	tr	—	—	—	33	14	1.1	782	tr	0.15	0.07	2.7	31
	Boiled (about 3 per lb, raw)																		
646	Peeled after boiling	1 potato	137	80	105	3	tr	—	—	—	23	10	0.8	556	tr	0.12	0.05	2.0	22
647	Peeled before boiling	1 potato	135	83	90	3	tr	—	—	—	20	8	0.7	385	tr	0.12	0.05	1.6	22
	French-fried, strip (2 to 3½" long)																		
648	Prepared from raw	10 strips	50	45	135	2	7	1.7	1.2	3.3	18	8	0.7	427	tr	0.07	0.04	1.6	11
649	Frozen, oven-heated	10 strips	50	53	110	2	4	1.1	0.8	2.1	17	5	0.9	326	tr	0.07	0.01	1.3	11
650	Hashed brown, prepared from frozen	1 c.	155	56	345	3	18	4.6	3.2	9.0	45	28	1.9	439	tr	0.11	0.03	1.6	12
	Mashed, prepared from— Raw																		
651	Milk added	1 c.	210	83	135	4	2	0.7	0.4	tr	27	50	0.8	548	40	0.17	0.11	2.1	21
652	Milk and butter added	1 c.	210	80	195	4	9	5.6	2.3	0.2	26	50	0.8	525	360	0.17	0.11	2.1	19
653	Dehydrated flakes (without milk), water, milk, butter, and salt added	1 c.	210	79	195	4	7	3.6	2.1	0.2	30	65	0.6	601	270	0.08	0.08	1.9	11
654	Potato chips (1¾" × 2½" oval cross section)	10 chips	20	2	115	1	8	2.1	1.4	4.0	10	8	0.4	226	tr	0.04	0.01	1.0	3
655	Potato salad, made with cooked salad dressing	1 c.	250	76	250	7	7	2.0	2.7	1.3	41	80	1.5	798	350	0.20	0.18	2.8	28
656	Pumpkin, canned	1 c.	245	90	80	2	1	—	—	—	19	61	1.0	588	15,680	0.07	0.12	1.5	12
657	Radishes, raw (prepackaged) stem ends, rootlets cut off	4 radishes	18	95	5	tr	tr	—	—	—	1	5	0.2	58	tr	0.01	0.01	0.1	5
658	Sauerkraut, canned, solids and liquid	1 c.	235	93	40	2	tr	—	—	—	9	85	1.2	329	120	0.07	0.09	0.5	33
	Southern peas (see Blackeye peas, items 585–586) Spinach																		
659	Raw, chopped	1 c.	55	91	15	2	tr	—	—	—	2	51	1.7	259	4460	0.06	0.11	0.3	28
	Cooked, drained																		
660	From raw	1 c.	180	92	40	5	1	—	—	—	6	167	4.0	583	14,580	0.13	0.25	0.9	50
	From frozen																		
661	Chopped	1 c.	205	92	45	6	1	—	—	—	8	232	4.3	683	16,200	0.14	0.31	0.8	39
662	Leaf	1 c.	190	92	45	6	1	—	—	—	7	200	4.8	688	15,390	0.15	0.27	1.0	53
663	Canned, drained solids	1 c.	205	91	50	6	1	—	—	—	7	242	5.3	513	16,400	0.04	0.25	0.6	29
	Squash, cooked																		
664	Summer (all varieties), diced, drained	1 c.	210	96	30	2	tr	—	—	—	7	53	0.8	296	820	0.11	0.17	1.7	21
665	Winter (all varieties), baked, mashed	1 c.	205	81	130	4	1	—	—	—	32	57	1.6	945	8610	0.10	0.27	1.4	27

(continued)

APPENDIX 1. (continued)

Item No. (A)	Foods, Approximate Measures, Units, and Weight (Edible Part Unless Footnotes Indicate Otherwise) (B)	g	Water Per-cent (C)	Food Energy Cal-ories (D)	Protein (E)	Fat (F)	Fatty Acids Saturated (Total) (G)	Unsaturated Oleic (H)	Unsaturated Linoleic (I)	Carbohydrate (J)	Calcium (K)	Phosphorus (L)	Iron (M)	Potassium (N)	Vitamin A Value (O)	Thiamine (P)	Riboflavin (Q)	Niacin (R)	Ascorbic Acid (S)
		g			g	g	g	g	g	g	mg	mg	mg	mg	IU	mg	mg	mg	mg
	Sweet potatoes																		
	Cooked (raw, 5" × 2", about 2½ per lb)																		
666	Baked in skin, peeled ....1 potato	114	64	160	2	1	—	—	—	37	46	66	1.0	342	9230	0.10	0.08	0.8	25
667	Boiled in skin, peeled ....1 potato	151	71	170	3	1	—	—	—	40	48	71	1.1	367	11,940	0.14	0.09	0.9	26
668	Candied, 2½" × 2" piece .....1 piece	105	60	175	1	3	2.0	0.8	0.1	36	39	45	0.9	200	6620	0.06	0.04	0.4	11
	Canned																		
669	Solid pack (mashed) ....1 c.	255	72	275	5	1	—	—	—	63	64	105	2.0	510	19,890	0.13	0.10	1.5	36
670	Vacuum pack, piece (2¾" × 1")........1 piece	40	72	45	1	tr	—	—	—	10	10	16	0.3	80	3120	0.02	0.02	0.2	6
	Tomatoes																		
671	Raw (2⅗" diam, 3 per 12 oz pkg).........1 tomato[66] ..	135	94	25	1	tr	—	—	—	6	16	33	0.6	300	1110	0.07	0.05	0.9	28[67]
672	Canned, solids and liquid ....1 c.	241	94	50	2	tr	—	—	—	10	14[68]	46	1.2	523	2170	0.12	0.07	1.7	41
673	Tomato catsup ....1 c.	273	69	290	5	1	—	—	—	69	60	137	2.2	991	3820	0.25	0.19	4.4	41
674	1 tbsp.	15	69	15	tr	tr	—	—	—	4	3	8	0.1	54	210	0.01	0.01	0.2	2
	Tomato juice, canned																		
675	Cup ....1 c.	243	94	45	2	tr	—	—	—	10	17	44	2.2	552	1940	0.12	0.07	1.9	39
676	Glass (6 fl oz) ....1 glass	182	94	35	2	tr	—	—	—	8	13	33	1.6	413	1460	0.09	0.05	1.5	29
677	Turnips, cooked, diced ....1 c.	155	94	35	1	tr	—	—	—	8	54	37	0.6	291	tr	0.06	0.08	0.5	34
	Turnip greens, cooked, drained																		
678	From raw (leaves and stems) ...1 c.	145	94	30	3	tr	—	—	—	5	252	49	1.5	—	8270	0.15	0.33	0.7	68
679	From frozen (chopped).........1 c.	165	93	40	4	tr	—	—	—	6	195	64	2.6	246	11,390	0.08	0.15	0.7	31
680	Vegetables, mixed, frozen, cooked ....1 c.	182	83	115	6	1	—	—	—	24	46	115	2.4	348	9010	0.13	0.22	2.0	15

MISCELLANEOUS ITEMS

No.	Food, approximate measure, and weight	Grams	Water (%)	Food energy	Protein	Fat	Saturated	Monounsat.	Polyunsat.	Carbohydrate	Calcium	Phosphorus	Iron	Potassium	Vitamin A	Thiamin	Riboflavin	Niacin	Ascorbic acid
	Baking powders for home use																		
	Sodium aluminum sulfate																		
681	With monocalcium phosphate monohydrate ... 1 tsp	3.0	2	5	tr	0	0	0	0	1	58	87	—	5	0	0	0	0	0
682	With monocalcium phosphate monohydrate, calcium sulfate ... 1 tsp	2.9	1	5	tr	0	0	0	0	1	183	45	—	—	0	0	0	0	0
683	Straight phosphate ... 1 tsp	3.8	2	5	tr	0	0	0	0	1	239	359	—	6	0	0	0	0	0
684	Low-sodium ... 1 tsp	4.3	2	5	tr	0	0	0	0	2	207	314	—	471	0	0	0	0	0
685	Barbecue sauce ... 1 c.	250	81	230	4	17	2.2	4.3	10.0	20	53	50	2.0	435	900	0.03	0.03	0.8	13
	Beverages, alcoholic																		
686	Beer ... 12 fl oz.	360	92	150	1	0	0	0	0	14	18	108	tr	90	—	0.01	0.11	2.2	—
	Gin, rum, vodka, whisky																		
687	80-proof ... 1½-fl oz jigger	42	67	95	—	0	0	0	0	tr	—	—	—	1	—	—	—	—	—
688	86-proof ... 1½-fl oz jigger	42	64	105	—	0	0	0	0	tr	—	—	—	1	—	—	—	—	—
689	90-proof ... 1½-fl oz jigger	42	62	110	—	0	0	0	0	tr	—	—	—	1	—	—	—	—	—
	Wines																		
690	Dessert ... 3½-fl oz glass	103	77	140	tr	0	0	0	0	8	8	8	—	27	—	0.01	0.02	0.2	—
691	Table ... 3½-fl oz glass	102	86	85	tr	0	0	0	0	4	9	10	0.4	94	—	tr	0.01	0.1	—
	Beverages, carbonated, sweetened, nonalcoholic																		
692	Carbonated water ... 12 fl oz.	366	92	115	0	0	0	0	0	29	—	—	—	—	0	0	0	0	0
693	Cola-type ... 12 fl oz.	369	90	145	0	0	0	0	0	37	—	—	—	—	0	0	0	0	0
694	Fruit-flavored sodas and Tom Collins mixer ... 12 fl oz.	372	88	170	0	0	0	0	0	45	—	—	—	—	0	0	0	0	0
695	Ginger ale ... 12 fl oz.	366	92	115	0	0	0	0	0	29	—	—	—	0	0	0	0	0	0
696	Root beer ... 12 fl oz.	370	90	150	0	0	0	0	0	39	—	—	—	0	0	0	0	0	0
	Chili powder (see Peppers, hot, red, item 642)																		
	Chocolate																		
697	Bitter or baking ... 1 oz	28	2	145	3	15	8.9	4.9	0.4	8	22	109	1.9	235	20	0.01	0.07	0.4	0
	Semisweet (see Candy, chocolate, item 539)																		
698	Gelatin, dry ... 1 7-g envelope	7	13	25	6	tr	0	0	0	0	—	—	—	—	—	—	—	—	—
699	Gelatin dessert prepared with gelatin dessert powder and water ... 1 c.	240	84	140	4	0	0	0	0	34	—	—	—	—	—	—	—	—	—

(continued)

APPENDIX 1. (continued)

Item No. (A)	Foods, Approximate Measures, Units, and Weight (Edible Part Unless Footnotes Indicate Otherwise) (B)	(C) Water Per-cent	(D) Food Energy Cal-ories	(E) Protein g	(F) Fat g	(G) Saturated (Total) g	(H) Oleic g	(I) Linoleic g	(J) Carbo-hydrate g	(K) Calcium mg	(L) Phos-phorus mg	(M) Iron mg	(N) Potassium mg	(O) Vitamin A Value IU	(P) Thiamine mg	(Q) Riboflavin mg	(R) Niacin mg	(S) Ascorbic Acid mg
700	Mustard, prepared, yellow . . . . . . 1 tsp or individual serving pouch or cup . . . . . . (5 g)	80	5	tr	tr	—	—	tr	tr	4	4	0.1	7	—	—	—	—	—
701	Olives, pickled, canned — Green . . . 4 medium, 3 extra large, or 2 giant[69] . . . (16 g)	78	15	tr	2	0.2	1.2	0.1	tr	8	2	0.2	7	40	—	—	—	—
702	Ripe, Mission . . . 3 small or 2 large[69] . . . (10 g)	73	15	tr	2	0.2	1.2	0.1	tr	9	1	0.1	2	10	tr	—	—	—
	Pickles, cucumber																	
703	Dill, medium, whole (3¾" long, 1¼" diam) . . . 1 pickle . . . (65 g)	93	5	tr	tr	—	—	—	1	17	14	0.7	130	70	tr	0.01	tr	4
704	Fresh-pack, slices (1½" diam, ¼" thick) . . . 2 slices . . . (15 g)	79	10	tr	tr	—	—	—	3	5	4	0.3	—	20	tr	tr	1	1
705	Sweet, gherkin, small, whole (about 2½" long, ¾" diam) . . . 1 pickle . . . (15 g)	61	20	tr	tr	—	—	—	5	2	2	0.2	—	10	tr	tr	1	—
706	Relish, finely chopped, sweet . . . 1 tbsp . . . (15 g)	63	20	tr	tr	—	—	—	5	3	2	0.1	—	—	—	—	—	—
	Popcorn (see items 476–478)																	
707	Popsicle, 3-fl oz size . . . 1 popsicle . . . (95 g)	80	70	0	0	0	0	0	18	0	tr	—	—	0	0	0	—	0
	Soups — Canned, condensed — Prepared with equal volume of milk																	

Item	Food	Measure	Grams	Water (%)	Cal.	Protein	Fat	Sat.	Mono	Poly	Carb.	Calcium	Phos.	Iron	Potas.	Vit. A	Thiamin	Ribo.	Niacin	Asc.
708	Cream of chicken	1 c	245	85	180	7	10	4.2	3.6	1.3	15	172	152	0.5	260	610	0.05	0.27	0.7	2
709	Cream of mushroom	1 c	245	83	215	7	14	5.4	2.9	4.6	16	191	169	0.5	279	250	0.05	0.34	0.7	1
710	Tomato	1 c	250	84	175	7	7	3.4	1.7	1.0	23	168	155	0.8	418	1200	0.10	0.25	1.3	15
	Prepared with equal volume of water																			
711	Bean with pork	1 c	250	84	170	8	6	1.2	1.8	2.4	22	63	128	2.3	395	650	0.13	0.08	1.0	3
712	Beef broth, bouillon, consommé	1 c	240	96	30	5	0	0	0	0	3	tr	31	0.5	130	tr	tr	0.02	1.2	—
713	Beef noodle	1 c	240	93	65	4	3	0.6	0.7	0.8	7	7	48	1.0	77	50	0.05	0.07	1.0	tr
714	Clam chowder, Manhattan-type (with tomatoes, without milk)	1 c	245	92	80	2	3	0.5	0.4	1.3	12	34	47	1.0	184	880	0.02	0.02	1.0	—
715	Cream of chicken	1 c	240	92	95	3	6	1.6	2.3	1.1	8	24	34	0.5	79	410	0.02	0.05	0.5	tr
716	Cream of mushroom	1 c	240	90	135	2	10	2.6	1.7	4.5	10	41	50	0.5	98	70	0.02	0.12	0.7	tr
717	Minestrone	1 c	245	90	105	5	3	0.7	0.9	1.3	14	37	59	1.0	314	2350	0.07	0.05	1.0	—
718	Split pea	1 c	245	85	145	9	3	1.1	1.2	0.4	21	29	149	1.5	270	440	0.25	0.15	1.5	1
719	Tomato	1 c	245	91	90	2	3	0.5	0.5	1.0	16	15	34	0.7	230	1000	0.05	0.05	1.2	12
720	Vegetable beef	1 c	245	92	80	5	2	—	—	—	10	12	49	0.7	162	2700	0.05	0.05	1.0	—
721	Vegetarian	1 c	245	92	80	2	2	—	—	—	13	20	39	1.0	172	2940	0.05	0.05	1.0	—
	Dehydrated																			
722	Bouillon cube (½")	1 cube	4	4	5	1	tr	—	—	—	tr	—	—	—	4	—	—	—	—	—
	Mixes																			
	Unprepared																			
723	Onion	1½-oz pkg	43	3	150	6	5	1.1	2.3	1.0	23	42	49	0.6	238	30	0.05	0.03	0.3	6
	Prepared with water																			
724	Chicken noodle	1 c	240	95	55	2	1	—	—	—	8	7	19	0.2	19	50	0.07	0.05	0.5	tr
725	Onion	1 c	240	96	35	1	1	—	—	—	6	10	12	0.2	58	tr	tr	tr	tr	2
726	Tomato vegetable with noodles	1 c	240	93	65	1	1	—	0	0	12	7	19	0.2	29	480	0.05	0.02	0.5	5
727	Vinegar, cider	1 tbsp	15	94	tr	tr	tr	—	0	0	1	1	1	0.1	15	—	—	—	—	—
728	White sauce, medium, with enriched flour	1 c	250	73	405	10	31	19.3	7.8	0.8	22	288	233	0.5	348	1150	0.12	0.43	0.7	2
	Yeast																			
729	Baker's, dry, active	1 pkg	7	5	20	3	tr	—	—	—	3	3	90	1.1	140	tr	0.16	0.38	2.6	tr
730	Brewer's, dry	1 tbsp	8	5	25	3	tr	—	—	—	3	17[7]	140	1.4	152	tr	1.25	0.34	3.0	tr

(continued)

[1] Vitamin A value is largely from beta-carotene used for coloring. Riboflavin value for items 40–41 applies to products with added riboflavin.
[2] Applies to product without added vitamin A. With added vitamin A, value is 500 International Units (IU).
[3] Applies to product without vitamin A added.
[4] Applies to product with added vitamin A. Without added vitamin A, value is 20 IU.
[5] Yields 1 qt fluid milk when reconstituted according to package directions.
[6] Applies to product with added vitamin A.
[7] Weight applies to product with label claim of 1⅓ cups equal 3.2 oz.

[8] Applies to products made from thick shake mixes and those that do not contain added ice cream. Products made from milk shake mixes are higher in fat and usually contain added ice cream.

[9] Content of fat, vitamin A, and carbohydrate varies. Consult the label when precise values are needed for special diets.

[10] Applies to product made with milk containing no added vitamin A.

[11] Based on year-round average.

[12] Based on average vitamin A content of fortified margarine. Federal specifications for fortified margarine require a minimum of 15,000 IU vitamin A per pound.

[13] Fatty acid values apply to product made with regular-type margarine.

[14] Dipped in egg, milk or water, and breadcrumbs; fried in vegetable shortening.

[15] If bones are discarded, value for calcium will be greatly reduced.

[16] Dipped in egg, breadcrumbs, and flour or batter.

[17] Prepared with tuna, celery, salad dressing (mayonnaise type) pickle, onion, and egg.

[18] Outer layer of fat on the cut was removed to within approximately ½" of the lean. Deposits of fat within the cut were not removed.

[19] Crust made with vegetable shortening and enriched flour.

[20] Regular-type margarine used.

[21] Value varies widely.

[22] About one-fourth of the outer layer of fat on the cut was removed. Deposits of fat within the cut were not removed.

[23] Vegetable shortening used.

[24] Also applies to pasteurized apple cider.

[25] Applies to product without added ascorbic acid. For value of product with added ascorbic acid, refer to label.

[26] Based on product with label claim of 45% of U.S. RDA in 6 fl oz.

[27] Based on product with label claim of 100% of U.S. RDA in 6 fl oz.

[28] Weight includes peel and membranes between sections. Without these parts the weight of the edible portion is 123 g for item 246 and 118 g for item 247.

[29] For white-fleshed varieties, value is about 20 IU per cup; for red-fleshed varieties, 1080 IU.

[30] Weight includes seeds. Without seeds, weight of the edible portion is 57 g.

[31] Applies to product without added ascorbic acid. With added ascorbic acid, based on claim that 6 fl oz of reconstituted juice contains 45% or 50% of the U.S. RDA, value is 108 mg or 120 mg for a 6-fl-oz can (item 258), 36 or 40 for 1 cup of diluted juice (item 259).

[32] For products with added thiamin and riboflavin but without added ascorbic acid, values would be 0.60 mg for thiamin, 0.80 mg for riboflavin, and trace for ascorbic acid. For products with only ascorbic acid added, value varies with the brand. Consult the label.

[33] Weight includes rind. Without rind, the weight of the edible portion is 272 g for item 271 and 149 g for item 272.

[34] Represents yellow-fleshed varieties. For white-fleshed varieties, value is 50 IU for 1 peach, 90 IU for 1 cup of slices.

[35] Value represents products with added ascorbic acid. For products without added ascorbic acid, value is 116 mg for a 10-oz container; 103 mg for 1 cup.

[36] Weight includes pits. After removal of the pits, the weight of the edible portion is 258 g for item 302, 133 g for item 303, 43 g for item 304, and 213 g for item 305.

[37] Weight includes rind and seeds. Without rind and seeds, weight of the edible portion is 426 g.

[38] Made with vegetable shortening.

[39] Applies to product made with white cornmeal. With yellow cornmeal, value is 30 IU.

[40] Applies to white varieties. For yellow varieties, value is 150 IU.

[41] Applies to products that do not contain disodium phosphate. If disodium phosphate is an ingredient, value is 162 mg.

[42] Value may range from less than 1 mg to about 8 mg depending on the brand. Consult the label.

[43] Applies to product without added nutrient. Without added nutrient, value is trace.

[44] Value varies with the brand. Consult the label.

[45] Applies to product without added nutrient. Without added nutrient, value is trace.

[46] Excepting angel/food cake, cakes were made from mixes containing vegetable shortening; icings, with butter.

[47] Excepting spongecake, vegetable shortening was used for cake portion; butter, for icing. If butter or margarine was used for cake portion, vitamin A values would be higher.

[48] Applies to product made with a sodium aluminum-sulfate type baking powder. With a low-sodium-type baking powder containing potassium, value would be about twice the amount shown.

[49] Equal weights of flour, sugar, eggs, and vegetable shortening.

[50] Products are commercial unless otherwise specified.

[51] Made with enriched flour and vegetable shortening except for macaroons, which do not contain flour or shortening.

[52] Icing made with butter.

[53] Applies to yellow varieties; white varieties contain only a trace.

[54] Contains vegetable shortening and butter.

[55] Made with corn oil.

[56] Made with regular margarine.

[57] Applies to product made with yellow cornmeal.

[58] Made with enriched degermed cornmeal and enriched flour.

[59] Product may or may not be enriched with riboflavin. Consult the label.

[60] Value varies with the brand. Consult the label.

[61] Weight includes cob. Without cob, weight is 77 g for item 612, 126 g for item 613.

[62] Based on yellow varieties. For white varieties, value is trace.

[63] Weight includes refuse of outer leaves and core. Without these parts, weight is 163 g.

[64] Weight includes core. Without core, weight is 539 g.

[65] Value based on white-fleshed varieties. For yellow-fleshed varieties, value is 70 IU for item 633, 50 IU for item 634, and 80 IU for item 635.

[66] Weight includes cores and stem ends. Without these parts, weight is 123 g.

[67] Based on year-round average. For tomatoes marketed from November through May, value is about 12 mg; from June through October, 32 mg.

[68] Applies to product without calcium salts added. Value for products with calcium salts added may be as much as 63 mg for whole tomatoes, 241 mg for cut forms.

[69] Weight includes pits. Without pits, weight is 13 g for item 701, 9 g for item 702.

[70] Value may vary from 6 to 60 mg.

(From USDA Home and Garden Bulletin No. 72, Washington, DC, 1981)

APPENDIX 2. Food and Nutrition Board, National Academy of Sciences—National Research Council Recommended Dietary Allowances,* Revised 1989

Designed for the maintenance of good nutrition of practically all healthy people in the United States

Category	Age (years) or Condition	Weight (kg)	Weight (lb)	Height (cm)	Height (in)	Protein (g)	Fat-Soluble Vitamins				Water-Soluble Vitamins							Minerals						
							Vitamin A (µg R.E.)‡	Vitamin D (µg)§	Vitamin E (mg α-T.E.)∥	Vitamin K (µg)	Vitamin C (mg)	Thiamin (mg)	Riboflavin (mg)	Niacin (mg N.E.)¶	Vitamin B₆ (mg)	Folate (µg)	Vitamin B₁₂ (µg)	Calcium (mg)	Phosphorus (mg)	Magnesium (mg)	Iron (mg)	Zinc (mg)	Iodine (µg)	Selenium (µg)
INFANTS	0.0–0.5	6	13	60	24	13	375	7.5	3	5	30	0.3	0.4	5	0.3	25	0.3	400	300	40	6	5	40	10
	0.5–1.0	9	20	71	28	14	375	10	4	10	35	0.4	0.5	6	0.6	35	0.5	600	500	60	10	5	50	15
CHILDREN	1–3	13	29	90	35	16	400	10	6	15	40	0.7	0.8	9	1.0	50	0.7	800	800	80	10	10	70	20
	4–6	20	44	112	44	24	500	10	7	20	45	0.9	1.1	12	1.1	75	1.0	800	800	120	10	10	90	20
	7–10	28	62	132	52	28	700	10	7	30	45	1.0	1.2	13	1.4	100	1.4	800	800	170	10	10	120	30
MALES	11–14	45	99	157	62	45	1,000	10	10	45	50	1.3	1.5	17	1.7	150	2.0	1,200	1,200	270	12	15	150	40
	15–18	66	145	176	69	59	1,000	10	10	65	60	1.5	1.8	20	2.0	200	2.0	1,200	1,200	400	12	15	150	50
	19–24	72	160	177	70	58	1,000	10	10	70	60	1.5	1.7	19	2.0	200	2.0	1,200	1,200	350	10	15	150	70
	25–50	79	174	176	70	63	1,000	5	10	80	60	1.5	1.7	19	2.0	200	2.0	800	800	350	10	15	150	70
	51+	77	170	173	68	63	1,000	5	10	80	60	1.2	1.4	15	2.0	200	2.0	800	800	350	10	15	150	70
FEMALES	11–14	46	101	157	62	46	800	10	8	45	50	1.1	1.3	15	1.4	150	2.0	1,200	1,200	280	15	12	150	45
	15–18	55	120	163	64	44	800	10	8	55	60	1.1	1.3	15	1.5	180	2.0	1,200	1,200	300	15	12	150	50
	19–24	58	128	164	65	46	800	10	8	60	60	1.1	1.3	15	1.6	180	2.0	1,200	1,200	280	15	12	150	55
	25–50	63	138	163	64	50	800	5	8	65	60	1.1	1.3	15	1.6	180	2.0	800	800	280	15	12	150	55
	51+	65	143	160	63	50	800	5	8	65	60	1.0	1.2	13	1.6	180	2.0	800	800	280	10	12	150	55
PREGNANT						60	800	10	10	65	70	1.5	1.6	17	2.2	400	2.2	1,200	1,200	320	30	15	175	65
LACTATING	1st 6 months					65	1,300	10	12	65	95	1.6	1.8	20	2.1	280	2.6	1,200	1,200	355	15	19	200	75
	2nd 6 months					62	1,200	10	11	65	90	1.6	1.7	20	2.1	260	2.6	1,200	1,200	340	15	16	200	75

(Reprinted with permission from the National Academy of Sciences, Washington, DC.)

*The allowances, expressed as average daily intake over time, are intended to provide for individual variations among most normal persons as they live in the United States under usual environmental stresses. Diets should be based on a variety of common foods in order to provide other nutrients for which human requirements have been less well defined.

†Weights and heights of Reference Adults are actual medians for the U.S. population of the designated age, as reported by NHANES II. The use of these figures does not imply that the height-to-weight ratios are ideal.

‡Retinol equivalents. 1 retinol equivalent = 1 µg retinol or 6 µg β-carotene.

§As cholecalciferol. 10 µg cholecalciferol = 400 I.U. of vitamin D.

∥α-Tocopherol equivalents. 1 mg d-α tocopherol = 1 α-T.E.

¶1 N.E. (niacin equivalents) is equal to 1 mg of niacin or 60 mg of dietary tryptophan.

APPENDIX 3. Estimated Safe and Adequate Daily Dietary Intakes of Selected Vitamins and Minerals*

| | | Vitamins | | Trace Elements† | | | | | |
Category	Age (years)	Biotin (μg)	Pantothenic Acid (mg)	Copper (mg)	Manganese (mg)	Fluoride (mg)	Chromium (μg)	Molybdenum (μg)
INFANTS	0–0.5	10	2	0.4–0.6	0.3–0.6	0.1–0.5	10–40	15–30
	0.5–1	15	3	0.6–0.7	0.6–1.0	0.2–1.0	20–60	20–40
CHILDREN AND	1–3	20	3	0.7–1.0	1.0–1.5	0.5–1.5	20–80	25–50
ADOLESCENTS	4–6	25	3–4	1.0–1.5	1.5–2.0	1.0–2.5	30–120	30–75
	7–10	30	4–5	1.0–2.0	2.0–3.0	1.5–2.5	50–200	50–150
	11+	30–100	4–7	1.5–2.5	2.0–5.0	1.5–2.5	50–200	75–250
ADULTS		30–100	4–7	1.5–3.0	2.0–5.0	1.5–4.0	50–200	75–250

(Food and Nutrition Board, National Research Council. Recommended Dietary Allowances, 10th ed. Washington DC: National Academy Press, 1989)

* Because there is less information on which to base allowances, these figures are not given in the main table of RDA and are provided here in the form of ranges of recommended intakes.

† Since the toxic levels for many trace elements may be only several times usual intakes, the upper levels for the trace elements given in this table should not be habitually exceeded.

APPENDIX 4. *Estimated Sodium, Chloride, and Potassium Minimum Requirements of Healthy Persons**

Age	Weight (kg)*	Sodium (mg)*†	Chloride (mg)*†	Potassium (mg)‡
MONTHS				
0–5	4.5	120	180	500
6–11	8.9	200	300	700
YEARS				
1	11.0	225	350	1,000
2–5	16.0	300	500	1,400
6–9	25.0	400	600	1,600
10–18	50.0	500	750	2,000
>18§	70.0	500	750	2,000

(Food and Nutrition Board, National Research Council. Recommended Dietary Allowances, 10th ed. Washington DC: National Academy Press, 1989)

* No allowance has been included for large, prolonged losses from the skin through sweat.

† There is no evidence that higher intakes confer any health benefit.

‡ Desirable intakes of potassium may considerably exceed these values (~3,500 mg for adults).

§ No allowance included for growth. Values for those below 18 years assume a growth rate at the 50th percentile reported by the National Center for Health Statistics and averaged for males and females.

APPENDIX 5. *Diet and Drugs*

Many drugs have the potential to affect, and be affected by, nutrition. Sometimes, drug–nutrient interactions are the intended action of the drug; at other times, alterations in nutrient intake, metabolism, or excretion may be an unfortunate side effect of drug therapy.

Although well-nourished individuals on short-term drug therapy may easily withstand the negative effects of drug–nutrient interactions, malnourished clients or clients on long-term drug regimens may experience significant nutrient deficiencies and decreased tolerance to drug therapy. Although potential and actual drug–nutrient interactions vary considerably among specific drugs, clients at greatest risk for developing drug-induced nutrient deficiencies include those

- Whose diets are chronically inadequate.
- Who have increased nutritional needs, such as infants, adolescents, and pregnant and lactating women.
- Who are elderly.
- Who have chronic illnesses.
- On long-term or multiple drug regimens.
- Who self-medicate.
- Who are substance abusers.

The mechanisms by which drugs can affect food and nutrients are listed below.

Mechanism: Altered Food Intake Related to the Following:

Increased appetite: The following drugs may stimulate appetite:
- Antihistamines: cyproheptadine hydrochloride
- Psychotropic drugs: chlorpromazine, chlordiazepoxide, diazepam, meprobamate
- Some mild tranquilizers with antiemetic and antihistaminic properties (however, the elderly may experience decreased appetite and weight loss when given tranquilizers)
- Tricyclic antidepressants: amitriptyline hydrochloride
- Steriods: anabolic steroids like testosterone; glucocorticoids like prednisone

Anorexia: The following drugs may cause anorexia:
- Amphetamines
- Alcohol
- Anticancer agents

Increased satiety caused by delayed gastric emptying: Delayed gastric emptying may be caused by
- Beta-adrenergic stimulant: salbutamol
- Dopamine precursor: levodopa

Changes in the sense of taste or smell: The following drugs may alter taste or smell sensations:
- Local anesthetics: benzocaine, cocaine, procaine
- Antibiotics: amphotericin B, ampicillin, griseofulvin, lincomycin, streptomycin, tetracyclines

- Anticancer agents: methotrexate, doxorubicin hydrochloride
- Anticoagulant: phenindione
- Antihistamine: chlorpheniramine maleate
- Antihypertensive agents: captopril, diazoxide, ethacrynic acid
- Anti-infectious agent: metronidazole
- Chelating agent: D-penicillamine
- Cholesterol-lowering agent: clofibrate
- Hypoglycemia agent: glipizide
- Psychoactive agents: carbamazepine, lithium carbonate, phenytoin, amphetamines
- Toothpaste ingredient: sodium lauryl sulfate

Nausea or vomiting
- Almost all drugs have the potential to induce nausea and vomiting, depending on the dosage and length of time used.
- Nausea and vomiting are often the major side effects of anticancer drugs, such as alkylating agents, antimetabolites, and natural and synthetic agents.

Inflammation of the mouth: Sores in the mouth may be attributed to the use of:
- Anticancer agents: Mechlorethamine, mercaptopurine, methotrexate, bleomycin, vinblastine sulfate

Mechanism: Altered Nutrient Absorption Related to the Following:

Changes in the pH of the GI tract: The following drugs can change the GI pH:
- Antacids increase the pH of the GI tract and may thereby decrease the absorption of folic acid, iron (carbonate antacids), phosphate (aluminum antacids), or vitamin A (aluminum hydroxide).
- Potassium supplements can decrease the absorption of vitamin B_{12} by lowering ileal pH.

Increased GI motility
- Laxatives like bisacodyl, senna, and phenolphthalein speed the passage of food through the GI tract and thereby reduce the time available for nutrient absorption.

Damage to the intestinal mucosa: Drugs that can damage the intestinal mucosa include:
- Alcohol → malabsorption of vitamin B_{12} and folic acid
- Antibiotic: neomycin → malabsorption of fat, vitamin B_{12}, nitrogen, lactose, sucrose, sodium, potassium, iron, and calcium
- Antigout: colchicine → malabsorption of fat, vitamin B_{12}, carotene, lactose, sodium, and potassium
- Antimetabolite: methotrexate → malabsorption of calcium
- Non-narcotic analgesics: chronic use of aspirin and other salicylates can erode the lining of the stomach and intestine, leading to blood loss and iron deficiency.

Binding agents or physical barriers that prevent absorption: Binding agents or barriers include:

- Antacids: aluminum hydroxide antacids bind with phosphate to prevent its absorption.
- Anti-inflammatory: salicylazosulfapyridine blocks the absorption of folic acid.
- Antituberculosis agent: para-aminosalicylic acid blocks the absorption of vitamin B_{12}.
- Chelating agent: penicillamine binds with copper, iron, and zinc.
- Laxatives: mineral oil blocks the absorption of the fat-soluble vitamins.

Mechanism: Altered Nutrient Metabolism Related to the Following:

Drugs that function as nutrient antagonists

- Folic acid antagonists include: methotrexate, pyrimethamine, triamterene, trimethoprim.
- Vitamin B_6 antagonists include: isoniazid, hydralazine, cycloserine, levodopa.
- Vitamin B_{12} antagonist: nitrous oxide
- Vitamin K antagonists include coumarin anticoagulants.

Altered enzyme systems that metabolize nutrients

- Anticonvulsants: phenobarbital and phenytoin can cause vitamin D deficiency by altering enzyme systems that increase the inactivation of vitamin D.
- Antimalarial: pyrimethamine inhibits enzymes necessary for normal folic acid metabolism.

Increased/decreased nutrient degradation

- Antacid: aluminum hydroxide destroys thiamine.

Mechanism: Altered Nutrient Excretion Related to the Following:

Altered renal reabsorption

- Alcohol increases the excretion of magnesium and zinc.
- Antigout: probenecid decreases urinary excretion of pantothenic acid.
- Diuretics generally may increase urinary thiamine, vitamin B_6, calcium, magnesium, potassium, phosphate, and zinc. Specifically

    Acetazolamide increases urinary calcium and potassium.

    Chlorthalidone increases urinary zinc and potassium.

    Ethacrynic acid and furosemide increase urinary calcium, magnesium, and potassium.

    Mercurials increase urinary thiamine, magnesium, and calcium.

    Spironolactone increases urinary calcium and magnesium.

    Thiazides increase urinary potassium, magnesium, zinc, and riboflavin.

    Triamterene may increase urinary calcium.

Just as drugs can alter nutrients, food and nutrients can alter drug absorption, metabolism, and excretion. Specific mechanisms are listed below.

Mechanism: Altered Drug Absorption Related to the Following:

Altered secretion of digestive juices
Altered GI motility
Food-drug binding, which renders the drug incapable of being absorbed

Examples of drugs whose absorption is delayed by the presence of food include[3]

- Acetaminophen (pectin)
- Amoxicillin
- Aspirin
- Cephaloxin
- Digoxin
- Erythromycin
- Furosemide
- Potassium ion
- Sulfadiazine
- Sulfamethoxine
- Sulfamethoxypridazine
- Sulfanilamide
- Sulfasymazine
- Sulfisoxazole

Examples of drugs whose absorption is increased by the presence of food include

- Diazepam
- Griseofulvin (fat)
- Hydrochlorothiazide
- Metoprolol
- Nitrofurantoin
- Propranolol
- Riboflavin

Examples of drugs whose absorption is decreased by the presence of food include

- Amoxicillin
- Ampicillin
- Aspirin
- Demethylchlortetracycline
- Doxycycline
- Isoniazid
- Levodopa (protein, amino acids)
- Methacycline
- Methyldopa (protein, amino acids)
- Oxytetracycline
- Penicillamine
- Penicillin G
- Penicillin V (K)
- Phenethicillin
- Phenobarbital
- Propantheline
- Rifampin
- Tetracycline

Mechanism: Food May Alter Drug Metabolism By the Following:

Interfering with the action of a drug: Examples:
- A large intake of coffee, tea, or other caffeine-containing beverages may enhance the side effects of theophylline.
- Large amounts of natural licorice, which tends to increase potassium excretion and sodium retention, may interfere with the action of antihypertensive agents and diuretics. Clients who take digitalis and who experience licorice-induced hypokalemia are at increased risk of digitalis toxicity.
- A high-salt (sodium) intake reduces the therapeutic response to lithium; a low-salt diet may enhance drug activity.
- A high intake of vitamin K-rich vegetables (broccoli, turnip greens, lettuce, cabbage) may inhibit the action of the anticoagulant warfarin.

Contributing pharmacologically active substances: Example:
- Monoamine oxidase inhibitors (MAOIs) are antidepressants that potentiate the cardiovascular effect of tyramine and other vasoactive amines in food. A hypertensive crisis may occur within several hours after foods containing tyramine are ingested with MAOIs. Signs and symptoms include increased blood pressure, headache, pallor, nausea, vomiting, restlessness, dilated pupils, sweating, palpitations, angina, and fever. Death caused by intracranial bleeding occurs rarely. Tyramine-containing foods that are contraindicated during MAOI therapy include[1] the following:

  Dairy Products
  > Sharp or aged cheese like Bleu, Boursault, Brick, Brie, Camembert, Cheddar, Emmenthaler, Gruyère, Mozzarella, Parmesan, Romano, Roquefort, Stilton
  > Sour cream, yogurt

  Meats and Fish
  > Fermented meat, fish, poultry, and sausage
  > Caviar
  > Chicken liver
  > Pickled herring

  Fruits and Vegetables
  > Broad beans
  > Avocado
  > Bananas
  > Canned figs
  > Raisins

  Beverages
  > Beer
  > Chianti wine; other wine in large quantities
  > Sherry

  Miscellaneous
  > Active yeast preparations
  > Soy sauce
  > Coffee, cola, and chocolate contain other vasopressors and may also be contraindicated.

Mechanism: Food May Alter Drug Excretion By the Following:

Changing urinary pH: Example:
- An excess intake of citrus juices may increase the pH of the urine, and therefore increase blood levels of quinidine.

BIBLIOGRAPHY

1. American Dietetic Association: Manual of Clinical Dietetics. Developed by The Chicago Dietetic Association and The South Suburban Dietetic Association, 1988
2. Malseed, RT: Pharmacology Drug Therapy and Nursing Considerations, 3rd ed. Philadelphia: JB Lippincott, 1990

APPENDIX 6. *Test Diets*

Test diets vary among facilities, based on the laboratory's policies. Dietary modifications for common test diets are listed below.

Test	Purpose	Dietary Modifications

Fecal fat determination	To diagnose malabsorption, cystic fibrosis	100 g of fat/day (*i.e.,* a high-fat diet) is consumed for 3 days before stool collection. Recommended intake includes at least the followings foods or their equivalent:
		  2 c whole milk
		  8 oz lean meat
		  1 egg
		  4 or more servings of fruits and vegetables
		  4 or more servings of bread and cereals
		  10 servings of fat

Glucose tolerance test	To diagnose diabetes mellitus	A high-CHO diet containing at least 300 g of CHO is consumed for 3 days before the test. Some experts question the validity of the test, and contend that as long as an adequate amount of CHO is consumed (*i.e.,* 150 g/day), further modification is not necessary.
Calcium test	To diagnose hypercalciuria, which is detectable only at moderately high calcium intakes	An intake of 1000 mg of calcium is recommended. Of that, 400 mg is apt to be from dietary sources and the remaining 600 mg obtained from supplements.
Serotonin test (5 HIAA or 4 hydrosyin-doleacetic acid)	To determine the metabolite of malignant tumors of the intestinal tract	Eliminate the following foods for at least 24 hours before the test: walnuts, bananas, plantains, avocados, tomatoes, red plums, red blue plums, pineapples, pineapple juice, and passion fruit

Source: American Dietetic Association: Manual of Clinical Dietetics. Developed by The Chicago Dietetic Association and the South Suburban Dietetic Association, 1988

APPENDIX 7. Selected Enteral Formulas

	Manufacturer	Form	Major Nutrient Sources	Nutritional Considerations	Volume to Meet 100% USRDA
PART I. COMPLETE FORMULAS: FORMULAS THAT MAY BE USED AS THE SOLE SOURCE OF NUTRITION					
SECTION A. BLENDERIZED FORMULAS CONTAINING INTACT PROTEIN					
Compleat Regular Formula	Sandoz Nutrition	Ready to use	Protein: Beef, nonfat milk CHO: Fruits, vegetables, maltodextrin, nonfat milk Fat: Beef, corn oil	1.07 cal/ml 16% cal from protein 450 mOsm Contains lactose	1500 ml
Compleat Modified Formula	Sandoz Nutrition	Ready to use	Protein: Beef, calcium caseinate CHO: Maltodextrin, fruits, vegetables Fat: Beef, corn oil	1.07 cal/ml 16% cal from protein 300 mOsm Lactose free	1500 ml
Vitaneed	Sherwood Medical	Ready to use	Protein: Beef, sodium and calcium caseinates CHO: Maltodextrin, puréed fruit and vegetables Fat: Soy oil, beef	1.0 cal/ml 14% cal from protein 310 mOsm Lactose free Low sodium	2000 ml
SECTION B. PROTEIN ISOLATE FORMULAS CONTAINING LACTOSE					
Meritene Liquid	Sandoz Nutrition	Ready to use	Protein: Concentrated sweet skim milk CHO: Lactose, hydrolyzed cornstarch, sucrose Fat: Corn oil	0.96 cal/ml 24% cal from protein 510–570 mOsm Routine oral supplement	1250 ml
Meritene Powder	Sandoz Nutrition	Powder; mixes with milk	Protein: Nonfat milk, whole milk CHO: Lactose, sucrose, hydrolyzed cornstarch Fat: Milk fat	1.06 cal/ml 26% cal from protein 690 mOsm Routine oral supplement	1040 ml
Sustacal Powder	Mead Johnson	Powder; mixes with milk or water	Protein: Nonfat milk, whole milk CHO: Lactose, sugar, corn syrup solids Fat: Milk fat (when prepared according to directions with whole milk)	1.33 cal/ml 23% cal from protein (when prepared with whole milk) 899 mOsm Routine oral supplement	899 ml
Sustagen	Mead Johnson	Powder; mixes with water	Protein: Nonfat milk, powdered whole milk, calcium caseinate CHO: Corn syrup solids, lactose, dextrose Fat: Milk fat	1.9 cal/ml 24% cal from protein 1100 mOsm Routine oral supplement	1030 ml

Ensure	Ross Laboratories	Ready to use	Protein: Sodium and calcium caseinates, soy protein isolates CHO: Corn syrup, sucrose Fat: Corn oil	1.06 cal/ml 14% cal from protein 450 mOsm Low residue	1887 ml
Ensure HN	Ross Laboratories	Ready to use	Protein: Sodium and calcium caseinates, soy protein isolate CHO: Corn syrup, sucrose Fat: Corn oil	1.06 cal/ml 16.7% cal from protein 470 mOsm Higher in protein than Ensure	1321 ml
Ensure Plus	Ross Laboratories	Ready to use	Protein: Sodium and calcium caseinates, soy protein isolate CHO: Corn syrup, sucrose Fat: Corn oil	1.5 cal/ml 14.7% cal from protein 690 mOsm Low residue Higher in protein and calories than Ensure	1420 ml
Impact	Sandoz	Ready to use	Protein: sodium and calcium caseinates, L-arginine CHO: Hydrolyzed cornstarch Fat: Structured lipids from palm kernel oil and sunflower oil, refined menhaden oil	1.0 cal/ml 22% cal from protein 375 mOsm Low residue Enriched with arginine, RNA, and omega-3 fatty acids Designed for critically ill patients	1500 ml
Isocal	Mead Johnson	Ready to use	Protein: Calcium and sodium caseinates, soy protein isolates CHO: Maltodextrin Fat: Soy oil, MCT	1.06 cal/ml 13% cal from protein 270 mOsm Low residue Low sodium Standard tube feeding	1890 ml
Isocal HCN	Mead Johnson	Ready to use	Protein: Calcium and sodium caseinates CHO: Corn syrup Fat: Soybean oil, MCT	2.0 cal/ml 15% cal from protein 640 mOsm Low residue Low sodium High protein, high calorie, tube feeding	1000 ml
Isosource	Sandoz	Ready to use	Protein: Sodium and calcium caseinates, soy protein isolates CHO: Hydrolyzed cornstarch Fat: MCT (50% of fat calories), canola oil	1.2 cal/ml 14% cal from protein 360 mOsm Low residue	1500 ml

(continued)

APPENDIX 7. Selected Enteral Formulas (continued)

	Manufacturer	Form	Major Nutrient Sources	Nutritional Considerations	Volume to Meet 100% USRDA
Isotein HN	Sandoz Nutrition	Powder; mixes with water	Protein: Delactosed lactalbumin CHO: Hydrolyzed cornstarch, monosaccharides Fat: Partially hydrogenated soybean oil, MCT	1.2 cal/ml 23% cal from protein 300 mOsm Low residue High protein	1770 ml
Magnacal	Sherwood Medical	Ready to use	Protein: Calcium and sodium caseinates CHO: Maltodextrin, sucrose Fat: Partially hydrogenated soy oil	2.0 cal/ml 14% cal from protein 590 mOsm Low residue High calorie	1000 ml
Osmolite	Ross Laboratories	Ready to use	Protein: Sodium and calcium caseinates, soy protein isolate CHO: Hydrolyzed cornstarch Fat: MCT, corn oil, soy oil	1.06 cal/ml 14% cal from protein 290 mOsm Low residue Low sodium, low potassium	1887 ml
Osmolite HN	Ross Laboratories	Ready to use	Protein: Sodium and calcium caseinates, soy protein isolate CHO: Hydrolyzed cornstarch Fat: MCT, corn oil, soy oil	1.06 cal/ml 16.7% cal from protein 310 mOsm Low residue Higher in protein than Osmolite	1320 ml
Pulmocare	Ross Laboratories	Ready to use	Protein: Sodium and calcium caseinates CHO: Hydrolyzed cornstarch and sucrose Fat: Corn oil	1.5 cal/ml 16.7% cal from protein 490 mOsm High-fat, low-CHO formula designed to reduce carbon dioxide production in clients with respiratory disease	947 ml
Resource Liquid	Sandoz Nutrition	Ready to use	Protein: Sodium and calcium caseinates, soy protein isolate CHO: Hydrolyzed cornstarch, sucrose Fat: Corn oil	1.06 cal/ml 14% cal from protein 430 mOsm Routine oral supplement	1890 ml
Sustacal Liquid	Mead Johnson	Ready to use	Protein: Calcium caseinates, soy protein isolate, sodium caseinates	1.0 cal/ml 24% cal from protein 620 mOsm	1080 ml

Product	Company	Preparation	Composition	Characteristics	Volume to meet RDA
(continued from previous page)			CHO: Sucrose, corn syrup; Fat: Partially hydrogenated soy oil		
Sustacal HC	Mead Johnson	Ready to use	Protein: Calcium and sodium caseinates; CHO: Corn syrup solids, sugar; Fat: Corn oil	Low residue; High protein; Routine oral supplement; 1.5 cal/ml; 16% cal from protein; 650 mOsm	1200 ml
Traumacal	Mead Johnson	Ready to use	Protein: Calcium and sodium caseinates; CHO: Corn syrup, sugar; Fat: Soybean oil, MCT	Low residue; Intended as high-calorie oral supplement; 1.5 cal/ml; 22% cal from protein; 490 mOsm; High in protein and calories; Designed for metabolic stress	2000 ml
Travasorb	Clintec Nutrition Company	Ready to use	Protein: Sodium caseinates, soy protein isolate, calcium caseinates; CHO: Sucrose, corn syrup solids; Fat: Corn oil, partially hydrogenated soy oil	1.06 cal/ml; 14% cal from protein; 488 mOsm	1896 ml
Travasorb MCT	Clintec Nutrition Company	Powder; mixes with water	Protein: Lactalbumin, potassium caseinates; CHO: Corn syrup solids; Fat: MCT, sunflower oil	1.0–2.0 cal/ml, depending on dilution; 20% cal from protein; 400 mOsm; Intended for clients with fat maldigestion or fat malabsorption (approx. 80% of the fat is provided as MCT)	2000 ml
SECTION D. FIBER-CONTAINING PROTEIN ISOLATE FORMULAS					
Enrich	Ross Laboratories	Ready to use	Protein: Sodium and calcium caseinates, soy protein isolate; CHO: Hydrolyzed cornstarch, sucrose, soy fiber (fiber source); Fat: Corn oil	1.1 cal/ml; 14.5% cal from protein; 480 mOsm; 3.4 g of added fiber/8 oz. serving; Oral supplement	1391 ml
Fibersource	Sandoz	Ready to use	Protein: Sodium and calcium caseinates; CHO: Hydrolyzed cornstarch, soy fiber; Fat: MCT (50% of fat calories), canola oil	1.2 cal/ml; 14% cal from protein; 390 mOsm; 2.5 g fiber/250 ml	1500 ml

(continued)

APPENDIX 7. Selected Enteral Formulas (continued)

	Manufacturer	Form	Major Nutrient Sources	Nutritional Considerations	Volume to Meet 100% USRDA
Fibersource HN	Sandoz	Ready to use	Protein: Sodium and calcium caseinates CHO: Hydrolyzed cornstarch, soy fiber Fat: MCT (50% of fat calories), canola oil	1.2 cal/ml 18% cal from protein 390 mOsm 1.7 g fiber/250 ml	1500 ml
Jevity	Ross Laboratories	Ready to use	Protein: Sodium and calcium caseinates CHO: Hydrolyzed cornstarch, soy fiber Fat: MCT (50% of fat calories), corn oil, soy oil	1.06 cal/ml 16.7% cal from protein 300 mOsm 3.4 g fiber/8 fl oz	1321 ml
Sustacal with Fiber	Mead Johnson	Ready to use	Protein: Sodium and calcium caseinates, soy protein isolate CHO: Maltodextrin, sugar Fat: Corn oil	1.06 cal/ml 17% cal from protein 480 mOsm 8.4 g dietary fiber/1500 cal	1420 ml
Ultracal	Mead Johnson	Ready to use	Protein: Sodium and calcium caseinate CHO: Maltodextrin, oat fiber, soy fiber Fat: Soy oil, MCT	1.06 cal/ml 17% cal from protein 310 mOsm 13.6 g dietary fiber/1000 cal	1180 ml

SECTION E. DEFINED FORMULAS CONTAINING HYDROLYZED PROTEINS AND/OR AMINO ACIDS THAT ARE LACTOSE-FREE AND CONTAIN MINIMAL RESIDUE

	Manufacturer	Form	Major Nutrient Sources	Nutritional Considerations	Volume to Meet 100% USRDA
Criticare HN	Mead Johnson	Ready to use	Protein: Enzymatically hydrolyzed casein CHO: Maltodextrin, modified cornstarch Fat: Safflower oil, soy oil	1.06 cal/ml 14% cal from protein 650 mOsm	1890 ml
Reabilan	O'Brien/KMI	Ready to use	Protein: Small peptides derived from the hydrolysis of casein and whey CHO: Maltodextrin, tapioca starch Fat: MCT, soy oil	1.0 cal/ml 13% cal from protein 350 mOsm	2250 ml
Reabilan HN	O'Brien/KMI	Ready to use	Protein: Small peptides derived from the hydrolysis of casein and whey CHO: Maltodextrin, tapioca starch Fat: MCT, soy oil	1.33 cal/ml 17% cal from protein 490 mOsmo Semielemental diet for hypermetabolic patients; high nitrogen	1875 ml

Stressstein	Sandoz Nutrition	Powder; mixes with water	Protein: Free amino acids (44% branched-chain amino acids) CHO: Maltodextrin Fat: MCT, soybean oil	1.2 cal/ml 23% cal from protein 910 mOsm Modified amino acid, branched-chain enriched formula specifically designed for patients with severe metabolic stress and trauma	2000 ml
Tolerex	Norwich–Eaton Pharmaceuticals	Powder; mixes with water	Protein: Free amino acids CHO: Glucose oligosaccharides Fat: Safflower oil	1.0 cal/ml 8.2% cal from protein 550 mOsm	1800 ml
Travasorb HN	Clintec Nutrition Company	Powder; mixes with water	Protein: Enzymatically hydrolyzed lactalbumin CHO: Glucose oligosaccharides Fat: MCT, safflower oil	1.0 cal/ml 18% cal from protein 560 mOsm High protein Low fat	2000 ml
Travasorb STD	Clintec Nutrition Company	Powder; mixes with water	Protein: Hydrolyzed lactalbumin CHO: Glucose oligosaccharides Fat: MCT, sunflower oil	1.0 cal/ml 12% cal from protein 560 mOsm	2000 ml
Vital HN	Ross Laboratories	Powder; mixes with water	Protein: Peptides from partially hydrolyzed whey, soy, and meat protein, with added free essential amino acids CHO: Hydrolyzed cornstarch, sucrose Fat: Safflower oil, MCT	1.0 cal/ml 16.7% cal from protein 500 mOsm High protein Low sodium	1500 ml
Vivonex T.E.N.	Sandoz Nutrition	Powder; mixes with water	Protein: Free amino acids (33% branched-chain amino acids) CHO: Maltodextrins Fat: Safflower oil	1.0 cal/ml 15.3% cal from protein 630 mOsm Modified amino acid, enriched branched-chain formula designed for stressed, catabolic patients	2000 ml

PART II. SPECIALLY DEFINED FORMULAS: DIET SUPPLEMENTS (INCOMPLETE FORMULAS) DESIGNED FOR PATIENTS WITH SPECIFIC METABOLIC DISORDERS

SECTION A. SUPPLEMENTS DESIGNED FOR PATIENTS WITH LIVER FAILURE

Hepatic–Aid II	Kendall McGaw	Powder; mixes with water	Protein: Free amino acids (46% branched-chain amino acids) CHO: Maltodextrin, sucrose	1.1 cal/ml 15% cal from protein 560 mOsm	

(continued)

APPENDIX 7. Selected Enteral Formulas (continued)

	Manufacturer	Form	Major Nutrient Sources	Nutritional Considerations	Volume to Meet 100% USRDA
			Fat: Partially hydrogenated soybean oil	Altered amino acid pattern; does not contain vitamins, minerals, or electrolytes	
Travasorb Hepatic	Clintec Nutrition Company	Powder; mixes with water	Protein: Free amino acids (50% branched-chain amino acids) CHO: Glucose oligosaccharides Fat: MCT, sunflower oil	1.1 cal/ml 10.6% cal from protein 560 mOsm Altered amino acid pattern; includes vitamins, minerals, and electrolytes Flavors available	

SECTION B. SUPPLEMENTS DESIGNED FOR PATIENTS WITH RENAL FAILURE

	Manufacturer	Form	Major Nutrient Sources	Nutritional Considerations	Volume to Meet 100% USRDA
AminAid	Kendall McGaw	Powder; mixes with water	Protein: Free essential amino acids plus histidine CHO: Maltodextrin, sucrose Fat: Partially hydrogenated soybean oil	2.0 cal/ml 4% cal from protein 700 mOsm Essential amino acids in a high-calorie, low-electrolyte supplement. Does not contain vitamins or minerals	
Travasorb Renal	Clintec Nutrition Company	Powder; mixes with water	Protein: Crystalline L-amino acids CHO: Glucose oligosaccharides, sucrose Fat: MCT, sunflower oil	1.4 cal/ml 6.9% cal from protein 590 mOsm Essential amino acids in a high-calorie, electrolyte-free supplement. Does not contain fat-soluble vitamins Flavors available	

PART III. MODULAR COMPONENTS (INCOMPLETE DIET SUPPLEMENTS) Intended for oral use; may be mixed with food or enteral formulas

SECTION A. PROTEIN MODULES

	Manufacturer	Form	Major Nutrient Sources	Nutritional Considerations	Volume to Meet 100% USRDA
Casec	Mead Johnson	Powder	Major protein source: calcium caseinate	3.7 cal/g	
Nutrisource Protein	Sandoz Nutrition	Powder	Major protein source: lactalbumin, egg white solids	4.0 cal/g	

Product	Manufacturer	Form	Composition	Value
Propac	Sherwood Medical	Powder	Major protein source: whey protein concentrate	4.0 cal/g
RDP (Rapid Dispersing Protein)	Corpak, Inc.	Powder	Major protein source: whey protein caseinate	3.6 cal/g

SECTION B. CHO MODULES

Product	Manufacturer	Form	Composition	Value
Liquid CHO Supplement	Corpak, Inc.	Liquid	Major CHO source: glucose polymers	2.5 cal/g
Moducal	Mead Johnson	Powder	Major CHO source: maltodextrins	3.8 cal/g
Nutrisource Carbohydrate	Sandoz Nutrition	Liquid	Major CHO source: deionized corn syrup solids	3.2 cal/ml
Polycose Liquid	Ross Laboratories	Liquid	Major CHO source: hydrolyzed cornstarch	2.0 cal/ml
Polycose Powder	Ross Laboratories	Powder	Major CHO source: hydrolyzed cornstarch	3.8 cal/g
Pure Carbohydrate Supplement	Corpak, Inc.	Powder	Major CHO source: glucose polymers	4.0 cal/g
Sumacal	Sherwood Medical	Powder	Major CHO source: maltodextrins	3.8 cal/g

SECTION C. FAT MODULES

Product	Manufacturer	Form	Composition	Value
High Fat Supplement	Corpak, Inc.	Powder	Major fat source: partially hydrogenated coconut oil	6.12 cal/g
MCT Oil	Mead Johnson	Liquid	Major fat source: coconut oil	7.7 cal/ml
Microlipid	Sherwood Medical	Liquid	Major fat source: safflower oil	4.5 cal/ml
Nutrisource Lipid—Long Chain Triglycerides	Sandoz Nutrition	Liquid	Major fat source: soybean oil	2.2 cal/ml
Nutrisource Lipid—Medium Chain Triglycerides	Sandoz Nutrition	Liquid	Major fat source: coconut oil	2.0 cal/ml

SECTION D. MIXED MODULES

Product	Manufacturer	Form	Composition	Value
Citrotein	Sandoz Nutrition	Powder	Major protein source: egg white solids (25% of total calories) Major CHO source: Sucrose, maltodextrin (73% of total calories) Major fat source: partially hydrogenated soybean oil (2% of total calories)	0.66 cal/ml Oral supplement appropriate for clear liquid diets

SECTION E. FIBER MODULES

Product	Manufacturer	Form	Composition	Value
Fibrad	Ross Laboratories	Powder	Fiber sources: Pea fiber, oat fiber, sugar-beet fiber, xanthan gum	0.55 cal/g 0.77 g fiber/g

APPENDIX 8. *Caffeine Content of Selected Beverages and Foods*

Source	Average mg of caffeine
Coffee (6 oz cup)	
• Brewed	103
• Instant	57
Flavored coffee from instant mixes (6 oz)	
• Cafe amaretto	60
• Cafe francais	53
• Cafe vienna	56
• Irish mocha mint	27
• Orange cappuccino	73
• Suisse mocha	41
Coffee, instant dry powder (1 teaspoon)	
• Regular	57
• Coffee with chicory	37
• Decaffeinated	2
Tea beverage	
• Brewed 3 min (6 fl oz)	36
• Instant powder (1 tsp)	31
Soft drinks containing caffeine (12 fl oz)	
• Coca-Cola	46
• Cola soda, decaffeinated	tr
• Diet Coke	46
• Diet RC	48
• Mountain Dew	54
• Mr. Pibb	40
• Mello Yello	52
• Pepsi Cola	38
• Diet Pepsi	36
• RC Cola	36
Chocolate products	
• Baking chocolate, 1 oz unsweetened	25
• Chocolate frozen pudding pop, 1 pop	2
• Chocolate milk, 8 fl oz	8
• Chocolate powder for milk, 1 T	8
• Chocolate syrup, 2 T	5
• Chocolate pudding, ½ c	5
• Cocoa beverage, 6 fl oz	4
• Cocoa, mix powder, 1 oz	5

Source: Pennington JAT: Bowes and Church's Food Values of Portions Commonly Used, 15th ed. Philadelphia: JB Lippincott, 1989

APPENDIX 9. *Sources of Potassium*

Fruit and Fruit Juices

- Apple juice, apricots and apricot nectar, avocado, banana, cantaloupe, dates, figs, grapefruit and grapefruit juice, honeydew melons, nectarines, oranges and orange juice, papayas, dried and fresh peaches, pears, plums, prunes and prune juice, raisins, strawberries, tangerines and tangerine juice, watermelon
- Contain negligible amounts of sodium, and except for dried fruits, are generally low in calories

Vegetables and Vegetable Juices

- Artichokes, asparagus, broccoli, brussel sprouts, cooked dried beans (lima, kidney, navy, pinto, soybeans), cauliflower, eggplant, "greens" (beet greens, collard leaves, spinach, Swiss chard leaves*), green pepper, mushrooms, okra, parsnips, peas, potatoes (especially baked in the skin), pumpkins, rhubarb, rutabagas, sweet potatoes (baked), tomatoes, tomato juice (canned* and low-sodium canned), turnips, canned vegetable juice cocktail,* winter squash, yams, zucchini
- Generally low in sodium if prepared without salt and used fresh, frozen, and low-sodium canned (exception: those items starred contain more than 100 mg of sodium per average serving).
- Fresh and frozen vegetables are higher in potassium than canned; baking retains potassium content, boiling leaches potassium

Meats

- Beef, chicken, clams,* cod,* flounder,* haddock,* halibut,* fresh ham, beef kidney,* liver,* fresh lobster,* pork loin chops, salmon (canned,* low-sodium canned, fresh*), scallops,* beef sweetbreads, tuna (canned,* low-sodium canned), and turkey
- Calorie content depends on fat content and method of preparation; those items starred contain more than 100 mg of sodium per average serving (3 oz cooked)

Dairy Products

- Whole, low-fat, skim, and evaporated milk; buttermilk, chocolate milk, hot chocolate, hot cocoa, low-fat yogurt
- Calorie content largely depends on the fat content; all items contain more than 100 mg of sodium per 1 cup serving (exception: low-sodium milk)

(Adapted from United States Department of Agriculture, Agricultural Research Service: Nutritive Value of American Foods in Common Units. In Agricultural Handbook No. 456. Washington, DC, Superintendent of Documents, 1975, and Whitney EN, Cataldo CB: Understanding Normal and Clinical Nutrition. St Paul, MN: West Publishing, 1983)

APPENDIX 10. *Procedure for Determining Calorie Requirements*

I. *Calculate "Ideal" Body Weight Based on Height*

- Females: Allow 100 lb for the first 5 ft.
  Add 5 lb for each inch over 5 ft.
- Males: Allow 106 lb for the first 5 ft.
  Add 6 lb for each inch over 5 ft.
- Children: Based on growth charts showing weight for age

II. *Assess Weight Status*

Underweight	Ideal Weight Range	Overweight	Obese
>10% under ideal	±10% of ideal depending on size of body frame	10%–20% over ideal	>20% over ideal

III. *Calculate Calorie Requirements Based on Sex and Activity*

Adults

Multiply IBW (kg) × 24 hours × 1.0 cal/kg (men) or 0.9 cal/kg (women) to determine basal calorie requirements. Depending on activity level, multiply basal energy requirements by the appropriate number below

Activity	*Calories*
Sedentary	Basal calorie needs × 1.3
Moderate	Basal calorie needs × 1.5
Heavy	Basal calorie needs × 1.75

	To gain	*To lose*
1 lb/week	Add 500 cal/day	Subtract 500 cal/day
2 lb/week	Add 1000 cal/day	Subtract 1000 cal/day

Children (under 12 years old)
- Calorie needs vary according to rate of growth and activity levels.
- Generally, allow 1000 calories plus 100 cal/year of age.
- Monitor and adjust calorie allowance as needed to maintain normal growth.

Example: A 5'6" female weighs 150 pounds and is sedentary.

I. Her "ideal" body weight is:

$$100 \text{ pounds} + (5 \text{ pounds} \times 6 \text{ inches})$$
$$= 100 \text{ pounds} + 30 \text{ pounds}$$
$$= 130 \text{ pounds}$$

II. Her weight status is *overweight*

130 pound ±13 pounds (10%) = 117–143 for ideal weight range

III. Calorie requirements

130 pounds ÷ 2.2 pounds/kg = 59 kg

Basal energy requirements = 59 kg × 24 hours × 0.9 cal/kg = 1274

= 1274 calories

Total calories based on sedentary activity = 1274 × 1.3 = 1652

If a 1-pound weight loss/week is desired, the woman needs to restrict calorie intake to 1652 calories − 500 calories = 1152 calories/day.

APPENDIX 11. *Exchange List**

List 1: Starch/Bread List

Each item in this list contains approximately 15 g of CHO, 3 g of protein, a trace of fat, and 80 calories. Whole grain products average about 2 g of fiber per serving. Items appearing in **boldface** contain 3 or more g of fiber.

Food	Amount
CEREALS/GRAINS/PASTA	
Bran cereals, concentrated	⅓ c
Bran cereals, flaked (such as Bran Buds, All Bran)	½ c
Bulgur, cooked	½ c
Cooked cereals	½ c
Cornmeal, dry	2½ tbsp
Grapenuts	3 tbsp
Grits, cooked	½ c
Other ready-to-eat unsweetened cereals	¾ c
Pasta, cooked	½ c
Puffed cereal	1½ c
Rice, white or brown, cooked	⅓ c
Shredded wheat	½ c
Wheat germ	**3 tbsp**
DRIED BEANS/PEAS/LENTILS	
Beans and peas, cooked (such as kidney, white, split, blackeye)	⅓ c
Lentils, cooked	⅓ c
Baked beans	¼ c
STARCHY VEGETABLES	
Corn	½ c
Corn on cob, 6″ long	**1**
Lima beans	½ c
Peas, green, canned or frozen	½ c
Plantain	½ c
Potato, baked	1 small (3 oz)
Potato, mashed	½ c
Squash, winter (acorn, butternut)	¾ c
Yam, sweet potato, plain	⅓ c
BREAD	
Bagel	½ (1 oz)
Bread sticks, crisp, 4″ long × ½″	2 (⅔ oz)
Croutons, low-fat	1 c
English muffin	½
Frankfurter or hamburger bun	½ (1 oz)
Pita, 6″ across	½
Plain roll, small	1 (1 oz)
Raisin, unfrosted	1 slice (1 oz)
Rye, pumpernickel	**1 slice (1 oz)**
Tortilla, 6″ across	1
White (including French, Italian)	1 slice (1 oz)
Whole-wheat	1 slice (1 oz)

(continued)

Food	Amount
CRACKERS/SNACKS	
Animal crackers	8
Graham crackers, 2½″ square	3
Matzos	¾ oz
Melba toast	5 slices
Oyster crackers	24
Popcorn, popped, no fat added	3 c
Pretzels	¾ oz
Rye crisp, 2″ × 3½″	4
Saltine-type crackers	6
Whole-wheat crackers, no fat added (crisp breads, such as Finn, Kavli, Wasa)	2–4 slices (¾ oz)
STARCH FOODS PREPARED WITH FAT	
(count as 1 starch/bread serving plus 1 fat serving)	
Biscuit, 2½″ across	1
Chow mein noodles	½ c
Corn bread, 2″ cube	1 (2 oz)
Cracker, round butter-type	6
French fried potatoes, 2″ to 3½″ long	10 (1½ oz)
Muffin, plain, small	1
Pancake, 4″ across	2
Stuffing, bread, prepared	¼ c
Taco shell, 6″ across	2
Waffle, 4½″ square	1
Whole-wheat crackers, fat added (such as Triscuits)	4–6 (1 oz)

List 2: Meat List

Each serving of meat and substitutes on this list contains about 7 g of protein. The amount of fat and number of calories vary, depending on what kind of meat or substitute you choose. The list is divided into three parts based on the amount of fat and calories: lean meat, medium-fat meat, and high-fat meat. One ounce (one meat exchange) of each of these includes

	CHO (g)	Protein (g)	Fat (g)	Calories
Lean	0	7	3	55
Medium-fat	0	7	5	75
High-fat	0	7	8	100

Meats and meat substitutes that have 400 milligrams or more of sodium per exchange are indicated by this symbol #.

Food	Amount
LEAN MEAT AND SUBSTITUTES	
(one exchange is equal to any one of the following items)	
Beef: USDA Good or Choice grades of lean beef, such as round, sirloin, and flank steak; tenderloin and chipped beef #	1 oz
Pork: Lean pork, such as fresh ham: canned, cured, or boiled ham,# Canadian bacon,# tenderloin	1 oz

Food	Amount
Veal: All cuts are lean except for veal cutlets (ground or cubed). Examples of lean veal are chops and roasts.	1 oz
Poultry: Chicken, turkey, Cornish hen (without skin)	1 oz
Fish: All fresh and frozen fish	1 oz
Crab, lobster, scallops, shrimp, clams (fresh or canned in water*)	2 oz
Oysters	6 medium
Tuna* (canned in water)	¼ c
Herring (uncreamed or smoked)	1 oz
Sardines (canned)	2 medium
Wild Game: Venison, rabbit, squirrel	1 oz
Pheasant, duck, goose (without skin)	1 oz
Cheese: Any cottage cheese	¼ c
Grated parmesan	2 tbsp
Diet cheese* (with less than 55 cal/oz)	1 oz
Other: 95% fat-free luncheon meat	1 oz
Egg whites	3 whites
Egg substitutes with less than 55 cal/¼ c	¼ c

MEDIUM-FAT MEAT AND SUBSTITUTES
(one exchange is equal to any one of the following items)

Food	Amount
Beef: Most beef products fall into this category. Examples are all ground beef, roast (rib, chuck, rump), steak (cubes, Porterhouse, T-bone), and meatloaf.	1 oz
Pork: Most pork products fall into this category. Examples are chops, loin roast, Boston butt, cutlets.	1 oz
Lamb: Most lamb products fall into this category. Examples are chops, leg, and roast	1 oz
Veal: Cutlet (ground or cubed, unbreaded)	1 oz
Poultry: Chicken (with skin), domestic duck or goose (well drained of fat), ground turkey	1 oz
Fish: Tuna* (canned in oil and drained)	¼ c
Salmon* (canned)	¼ c
Cheese: Skim or part-skim milk cheeses, such as	
Ricotta	¼ c
Mozzarella	1 oz
Diet cheese* (with 56–80 cal/oz)	1 oz
Other: 86% fat-free luncheon meat*	1 oz
Egg (high in cholesterol, limit to 3/week)	1
Egg substitutes with 56–80 cal/¼ c	¼ c
Tofu (2½″ × 2¾″ × 1″)	4 oz
Liver, heart, kidney, sweetbreads (high in cholesterol)	1 oz

HIGH-FAT MEAT AND SUBSTITUTES
(Remember, these items are high in saturated fat, cholesterol, and calories, and should be used only three [3] times per week. One exchange is equal to any one of the following items)

Food	Amount
Beef: Most USDA Prime cuts of beef, such as ribs, corned beef*	1 oz
Pork: Spareribs, ground pork, pork sausage* (patty or link)	1 oz
Lamb: Patties (ground lamb)	1 oz
Fish: Any fried fish product	1 oz
Cheese: All regular cheeses,* such as American, blue, cheddar, Monterey, Swiss	1 oz
Other: Luncheon meat,* such as bologna, salami, pimento loaf	1 oz
Sausage,* such as Polish, Italian	1 oz

Food	Amount
Knockwurst, smoked	1 oz
Bratwurst[#]	1 oz
Frankfurter[#] (turkey or chicken)	1 frank (10/lb)
Peanut butter (contains unsaturated fat)	1 tbsp
Frankfurter[#] (beef, pork, or combination) (count as one high-fat meat plus one fat exchange)	1 frank (10/lb)

List 3: Vegetable List

Each vegetable serving on this list contains about 5 g of CHO, 2 g of protein, and 25 calories. Vegetables contain 2 to 3 g of dietary fiber. Vegetables that contain 400 mg of sodium per serving are indicated by this symbol [#].

Unless otherwise noted, the serving size for vegetables (one vegetable exchange) is ½ c of cooked vegetables or vegetable juice or 1 c of raw vegetables

Starchy vegetables such as corn, peas, and potatoes are found in the Starch/Bread List. For free vegetables, see Free Foods List.

Artichoke (½ medium)
Asparagus
Beans (green, wax, Italian)
Bean sprouts
Beets
Broccoli
Brussels sprouts
Cabbage, cooked
Carrots
Cauliflower
Eggplant
Greens (collard, mustard, turnip)
Kohlrabi
Leeks

Mushrooms, cooked
Okra
Onions
Pea pods
Peppers (green)
Rutabaga
Sauerkraut[#]
Spinach, cooked
Summer squash (crookneck)
Tomato (one large)
Tomato/vegetable juice[#]
Turnips
Water chestnuts
Zucchini, cooked

List 4: Fruit List

Each item in this list contains about 15 g of CHO, and 60 calories. Fresh, frozen, and dry fruits have about 2 g of fiber per serving. Fruits that have 3 or more g of fiber per serving appear in **boldface**. Fruit juices contain very little dietary fiber. Unless otherwise noted, the serving size for one fruit serving is ½ c of fresh fruit or fruit juice or ¼ c of dried fruit.

Food	Amount
Apple (raw, 2″ across)	1 apple
Applesauce (unsweetened)	½ c
Apricots (medium, raw) or	1 apricot
Apricots (canned)	½ c or 4 halves
Banana (9″ long)	½ banana

Food	Amount
Blackberries (raw)	**¾ c**
Blueberries (raw)	**¾ c**
Cantaloupe (5″ across)	⅓ melon
(cubes)	1 c
Cherries (large, raw)	½ c
Figs (raw, 2″ across)	2 figs
Fruit cocktail (canned)	½ c
Grapefruit (medium)	½ grapefruit
Grapefruit (segments)	¾ c
Grapes (small)	15 grapes
Honeydew melon (medium)	⅛ melon
(cubes)	1 c
Kiwi (large)	1 kiwi
Mandarin oranges	¾ c
Mango (small)	½ mango
Nectarine (1½″ across)	**1 nectarine**
Orange (2½″ across)	1 orange
Papaya	1 c
Peach (2¾″ across)	1 peach or ¾ c
Peaches (canned)	½ c or 2 halves
Pear	½ large or 1 small
Pears (canned)	½ c or 2 halves
Persimmon (medium, native)	2 persimmons
Pineapple (raw)	¾ c
Pineapple (canned)	⅓ c
Plum (raw, 2″ across)	2 plums
Pomegranate	**½ pomegranate**
Raspberries (raw)	**1 c**
Strawberries (raw, whole)	**1¼ c**
Tangerine (2½″ across)	2 tangerines
Watermelon (cubes)	1¼ c
DRIED FRUIT	
Apples	**4 rings**
Apricots	**7 halves**
Dates	2½ medium
Figs	**1½**
Prunes	**3 medium**
Raisins	2 tbsp
FRUIT JUICE	
Apple juice/cider	½ c
Cranberry juice cocktail	⅓ c
Grapefruit juice	½ c
Grape juice	⅓ c
Orange juice	½ c
Pineapple juice	½ c
Prune juice	⅓ c

List 5: Milk List

Each serving of milk or milk products on this list contains about 12 g CHO and 8 g of protein. The amount of fat in milk is measured in percent (%) of butterfat. The calories vary, depending on what kind of milk you choose. The list is divided into three parts based on the amount of fat and calories: skim/very lowfat milk, lowfat milk, and whole milk. One serving (one milk exchange) of each of these includes

	CHO (g)	Protein (g)	Fat (g)	Calories
Skim/very lowfat	12	8	trace	90
Lowfat	12	8	5	120
Whole	12	8	8	150

Food	Amount
SKIM AND VERY LOWFAT MILK	
Skim milk	1 c
½% milk	1 c
1% milk	1 c
Lowfat buttermilk	1 c
Evaporated skim milk	½ c
Dry nonfat milk	⅓ c
Plain nonfat yogurt	8 oz
LOWFAT MILK	
2% milk	1 c fluid
Plain lowfat yogurt (with added nonfat milk solids)	8 oz
WHOLE MILK	
Whole milk	1 c
Evaporated whole milk	½ c
Whole plain yogurt	8 oz

List 6: Fat List

Each serving on the fat list contains about 5 g of fat and 45 calories. Foods that contain 400 mg of sodium if more than one or two servings are eaten are indicated by this symbol #. Foods that contain 400 mg or more of sodium per serving are indicated by this symbol †.

Food	Amount
UNSATURATED FATS	
Avocado	⅛ medium
Margarine	1 tsp
Margarine, diet#	1 tbsp
Mayonnaise	1 tsp
Mayonnaise, reduced-calorie#	1 tbsp
Nuts and Seeds:	
Almonds, dry roasted	6 whole
Cashews, dry roasted	1 tbsp
Pecans	2 whole
Peanuts	20 small or 10 large
Walnuts	2 whole
Other nuts	1 tbsp
Seeds, pine nuts, sunflower (without shells)	1 tbsp
Pumpkin seeds	2 tsp
Oil (corn, cottonseed, safflower, soybean, sunflower, olive, peanut)	1 tsp
Olives#	10 small or 5 large

Food	Amount
Salad dressing, mayonnaise-type	2 tsp
Salad dressing, mayonnaise-type, reduced-calorie	1 tbsp
Salad dressing (all varieties)#	1 tbsp
Salad dressing, reduced-calorie† (Two tablespoons of low-calorie salad dressing is a free food.)	2 tbsp
SATURATED FATS	
Butter	1 tsp
Bacon#	1 slice
Chitterlings	½ oz
Coconut, shredded	2 tbsp
Coffee whitener, liquid	2 tbsp
Coffee whitener, powder	4 tsp
Cream (light, coffee, table)	2 tbsp
Cream, sour	2 tbsp
Cream (heavy, whipping)	1 tbsp
Cream cheese	1 tbsp
Salt pork#	¼ oz

Free Foods List

A *free food* is any food or drink that contains less than 20 calories per serving. You can eat as much as you want of those items that have no serving size specified. You may eat two or three servings per day of those items that have a specific serving size. Be sure to spread them out through the day. Foods containing 3 g or more of fiber are listed in **boldface.** Foods with 400 mg or more of sodium are indicated with this symbol #.

Drinks
  Bouillon# or broth without fat
  Bouillon, low-sodium
  Carbonated drinks, sugar-free
  Carbonated water
  Club soda
  Cocoa powder, unsweetened (1 tbsp)
  Coffee/tea
  Drink mixes, sugar-free
  Tonic water, sugar-free
Nonstick pan spray
Fruit
  Cranberries, unsweetened (½ c)
  Rhubarb, unsweetened (½ c)
Vegetables (raw, 1 c)
  Cabbage
  Celery
  Chinese cabbage
  Cucumber
  Green onion
  Hot peppers
  Mushrooms

Radishes
Zucchini
Salad greens
　Endive
　Escarole
　Lettuce
　Romaine
　Spinach
Sweet substitutes
　Candy, hard, sugar-free
　Gelatin, sugar-free
　Gum, sugar-free
　Jam/jelly, sugar-free (2 tsp)
　Pancake syrup, sugar-free (1–2 tbsp)
　Sugar substitutes (saccharin, aspartame)
　Whipped topping (2 tbsp)
Condiments
　Catsup (1 tbsp)
　Horseradish
　Mustard
　Pickles,# dill, unsweetened
　Salad dressing, low-calories (2 tbsp)
　Taco sauce (1 tbsp)
　Vinegar

Seasonings can be very helpful in making food taste better. Be careful of how much sodium you use. Read the label, and choose those seasonings that do not contain sodium or salt.

Basil (fresh)
Celery seeds
Cinnamon
Chili powder
Chives
Curry
Dill
Flavoring extracts (vanilla, almond, walnut, peppermint, butter, lemon, etc.)
Garlic
Garlic powder
Herbs
Hot pepper sauce
Lemon
Lemon juice
Lemon pepper
Lime
Lime juice
Mint
Onion powder
Oregano
Paprika
Pepper
Pimento
Spices
Soy sauce#
Soy sauce, low sodium ("lite")
Wine, used in cooking (¼ c)
Worcestershire sauce

The exchange lists are the basis of a meal planning system designed by a committee of the American Diabetes Association and the American Dietetic Association. While designed primarily for people with diabetes and others who must follow special diets, the exchange lists are based on principles of good nutrition that apply to everyone. © 1986 American Diabetes Association, American Dietetic Association.

APPENDIX 12. *Foods for Occasional Use**

Moderate amounts of some foods can be used in your meal plan, in spite of their sugar or fat content, as long as you can maintain blood-glucose control. The following table includes average exchange values for some of these foods. Because they are concentrated sources of carbohydrate, you will notice that the portion sizes are very small. Check with your dietitian for advice on how often and when you can eat them.

Food	Amount	Exchange
Angel food cake	¹⁄₁₂ cake	2 starch
Cake, no icing	¹⁄₁₂ cake, or a 3″ square	2 starch, 2 fat
Cookies	2 small (1¾″ across)	1 starch, 1 fat
Frozen fruit yogurt	⅓ c	1 starch
Gingersnaps	3	1 starch
Granola	¼ c	1 starch, 1 fat
Granola bars	1 small	1 starch, 1 fat
Ice cream, any flavor	½ c	1 starch, 2 fat
Ice milk, any flavor	½ c	1 starch, 1 fat
Sherbet, any flavor	¼ c	1 starch
Snack chips,* all varieties	1 oz	1 starch, 2 fat
Vanilla wafers	6 small	1 starch, 1 fat

If more than one serving is eaten, these foods have 400 mg or more of sodium.

APPENDIX 13. *Calcium and Phosphorus Content of Selected Foods*

Item	Amount	Calcium (mg)	Phosphorus (mg)
MILK AND MILK BEVERAGES			
Skim	1 cup	302	247
1%	1 cup	300	235
2%	1 cup	297	232
Whole	1 cup	291	228
Goat milk	1 cup	326	270
Chocolate milk (with 1% milk)	1 cup	287	256
YOGURT			
Plain low-fat with nonfat dry milk	1 cup	415	326
Plain whole milk	1 cup	274	215
Low-fat fruit-flavored	1 cup	314	247
CHEESE			
Cheddar	1 oz	214	145
Cottage cheese, lowfat	½ cup	78	170
Mozarella	1 oz	147	105
Ricotta, part skim	½ cup	337	226
Swiss	1 oz	272	171
Processed American	1 oz	184	211
American cheese food	1 oz	163	130
DESSERTS			
Ice cream, chocolate	1 cup	186	168
Ice cream, vanilla, reg	1 cup	176	134
Ice milk, vanilla	1 cup	176	129
Ice milk, vanilla soft serve	1 cup	274	202
Pudding, instant vanilla from skim milk	½ cup	157	314
Orange sherbet	1 cup	103	74
FISH AND SHELLFISH			
Oysters	¾ cup	129	204
Salmon, chinook, cnd	⅔ cup	154	289
Sardines, cnd in brine	3½ oz	303	354
Scallops, steamed	3½ oz	115	338
Shrimp, cnd, dry pack	3½ oz	115	263
Tuna, cnd, in oil	6½ oz	61	3
"GREENS"			
Collard	½ cup	179	50
Dandelion	½ cup	147	44
Turnip	½ cup	134	27
Mustard	½ cup	97	23
Spinach	½ cup	84	34

Index

Page numbers followed by f *indicate figures; those followed by* t *indicate tabular material.*
Page numbers followed by b *indicate boxed material.*

Absorption. *See also*
  Digestion
  of food, 406, 406f
  drugs affecting,
    650–651
Accutane. *See* Istretinoin
Acesulfame-K (Sunette),
    24b
Acetaminophen
  absorption of
    food effect on, 652
Acetazolamide
  effect of
    on calcium, 146
    on nutrient excretion,
      651
Acetyl coenzyme A, 27
Achlorhydria, 431, 496
Acid ash diet, 552–553
Acid–base balance,
    173–175
  regulation of, 33, 173,
    533
Acid–base imbalances,
    175–176
Acid-forming foods, 176,
    552–553, 553b
Acidophilus milk, 447
Acidosis
  metabolic, 175
  respiratory, 175
Acids, 173
Acne, 115, 314
Addison's disease. *See*
    Adrenocortical

  insufficiency,
    primary
Additives, 310
Adolescent nutrition
  assessment in, 313
    criteria for, 313b
  daily food guide for, 277t
  diagnosis in: Health
    Seeking Behav-
    iors, as evi-
    denced by lack of
    knowledge of nor-
    mal nutritional
    requirements for
    adolescents and
    the desire to
    learn, 313
  goals in, 315
  growth characteristics
    and implications
    of, 312
  in pregnancy
    counseling in, 255
    requirements in, 255
    risks in, 254
  interventions in, 315, 317
    monitoring of, 315
    teaching for, 315
  RDA in, 277t, 646
Adrenal cortex
  disorders of, 527–531.
    See Adrenocortical
    insufficiency
Adrenal corticosteroids
  effect of

    on calcium, 146, 582t
    on nitrogen balance,
      582t
    on potassium, 169,
      582t
    on vitamin B$_6$, 133
    on vitamin C, 127
    on vitamin D, 118
    on zinc and, 157
  side effects of, 582t
Adrenocortical insufficiency
  complications of, 527
  definitions of, 517
  etiology of, 527
  fluid volume deficit in,
    530
  hypoglycemia in,
    529–530
  nursing interventions in,
    527
  primary
    assessment in,
      529–530
    complications of, 527,
      529
    definition of, 527
    diagnosis in: Fluid Vol-
      ume Deficit,
      related to abnor-
      mal fluid loss
      (increased excre-
      tion) secondary to
      primary adreno-
      cortical insuffi-
      ciency, 530

681